Systematic Reviews
in Health Research

Systematic Reviews in Health Research

Meta-Analysis in Context

THIRD EDITION

Edited by

Matthias Egger

Professor of Epidemiology and Public Health
Institute for Social and Preventive Medicine (ISPM)
University of Bern, Bern, Switzerland
&
Centre for Infectious Diseases Epidemiology and Research
University of Cape Town, South Africa

Julian P.T. Higgins

Professor of Evidence Synthesis
Population Health Sciences
Bristol Medical School
University of Bristol, Bristol, UK

George Davey Smith

Professor of Clinical Epidemiology and Director of the MRC
Integrative Epidemiology Unit
University of Bristol, Bristol, UK

WILEY Blackwell   BMJ|Books

Library of Congress Cataloging-in-Publication Data

Names: Egger, Matthias, editor. | Higgins, Julian P. T., editor. | Davey
  Smith, George, editor.
Title: Systematic reviews in health research : meta-analysis in context /
  edited by Matthias Egger, Julian P. T. Higgins, George Davey Smith.
Other titles: Systematic reviews in health care (Egger)
Description: Third edition. | Hoboken, NJ : John Wiley & Sons, Inc., 2022.
  | Prev. ed.: Systematic reviews in health care / edited by Matthias
  Egger, George Davey Smith and Douglas G. Altman. 2nd ed. 2001.
Identifiers: LCCN 2021049316 (print) | LCCN 2021049317 (ebook) | ISBN
  9781405160506 (hardback) | ISBN 9781119099376 (adobe pdf) | ISBN
  9781119099383 (epub)
Subjects: MESH: Systematic Reviews as Topic | Meta-Analysis as Topic |
  Research Design | Evidence-Based Medicine | Controlled Clinical Trials
  as Topic
Classification: LCC R853.S94 (print) | LCC R853.S94 (ebook) | NLM W 20.5
  | DDC 610/.7/2–dc23/eng/20211029
LC record available at https://lccn.loc.gov/2021049316
LC ebook record available at https://lccn.loc.gov/2021049317

Contents

Preface

Iain Chalmers and Doug Altman edited the first edition of this book, which was published in 1995 and called simply *Systematic Reviews*. Their foreword focused on the "poor scientific quality of [traditional] reviews of clinical research" and the "disregard of scientific principles," which may harm decision-making and patient outcomes [1]. Systematic reviews allow a more objective appraisal by systematically identifying, scrutinizing, and synthesizing the relevant studies. Today, more than a quarter of a century and two editions later [1, 2], systematic reviews and meta-analyses have become widely established, with thousands of such studies published every year. Also, their function has broadened, from the scientific synthesis of evidence to inform clinical practice, the main concern in 1995, to becoming part of the methods toolkit to address a wide range of questions, including evaluation of interventions, diagnosis and prognosis, prevalence and burden of disease, and discovery research.

This broader role is reflected in the current third edition. Of the 27 chapters, 12 are new, covering systematic reviews of prediction models, genetic association studies, and prevalence studies. The focus on methods has become stronger too, with new chapters dealing with missing data, network meta-analysis, and dose–response meta-analysis. These changes explain the book's new title (*Systematic Reviews in Health Research*, rather than in Health Care) and revised structure. The first chapter discusses the rationale, history, and strengths and limitations of systematic reviews and meta-analysis. This introductory chapter is followed by a section on principles and procedures (six chapters), a section on meta-analysis (seven chapters), and one on systematic reviews and meta-analysis of specific study designs (six chapters). Two chapters cover Cochrane (formerly the Cochrane Collaboration) and systematic reviews and meta-analyses in guideline development and the *GRADE* approach (Grading of Recommendations Assessment, Development and Evaluation). The book ends with an outlook on innovations in and the future of systematic reviews and meta-analysis (two chapters) and a section on software (three chapters). The 15 chapters that made the journey from the second to the third edition have all been thoroughly updated. Nevertheless, all chapters will age, some more quickly than others. The book's website (www.systematic-reviews3.org) will be our antidote to premature aging, by offering updates of some chapters (for example, those on software packages) and highlighting references to recent critical articles and instruments, new software, and other developments.

The intended audience will be similar to that for the popular second edition [2]: methodologically inclined clinicians, epidemiologists, health services researchers, and public health specialists interested in conducting high-quality systematic reviews and meta-analyses. The book will also be of interest to doctoral and other students in the health sciences. Indeed, we see this book as an excellent resource for teaching and will provide exercises and computer practicals on the companion website.

On the long journey from the second to the third edition, we lost our dear friend, collaborator, and co-editor, Douglas Graham Altman. Doug sadly died, aged 69, on June 3, 2018. He made essential contributions to this third edition, helping define focus and content and co-authoring several chapters. On the following pages, we reprint Iain Chalmers' wonderful tribute to Doug's visionary role in developing systematic reviews and clarifying the role of meta-analysis [3]. We miss you very much, Doug, and dedicate this book to you.

Last but not least, huge thanks to all contributors to this book. They made it possible by patiently and stoically updating their chapters over several years. Many thanks to our project managers and editors in Bern, Carole Dupont, Chris Ritter, and Geraldine Wong, who supported us so well on this long journey. A big thank-you also to the editors at Wiley, Jennifer Seward, Samras Johnson V, and Ella Elliot, for their brilliant help and their patience.

The first edition of this book was applauded for its "simple and often humorous" discussion and its "intuitively appealing explanations" [4]. We hope you will agree that the third edition continues in this tradition.

Bern and Bristol, April 2022
Matthias Egger, Julian P.T. Higgins, George Davey Smith

REFERENCES

1. Chalmers, I. and Altman, D. (1995). Foreword. In: *Systematic Reviews* (ed. I. Chalmers and D. Altman). London: BMJ Publishing Group.

2. Egger, M., Davey Smith, G., Altman, D.G. et al. (ed.) (2001). *Systematic Reviews in Health Care: Meta-Analysis in Context*, 2e. London: BMJ Books.

3. Chalmers, I. (2020). Doug Altman's prescience in recognising the need to reduce biases before tackling imprecision in systematic reviews. *J. R. Soc. Med.* 113: 119–122. https://doi.org/10.1177/0141076820908496.

4. DerSimonian, R. (1997). Book Review: Systematic Review. I. Chalmers and D. G. Altman (eds), BMJ Publishing Group, London, 1995. No. of pages: 117. ISBN 0-7279-0904-5. *Stat. Med.* 16: 2930–2930.

Tribute

Professor Doug Altman (1948–2018) co-edited the first and second editions of this book. Here, Sir Iain Chalmers, founder of The Cochrane Collaboration and the James Lind Alliance, reflects on Altman's seminal contributions to the concept of systematic reviews and the role of meta-analysis.

Doug Altman's Prescience in Recognizing the Need to Reduce Biases before Tackling Imprecision in Systematic Reviews

Iain Chalmers

RECOGNITION OF SHARED INTERESTS AND THE ORIGINS OF A FRIENDSHIP

I came to know Doug Altman during the 1980s when we were both members of the editorial team at the *British Journal of Obstetrics and Gynaecology*. I was working at the National Perinatal Epidemiology Unit at that time; Doug was at the Division of Medical Statistics at the Medical Research Council's Clinical Research Centre. Our meeting at the *BJOG* was the beginning of what became a very close friendship.

Doug and I shared an interest in trying to improve the quality of the manuscripts submitted to the *BJOG*. We commissioned three papers providing reporting guidelines for those submitting reports of controlled trials, assessments of screening and diagnostic tests, and observational studies – early examples of an interest that would become manifested in Doug's creation of the *EQUATOR* Network (Enhancing the QUAlity and Transparency Of health Research).

We also discovered that we had both become interested in the scientific quality of reviews of research evidence, and the potential for statistical synthesis of estimates derived from several similar studies. I had used this approach in a review of four randomized comparisons of different ways of monitoring fetuses during labour [1], the results of which prompted a very large further controlled trial that confirmed the results of the meta-analysis [2].

Doug's interest in the scientific quality of reviews of research evidence had been stimulated by two papers published in the late 1970s by Richard Peto [3, 4]. These led Doug to prepare a seven-page typescript entitled "Evaluating a series of clinical trials of the same treatment" for presentation at the 1981 meeting of the International Epidemiological Association in Edinburgh [5]. Over the next two years Doug extended the material in the 7-page typescript to a 40-page typescript with the same title [6].

DOUG'S PIONEERING CONCEPTUALIZATION OF SYSTEMATIC REVIEWS AND THE ROLE OF META-ANALYSIS

Doug's 1983 paper is important in the history of systematic reviews because of his prescience of what is important in the science of research synthesis. Unfortunately, it has been hidden from view because it was never formally published. I think Doug first showed me "the almost final version of [his] 1983 paper (complete with handwritten corrections)" at the end of 1986. He said he intended to finalize and submit it for publication, but that did not happen. As he admitted more than two decades later, "I wish I had published my ideas back in 1983" [7]. Since 2011, the typescripts of both papers [5, 6] have been available in the James Lind Library, and the shorter paper, with an accompanying commentary by Doug, is also available in the *Cochrane Methods* supplement to the *Cochrane Database of Systematic Reviews* [8].

In both these papers Doug touched on issues that would become more widely recognized as important by the 1990s. In particular, he made clear that techniques of statistical synthesis – "meta-analysis" – were but one element in a science of research synthesis, and usually not the most important. He made clear that, although statistical synthesis could address those elements of between-study variability due to random variation, it could not deal with other sources of variability – differences in entry criteria, study populations, the methods used to generate comparison groups, baseline differences between treatment groups, degrees of blindness achieved, and variations in and deviations from treatment protocols. Doug comments at the beginning of a nine-page section on "Combining the data" in the longer paper that "Since the main purpose of the paper is to discuss the whole issue of whether or not to combine trials rather than to carry out a comparison of the available methods, not all of the possible statistical methods will be described" [6]. Both his papers stressed the likely importance of publication bias and he regretted the lack (then) of hard evidence of the bias and the challenges this posed. He makes the important and too often neglected point:

> *Although the problem of possible publication bias may appear to be a major restriction on the validity of combining the results from several trials, it is important to realise that any such bias applies to the interpretation of individual studies, although this is always ignored and each study's results taken at face value. ([6], p. 25)*

Toward the end of his 1983 paper, Doug presciently identified two desirable developments that would become widely appreciated by the end of the decade. First, the use of individual patient data:

> *In view of the non-statistical problems in the combination of results from different trials, the choice of statistical method is unlikely to matter greatly, but methods*

which make use of the raw data are definitely preferable to the combination of probabilities. The pooled estimate of relative risk should be presented with its confidence interval. ([6], p. 33)

Secondly, there is a paragraph in a section of the paper entitled "Ethical considerations" that anticipates developments in thinking and practice during the 1980s and 1990s, which Doug selected for attention after re-reading his paper over 30 years after drafting it [8]. Here's the paragraph that had struck him:

[it] is important to consider whether the results of a series of studies of the same treatment should be accumulated on a regular basis in order to monitor the current state of knowledge about those treatments. Further trials might then be dependent on the combined significance of already completed trials but using a stricter level of statistical significance (say P < 0.001) than is usually applied in single trials. Even without such information trials should perhaps not be given ethical committee approval unless the researchers had analysed the results of published trials in the way suggested in order to demonstrate that there was still uncertainty about the efficacy of the treatment, and the range of uncertainty encompassed clinically relevant benefit. Further, power calculations for a new trial could be conditional on the results of published trials. ([6], p. 27)

THE ORIGINS OF SYSTEMATIC REVIEWS IN HEALTH RESEARCH: META-ANALYSIS IN CONTEXT

Following wider recognition of the need to improve the scientific quality of reviews [9–11], the opening of the Cochrane Centre in Oxford in October 1992 helped to generate interest in the science of research synthesis [12]. I was delighted that Richard Smith, editor of the *British Medical Journal*, recognized this and proposed an all-day meeting run jointly by the *BMJ* and The Cochrane Centre. I was very glad that he accepted that the title of the meeting would refer to systematic reviews, and not to meta-analysis, as had been proposed originally. The meeting was held at the Royal Institution on 7 July 1993. Eight presentations covered the development of systematic reviews; doubts about them and the challenge of finding relevant studies; rationale and practicalities; and assessing, updating, and disseminating systematic reviews.

Based on the presentations made at the meeting, a series of articles about systematic reviews began in the 3 September 1994 issue of the *BMJ*. In his "Editor's Choice" column, Richard Smith noted that systematic review was "one of the most valuable tools in assessing new treatments and technologies" [13]. He was even more supportive in his Editor's Choice column a few weeks later:

Systematic reviews provide the highest quality evidence on treatment. . . The author of a systematic review poses a clear question, gathers all relevant trials (whether published or not), weeds out the scientifically flawed, and then

amalgamates the remaining trials to reach a conclusion. Every stage in the pro-
cess is crucial, and an article in the journal by Kay Dickersin and her colleagues
shows how a careful Medline search for randomised controlled trials will not
detect all such trials even in the journals indexed in Medline. [14]

Richard Smith went on to point out that systematic reviews are also important because – by amalgamating data from similar trials – they can increase the statistical power of treatment comparisons [14]. These succinct explanations of the rationale for systematic reviews made by the Editor-in-Chief of one of the world's most prominent medical journals were heartening to those of us calling for improvements in the scientific quality of reviews of research.

The *BMJ*'s series of articles on systematic reviews was well received and Richard Smith proposed that I should edit a compilation of the articles as a book. I accepted, on condition that Doug Altman would co-edit it with me, and I was very glad that both Richard and Doug agreed [15]. The contents and contributors to the book are shown in Figure T.1 and in the James Lind Library at https://www.jameslindlibrary.org/chalmers-i-altman-dg-1995. The book introduces and illustrates systematic reviews; discusses data collection for them; presents contrary stances on the value of using meta-analysis to generate overall summary statistics; provides guidelines for assessing the trustworthiness of reviews; describes how systematic reviews are being prepared, updated, and disseminated by the international network of people who together constitute the Cochrane Collaboration; and concludes with a classified bibliography for further reading. The book is dedicated to Thomas C. Chalmers, "in appreciation of his many pioneering contributions to the science of reviewing health research, and in particular, for the first clear demonstration of the dangers of relying on traditional reviews of research to guide clinical practice."

Doug's and my Preface in the book provided an opportunity to explain why we had used the term "systematic review" rather than the more technical neologism "meta-analysis":

Use of the term 'systematic review' implies only that a review has been prepared using some kind of systematic approach to minimising biases and random errors, and that the components of the approach will be documented in a materials and methods section. Other terms – particularly 'meta-analysis' – have caused confusion because of the implication that a systematic approach to reviews must entail quantitative synthesis of primary data to yield an overall summary statistic (meta-analysis). As we hope this book will help to make clear, this is not the case. In addition to those circumstances in which statistical synthesis (meta-analysis) of results of primary research is not advisable, there will be others in which it is quite simply impossible. It is just as important to take steps to control biases in reviews in these circumstances as it is to do so in circumstances in which meta-analysis is both indicated and possible. [15]

Doug reiterated this point in his 2013 commentary on "Twenty years of meta-analysis and evidence synthesis methods." He wrote:

FIGURE T.1   The contents and contributors to the first edition of the book on systematic reviews

As time went on we have realized that there are many hidden problems, nuances, extensions, and so on. And there have been big changes in strategy. The biggest impact probably came from the early realization that the statistical analysis is a relatively simple part of a rather complex set of actions which we now label as a systematic review. [8]

The issue was dealt with nicely in the title chosen for the second edition of the book, namely *Systematic Reviews in Health Care: Meta-Analysis in Context* [16]. I am grateful to the editors of the third edition of the book (Egger, Davey Smith, and Higgins) for inviting me to draw attention to the pioneering thinking and unpublished writing about research synthesis by their and my much-loved, late-lamented co-editorial colleague, Doug Altman.

Note

This text was published previously as Chalmers I. Doug Altman's prescience in recognising the need to reduce biases before tackling imprecision in systematic reviews. *Journal of the Royal Society of Medicine* 2020; 113:119–122.

ACKNOWLEDGMENTS

I am grateful to Mike Clarke, George Davey Smith, Anne Eisinga, Julian Higgins, and Richard Smith for comments on an earlier draft of this text.

REFERENCES

1. Chalmers, I. (1979). Randomised controlled trials of fetal monitoring 1973-1977. In: *Perinatal Medicine* (ed. O. Thalhammer, K. Baumgarten and A. Pollak), 260–265. Stuttgart: George Thieme.

2. MacDonald, D., Grant, A., Sheridan-Pereira, M. et al. (1985). The Dublin randomized controlled trial of intrapartum fetal heart rate monitoring. *Am. J. Obstet. Gynecol.* 152: 524–539.

3. Peto, R. (1978). Clinical trial methodology. *Biomedicine* 28 (special issue): 24–36.

4. Peto, R., Pike, M.C., Armitage, P. et al. (1977). Design and analysis of randomized clinical trials requiring prolonged observation of each patient. II. Analysis and examples. *Br. J. Cancer* 35: 1–39.

5. Altman, D.G. (1981). Evaluating a series of clinical trials of the same treatment. Unpublished seven-page summary of the author's presentation at a meeting of the International Epidemiological Association in Edinburgh, August 1981. Available from jameslindlibrary.org/altman-dg-1981.

6. Altman, D.G. (1983). Evaluating a series of clinical trials of the same treatment. Unpublished 40-page development of the author's seven-page summary of his presentation at a meeting of the International Epidemiological Association in Edinburgh, August 1981. Available from jameslindlibrary.org/altman-dg-1983.

7. Altman, D.G. (2015). Some reflections on the evolution of meta-analysis. *Res. Synth. Methods* 6: 265–267.

8. Altman, D. (2013). Twenty years of meta-analysis and evidence synthesis methods: a personal reflection. Cochrane methods. *Cochrane Database Syst. Rev.* 2013 (Suppl 1): 2–11. https://www.cochranelibrary.com/documents/20182/64256496/ Cochrane+Methods+2013/0f6dc933-5d27-fe40-6bd9-dfad13e08e50.

9. Jenicek, M. (1987). *Méta-analyse en médecine. Évaluation et synthèse de l'information clinique et épidémiologique* [Meta-analysis in Medicine: Evaluation and Synthesis of Clinical and Epidemiological Information]. St. Hyacinthe and Paris: EDISEM and Maloine Éditeurs.

10. Mulrow, C.D. (1987). The medical review article: state of the science. *Ann. Intern. Med.* 106: 485–488.

11. Oxman, A.D. and Guyatt, G.H. (1988). Guidelines for reading literature reviews. *Can. Med. Assoc. J.* 138: 697–703.

12. Chalmers, I., Dickersin, K., and Chalmers, T.C. (1992). Getting to grips with Archie Cochrane's agenda: all randomised controlled trials should be registered and reported. *BMJ* 305: 786–788.

13. Smith, R. (1994a). Hearts and minds. *BMJ* 309: 3 September.

14. Smith, R. (1994b). Systematic reviews, stupid doctors, and red meat. *BMJ* 309: 12 November.

15. Chalmers, I. and Altman, D.G. (1995). *Systematic Reviews*. London: BMJ Books.

16. Egger, M., Davey Smith, G., and Altman, D.G. (2001). *Systematic Reviews in Health Care: Meta-Analysis in Context*, 2e. London: BMJ Books.

List of Contributors

Douglas G. Altman
Centre for Statistics in Medicine
Nuffield Department of
Orthopaedics
Rheumatology and Musculoskeletal
Sciences
University of Oxford
Oxford, UK

Gerd Antes
Cochrane Germany (1997–2018)
University of Freiburg
Freiburg, Germany

Julia Bohlius
Institute of Social and Preventive Medicine
University of Bern
Bern, Switzerland;
Swiss Tropical and Public
Health Institute
Basel, Switzerland
and
University of Basel
Basel, Switzerland

Michael Borenstein
Director of Biostatistics
Biostat, Inc., Englewood
NJ, USA

Diana Buitrago-Garcia
Institute of Social and Preventive Medicine
University of Bern
Bern, Switzerland

Iain Chalmers
Centre for Evidence-Based Medicine
University of Oxford
Oxford, UK

Gary S. Collins
Centre for Statistics in Medicine
Nuffield Department of
Orthopaedics
Rheumatology and Musculoskeletal Sciences
University of Oxford, Oxford, UK

Bruno R. da Costa
Institute of Health Policy
Management and Evaluation
University of Toronto
Toronto, Canada
and
Applied Health Research
Centre (AHRC)
St. Michael's Hospital
Toronto, Canada

Thomas P.A. Debray
Julius Center for Health Sciences
and Primary Care; Cochrane
Netherlands
University Medical Center Utrecht
Utrecht University
Utrecht, The Netherlands

George Davey Smith
Medical Research Council Integrative Epidemiology Unit
Population Health Sciences
Bristol Medical School
University of Bristol
Bristol, UK

Jonathan J. Deeks
Test Evaluation Research Group
Institute of Applied Health Research
University of Birmingham
Birmingham, UK

Olaf M. Dekkers
Department of Clinical
Epidemiology
Aarhus University Hospital
Aarhus, Denmark
and
Department of Clinical Epidemiology
Leiden University Medical Centre
Leiden, The Netherlands

Shah Ebrahim
Co-ordinating Editor, Cochrane
Heart Group (1995–2014)
and
London School of Hygiene &
Tropical Medicine
University of London
London, UK

Matthias Egger
Institute of Social and Preven-
tive Medicine
University of Bern
Bern, Switzerland
and
Centre for Infectious Diseases
Epidemiology and Research
University of Cape Town
South Africa

Julian Elliott
Cochrane Australia
School of Public Health and Preven-
tive Medicine
Monash University
Melbourne, Australia

David J. Fisher
Medical Research Council Clinical
Trial Unit
University College London
London, UK

Julie Glanville
Glanville.info
York, UK

Gibran Hemani
Medical Research Council Integra-
tive Epidemiology Unit
Population Health Sciences
Bristol Medical School
University of Bristol
Bristol, UK

Julian P.T. Higgins
Population Health Sciences
Bristol Medical School
University of Bristol
Bristol, UK
and
National Institute of Health
Research Applied Research Collabo-
ration West
University Hospitals Bristol and
Weston NHS Foundation Trust
Bristol, UK

Mark D. Huffman
Northwestern University Feinberg
School of Medicine
Chicago, IL, USA
and
The George Institute for
Global Health
University of New South Wales
Sydney, Australia

Brian Hutton
School of Epidemiology and
Public Health
University of Ottawa
Ottawa, Canada
and
Clinical Epidemiology Program
Ottawa Hospital Research Institute
Ottawa, Canada

Susanna C. Larsson
Institute of Environmental Medicine
Karolinska Institutet
Stockholm, Sweden

and
Department of Surgical Sciences
Uppsala University
Uppsala, Sweden

Carol Lefebvre
Lefebvre Associates Ltd
Oxford, UK

Tianjing Li
Department of Ophthalmology
School of Medicine
University of Colorado Anschutz
Medical Campus
Aurora, CO, USA

Dimitris Mavridis
Department of Primary Education,
University of Ioannina
Ioannina, Greece

David Moher
Centre for Journalology
Clinical Epidemiology Program
Ottawa Hospital Research Institute
Ottawa, Canada
and
School of Epidemiology and
Public Health
University of Ottawa
Ottawa, Canada

Karel G.M. Moons
Julius Center for Health Sciences
and Primary Care; Cochrane
Netherlands
University Medical Center Utrecht
Utrecht University
Utrecht, The Netherlands

Nicola Orsini
Department of Global Public Health
Karolinska Institutet
Stockholm, Sweden

Nancy Owens
Cochrane Central Executive Team
(2001–2018)
Fairfax, VA, USA

Matthew J. Page
School of Public Health and
Preventive Medicine
Monash University
Melbourne, Australia

Richard D. Riley
Centre for Prognosis Research
School of Medicine
Keele University
Newcastle-under-Lyme, UK

Eliane Rohner
Institute of Social and Preventive
Medicine
University of Bern
Bern, Switzerland

Georgia Salanti
Institute of Social and Preventive
Medicine
University of Bern
Bern, Switzerland

Jelena Savović
Population Health Sciences
Bristol Medical School
University of Bristol
Bristol, UK
and
National Institute of Health
Research Applied Research
Collaboration West
University Hospitals Bristol and
Weston NHS Foundation Trust
Bristol, UK

Guido Schwarzer
Faculty of Medicine and Medical
Center
Institute of Medical Biometry and
Statistics
University of Freiburg
Freiburg, Germany

Holger J. Schünemann
Department of Health Research
Methods, Evidence, and Impact and
Department of Medicine
McMaster University
Hamilton, Ontario, Canada

Larissa Shamseer
Knowledge Translation Program
Li Ka Shing Knowledge Institute
St. Michael's Hospital
Unity Health Toronto
Toronto, Canada

Mark C. Simmonds
Centre for Reviews and
Dissemination
University of York
York, UK

Beverley Shea
Centre for Journalology
Clinical Epidemiology Program
Ottawa Hospital Research Institute
Ottawa, Canada
and
School of Epidemiology and
Public Health
University of Ottawa
Ottawa, Canada

Jonathan A.C. Sterne
Population Health Sciences
Bristol Medical School
University of Bristol
Bristol, UK

Lesley A. Stewart
Centre for Reviews and Dissemination
University of York
York, UK

Yemisi Takwoingi
Test Evaluation Research Group
Institute of Applied Health Research
University of Birmingham
Birmingham, UK

David Tovey
Editor in Chief, The Cochrane
Library (2009–2019)
Sussex, UK

Sven Trelle
CTU Bern, University of Bern
Bern, Switzerland

Tari Turner
Cochrane Australia
School of Public Health and Preventive Medicine
Monash University
Melbourne, Australia

Ian R. White
MRC Clinical Trials Unit at UCL
London, UK

Penny F. Whiting
Population Health Sciences
Bristol Medical School
University of Bristol
Bristol, UK

Marcel Zwahlen
Institute of Social and Preventive Medicine
University of Bern
Bern, Switzerland

About the Companion Website

This book is accompanied by a website offering supplementary materials:

www.systematic-reviews3.org

CHAPTER 1

Systematic Reviews in Health Research

An Introduction

Matthias Egger, Julian P.T. Higgins, and George Davey Smith

The volume of data that needs to be considered by practitioners and researchers is constantly expanding. In most areas, it has become impossible for the individual to read, critically evaluate, and synthesize the state of current knowledge, let alone keep updating this on a regular basis. Reviews have become essential tools for anybody who wants to keep up with the new evidence that is accumulating in their field of interest. Reviews are also required to identify areas where the available evidence is insufficient and further studies are needed. In 1987, Cynthia Mulrow drew attention to the poor quality of traditional reviews, pointing out that "current medical reviews do not routinely use scientific methods to identify, assess, and synthesize information" [1]. In response to this situation, methods and guidance on systematically reviewing studies were developed to produce explicitly formulated, reproducible, and up-to-date summaries of the effects of health care interventions. The focus was initially on randomized controlled trials (RCTs), but soon expanded to other study designs. This is illustrated by the sharp increase, since around 2005, in the number of reviews that used formal methods to synthesize evidence (Figure 1.1).

This chapter aims to clarify terminology and scope, provide some historical background, introduce the potentials, promise, and limitations of systematic reviews and meta-analysis, and give an overview of the topics covered in this book.

1.1 SYSTEMATIC REVIEW, META-ANALYSIS, OR EVIDENCE SYNTHESIS?

A number of terms are used to describe the process of systematically reviewing and integrating research evidence, including "systematic review," "meta-analysis," "overview," and "pooling." In the foreword to the first edition of this book, Chalmers and

Systematic Reviews in Health Research: Meta-Analysis in Context, Third Edition. Edited by Matthias Egger, Julian P.T. Higgins, and George Davey Smith.
© 2022 John Wiley & Sons Ltd. Published 2022 by John Wiley & Sons Ltd.
Companion website: www.systematic-reviews3.org

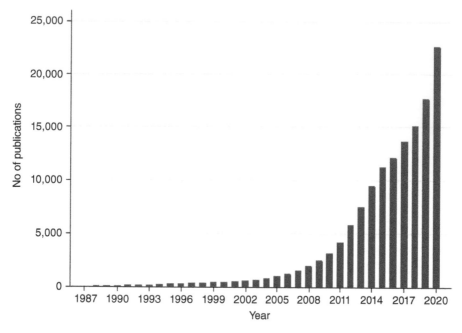

FIGURE 1.1   Number of publications concerning meta-analysis, 1987–2020. Results from MEDLINE search using text word and medical subject heading (MESH) "meta-analysis" and text word "systematic review."

Altman [2] defined systematic review as a review that was prepared using a "systematic approach to minimizing biases and random errors documented in a materials and methods section." A systematic review may, or may not, include a meta-analysis: "a statistical analysis of the results from independent studies, which generally aims to produce a single, typical estimate of a treatment effect" [3].

The distinction between systematic review and meta-analysis is essential because it is always appropriate and desirable to review a body of data systematically. In contrast, it may sometimes be inappropriate, or even misleading, to pool results from separate studies statistically [4]. Indeed, reviewers often find it hard to resist the temptation of combining studies even when such meta-analysis is questionable or inappropriate. According to the Royal Society [5], "evidence synthesis" describes the process of synthesizing information from a range of sources and disciplines to inform policymaking. Such an evidence synthesis typically includes several systematic reviews and meta-analyses, or may involve the statistical synthesis of a range of different types of evidence (see also discussion of triangulation of evidence in Chapter 19).

Other types of reviews that have emerged in recent years include "scoping reviews," "rapid reviews," and "umbrella reviews" [6]. Scoping reviews describe or map key concepts, types of evidence, and gaps in a defined research area [7]. In rapid reviews, time is gained by using less rigorous processes to identify studies [8]. Umbrella reviews, which are meta-reviews (or "overviews") of systematic reviews and meta-analyses, reflect the explosion in the number of such publications and address the fact that systematic reviews and meta-analyses addressing the same question may reach opposite conclusions [9] (see also Chapter 7).

1.2   THE SCOPE OF META-ANALYSIS

An important distinction can be made between meta-analysis of RCTs and meta-analysis of observational studies of interventions (Chapter 15) or etiology (Chapter 19). Consider a set of high-quality trials that examined the same intervention in comparable patient populations: each trial should provide an unbiased estimate of the same underlying treatment effect. The variability observed between the trials can be attributed to random variation, and meta-analysis should provide an equally unbiased estimate of the treatment effect with increased precision. A fundamentally different situation typically arises in observational epidemiological studies, for example case–control studies, cross-sectional studies, or cohort studies. Due to confounding and selection bias, these studies may produce estimates of causal associations that deviate from the underlying causal associations beyond what can be attributed to chance. Combining a set of observational studies will thus often provide spuriously precise, biased estimates of causal associations. The thorough consideration of heterogeneity between observational study results, particularly of possible confounding and bias, will generally provide more insights than the mechanical calculation of an overall measure of effect.

The fundamental difference between observational studies and RCTs does not mean that the latter are immune to bias. Publication bias and other reporting biases (see Chapter 5) may distort the evidence from both trials and observational studies [10]. Bias may also be introduced if trials' methodological quality is inadequate (Chapter 4) [11]. For both RCTs and observational studies, it is crucial to understand the limitations of meta-analysis and the importance of exploring heterogeneity and sources of bias.

1.3   HISTORICAL NOTES

Efforts to compile summaries of research for medical practitioners are not new [12–14]. In 1753, James Lind included a "Critical and Chronological View of what has been published on the subject" in his "Treatise of the Scurvy." He argued:

> *Before the subject could be set in a clear and proper light, it was necessary to remove a great deal of rubbish. [15]*

This illustrates an important function of systematic reviews, namely the central role of sound eligibility criteria for the studies to be included, the critical appraisal of studies (see Chapter 4), and, more generally, the problem of research waste created by poor-quality studies [14, 16].

The statistical basis of meta-analysis reaches back to the seventeenth century when, in astronomy and geodesy, intuition and experience suggested that combinations of data might be better than attempts to choose among them (Box 1.1). In the twentieth century, the distinguished statistician Karl Pearson (Figure 1.3) was, in 1904, the first medical researcher reporting the use of formal techniques to combine data from different studies. The rationale for pooling studies put forward by Pearson in his account on serum inoculations against enteric fever is still one of the main reasons for undertaking meta-analysis today:

Box 1.1   From Laplace and Gauss to the First Textbook
of Meta-Analysis

Keith O'Rourke

Astronomers long ago noticed that observations of the same objects differed even
when made by the same observers under similar conditions. The calculation of the
mean as a more precise value than a single measurement appeared by the end of the
seventeenth century [17]. By the late 1700s probability models were used to represent
the uncertainty of observations. Laplace decided to report these models as the truth,
together with the "probability of some error," the concept at the heart of maximum
likelihood estimation [18]. Laplace's method of combining and quantifying uncertainty in the combination of observations required an explicit probability distribution for errors. Gauss drew on empirical experience and argued that a probability
distribution corresponding to what is today referred to as the Normal or Gaussian
distribution would be best. This remained speculative until Laplace's discovery of
the central limit theorem – that for large sample sizes the error distribution will
always be close to Normally distributed. Most statistical techniques used today
in meta-analysis follow from Gauss's and Laplace's work. Airy disseminated their
work in his 1861 "textbook" on "meta-analysis" for astronomers (Figure 1.2), which
included the first formulation of a random effects model to allow for heterogeneity
in the results [19]. Airy offered practical advice and argued for the use of judgment
to determine what type of statistical model should be used.

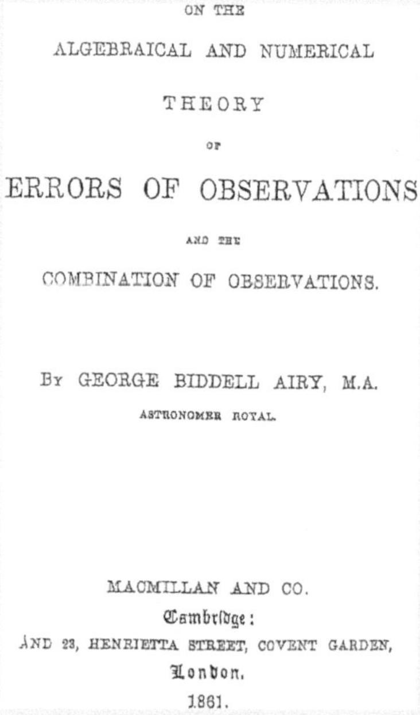

ON THE

ALGEBRAICAL AND NUMERICAL

THEORY

OF

ERRORS OF OBSERVATIONS

AND THE

COMBINATION OF OBSERVATIONS.

By GEORGE BIDDELL AIRY, M.A.

ASTRONOMER ROYAL.

MACMILLAN AND CO.
Cambridge:
AND 23, HENRIETTA STREET, COVENT GARDEN,
London.
1861.

FIGURE 1.2   Title page of the first "textbook" of meta-analysis, 1861.

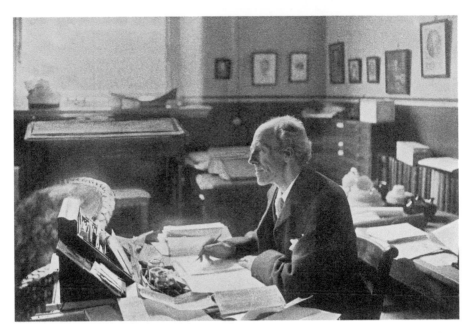

FIGURE 1.3   Distinguished statistician Karl Pearson (1857–1936) is seen as the first medical researcher to use formal techniques to combine data from different studies. *Source*: Wikimedia Commons / CC BY 4.0.

Many of the groups . . . are far too small to allow of any definite opinion being formed at all, having regard to the size of the probable error involved. [20]

Such techniques were not widely used in medicine for many years to come. In contrast to medicine, the social sciences and, in particular, psychology and educational research soon became interested in the synthesis of research findings. In the 1930s, 80 experiments examining the "potency of moral instruction in modifying conduct" were systematically reviewed [21]. In 1976 the psychologist Glass coined the term "meta-analysis" in a classic paper entitled "Primary, secondary and meta-analysis of research" [22]. Three years later, the British physician and epidemiologist Archie Cochrane drew attention to the fact that people who want to make informed health care decisions do not have ready access to reliable reviews of the available evidence [23]. In the 1980s, meta-analysis became increasingly popular in medicine, particularly in cardiovascular disease [24, 25], oncology [26], and perinatal care [27]. In the 1990s, the foundation of the Cochrane Collaboration (see Chapter 21) facilitated numerous developments, many of which are covered in this book.

1.4   WHY DO WE NEED SYSTEMATIC REVIEWS? THE SITUATION IN THE 1980s

A likely scenario in the 1980s, when discussing the discharge of a patient who had suffered an uncomplicated myocardial infarction, is as follows: a keen junior doctor asks whether the patient should receive a beta-blocker for secondary prevention of

TABLE 1.1   Conclusions from four randomized controlled trials of beta-blockers in secondary prevention after myocardial infarction.

"The mortality and hospital readmission rates were not significantly different in the two groups. This also applied to the incidence of cardiac failure, exertional dyspnoea, and frequency of ventricular ectopic beats." Reynolds (1972) [28]
"Until the results of further trials are reported long-term beta-adrenoceptor blockade (possibly up to two years) is recommended after uncomplicated anterior myocardial infarction." Multicentre International Study (1977) [29]
"The trial was designed to detect a 50% reduction in mortality and this was not shown. The non-fatal reinfarction rate was similar in both groups." Baber et al. (1981) [30]
"We conclude that long-term treatment with timolol in patients surviving acute myocardial infarction reduces mortality and the rate of reinfarction." Norwegian Multicenter Study Group (1981) [31]

a future cardiac event. After a moment of silence, the consultant decides that this question should be discussed in detail at the Journal Club on Thursday. The junior doctor (who now regrets that he asked the question) is told to present the relevant literature. It is late in the evening when he makes his way to the library. The MEDLINE search identifies four clinical trials [28–31]. When reviewing the conclusions from these trials (Table 1.1), the doctor finds them to be confusing and contradictory. His consultant points out that the sheer amount of research published makes it impossible to keep track of and critically appraise individual studies. She recommends a good review article. Back in the library, the junior doctor finds a report that the *BMJ* published in 1981 in a "Regular Reviews" section [32]. This review concluded:

> *Thus, despite claims that they reduce arrhythmias, cardiac work, and infarct size, we still have no clear evidence that beta-blockers improve long-term survival after infarction despite almost 20 years of clinical trials. [32]*

The junior doctor is relieved. He summarizes the article in the Journal Club, and the patient is discharged without a beta-blocker.

1.5   TRADITIONAL REVIEWS

Traditional reviews have several disadvantages. First, the classical review is subjective and prone to bias and error [33]. Mulrow showed that among 50 reviews published in the mid-1980s in prominent general medicine journals, 49 did not specify the sources of information used and failed to perform a standardized assessment of the studies' methodological quality [1]. Indeed, our junior doctor could have consulted a review published in the *European Heart Journal* in the same year. This one concluded that "it seems perfectly reasonable to treat patients who have survived an infarction with timolol" [34]. Without being guided by a formal framework, reviewers will inevitably disagree about issues as basic as what types of studies it is appropriate to include and how to balance the quantitative evidence they provide. Selective inclusion of studies that support the author's view is common. In controversial areas, the conclusions drawn from a given body of evidence may be associated more with the specialty of the reviewer than with the available data [35]. Also, studies supporting prevailing opinion and positive studies are cited more frequently than unsupportive studies [36–38].

Once a set of studies has been assembled, authors might count the number of studies supporting various sides of an issue and choose the view receiving the most votes. Such "vote counting" is problematic, since it ignores sample size, the size of the effect or association, and sometimes even the research design. Thus, it is hardly surprising that reviewers using traditional methods often reach opposite conclusions [1] and miss small but potentially relevant differences [39]. By systematically identifying, scrutinizing, tabulating, and perhaps integrating all relevant studies using meta-analysis, systematic reviews allow a more objective appraisal, which can help resolve uncertainties when the original research, classical reviews, and editorial comments disagree.

The advent of systematic reviews and meta-analyses does not mean that narrative reviews and opinion pieces have no place [40]. Narrative reviews can be helpful to provide clarification, insight, and opinion on broader (policy) issues [41], to develop a conceptual framework, or to track the development of an idea (as we do in this chapter) [42]. However, whenever possible, they should draw on well-conducted systematic reviews.

1.6   LIMITATIONS OF A SINGLE STUDY

A single study often fails to detect or exclude a modest but relevant difference in the effects of two therapies. A trial may thus show no statistically significant treatment effect when, in reality, such an effect exists – it may produce a false-negative result. A classic study from the 1970s found that so-called negative RCTs often lack the statistical power to exclude meaningful clinical effects [43]. Although sample sizes have increased [44], the problem of underpowered clinical trials continues [45]. Often the required sample size may be difficult to achieve. An intervention that reduces mortality from myocardial infarction by 10% could delay thousands of deaths each year in the UK alone. Over 10000 patients in each treatment group would be needed to detect such an effect with high certainty [46].

The meta-analytic approach is an attractive alternative to such a large, expensive study. Data from patients in trials evaluating the same or a similar drug in several smaller, but comparable, studies are considered. Methods used for meta-analysis employ a weighted average of the results in which the larger trials have more influence than the smaller ones (Chapter 9). Comparisons are made exclusively between patients enrolled in the same study. In this way, the necessary number of patients may be reached, and relatively small effects can be detected or excluded with confidence.

Systematic reviews also contribute to gauging the applicability of study results. The findings of a particular study will, a priori, apply only to patients with the same characteristics as those investigated in the trial. If several trials in different groups of participants show similar results, we can conclude that the effect of the intervention under study has some generality. Meta-analyses of the individual participant data (**IPD meta-analysis**, see Chapter 12) from several trials are particularly useful to answer questions about whether effects vary among subgroups – e.g. among men and women, older and younger patients, or participants with different severities of the disease. Further, a single trial typically will examine the efficacy of one or two interventions. However, for a given condition, for example depression, several treatment options will be available, and doctors need to choose between them. **Network meta-analysis** (see Chapter 13) allows the simultaneous comparison of multiple interventions.

1.7 A MORE TRANSPARENT AND THOROUGH APPRAISAL

An important advantage of systematic reviews is that they render the review process transparent. In traditional reviews, it is often not clear how the conclusions follow from the data examined. In a well-presented systematic review, it should be possible for readers to replicate the quantitative component of the argument. The data included in meta-analyses must be presented in full or made available to facilitate this. The increased openness required leads to the replacement or underpinning of vague descriptors such as "some evidence of a trend," "a weak relationship," and "a strong relationship with reproducible estimates and their confidence intervals" [47]. Performing a systematic review mandates a thorough examination of studies' quality or risk of bias (see Chapters 4 and 5), and meta-analysis forces reviewers to scrutinize the data.

1.8 THE EPIDEMIOLOGY OF RESULTS

The tabulation, exploration, and evaluation of results are important components of systematic reviews (see Chapter 2). This can be taken further to explore sources of heterogeneity and test new hypotheses that were not posed in individual studies, for example using meta-regression techniques (see Chapter 10). In such "meta-epidemiology of results," the findings of an original study replace the individual as the unit of analysis [48, 49]. For example, a meta-regression analysis of RCTs of preventive home visits in older people showed that functional decline was reduced in trials that used comprehensive geriatric assessments but not in other trials [50]. However, although the studies included may be controlled experiments, the meta-analysis itself is subject to many biases inherent in observational studies. Aggregation or ecological bias is also a problem unless IPD are available (see Chapter 12). Nevertheless, systematic reviews can lead to the most promising or urgent research question and may permit a more accurate calculation of the sample sizes needed in future studies (see Chapter 24).

1.9   WHAT WAS THE EVIDENCE IN 1981?

What conclusions would our junior doctor have reached had he had access to a meta-analysis? Figure 1.4 shows the results from a meta-analysis that included 33 randomized comparisons of beta-blockers versus placebo or alternative treatment in patients with myocardial infarction [51]. These trials were published from 1967 to 1997. The combined risk ratio indicates that beta-blockade starting after the acute infarction reduced subsequent premature mortality by an estimated 20% (risk ratio 0.80). **Cumulative meta-analysis** is a useful way to show the evidence available in 1981 and at other points

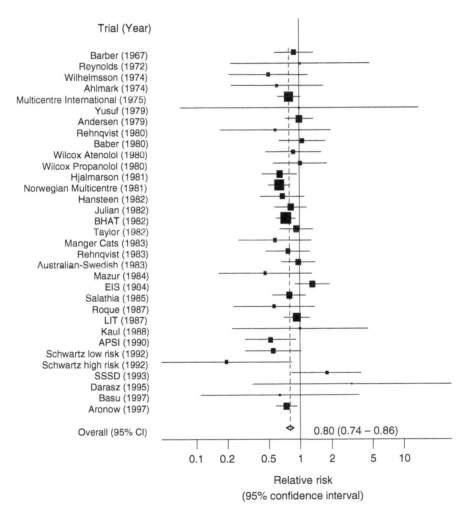

FIGURE 1.4   Forest plot showing mortality results from trials of beta-blockers in secondary prevention after myocardial infarction. Trials are ordered by year of publication. The black square and horizontal line correspond to the trials' risk ratio and 95% confidence intervals. The area of the black squares reflects the weight each trial contributes in the meta-analysis. The diamond represents the combined relative risk with its 95% confidence interval, indicating a 20% reduction in the odds of death. See Chapter 2 for a detailed description of forest plots. *Source*: Adapted from Freemantle et al. [51].

in time: the meta-analysis is updated whenever a new relevant trial becomes available. This allows the retrospective identification of the point in time when a treatment effect first became convincing. Here a beneficial effect became evident by 1981 (Figure 1.5). Subsequent trials in a further 15 000 patients simply confirmed this result, suggesting that the further studies may have been superfluous if not unethical [50].

Similarly, Lau et al. showed that for the trials of intravenous streptokinase in acute myocardial infarction, a convincing reduction in total mortality was demonstrated already by 1973 [49] (Figure 1.6). At that time, 2432 patients had been randomized in eight small trials. The results of the subsequent 25 studies, which included the very large GISSI-1 and ISIS-2 trials [51, 52] and enrolled a total of 34 542 additional patients, increased the strength of the evidence until the first mega-trial appeared in 1986, narrowing the confidence intervals around an essentially unchanged estimate of about 20% reduction in the risk of death. Interestingly, at least one country licensed streptokinase for use in myocardial infarction before GISSI-1 [51] was published, whereas many national authorities waited for this trial to appear, and some waited a further two years for the results of ISIS-2 [52] (Figure 1.6).

The concept of cumulative meta-analysis has since been expanded to "living systematic reviews," where a review is continually updated as new relevant evidence becomes available (Chapter 23). The approach may be applied to any systematic review and may involve updating meta-analyses. Living systematic reviews require a longer-term commitment and appropriate funding. They became essential in the response to the COVID-19 pandemic, with many such reviews and updates published in 2020 and 2021 [52, 53].

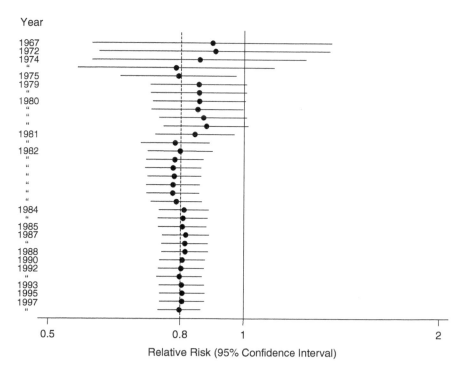

FIGURE 1.5   Cumulative meta-analysis of controlled trials of beta-blockers after myocardial infarction. The data correspond to Figure 1.4. A statistically significant (P < 0.05) beneficial effect on mortality became evident in 1981.

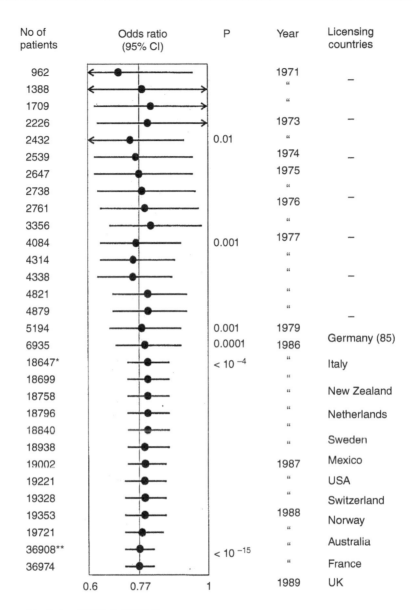

No of patients	Odds ratio (95% CI)	P	Year	Licensing countries
962			1971	
1388			"	
1709			"	–
2226			1973	
2432		0.01	"	–
2539			1974	
2647			1975	–
2738			"	
2761			1976	–
3356			"	
4084		0.001	1977	–
4314			"	
4338			"	–
4821			"	
4879			"	–
5194		0.001	1979	
6935		0.0001	1986	Germany (85)
18647*		< 10⁻⁴	"	Italy
18699			"	
18758			"	New Zealand
18796			"	Netherlands
18840			"	
18938			"	Sweden
19002			1987	Mexico
19221			"	USA
19328			"	Switzerland
19353			1988	Norway
19721			"	
36908**		< 10⁻¹⁵	"	Australia
36974			"	France
	0.6 0.77 1		1989	UK

* includes GISSI-1, **ISIS-2

FIGURE 1.6 Cumulative meta-analysis of randomized controlled trials of intravenous streptokinase in myocardial infarction. The number of patients randomized in a total of 33 trials and national authorities licensing streptokinase for use in myocardial infarction are also shown.

1.10   AN EXERCISE IN MEGA-SILLINESS?

Systematic reviews and, in particular, meta-analysis received a mixed reception initially. In 1978, the controversial psychologist Hans Eysenck [54] described an early meta-analysis of psychotherapy trials as an "exercise in mega-silliness" [55]. The authors of meta-analyses of perinatal care were dismissed as terrorists ("an obstetrical Baader-Meinhof gang") [56].

To some clinicians objecting to the findings of meta-analyses, "a tool has become a weapon" [57], while others "still prefer the conventional narrative review article" [58]. On closer inspection, many of the criticisms concerned shortcomings in the dissemination and quality of medical research, including publication bias and other reporting biases (see Chapter 5), or the low quality of the studies included in meta-analyses, the "garbage in, garbage out" problem (Chapter 4). These problems affect any review [59], but well-conducted systematic reviews and meta-analyses make them visible and address them (see Chapters 4 and 5). Another common criticism is the lack of attention to heterogeneity in the results of studies included in meta-analyses, followed by the uncritical calculation of a summary effect. We share this concern, but emphasize that some practitioners' inappropriate use of a method does not mean the method itself is flawed.

The misguided "mass production" of systematic reviews and meta-analyses is a serious threat to evidence synthesis [60]. In 2010, Bastian and colleagues asked "How will we ever keep up?" and pointed out that 75 trials and 11 systematic reviews are published each day [40]. Since then, the problem has become much worse (Figure 1.1). The quality of many reviews is poor and some duplicate the work of others, contributing to research waste [61]. A study of systematic reviews indexed in MEDLINE in 2014 found that the majority did not consider the risk of biases when interpreting results, and about a third used inappropriate statistical methods [62]. The pressure to publish (or perish) and the fact that systematic reviews and meta-analyses are popular with editors undoubtedly contributes to this situation. Systematic reviews and meta-analyses are cited more than other studies and help increase a journal's impact factor [63]. There is agreement that the incentive structure in academia and culture must change. The San Francisco Declaration on Research Assessment (DORA), which many academic institutions have signed, calls for the journal impact factor to be abandoned, emphasizing the content of a paper rather than publication metrics [64]. With this book, we want to help improve systematic reviews and meta-analyses and support DORA's emphasis on content and quality.

1.11 CONCLUSIONS

For many questions, systematic reviews, including if appropriate a formal meta-analysis, are superior to the narrative approach to reviewing research. In addition to providing a precise estimate of the overall effect of interventions in some instances, appropriate examination of heterogeneity across individual studies can produce useful information to guide rational and cost-effective decisions. Systematic reviews are also important to demonstrate areas where the available evidence is insufficient and where new, adequately sized trials are required.

ACKNOWLEDGMENTS

We are grateful to Sir David Cox for providing key references to early statistical work. We thank Dr. T Johansson and G Enocksson (Pharmacia AB, Stockholm) and Dr. A Schirmer and Dr. M Thimme (Behring AG, Marburg) for providing data on licensing of streptokinase in different countries.

REFERENCES

1. Mulrow, C.D. (1987). The medical review article: state of the science. *Ann. Intern. Med.* 106: 485–488. https://doi.org/10.7326/0003-4819-106-3-485.

2. Chalmers, I. and Altman, D. (1995). *Systematic Reviews*. London: BMJ Publishing Group.

3. Huque, M.F. (1988). Experiences with meta-analysis in NDA submissions. *Proc. Biopharm. Sect. Am. Stat. Assoc.* 2: 28–33.

4. Egger, M. and Davey, S.G. (1995). Misleading meta-analysis. *Br. Med. J.* 311: 753–754.

5. Royal Society (2018). Evidence synthesis. September 19. https://royalsociety.org/topics-policy/projects/evidence-synthesis (accessed February 21, 2022).

6. Grant, M.J. and Booth, A. (2009). A typology of reviews: an analysis of 14 review types and associated methodologies. *Health Info. Libr. J.* 26: 91–108.

7. Colquhoun, H.L., Levac, D., O'Brien, K.K. et al. (2014). Scoping reviews: time for clarity in definition, methods, and reporting. *J. Clin. Epidemiol.* 67: 1291–1294. https://doi.org/10.1016/j.jclinepi.2014.03.013.

8. Tricco, A.C., Antony, J., Zarin, W. et al. (2015). A scoping review of rapid review methods. *BMC Med.* 13: 224. https://doi.org/10.1186/s12916-015-0465-6.

9. Papatheodorou, S. (2019). Umbrella reviews: what they are and why we need them. *Eur. J. Epidemiol.* 34: 543–546. https://doi.org/10.1007/s10654-019-00505-6.

10. Page, M.J., Sterne, J.A.C., Higgins, J.P.T., and Egger, M. Investigating and dealing with publication bias and other reporting biases in meta-analyses of health research: a review. *Res. Synth. Methods* https://doi.org/10.1002/jrsm.1468.

11. Page, M.J., Higgins, J.P.T., Clayton, G. et al. (2016). Empirical evidence of study design biases in randomized trials: systematic review of meta-epidemiological studies. *PLoS One* 11: e0159267. https://doi.org/10.1371/journal.pone.0159267.

12. Chalmers, I., Hedges, L.V., and Cooper, H. (2002). A brief history of research synthesis. *Eval. Health Prof.* 25: 12–37.

13. Clarke, M. (2016). History of evidence synthesis to assess treatment effects: personal reflections on something that is very much alive. *J. R. Soc. Med.* 109: 154–163. https://doi.org/10.1177/0141076816640243.

14. Clarke, M. and Chalmers, I. (2018). Reflections on the history of systematic reviews. *Br. Med. J. Evid. Based Med.* 23: 121–122. https://doi.org/10.1136/bmjebm-2018-110968.

15. Lind, J. (1753). *A Treatise of the Scurvy. In Three Parts*. Edinburgh: A. Kincaid & A. Donaldson. Available at The James Lind Library, https://www.jameslindlibrary.org/lind-j-1753 (accessed February 21, 2022).

16. Ioannidis, J.P.A., Greenland, S., Hlatky, M.A. et al. (2014). Increasing value and reducing waste in research design, conduct, and analysis. *Lancet* 383: 166–175. https://doi.org/10.1016/S0140-6736(13)62227-8.

17. Plackett, R.L. (1958). Studies in the history of probability and statistics: VII. The principle of the arithmetic mean. *Biometrika* 45: 130–135.

18. Stigler, S.M. (1990). *The History of Statistics: The Measurement of Uncertainty Before 1900*. Cambridge, MA: Belknap Press of Harvard University Press.

19. Airy, G.B. (1861). *On the Algebraical and Numerical Theory of Errors of Observations and the Combinations of Observations*. London: Macmillan.

20. Pearson, K. (1904). Report on certain enteric fever inoculation statistics. *Br. Med. J.* 3: 1243–1246.

21. Peters, C.C. (1933). Summary of the Penn State experiments on the influence of instruction in character education. *J. Educ. Sociol.* 7: 269–272.

22. Glass, G.V. (1976). Primary, secondary and meta-analysis of research. *Educ. Res.* 5: 3–8.

23. Cochrane, A.L. (1979). *1931–1971: A Critical Review, with Particular Reference to the Medical Profession. In: Medicines for the Year 2000.* London: Office of Health Economics.

24. Baber, N.S. and Lewis, J.A. (1982). Confidence in results of beta-blocker postinfarction trials. *Br. Med. J.* 284: 1749–1750.

25. Yusuf, S., Peto, R., Lewis, J. et al. (1985). Beta blockade during and after myocardial infarction: an overview of the randomized trials. *Prog. Cardiovasc. Dis.* 17: 335–371.

26. Early Breast Cancer Trialists' Collaborative G (1988). Effects of adjuvant tamoxifen and of cytotoxic therapy on mortality in early breast cancer. An overview of 61 randomized trials among 28,896 women. *N. Engl. J. Med.* 319: 1681–1692.

27. Chalmers, I., Enkin, M., and Keirse, M.J.N.C. (1989). *Effective Care during Pregnancy and Childbirth.* Oxford: Oxford University Press.

28. Reynolds, J.L. and Whitlock, R.M.L. (1972). Effects of a beta-adrenergic receptor blocker in myocardial infarction treated for one year from onset. *Br. Heart J.* 34: 252–259.

29. Supplementary Report Multicentre International Study (1977). Reduction in mortality after myocardial infarction with long-term beta-adrenoceptor blockade. *Br. Med. J.* 2: 419–421.

30. Baber, N.S., Wainwright Evans, D., Howitt, G. et al. (1980). Multicentre post-infarction trial of propranolol in 49 hospital in the United Kingdom, Italy and Yugoslavia. *Br. Heart J.* 44: 96–100.

31. Norwegian Multicenter Study Group (1981). Timolol-induced reduction in mortality and reinfarction in patients surviving acute myocardial infarction. *N. Engl. J. Med.* 304: 801–807.

32. Mitchell, J.R.A. (1981). Timolol after myocardial infarction: an answer or a new set of questions? *Br. Med. J.* 282: 1565–1570.

33. Teagarden, J.R. (1989). Meta-analysis: whither narrative review? *Pharmacotherapy* 9: 274–284.

34. Hampton, J.R. (1981). The use of beta blockers for the reduction of mortality after myocardial infarction. *Eur. Heart J.* 2: 259–268.

35. Chalmers, T.C., Frank, C.S., and Reitman, D. (1990). Minimizing the three stages of publication bias. *J. Am. Med. Assoc.* 263: 1392–1395.

36. Ravnskov, U. (1992). Cholesterol lowering trials in coronary heart disease: frequency of citation and outcome. *Br. Med. J.* 305: 15–19.

37. Chapman, S., Ragg, M., and McGeechan, K. (2009). Citation bias in reported smoking prevalence in people with schizophrenia. *Austral. N. Zeal. J. Psychiatr.* 43: 277–282. https://doi.org/10.1080/00048670802653372.

38. Frank, R.A., Sharifabadi, A.D., Salameh, J.-P. et al. (2019). Citation bias in imaging research: are studies with higher diagnostic accuracy estimates cited more often? *Eur. Radiol.* 29: 1657–1664. https://doi.org/10.1007/s00330-018-5801-8.

39. Cooper, H. and Rosenthal, R. (1980). Statistical versus traditional procedures for summarising research findings. *Psychol. Bull.* 87: 442–449.

40. Bastian, H., Glasziou, P., and Chalmers, I. (2010). Seventy-five trials and eleven systematic reviews a day: how will we ever keep up? *PLoS Med.* 7: e1000326. https://doi.org/10.1371/journal.pmed.1000326.

41. Greenhalgh, T., Thorne, S., and Malterud, K. (2018). Time to challenge the spurious hierarchy of systematic over narrative reviews? *Eur. J. Clin. Invest.* 48: e12931. https://doi.org/10.1111/eci.12931.

42. Gurevitch, J., Koricheva, J., Nakagawa, S., and Stewart, G. (2018). Meta-analysis and the science of research synthesis. *Nature* 555: 175–182. https://doi.org/10.1038/nature25753.

43. Freiman, J.A., Chalmers, T.C., Smith, H., and Kuebler, R.R. (1992). The importance of beta, the type II error, and sample size in the design and interpretation of the randomized controlled trial. In: *Medical Uses of Statistics*, vol. 2 (eds. J.C. Bailar and F. Mosteller), 357–373. Boston, MA: NEJM Books.

44. Lamberink, H.J., Otte, W.M., Sinke, M.R.T. et al. (2018). Statistical power of clinical trials increased while effect size remained stable: an empirical analysis of 136,212 clinical trials between 1975 and 2014. *J. Clin. Epidemiol.* 102: 123–128. https://doi.org/10.1016/j.jclinepi.2018.06.014.

45. Boulos, M.I., Dharmakulaseelan, L., Brown, D.L., and Swartz, R.H. (2021). Trials in sleep apnea and stroke: learning from the past to direct future approaches. *Stroke* 52: 366–372. https://doi.org/10.1161/STROKEAHA.120.031709.

46. Collins, R., Keech, A., Peto, R. et al. (1992). Cholesterol and total mortality: need for larger trials. *Br. Med. J.* 304: 1689.

47. Rosenthal, R. (1990). An evaluation of procedures and results. In: *The Future of Meta-Analysis* (eds. K.W. Wachter and M.L. Straf), 123–133. New York: Russel Sage Foundation.

48. Jenicek, M. (1989). Meta-analysis in medicine. Where we are and where we want to go. *J. Clin. Epidemiol.* 42: 35–44. https://doi.org/10.1016/0895-4356(89)90023-1.

49. Naylor, C.D. (1997). Meta-analysis and the meta-epidemiology of clinical research. *Br. Med. J.* 315: 617–619.

50. Stuck, A.E., Egger, M., Hammer, A. et al. (2002). Home visits to prevent nursing home admission and functional decline in elderly people – systematic review and meta-regression analysis. *J. Am. Med. Assoc.* 287: 1022–1028. https://doi.org/10.1001/jama.287.8.1022.

51. Freemantle, N., Cleland, J., Young, P. et al. (1999). Beta blockade after myocardial infarction: systematic review and meta regression analysis. *Br. Med. J.* 318: 1730–1737. https://doi.org/10.1136/bmj.318.7200.1730.

52. Negrini, S., Mg, C., Côté, P., and Arienti, C. (2021). A systematic review that is "rapid" and "living": a specific answer to the COVID-19 pandemic. *J. Clin. Epidemiol.* https://doi.org/10.1016/j.jclinepi.2021.05.025.

53. Buitrago-Garcia, D., Egli-Gany, D., Counotte, M.J. et al. (2020). Occurrence and transmission potential of asymptomatic and presymptomatic SARS-CoV-2 infections: a living systematic review and meta-analysis. *PLoS Med.* 17: e1003346. https://doi.org/10.1371/journal.pmed.1003346.

54. Pelosi, A.J. (2019). Personality and fatal diseases: revisiting a scientific scandal. *J. Health Psychol.* 24: 421–439. https://doi.org/10.1177/1359105318822045.

55. Eysenck, H.J. (1978). An exercise in mega-silliness. *Am. Psychol.* 33: 517–517. https://doi.org/10.1037/0003-066X.33.5.517.a.

56. Mann, C. (1990). Meta-analysis in the breech. *Science* 249: 476–480. https://doi.org/10.1126/science.2382129.

57. Boden, W.E. (1992). Meta-analysis in clinical trials reporting: has a tool become a weapon? *Am. J. Cardiol.* 69: 681–686.

58. Bailar, J.C. (1997). The promise and problems of meta-analysis. *N. Engl. J. Med.* 337: 559–561.

59. Borenstein, M., Hedges, L.V., Higgins, J.P.T., and Rothstein, H.R. (2009). *Chapter 43. Criticisms of Meta-Analysis. Introduction to Meta-Analysis*, 1e, 377–387. Chichester: Wiley.

60. Page, M.J. and Moher, D. (2016). Mass production of systematic reviews and meta-analyses: an exercise in mega-silliness? *Milbank Q.* 94: 515–519. https://doi.org/10.1111/1468-0009.12211.

61. Helfer, B., Prosser, A., Samara, M.T. et al. (2015). Recent meta-analyses neglect previous systematic reviews and meta-analyses about the same topic: a systematic examination. *BMC Med.* 13: 82. https://doi.org/10.1186/s12916-015-0317-4.

62. Page, M.J., Shamseer, L., Altman, D.G. et al. (2016). Epidemiology and reporting characteristics of systematic reviews of biomedical research: a cross-sectional study. *PLoS Med.* 13: e1002028. https://doi.org/10.1371/journal.pmed.1002028.

63. Tahamtan, I., Afshar, A.S., and Ahamdzadeh, K. (2016). Factors affecting number of citations: a comprehensive review of the literature. *Scientometrics* 107: 1195–1225. https://doi.org/10.1007/s11192-016-1889-2.

64. DORA (2012) San Francisco Declaration on Research Assessment. https://sfdora.org (accessed February 21, 2022).

PART I

PRINCIPLES AND PROCEDURES

CHAPTER 2

Principles of Systematic Reviewing

Julian P.T. Higgins, George Davey Smith, Douglas G. Altman, and Matthias Egger

Systematic reviews allow a more objective appraisal of the evidence than narrative reviews and may thus contribute to resolving uncertainty when original research, experts, and commentators disagree. Systematic reviews are also essential to decide whether new research studies are warranted and to identify specific questions to be addressed in future studies. As will be discussed in subsequent chapters, poorly conducted reviews and meta-analyses may be biased due to exclusion of relevant studies, the inclusion of inadequate studies, or the inappropriate statistical combination of studies. Such bias can be minimized if a few basic principles are observed. This chapter introduces these principles and gives an overview of the practical steps involved in performing a systematic review. We will focus on systematic reviews of controlled trials, although the principles apply equally to other quantitative research studies such as cohort studies, case–control studies, and cross-sectional studies. We stress that the present chapter can only serve as an elementary introduction. Readers who want to perform systematic reviews should consult the ensuing chapters and consider working with a major research synthesis organization like Cochrane (see Chapter 21).

2.1   DEVELOPING A REVIEW PROTOCOL

Systematic reviews should be viewed as observational studies of the evidence. The steps involved, summarized in Box 2.1, are similar to any other research undertaking: formulation of the problem to be addressed, collection and analysis of the data, and interpretation of the results. Likewise, a detailed study protocol that clearly states the

Systematic Reviews in Health Research: Meta-Analysis in Context, Third Edition. Edited by Matthias Egger, Julian P.T. Higgins, and George Davey Smith.
© 2022 John Wiley & Sons Ltd. Published 2022 by John Wiley & Sons Ltd.
Companion website: www.systematic-reviews3.org

Box 2.1   Steps in Conducting A Systematic Review

1. Formulate review question
2. Define inclusion and exclusion criteria
   Consider PICO and other criteria:
   - **P**articipants
   - **I**nterventions, exposures, tests, or other factors of interest
   - **C**omparators
   - **O**utcomes
   - Study designs and methodological features
3. Prepare protocol
   - Cover points 1–2 and methods for 4–8 in as much detail as possible
   - Prespecify potential sources of heterogeneity to be explored
4. Locate studies (see also Chapter 3)
   Develop search strategy considering the following sources:
   - Electronic databases
   - Checking of reference lists
   - Handsearching of key journals
   - Personal communication with experts in the field
5. Select studies
   - Have eligibility assessed by >1 observer
   - Develop strategy to resolve disagreements
   - Keep log of excluded studies, with reasons for exclusions
6. Assess risk of bias or study quality (see also Chapter 4)
   - Consider assessment by >1 observer
   - Use domain-based assessments or simple checklists rather than numeric scales
7. Collect data
   - Design and pilot data collection form
   - Consider data extraction from reports by >1 observer
   - Consider possibility of collating individual participant data
8. Analyze and present results (see also Chapters 8–14)
   - Tabulate characteristics and results of individual studies
   - Examine forest plot
   - Explore possible sources of heterogeneity
   - Consider meta-analysis of all studies or subsets of studies
   - Perform sensitivity analyses, examine funnel plots
   - Make list of excluded studies available to interested readers

9. Interpret results (see also Chapter 21)
   - Consider limitations, including publication and related biases
   - Consider strength of evidence, including amount of evidence and quality of studies
   - Consider consistency of evidence across studies
   - Consider applicability
   - Consider meaningful presentation of findings (e.g. using absolute risks rather than relative risks)
   - Consider economic implications
   - Consider implications for future research

question to be addressed, the criteria for selecting relevant studies, and the methods to identify and analyze information should be written in advance. This is important to avoid bias being introduced by decisions that are influenced by the data. For example, studies that produced unexpected or undesired results might be inappropriately excluded by post hoc changes to the inclusion criteria. Similarly, unplanned data-driven subgroup analyses are likely to produce spurious results [1–3], and lack of clarity on primary and secondary outcomes for the review leads to the possibility of selective reporting of those the reviewers consider as most favorable. The review protocol should ideally be written by a group of reviewers with expertise in the content area and the science of research synthesis, and should be registered on a publicly accessible resource such as PROSPERO [4].

2.1.1 Objectives and Eligibility Criteria

The formulation of detailed objectives is at the heart of any research project. For reviews on the effects of health care interventions, a review question is often articulated using a PICO framework. This mnemonic refers to specifying the participants (P), interventions (I), comparators (C), and outcomes (O) of interest. Variations of this framework are applicable to reviews of different types of questions. For example, an objective to summarize evidence on the prevalence of a particular disease may only need to specify the types of participants and the disease of interest (see also the chapters on systematic reviews of other specific study designs later in this book).

As with patient inclusion and exclusion criteria in clinical studies, eligibility criteria can then be defined for the types of studies to be included. These criteria relate to the review objectives (e.g. participants, interventions being compared) and to the kinds of studies to be included (e.g. study design, length of follow-up). They should be selected with a view to the combinability of studies in a synthesis. It is not always necessary to use every component of the review question (e.g. all elements of PICO) as criteria for including studies. The reporting of particular outcome measures from a controlled trial, for example, can be influenced by the results for that outcome. Thus specifying that outcome data must be available for the study to be eligible for the review may result in a biased subset of included studies. While it will not be possible to include the study in a meta-analysis, the potential impact of the study's omission can at least be considered.

Features of the design and rigor of research studies can influence the results [5–7], as discussed in Chapters 4 and 10. Questions about the effects of interventions would ideally be addressed only using controlled trials with proper randomization of interventions to participants that report on all initially included participants according to the intention-to-treat principle, and that use an objective, preferably blinded, outcome assessment. However, assessing whether studies were well performed can be a subjective process, especially since the information reported is often inadequate for this purpose [8–10]. Therefore, it may be preferable to define only basic inclusion criteria in relation to study design features and to perform a detailed assessment of each included study's merits as part of the review itself (see Section 2.1.3).

2.1.2   Literature Search

The search strategy for identification of the relevant studies should be clearly delineated. As discussed in Chapter 3, the starting point is usually a search of bibliographic databases. The main bibliographic databases in health research are MEDLINE and Embase, although regional databases and subject-specific databases may also be important. Conference proceedings, PhD theses, and the bibliographies of review articles, monographs, and the located studies should also be scrutinized, as should relevant online study registries (such as http://clinicaltrials.gov) where these are relevant to the research question. The search should be extended to include unpublished studies where possible, as their results may differ systematically from published studies. As discussed in Chapter 5, a systematic review that is restricted to published evidence may produce distorted results due to publication bias. Colleagues, experts in the field, contacts in relevant organizations, and other informal channels can be important sources of information on unpublished and ongoing studies.

Identifying controlled trials for systematic reviews is more straightforward than identifying other types of studies. Randomized trials and controlled trials are specifically tagged in MEDLINE and Embase, partly due to Cochrane's painstaking efforts to check the titles and abstracts of hundreds of thousands of MEDLINE and Embase records, which were then re-tagged as controlled trials if appropriate. Furthermore, Cochrane has identified thousands of reports of controlled trials by manual searches ("handsearching") of journals, conference proceedings, and other sources. All trials identified in the re-tagging and handsearching projects are included in the Cochrane Central Register of Controlled Trials (CENTRAL), which is available in the Cochrane Library (see Chapter 21). This register currently includes over a million records and is clearly the best single source of published trials for inclusion in systematic reviews. Searches of MEDLINE and Embase are, however, still required to identify trials that were published recently (see Chapter 3).

Registration of all research studies when they are established (and before their results become known) would reduce the risk of publication bias [11, 12]. Several registers are available for clinical trials (see Chapter 5) and these are an important source of information about ongoing and completed trials. One Cochrane group has proposed to include only trials that have been registered at inception, which should substantially reduce the risk of publication bias, although it may risk excluding relevant, high-quality studies that were not registered [13].

2.1.3   Selection of Studies, Assessment of Methodological Quality, and Data Extraction

Decisions regarding the inclusion or exclusion of individual studies often involve some degree of subjectivity. Therefore, it is useful to have two observers checking the eligibility of candidate studies, with disagreements being resolved by discussion or a third reviewer.

Before incorporating individual studies into syntheses, it is important to consider the extent to which their results can be trusted. Even though randomized controlled trials provide the best evidence of the effects of medical interventions, they are not immune to bias. Studies relating methodological features of trials to their results have shown that several features can be associated with effect sizes [7]. Inadequate concealment of treatment allocation, resulting, for example, from the use of open random number tables, is on average associated with larger treatment effects, as is a lack of blinding of outcome assessors, particularly when the outcome assessment involves judgment [14].

Many tools are available to assess the risk of bias or the methodological quality of research studies, particularly for controlled trials [15] and epidemiological association studies [16]. Empirical evidence [17, 18] and theoretical considerations [19] suggest that although summary quality scores may in some circumstances provide a useful overall assessment, numeric scales should not generally be used to assess the quality of trials in systematic reviews. Rather, as discussed in Chapter 4, the relevant methodological aspects should be identified and assessed individually. Again, independent assessment by more than one observer is desirable.

Two independent observers should extract data from reports of studies so that errors can be avoided. A standardized data extraction form is needed for this purpose. Data extraction forms should be carefully designed, piloted, and revised if necessary. Electronic data collection forms are the norm these days. They facilitate the combination of data extraction and entry into one step and the automatic detection of inconsistencies between data recorded by different observers. However, programming and revising electronic forms can be time-consuming, although a growing number of systematic review software systems are now available to support this process (see Chapters 6 and 23).

Direct contact with the authors of the included studies is a useful supplement to extracting data from study reports. Such contacts may lead to the collation of individual participant data and a collaborative re-analysis of the original data. This approach is widely considered to be the gold standard approach to meta-analysis and is discussed in Chapter 12.

2.2   PRESENTING, COMBINING, AND INTERPRETING RESULTS

Once studies have been selected, critically appraised, and data extracted, the characteristics of included studies should be presented in tabular form. Table 2.1 shows the characteristics of the long-term trials included in a systematic review of the effect of beta-blockade in secondary prevention after myocardial infarction (we mentioned

TABLE 2.1 Characteristics of long-term trials comparing beta-blockers with control.

Author	Year	Drug	Study duration (years)	Concealment of treatment allocation	Double-blind	Mortality (No./total no.)	
						Beta-blocker	Control
Barber	1967	Practolol	2	Unclear	Unclear	33/207	38/213
Reynolds	1972	Alprenolol	1	Yes	Yes	3/38	3/39
Ahlmark	1974	Alprenolol	2	Unclear	Unclear	5/69	11/93
Wilhelmsson	1974	Alprenolol	2	Unclear	Yes	7/114	14/116
Multicentre International	1975	Practolol	2	Unclear	Yes	102/1533	127/1520
Yusuf	1979	Atenolol	1	Unclear	Yes	1/11	1/11
Andersen	1979	Alprenolol	1	Unclear	Yes	61/238	62/242
Rehnqvist	1980	Metroprolol	1	Unclear	Unclear	4/59	6/52
Baber	1980	Propranolol	0.75	Unclear	Yes	28/355	27/365
Wilcox (atenolol)	1980	Atenolol	1	Yes	Yes	17/132	19/129
Wilcox (propanolol)	1980	Propranolol	1	Yes	Yes	19/127	19/129
Hjalmarson	1981	Metoprolol	2	Unclear	No	40/698	62/697
Norwegian Multicentre	1981	Timolol	1.4	Unclear	Yes	98/945	152/939
Hansteen	1982	Propranolol	1	Unclear	Yes	25/278	37/282
Julian	1982	Sotalol	1	Yes	Yes	64/873	52/583
BHAT	1982	Proprcnolol	2.1	Yes	Yes	138/1916	188/1921
Taylor	1982	Oxprenolol	4	Done	Yes	60/632	48/471
Manger Cats	1983	Metoprolol	1	Unclear	Yes	9/273	16/280
Rehnqvist	1983	Metroprolol	3	Unclear	Yes	25/154	31/147

Australian-Swedish	1983	Pindolol	2	Unclear	Yes	45/263	47/266
Mazur	1984	Propranolol	1.5	Unclear	No	5/101	11/103
EIS	1984	Oxprenolol	1	Unclear	Yes	57/853	45/883
Salathia	1985	Metoprolol	1	Unclear	Yes	49/416	52/348
Roqué	1987	Timolol	2	Unclear	Yes	7/102	12/98
LIT	1987	Metoprolol	1.5	Unclear	Yes	86/1195	93/1200
Kaul	1988	Propranolol	0.5	Unclear	Yes	3/25	3/25
ASPI	1990	Acebutolol	0.87	Yes	Yes	17/298	34/309
Schwartz (high risk)	1992	Oxprenolol	1.8	Unclear	No	2/48	12/56
Schwartz (low risk)	1992	Oxprenolol	1.8	Unclear	Yes	15/437	27/432
SSSD	1993	Metoprolol	3	Unclear	No	17/130	9/123
Darasz	1995	Xamoterol	0.5	Unclear	Yes	3/23	1/24
Basu	1997	Carvedilol	0.5	Unclear	Yes	2/75	3/71
Aronow	1997	Propranolol	1	Unclear	Unclear	44/79	60/79

Source: Adapted from Gøtzsche [24].

this example in Chapter 1 and will return to it later in this chapter) [20]. The review included all parallel-group, randomized trials that examined the effectiveness of beta-blockers versus placebo or alternative treatment in patients with myocardial infarction. The authors searched 11 bibliographic databases, including dissertation abstracts and gray literature databases, examined existing reviews, and checked the reference lists of each identified study. They identified 31 trials of at least six months' duration, which contributed 33 comparisons of beta-blockers with control groups (Table 2.1) [20].

2.2.1   Standardized Outcome Measure

Individual results must be expressed in a standardized format to allow for comparison between studies. Risk ratios or odds ratios are often calculated in controlled trials with a binary endpoint (e.g. disease versus no disease, or dead versus alive). The odds ratio has convenient mathematical properties, which allow for ease in combining data and testing the overall effect for statistical significance. Still, the odds ratio will differ from the risk ratio if the outcome is common (see Box 8.1 in Chapter 8). Risk ratios are frequently preferred over odds ratios because they are more intuitively understandable to most people [21, 22]. Absolute measures such as the absolute risk reduction or the number of patients who need to be treated for one person to benefit [23] are more helpful when applying results of trials in clinical practice (see below). If the outcome in a controlled trial is continuous and measurements are made on the same scale (e.g. blood pressure measured in mm Hg), the mean difference between the treatment and control groups is commonly used. If trials measured outcomes differently, any differences between intervention groups may be presented in standard deviation units rather than as absolute differences. For example, the efficacy of nonsteroidal anti-inflammatory drugs for reducing pain in patients with rheumatoid arthritis was measured using different scales [24]. The choice and calculation of appropriate summary statistics from controlled trials are covered in detail in Chapter 8.

Similar options are available in observational studies of the association between an exposure and an outcome. However, in case–control studies, the odds ratio should be used as an approximation to the risk ratio. It is common for statistical adjustments to be made to these associations to control for potential confounding factors. These adjustments might be made, for example, using logistic regression for a binary endpoint or using linear regression for a continuous outcome. The reviewer may not have much choice over the measure used and the adjustments made, but will generally have access to results that are unadjusted or adjusted for different potential confounders (see Chapters 15 and 19).

2.2.2   Graphical Display

Results from each trial are usefully graphically displayed together with their confidence intervals in a "forest plot," a form of presentation developed in the 1980s by Sir Richard Peto's group in Oxford [25]. Figure 2.1 provides the forest plot for the trials of beta-blockers in secondary prevention after myocardial infarction, which we discussed in Chapter 1 [20]. Each study is represented by a black square and a horizontal line that

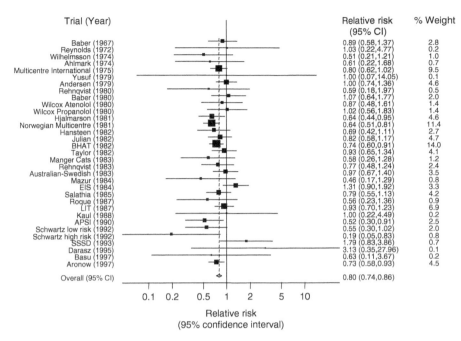

FIGURE 2.1 Forest plot showing total mortality from trials of beta-blockers in secondary prevention after myocardial infarction. The black square and horizontal line correspond to the risk ratio and 95% confidence intervals (CIs), respectively. The area of the black squares reflects the weight each trial contributes to the meta-analysis. The diamond at the bottom of the graph represents the combined risk ratio and its 95% CI, indicating a 20% reduction in the risk of death. The solid vertical line corresponds to no effect of treatment (risk ratio 1.0), the dotted vertical line to the combined risk ratio (0.8). The risk ratio, 95% CI, and weights are also given in tabular form. The graph was produced in STATA (see Chapter 25). *Source*: Adapted from Freemantle et al. [20].

correspond to the point estimate of the risk ratio and its 95% confidence interval. The 95% confidence intervals would contain the true underlying effect on 95% of the occasions, if the study were repeated again and again. The solid vertical line corresponds to no effect of treatment (a risk ratio of exactly 1). The confidence intervals of most studies cross this line. The area of the black squares reflects the weight of the study in the meta-analysis (see Section 2.2.4).

A logarithmic scale was used for plotting the risk ratios in Figure 2.1. There are several reasons why ratio measures are best plotted on logarithmic scales [26]. Most importantly, the value of a risk ratio and its reciprocal, for example 0.5 and 2, which represent risk ratios of the same magnitude but opposite directions, will be equidistant from 1. Studies with risk ratios below and above 1 will take up equal space on the graph and thus visually appear to be equally important. Also, confidence intervals will be symmetric around the point estimate.

2.2.3   Heterogeneity Between Study Results

The thoughtful consideration of heterogeneity between study results is an important aspect of systematic reviews (Chapter 10). As already mentioned, this should start when writing the review protocol by defining potential sources of heterogeneity and planning appropriate subgroup analyses. Once the data have been assembled, a simple inspection of the forest plot is informative. The results from the beta-blocker trials are fairly homogeneous, clustering between risk ratios of 0.5 and 1, with widely overlapping confidence intervals (Figure 2.1). In contrast, trials of BCG vaccination for the prevention of tuberculosis [27] (Figure 2.2) are clearly heterogeneous. The findings of the UK trial, which indicate a substantial benefit of BCG vaccination, are not compatible with those from the Madras or Puerto Rico trials, which suggest little effect or only a modest benefit. There is no overlap in the confidence intervals of the three trials. Other graphical representations are particularly useful to detect and investigate heterogeneity. These include funnel plots [28] (Chapter 5), L'Abbé plots [29] (see Chapter 8), and Galbraith plots [26].

Statistical measures of heterogeneity assess the extent to which the individual study results reflect a single underlying effect, as opposed to a distribution of effects. A direct measure of the variability in underlying effects across studies is the heterogeneity variance (often represented by tau^2, or τ^2). A commonly used alternative is the I^2 statistic, which measures approximately the proportion of variability in individual study results that is due to true effect differences (heterogeneity) rather than chance [30, 31]. Tests of homogeneity (also called tests for heterogeneity) are also available (see Chapter 9). If these measures fail to detect heterogeneity among results, then it is assumed that the differences observed between individual studies are a consequence of sampling variation and simply due to chance. The I^2 statistic for the beta-blocker trials is 13.6% and a τ^2 test of homogeneity gives P = 0.25; the corresponding statistics for the BCG trials are $I^2 = 92.1\%$ and P < 0.001. Substantial heterogeneity between study results, such as is observed here for the BCG trials, should not necessarily be seen as a problem for systematic reviews since it provides an opportunity for examining why treatment effects differ in different circumstances, as discussed below and in Chapter 10.

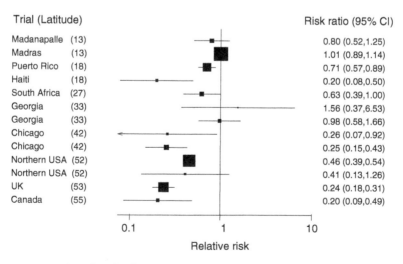

FIGURE 2.2   Forest plot of trials of BCG vaccine to prevent tuberculosis. Trials are ordered according to the latitude of the study location, expressed as degrees from the equator. No meta-analysis is shown. CI, confidence interval. *Source*: Adapted from Colditz et al. [27].

2.2.4   Methods for Estimating A Typical Effect

If, after careful consideration, a meta-analysis is deemed appropriate, the last step consists of estimating a typical effect by combining the data. Two principles are important. First, simply pooling the data from different studies and treating them as one large study would fail to preserve the integrity of each individual study and may introduce bias and confounding. In particular, pooling participants across randomized trials may remove all the benefits of randomization. An interesting example of the bias this pooling can introduce appeared in a review and "meta-analysis" of observational studies of the role of male circumcision in HIV transmission. The reviewers concluded that the risk of HIV infection was lower in uncircumcised men [32]. However, the analysis was performed by simply pooling the data from 33 diverse studies. A re-analysis stratifying the data by study found that an intact foreskin was in fact associated with an increased risk of HIV infection [33]. Confounding by study thus led to a change in the direction of the association (a case of "Simpson's paradox," in epidemiological parlance [34, 35]). The unit of the study must, therefore, always be maintained when combining data.

Second, simply calculating an arithmetic mean would be inappropriate. The results from small studies are more subject to the play of chance and should be given less weight. Methods used for meta-analysis employ a weighted average of the results, in which the larger trials generally have more influence than the smaller ones. A variety of statistical techniques are available for this purpose (see Chapter 9), which can be broadly classified into two approaches [36]. The difference is in whether the variability of the results *between* the studies is considered. The *fixed-effect* approach considers only random variation within studies, and individual studies are weighted solely by their precision [37]. The main alternative, the *random-effects* approach [38, 39], assumes a model in which different effects underlie the different studies, and these differences are taken into consideration as an additional source of variation. Effects are assumed to be randomly distributed, and the central point of this distribution is the focus of the combined effect estimate. Random-effects approaches generally give relatively more weight to smaller studies and lead to wider confidence intervals than fixed-effects approaches. The use of random-effects models has been advocated if there is heterogeneity between study results. This is problematic, however. Rather than simply ignoring it after applying some statistical model, the approach to heterogeneity should be to scrutinize and attempt to explain it (see Chapter 10).

While neither of the two approaches can be said to be "correct," a substantial difference in the combined effect calculated by the fixed- and random-effects approaches will be seen only if studies are markedly heterogeneous, as in the case of the BCG trials (Table 2.2). Combining trials using a random-effects model indicates that BCG vaccination halves the risk of tuberculosis, whereas fixed-effects analysis indicates that the risk is only reduced by 35%. The difference is explained by the different weight given to the large Madras trial, which showed no protective effect of vaccination (41% of the total weight with the fixed-effects model, 10% with the random-effects model, Table 2.2). Both analyses are probably misguided. As shown in Figure 2.2, BCG vaccination appears to be effective in cooler regions but not in warmer regions. This could be due to exposure to certain mycobacteria in the environment acting like "natural" BCG vaccination in warmer regions [40]. In this situation, it is more

TABLE 2.2   Meta-analysis of trials of BCG vaccination to prevent tuberculosis using a fixed-effects and random-effects model (inverse variance method). Note the differences in the weights allocated to individual studies.

Trial	Risk ratio (95% confidence interval)	Fixed-effects weight (%)	Random-effects weight (%)
Madanapalle	0.80 (0.52 to 1.25)	3.20	8.88
Madras	1.01 (0.89 to 1.14)	41.40	10.22
Puerto Rico	0.71 (0.57 to 0.89)	13.21	9.93
Haiti	0.20 (0.08 to 0.50)	0.73	6.00
South Africa	0.63 (0.39 to 1.00)	2.91	8.75
Georgia	0.98 (0.58 to 1.66)	0.31	3.80
Georgia	1.56 (0.37 to 6.53)	2.30	8.40
Chicago	0.26 (0.07 to 0.92)	0.40	4.40
Chicago	0.25 (0.15 to 0.43)	2.25	8.37
Northern USA	0.41 (0.13 to 1.26)	23.75	10.12
Northern USA	0.46 (0.39 to 0.54)	0.50	5.05
UK	0.24 (0.18 to 0.31)	8.20	9.71
Canada	0.20 (0.09 to 0.49)	0.84	6.34
Combined relative risks		0.65 (0.60 to 0.70)	0.49 (0.35 to 0.70)

Source: Adapted from Colditz et. al [27].

meaningful to quantify how the effect varies according to latitude than to calculate an overall estimate of effect, which will be misleading for either of the approaches (see Chapter 10 for further analyses of the BCG trials).

2.2.5   Sensitivity Analysis

There will often be different opinions on the correct method for performing a particular meta-analysis. The robustness of the findings to different assumptions should therefore always be examined in a thorough sensitivity analysis. This is illustrated in Figure 2.3 for the beta-blockers after myocardial infarction meta-analysis [20]. First, the overall effect was calculated by different statistical methods, using fixed-effects and random-effects approaches. It is evident from the figure that the overall estimate is virtually identical and that confidence intervals are only slightly wider when using the random-effects approach. This is explained by the relatively small amount of between-trial variation present in this meta-analysis.

The methodological quality of the beta-blocker trials was assessed in terms of concealment of allocation of study participants to beta-blocker or control groups and blinding of patients and investigators (see also Chapter 4) [20]. Figure 2.3 shows that the estimated treatment effect was similar for studies with and without concealment of treatment allocation. The eight studies that were not described as

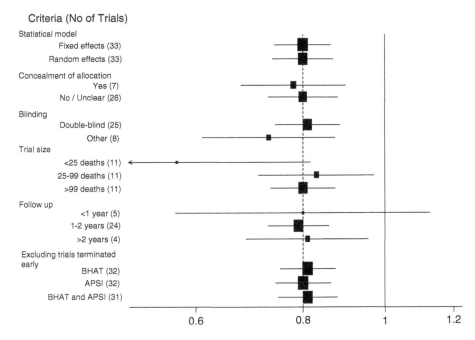

FIGURE 2.3   Sensitivity analyses examining the robustness of the effect on total mortality of beta-blockers in secondary prevention after myocardial infarction. The dotted vertical line corresponds to the combined relative risk from the fixed-effects model (0.8).

double-blind indicated more benefit than the 25 trials that were, but confidence intervals overlap widely.

Statistically significant results are more likely to get published than nonsignificant findings [41, 42], which can distort the findings of meta-analyses (see also Chapter 5). Whether such publication bias is plausible can be examined by stratifying the analysis by study size. If publication bias is present, it is expected that the larger published studies will report smaller effects because they are more likely to find that small estimates are statistically significant. Figure 2.3 shows that this is indeed the case in the beta-blocker example, with the 11 smallest trials (25 deaths or fewer) showing the largest effect. However, the exclusion of the smaller studies has little effect on the overall estimate. Studies varied in terms of length of follow-up, but this again had little effect on estimates. Finally, two trials [43, 44] were terminated earlier than anticipated based on the results from interim analyses [45]. The exclusion of these trials, however, again affects the overall estimate only marginally.

The sensitivity analysis thus shows that the results from this meta-analysis are robust to the choice of the statistical method and to the exclusion of trials of lesser quality or of studies terminated early. It also suggests that publication bias is unlikely to have distorted the findings.

2.3   INTERPRETING FINDINGS

The risk ratio of death associated with the use of beta-blockers after myocardial infarction is 0.80 (95% confidence interval 0.74 to 0.86) (Figure 2.1). The *relative risk reduction*, obtained by subtracting the risk ratio from 1 and expressing the result as a percentage,

TABLE 2.3   Beta-blockade in secondary prevention after myocardial infarction. Absolute risk reductions and numbers-needed-to-treat for one year to prevent one death, NNT(benefit), for different levels of control group mortality.

One-year mortality risk among controls (%)	Absolute risk reduction	NNT(benefit)
1	0.002	500
3	0.006	167
5	0.01	100
10	0.02	50
20	0.04	25
30	0.06	17
40	0.08	13
50	0.1	10

Calculations assume a constant relative risk reduction of 20%.

is 20% (95% confidence interval 14 to 26%). These relative measures of treatment effect ignore the underlying absolute risk. The risk of death among patients who have survived the acute phase of myocardial infarction varies widely [46]. For example, among patients with three or more cardiac risk factors, the probability of death at two years after discharge ranged from 24% to 60% [47]. Conversely, two-year mortality among patients with no risk factors was less than 3%. The *absolute risk reduction*, or risk difference, reflects both the underlying risk without therapy and the relative risk reduction associated with therapy.

For an underlying risk of 1% per year, the absolute risk reduction indicates that two deaths are prevented per 1000 treated patients (Table 2.3). This corresponds to 500 patients being treated for one year in order to prevent one death. Conversely, if the risk is above 10%, fewer than 50 patients have to be treated to prevent one death. Many clinicians would probably decide not to treat patients at very low risk, considering the large number of patients who would have to be exposed to the adverse effects of beta-blockade to prevent one death. Appraising the treatment effect in the form of a number needed to treat (NNT), derived from the combination of a patient's estimated risk without treatment with the relative risk reduction with treatment, is a helpful aid when making a decision with an individual patient.

This example illustrates the general principle that findings of meta-analyses may need to be re-expressed to assist with interpretation and application (see also Chapter 22). In this context, it is generally more meaningful to look at absolute rather than relative effects on risk when analyzing binary outcomes. A reasonable question is why we do not undertake the meta-analysis itself using an absolute effect measure such as the risk difference. The problem is that a *combined* risk difference (and the NNT calculated from it) will be essentially determined by the number and size of trials in low, intermediate, and high-risk patients. Combined results will thus apply only to patients at levels of risk corresponding to the average risk of the trial participants. Meta-analyses are generally therefore undertaken using relative effect measures, while absolute measures are used when applying the findings to a specific clinical or public health situation.

2.4   CONCLUSIONS

Systematic reviews are thorough reviews of previous research and are guided largely by methodological rigor, comprehensiveness, and transparency principles. The review processes are structured, such that issues of the completeness of the evidence identified, the methodological quality of component studies, and the combinability of evidence are made explicit. Nevertheless, the systematic reviewer must tackle several fundamental questions as part of the exercise. How likely is it that publication and related biases have been avoided? Is it sensible to combine the individual studies in meta-analysis, or is there heterogeneity between individual study results that renders the calculation of an overall estimate questionable? If meta-analysis was performed, how robust are the results to changes in assumptions? Finally, has the analysis contributed to the process of making rational health care decisions? These challenging issues will be considered in more depth in the following chapters.

REFERENCES

1. Oxman, A.D. and Guyatt, G.H. (1992). A consumer's guide to subgroup analyses. *Ann. Intern. Med.* 116: 78–84.

2. Brookes, S.T., Whitely, E., Egger, M. et al. (2004). Subgroup analyses in trials: risks of subgroup-specific analyses; power and sample size for the interaction test. *J. Clin. Epidemiol.* 57 (3): 229–236.

3. Assmann, S.F., Pocock, S.J., Enos, L.E., and Kasten, L.E. (2000). Subgroup analysis and other (mis)uses of baseline data in clinical trials. *Lancet* 355 (9209): 1064–1069.

4. Booth, A., Clarke, M., Dooley, G. et al. (2012). The nuts and bolts of PROSPERO: an international prospective register of systematic reviews. *Syst Rev.* 1: 2.

5. Sacks, H.S., Chalmers, T.C., and Smith, H. Jr. (1982). Randomized versus historical controls for clinical trials. *Am. J. Med.* 72: 233–240.

6. Schulz, K.F., Chalmers, I., Hayes, R.J., and Altman, D.G. (1995). Empirical evidence of bias: dimensions of methodological quality associated with estimates of treatment effects in controlled trials. *JAMA* 273: 408–412.

7. Page, M.J., Higgins, J.P.T., Clayton, G. et al. (2016). Empirical evidence of study design biases in randomized trials: systematic review of meta-epidemiological studies. *PLoS One* 11 (7): e0159267.

8. Moher, D., Hopewell, S., Schulz, K.F. et al. (2010). CONSORT 2010 explanation and elaboration: updated guidelines for reporting parallel group randomised trials. *BMJ* 340: c869.

9. Vandenbroucke, J.P., von Elm, E., Altman, D.G. et al. (2007). Strengthening the Reporting of Observational Studies in Epidemiology (STROBE): explanation and elaboration. *PLoS Med.* 4 (10): e297.

10. Bossuyt, P.M., Reitsma, J.B., Bruns, D.E. et al. (2003). The STARD statement for reporting studies of diagnostic accuracy: explanation and elaboration. *Ann. Intern. Med.* 138 (1): W1–W12.

11. De Angelis, C., Drazen, J.M., Frizelle, F.A. et al. (2004). Clinical trial registration: a statement from the International Committee of Medical Journal Editors. *Lancet* 364 (9438): 911–912.

12. Zarin, D.A., Tse, T., and Ide, N.C. (2005). Trial registration at ClinicalTrials.gov between May and October 2005. *N. Engl. J. Med.* 353 (26): 2779–2787.

13. Roberts, I., Ker, K., Edwards, P. et al. (2015). The knowledge system underpinning healthcare is not fit for purpose and must change. *BMJ* 350: h2463.

14. Savović, J., Jones, H.E., Altman, D.G. et al. (2012). Influence of reported study design characteristics on intervention effect estimates from randomized, controlled trials. *Ann. Intern. Med.* 157 (6): 426–438.

15. Moher, D., Jadad, A.R., Nichol, G. et al. (1995). Assessing the quality of randomized controlled trials: an annotated bibliography of scales and checklists. *Control. Clin. Trials.* 16 (1): 62–73.

16. Sanderson, S., Tatt, I.D., and Higgins, J.P.T. (2007). Tools for assessing quality and susceptibility to bias in observational studies in epidemiology: a systematic review and annotated bibliography. *Int. J. Epidemiol.* 36 (3): 666–676.

17. Jüni, P., Witschi, A., Bloch, R., and Egger, M. (1999). The hazards of scoring the quality of clinical trials for meta-analysis. *JAMA* 282 (11): 1054–1060.

18. da Costa, B.R., Hilfiker, R., and Egger, M. (2013). PEDro's bias: summary quality scores should not be used in meta-analysis. *J. Clin. Epidemiol.* 66 (1): 75–77.

19. Greenland, S. (1994). Quality scores are useless and potentially misleading. *Am. J. Epidemiol.* 140: 300–301.

20. Freemantle, N., Cleland, J., Young, P. et al. (1999). Beta blockade after myocardial infarction: systematic review and meta regression analysis. *BMJ* 318 (7200): 1730–1737.

21. Sackett, D.L., Deeks, J.J., and Altman, D.G. (1996). Down with odds ratios! *J. Evid. Based Med.* 1 (6): 164–166.

22. Davies, H.T., Crombie, I.K., and Tavakoli, M. (1998). When can odds ratios mislead? *BMJ* 316 (7136): 989–991.

23. Laupacis, A., Sackett, D.L., and Roberts, R.S. (1988). An assessment of clinically useful measures of the consequences of treatment. *N. Engl. J. Med.* 318: 1728–1733.

24. Gøtzsche, P.C. (1990). Sensitivity of effect variables in rheumatoid arthritis: a meta-analysis of 130 placebo controlled NSAID trials. *J. Clin. Epidemiol.* 43: 1313–1318.

25. Lewis, S. and Clarke, M. (2001). Forest plots: trying to see the wood and the trees. *BMJ* 322: 1479–1480.

26. Galbraith, R.F. (1988). A note on graphical presentation of estimated odds ratios from several clinical trials. *Stat. Med.* 7: 889–894.

27. Colditz, G.A., Brewer, T.F., Berkey, C.S. et al. (1994). Efficacy of BCG vaccine in the prevention of tuberculosis: meta- analysis of the published literature. *JAMA* 271 (9): 698–702.

28. Light, R.J. and Pillemer, D.B. (1984). *Summing up: The Science of Reviewing Research.* Cambridge, MA: Harvard University Press.

29. L'Abbe, K.A., Detsky, A.S., and O'Rourke, K. (1987). Meta-analysis in clinical research. *Ann. Intern. Med.* 107: 224–233.

30. Higgins, J.P.T. and Thompson, S.G. (2002). Quantifying heterogeneity in a meta-analysis. *Stat. Med.* 21 (11): 1539–1558.

31. Higgins, J.P.T., Thompson, S.G., Deeks, J.J., and Altman, D.G. (2003). Measuring inconsistency in meta-analysis. *BMJ* 327: 557–560.

32. Van Howe, R.S. (1999). Circumcision and HIV infection: review of the literature and meta-analysis. *Int. J. STD AIDS* 10 (1): 8–16.

33. O'Farrell, N. and Egger, M. (2000). Circumcision in men and the prevention of HIV infection: a 'meta-analysis' revisited. *Int. J. STD AIDS* 11 (3): 137–142.

34. Greenland, S., Robins, J.M., and Pearl, J. (1999). Confounding and collapsibility in causal inference. *Stat. Sci.* 14 (1): 29–46.

35. Rucker, G. and Schumacher, M. (2008). Simpson's paradox visualized: the example of the rosiglitazone meta-analysis. *BMC Med. Res. Methodol.* 8: 34.

36. Borenstein, M., Hedges, L.V., Higgins, J.P.T., and Rothstein, H. (2009). *Introduction to Meta-analysis*. Chichester: Wiley.

37. Rice, K., Higgins, J.P.T., and Lumley, T. (2018). A re-evaluation of fixed effect(s) meta-analysis. *J. R. Stat. Soc. Ser. A Stat. Soc.* 181 (1): 205–227.

38. DerSimonian, R. and Laird, N. (1986). Meta-analysis in clinical trials. *Control. Clin. Trials* 7: 177–188.

39. Higgins, J.P.T., Thompson, S.G., and Spiegelhalter, D.J. (2009). A re-evaluation of random-effects meta-analysis. *J. R. Stat. Soc. Ser. A. Stat. Soc.* 172 (1): 137–159.

40. Fine, P.E. (1995). Variation in protection by BCG: implications of and for heterologous immunity. *Lancet* 346 (8986): 1339–1345.

41. Easterbrook, P.J., Berlin, J.A., Gopalan, R., and Matthews, D.R. (1991). Publication bias in clinical research. *Lancet* 337: 867–872.

42. Dwan, K., Gamble, C., Williamson, P.R. et al. (2013). Systematic review of the empirical evidence of study publication bias and outcome reporting bias - an updated review. *PLoS One* 8 (7): e66844.

43. (1982). A randomized trial of propranolol in patients with acute myocardial infarction. I. Mortality results. *JAMA* 247 (12): 1707–1714.

44. Boissel, J.P., Leizorovicz, A., Picolet, H., and Ducruet, T. (1990). Efficacy of acebutolol after acute myocardial infarction (the APSI trial). The APSI Investigators. *Am. J. Cardiol.* 66 (9): 24C–31C.

45. Montori, V.M., Devereaux, P.J., Adhikari, N.K. et al. (2005). Randomized trials stopped early for benefit: a systematic review. *JAMA* 294 (17): 2203–2209.

46. Consortium TWTCC (2007). Genome-wide association study of 14,000 cases of seven common diseases and 3,000 shared controls. *Nature* 447 (7145): 661–678.

47. Multicenter Postinfarction Research G (1983). Risk stratification and survival after myocardial infarction. *N. Engl. J. Med.* 309 (6): 331–336.

CHAPTER 3

Identifying Randomized Controlled Trials

Julie Glanville and Carol Lefebvre

The chapter on "Identifying relevant studies for systematic reviews" in the first edition of this book, published in 1995, was a review of the evidence relating to the problems in identifying reports of randomized controlled trials (RCTs) for systematic reviews of health care interventions [1]. It focused on a particular difficulty that existed at that time in identifying such studies: only 19 000 reports of RCTs were readily identifiable, i.e. indexed as RCTs in MEDLINE, although records for many more reports of trials were already included in the database at that time.

By the second (2001) edition of this book [2], the situation had improved dramatically. Since 1994, Cochrane (see also Chapter 21) had, with the support of the US National Library of Medicine (NLM), systematically contributed to the re-tagging, as reports of trials, of nearly 100 000 additional records in MEDLINE. More importantly, the Cochrane Controlled Trials Register, subsequently known as the Cochrane Central Register of Controlled Trials (CENTRAL), was launched in 1996 and published and updated quarterly in the *Cochrane Library* [3, 4]. In 2001, CENTRAL contained records for more than 250 000 reports of controlled trials from MEDLINE, Embase, and other sources, and was recognized as "likely to be the best single source of published trials for inclusion in systematic reviews and meta-analyses" [5].

By the time of the third edition of this book, CENTRAL, which is now updated monthly, has reached nearly 2 million records or reports of trials [6, 7]. It includes all reports of trials that are readily identifiable in MEDLINE, i.e. indexed with Publication Type terms Randomized Controlled Trial or Controlled Clinical Trial (about 600 000 records in August 2021). Further, it includes about 700 000 additional trial records from Embase and/or MEDLINE; about 200 000 records from ClinicalTrials.gov; about 160 000 from the World Health Organization's International Clinical Trials Registry Platform (WHO ICTRP) not already included in ClinicalTrials.gov; and about 140 000 reports of trials from other sources (see Figure 3.1).

Systematic Reviews in Health Research: Meta-Analysis in Context, Third Edition. Edited by Matthias Egger, Julian P.T. Higgins, and George Davey Smith.
© 2022 John Wiley & Sons Ltd. Published 2022 by John Wiley & Sons Ltd.
Companion website: www.systematic-reviews3.org

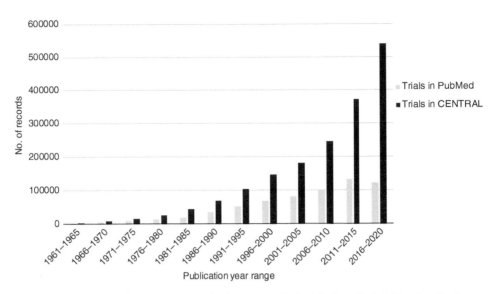

FIGURE 3.1   Number of randomized and other controlled trials in PubMed (Randomized Controlled Trials and Controlled Clinical Trials) and in CENTRAL (all records) 1961–2020 (data gathered August 2021).

This chapter describes sources that have contributed to CENTRAL and how they are still being searched. We outline some of the supplementary searches that should be undertaken in addition to searches of CENTRAL to identify studies for systematic reviews. We highlight some newer sources that have become available since the last edition of this book. We also provide information about where to identify guidance on identifying studies other than RCTs. We explore how searches are structured, how search terms are identified, and how interfaces allow search terms and concepts to be combined using Boolean operators. Finally, we describe how strategies can be tested and how to decide when to stop searching. We conclude with some evidence of the role and value of librarians and information specialists as part of the systematic review team.

3.1   SEARCHING CENTRAL TO IDENTIFY RANDOMIZED CONTROLLED TRIALS

As already noted, CENTRAL consists of records from a wide range of sources, including MEDLINE, Embase, CINAHL Plus, handsearching of journals and conference proceedings, trials register resources, and other sources. CENTRAL should, therefore, be searched as the "first port of call" to identify RCTs rapidly for systematic reviews. As the records come from various sources, they do not all have the same format and are indexed in various ways. Therefore, searches of CENTRAL should be carried out using a combination of Medical Subject Heading (*MeSH*) and free-text terms, including synonyms and related terms, aiming for a compromise between high sensitivity and adequate precision. Free-text terms are vital, since many thousands of records within

CENTRAL do not have MeSH terms and will not be retrieved if MeSH-only searches are conducted. While methodological search filters to identify specific study types can be useful in other databases [8], filters for RCTs should not be used in CENTRAL, nor should searches be limited to "human" studies. All records in CENTRAL should be reports of trials in humans, even though this may not be apparent from the records. Guidance on searching CENTRAL as part of the Cochrane Library is available from the Help section on the Cochrane Library home page (see Table 3.1).

TABLE 3.1   Key resources for identifying systematic reviews and reports of trials.

Resource	URL
AllTrials	https://www.alltrials.net
APA PsycINFO	https://www.apa.org/pubs/databases/psycinfo
ClinicalTrials.gov	https://clinicaltrials.gov
Cochrane Database of Systematic Reviews	https://www.cochranelibrary.com
Drugs@FDA	https://www.accessdata.fda.gov/scripts/cder/daf
EMA Online access to clinical data (clinical study reports)	https://clinicaldata.ema.europa.eu/web/cdp/home https://register.ema.europa.eu/identityiq/external/ registration.jsf#/register https://clinicaldata.ema.europa.eu/web/cdp/search
Epistemonikos	https://epistemonikos.org
EU Clinical Trials Register (EUCTR)	https://www.clinicaltrialsregister.eu/ctr-search/search https://www.clinicaltrialsregister.eu/about.html
FDA medical device databases	https://www.fda.gov/medical-devices/device-advice-comprehensive-regulatory-assistance/ medical-device-databases
Finding clinical trials, research registers and research results (trials registers resource)	https://sites.google.com/a/york.ac.uk/ yhectrialsregisters
Global Index Medicus	https://www.globalindexmedicus.net
Google Scholar	https://scholar.google.com
Health Canada info on drugs and medical devices	https://clinical-information.canada.ca/search/ci-rc
Health Systems Evidence	https://www.healthsystemsevidence.org/?lang=en
How CENTRAL is created	https://www.cochranelibrary.com/central/central-creation
International HTA database	https://www.inahta.org/hta-database
InterTASC Information Specialists' Sub-Group (ISSG) Search Filter Resource	https://sites.google.com/a/york.ac.uk/issg-search-filters-resource/home

TABLE 3.1   *(Continued)*

Resource	URL
Japanese Pharmaceuticals and Medical Devices Agency (PMDA)	https://www.pmda.go.jp/english/review-services/reviews/0001.html https://www.pmda.go.jp/english/review-services/reviews/approved-information/drugs/0001.html
KoreaMed	https://www.koreamed.org/SearchBasic.php
KSR Evidence	https://ksrevidence.com
Latin American and Caribbean Health Sciences Literature (LILACS)	https://lilacs.bvsalud.org/en
McMaster *PLUS*	https://plus.mcmaster.ca/mcmasterplusdb
OpenTrialsFDA	https://fda.opentrials.net/about
PDQ-Evidence	https://www.pdq-evidence.org/en
PROSPERO	https://www.crd.york.ac.uk/PROSPERO
PubMed PubReMiner	https://hgserver2.amc.nl/cgi-bin/miner/miner2.cgi
ScanMedicine	https://scanmedicine.com
Summarized Research in Information Retrieval for HTA (SuRe Info)	https://sure-info.org
SveMed+	https://svemedplus.kib.ki.se
Systematic Review Data Repository (SRDR+)	https://srdrplus.ahrq.gov
The Cochrane Handbook: Searching for Studies chapter – main text	https://training.cochrane.org/handbook/current/chapter-04
The Cochrane Handbook: Searching for Studies chapter – technical supplement	https://training.cochrane.org/handbook/current/chapter-04-technical-supplement-searching-and-selecting-studies
The Cochrane Handbook: Searching for Studies chapter – appendix of resources	https://training.cochrane.org/handbook/current/chapter-04-appendix-resources
The Cochrane Library	https://www.cochranelibrary.com
Trip and Trip Pro	https://www.tripdatabase.com
Web of Science	https://clarivate.com/webofsciencegroup/solutions/web-of-science
World Health Organization International Clinical Trials Registry Platform (ICTRP)	https://trialsearch.who.int

This table will be kept up to date on the book's website (www.systematic-reviews3.org).
Source: Based on [31] and [32].

3.1.1   Where Do CENTRAL Records Come From?

The justification for proposing that CENTRAL should be considered a key source for identifying trials for systematic reviews is based on the various projects that have been undertaken within Cochrane over the last 30 years to build CENTRAL. For further details, see the "How CENTRAL is created" webpage entry in Table 3.1.

3.1.2   The MEDLINE Re-tagging Project

In December 1993, NLM agreed to "re-tag" all MEDLINE records of randomized and quasi-randomized trial reports that were not already indexed as such in MEDLINE. The two terms for such trials (i.e. the Publication Type terms Randomized Controlled Trial and Controlled Clinical Trial) had only been introduced into MEDLINE in 1991 and 1995, respectively, and many records pre-dated this indexing. The re-tagging project resulted in more than 125 000 MEDLINE records, published between 1966 and 2004, being identified and included in CENTRAL [4, 9, 10]. Today, MEDLINE reports of RCTs continue to be identified for and included in CENTRAL.

3.1.3   The Embase Projects

In 1996, Elsevier agreed that reports of trials identified from Embase, whether or not they were indexed as trials, could be included in CENTRAL. As with MEDLINE, the relevant term for indexing RCTs had not been introduced into Embase until the early 1990s (1993). Many records pre-dated this indexing functionality, leading to the first Cochrane Embase project. More than a third of a million Embase records were scanned and about 100 000 additional trial reports, published between 1974 and 2010, were identified [10]. Only reports of trials in Embase, which were not already indexed as RCTs in MEDLINE, were of interest. These were then made available in CENTRAL. In 2013, a search filter to identify reports of RCTs using textual analysis of records was developed, which performs at over 97% sensitivity [11]. In January 2015, following an analysis of selected and rejected records, the search filter for Embase on Ovid was improved. It was later translated for Embase.com and implemented in 2018 [12].

3.1.4   Crowdsourcing and Other Initiatives

In an ongoing crowdsourcing project, volunteers assess records retrieved from databases such as Embase.com for relevance to CENTRAL. Two to six people assess whether a record is a report of an RCT. By November 2020, a "crowd" of approximately 19 000 volunteers had helped to identify more than 175 000 reports of RCTs [13]. The latest performance evaluation showed crowd sensitivity (the crowd's collective ability to identify reports of randomized trials correctly) and crowd specificity (correct identification of records to be rejected) to be 99.1% and 99.0%, respectively [13]. The Australasian Cochrane Centre identified RCTs from the Australasian Medical Index 1966–2009 [14]. A similar search was undertaken for KoreaMed up to March 2021. Searches are also ongoing for CINAHL Plus, ClinicalTrials.gov, and the WHO ICTRP. More than 3000 health care journals are being or have been handsearched, and records

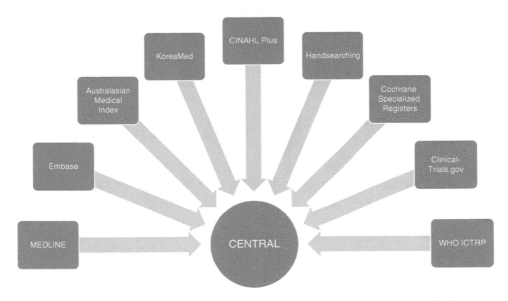

FIGURE 3.2   Sources contributing reports of randomized controlled trials to CENTRAL.

from the registers maintained by Cochrane Groups and Fields (see Chapter 21) are also added to CENTRAL monthly (see Figure 3.2).

3.2   SOURCES TO SEARCH IN ADDITION TO CENTRAL

In addition to searching CENTRAL to identify clinical trials for systematic reviews, it is necessary to search other sources. For an overview of these sources, see Box 3.1. This includes searching sources not (yet) searched for inclusion in CENTRAL and conducting supplementary searches of those already searched for CENTRAL. Even highly sensitive filters for study design, such as those used to identify RCTs in MEDLINE [1, 15], Embase [10, 12], and CINAHL Plus [16], can miss relevant studies. If there are not too many studies, it is preferable to search MEDLINE and Embase (and other databases) with subject searches only and omit study design filters. Reviewers should assess the yield of the subject searches to decide whether filters could be omitted to enhance sensitivity.

> **Box 3.1   Key Sources to Be Searched to Identify Randomized Controlled Trials for Systematic Reviews**
> - The Cochrane Central Register of Controlled Trials (CENTRAL) in the Cochrane Library
> - MEDLINE and Embase (with the provisos outlined in the text)
> - Other databases as appropriate
> - Sources of ongoing, completed, published, or unpublished studies, including trials registers and regulatory sources
> - Journals

- Gray literature, including conference abstracts, proceedings, dissertations and theses, etc.
- Websites and general web searching
- Citation sources and reference lists of included/excluded studies from related systematic views

There are many other sources in addition to CENTRAL, MEDLINE, Embase, and CINAHL Plus that should be searched. These include national, international, and regional databases; subject-specific databases; trials register resources and regulatory sources; gray literature including conference abstracts, dissertations, and theses; citation indexes; web searching; some newer sources focusing specifically on systematic reviews; and some newer document types such as pre-prints. Some of these sources are discussed below. They are discussed in detail in the *Cochrane Handbook* [17, 18].

3.2.1   Key Sources of Systematic Reviews

The sources listed below are collections of reviews, which in many cases provide access to lists of primary studies within those reviews. They offer helpful insights into the study identification methods used. See Table 3.1 for websites.

The **Cochrane Database of Systematic Reviews** (see also Chapter 21) contains the full text of systematic reviews of relevance to health care, including detailed information about the studies assessed as eligible for the reviews and studies assessed to be ineligible. The reviews also serve as a useful resource for highly sensitive search strategies.

Epistemonikos provides access to the reports of studies included in published systematic reviews, overviews, and structured summaries [19]. The reviews are identified from 10 databases, as well as other sources. Following a search query (which can be formulated in nine different languages), the user can select relevant reviews, and the system collects all eligible studies reported in those reviews. In August 2021, Epistemonikos contained nearly 400 000 systematic reviews identified from databases and other sources and classified by human screeners and a machine learning algorithm [19].

The **International HTA database** contains ongoing and published health technology assessments (HTAs) commissioned or undertaken by HTA organizations worldwide from 1996 to date.

KSR Evidence is a database of systematic reviews and meta-analyses published since 2015. In August 2021, it contained nearly 180 000 records, of which over 20 000 include a critical appraisal and a short summary with the key message of the review.

McMaster University offers a range of evidence databases (some focused on specific health care topics such as pain) containing reviews and critically appraised primary studies from its **McMaster PLUS** site. The university also provides **Health Systems Evidence**, a collection of research evidence about health systems and their management.

PDQ-Evidence is a resource providing access to evidence on health systems, which functions similarly to Epistemonikos in that it collects the eligible studies within systematic reviews.

PROSPERO is an international register of prospectively registered systematic reviews, rapid reviews, and umbrella reviews in health and social care.

The Agency for Healthcare Research and Quality (AHRQ) offers a **Systematic Review Data Repository (SRDR+)** [20] to support the production of systematic reviews. It also offers public access to the individual studies included in reviews and the data extracted from those studies.

Trip is a search engine for research evidence in PubMed, a range of evidence databases and websites. Trip presents search results in a hierarchical order, starting with systematic reviews, evidence summaries, guidelines and guidance, and moving to other evidence summaries and individual trials, and to other research.

3.2.2   Databases and Other Sources Not (Yet) Searched for Inclusion in CENTRAL

Despite the major efforts to identify and promote access to reports of RCTs from MEDLINE and Embase over the last 30 years, hundreds of health care databases and other sources (many in languages other than English) remain to be systematically searched. These include large multinational databases such as APA PsycINFO and Web of Science; language-specific or national research databases such as Global Index Medicus, LILACS, and SveMed+; and search engines such as Google Scholar (see Table 3.1 for websites). They are discussed in detail in the *Cochrane Handbook* [17, 18, 21].

3.2.3   Trials Registers, Regulatory Agency Sources, and Clinical Study Reports

Recent years have seen significant developments in the recording of information about ongoing trials. Many countries now have publicly accessible trials registers, and a dedicated website has been created by the authors of this chapter ("Finding clinical trials, research registers and research results"), which aims to list all international, national, and regional trials registers, together with some industry, subject-specific, and other registers (see Table 3.1). The WHO ICTRP provides access to a number of these resources, as does ScanMedicine, launched in May 2021 by the UK National Institute for Health Research (NIHR) Innovation Observatory (see Table 3.1).

Trials registers allow the prospective registration of trials, facilitate following the progress of a trial, and may facilitate access to trial results. They are a valuable resource for ongoing and completed trials, irrespective of whether the results are ever formally published, and can help address publication bias [22] (see also Chapter 5). In many countries, investigators are now obliged, by law or by their employers or funders, to register their trials in ClinicalTrials.gov (see Table 3.1) or other registers and to post their trial results. Trials registers, therefore, are an increasingly important source of information, including trial results. In 2011, over 12 000 ClinicalTrials.gov records had results in ClinicalTrials.gov, with many of these results not initially available from other sources [23]. By August 2021, over 50 000 of the 400 000 studies in ClinicalTrials.gov had results posted in the database.

There is extensive research into trial registration and its value and impact [24–26]. Trials registers are still developing, and at present there is no single resource providing access to all trials register records. Hence searching a range of resources is required. Of note is that even though ClinicalTrials.gov is part of the ICTRP, both resources need to be searched separately to ensure that relevant records are not missed due to differences in search interfaces and record content [26, 27]. The extent to which this might still be the case with the latest ICTRP interface, released in its final version in June 2021, and the current ClinicalTrials.gov interface remains to be ascertained. Further guidance on how to search these resources is available elsewhere [17, 18, 28].

Regulatory agencies are also an increasingly important source of information about trials and their results. Potentially relevant sources (see Table 3.1) include:

- *Canada*: in April 2019, Health Canada announced that it was starting to make clinical information about drugs and devices publicly available on its website.
- *European Union (EU)*: the EU Clinical Trials Register (EUCTR).
- *Japan*: the Japanese Pharmaceuticals and Medical Devices Agency (PMDA) provides access to internal reviews of approved drugs and medical devices (see the Reviews section of its website).
- *USA*: Drugs@FDA provides access to internal reviews by the Food and Drug Administration (FDA). Information on devices can be found in the FDA medical device databases.

Clinical study reports (CSRs) are the reports of clinical trials, providing detailed information on the methods and results of clinical trials submitted in support of marketing authorization applications. Sources include the European Medicines Agency (EMA).

Further information on the above is available in the *Cochrane Handbook* [17, 18, 21].

3.3   SEARCHING FOR STUDIES OTHER THAN RANDOMIZED CONTROLLED TRIALS

While considerable progress has been made in identifying studies for systematic reviews over recent decades [6, 9], particularly for identifying RCTs [17, 18, 21], identifying other types of studies has been less well developed. Detailed guidance exists for diagnostic accuracy studies [29], but widely accepted guidance is lacking for many study types. This book (see Chapters 15–19) and the *Cochrane Handbook* [30] include discussions of searching for various types of evidence. Summarized Research in Information Retrieval for HTA (SuRe Info, see Table 3.1) [31, 32] provides information relating to identifying all types of studies for systematic reviews and HTAs. It provides access to current information retrieval methods articles, including structured appraisals, and has a section on methods to search for specific aspects of health technologies.

3.4   BUILDING SEARCH STRATEGIES

Searches to inform systematic reviews usually aim to be extensive, i.e. to find as many relevant studies as possible. This emphasis on sensitivity intends to minimize publication and reporting biases (see also Chapter 5) and compensate for some researchers' failure to fully communicate all aspects of their research in titles and abstracts [22, 33–35]. As a consequence, reviewers will often tolerate low-precision searches to achieve sensitivity [36]. Low precision means looking at far more irrelevant records than relevant ones to avoid missing relevant ones. Sensitivity is achieved by using few search concepts but a wide range of search terms within each concept to capture reporting variation, and by searching a range of databases and other resources.

Searches should be developed to reflect the review question and the purpose and scope of the review, as the protocol is developed through discussions among the project team. Searches take account of the following:

- The concepts in the review question.
- The search terms that will capture the concepts.
- The bibliographic databases and other sources to be searched and their interfaces.

Reviewers should seek advice from a librarian or information specialist with experience in supporting systematic reviews. Librarians and information specialists offer advice and support in several areas, including the sources to search, designing search strategies, running the searches, saving, collating and de-duplicating search results, and obtaining copies of study reports. They support the use of reference management tools and other review production software, ensuring that retractions, errata, and comments are handled appropriately and that the study identification process is documented in compliance with current guidance [37–39]. They advise on the timing of any "update" or "top-up" searches to ensure that the review is as current as possible when published [17, 18].

3.4.1   Identifying the Concepts in the Review Question

Review questions are typically broken down into concepts, but only some of the concepts will inform the structure of the search strategy [17, 18, 29, 40]. PICO is a widely used model for effectiveness questions: Population, Intervention, Comparator, Outcomes [41]. Of the four concepts within PICO, only two are typically used for a systematic review search strategy, because using many concepts reduces the sensitivity of the search and risks missing relevant records. Most effectiveness reviews feature the Population and Intervention concepts. Comparators and Outcomes are usually left out. Comparators may be too diverse to specify and may involve the absence of treatment ("do nothing"). Outcomes may also vary widely, be challenging to capture, or not be fully reported. Questions that are not about effectiveness may use different or additional concepts (for example PICOTS for prognostic studies, see Chapters 17 and 18). A study design concept to capture RCTs may be added to the PICO for systematic reviews of RCTs, using tested and, ideally, validated search strategies [42–45]. The InterTASC

Information Specialists' Sub-Group (ISSG) Search Filter Resource (see Table 3.1) collates search filters grouped by study design and focus.

Searching databases efficiently requires knowledge of their design and content and the available search facilities. A search strategy for trials in CENTRAL via the Wiley interface to the Cochrane Library will differ from a search of MEDLINE via the Ovid interface, regarding both the concepts and the syntax used to structure searches. A Population and Intervention structured strategy combined with an RCT filter in MEDLINE will not need an RCT filter when it is run in CENTRAL, since CENTRAL only contains randomized or quasi-randomized studies.

3.4.2   Identifying the Search Terms to Capture the Concepts

For each concept, as many applicable search terms as possible should be collected [17, 18, 46]. Searchers typically build a list of relevant and related search terms that describe, for example, the Population and then assess whether any terms should be truncated (to capture term variations) or linked to other terms (phrases or words in proximity) [17, 18]. For example, a search designed to capture the Population concept of women with breast cancer will contain a range of search terms to reflect the ways in which the concept is described in the literature: "breast cancer", "breast neoplasms", "tumors of the breast", "mammary cancers", "mammary carcinoma", etc.

Reviewers can identify search terms in several ways. The records of key papers can be identified and scanned for search terms. The strategies from published reviews may be a valuable source of search terms. Searchers may also talk to experts or consult online thesauri, dictionaries, and web pages. Increasingly, searchers may use text mining (text analysis) tools to assess the concepts and identify search terms [47]. Text analysis packages, such as PubMed PubReMiner (Table 3.1), analyze the frequency of words and concepts in sets of records [18, 48, 49]. This can reveal frequently occurring words and phrases, which could be tested in search strategies, and identify concepts.

Searches make use of the title words, the abstract words, the author keywords, and any subject indexing (or thesaurus) terms that individual database producers have added to records, such as the MeSH terms added to MEDLINE records. Subject indexing schemes, such as MeSH, are often hierarchical, with broader (more general) indexing terms having one or more narrower (or more specific) term(s) below them. Subject indexing can increase search sensitivity by compensating for authors' variations when describing a concept, and can provide information in addition to that contained in the title, abstract, and author keywords. Subject indexing terms should not, however, be relied upon as the sole search option. Some databases, such as Science Citation Index, do not have a formal subject indexing scheme. Others, such as CENTRAL, have a mixed scheme in that many records are MeSH indexed, and others (including all those derived from non-MEDLINE sources) are not. In MEDLINE, there are always thousands of records that are awaiting indexing and so would not be retrieved by a search that relied solely on MeSH. These differences underpin the need for a strategy to search title and abstract fields as well as subject indexing terms.

When developing a search term list, it is helpful to collect related terms and broader or narrower terms and take account of differences in UK and US English spelling and national terminologies, for example "tumor" and "tumour." Abbreviated and unabbreviated terms and acronyms should feature, and both the generic and brand names of products, such as pharmaceuticals, pesticides, or chemicals, should be used. Searchers should consider whether vocabulary has changed over time (for example third world country, developing country, low-income country). Table 3.2 describes features such as truncation, wildcards, and proximity operators that should be considered, and gives examples for the Ovid and PubMed interfaces.

3.4.3   Combining Search Terms and Concepts

In many database interfaces, search terms and concepts are combined using Boolean operators (AND, OR, NOT). The OR operator gathers search terms within the same concept and identifies records containing one or more of those search terms. It makes the set of search results larger. A Population concept identifying breast cancer records will combine search terms as follows:

> breast cancer OR breast neoplasms OR mammary cancer OR mammary carcinoma (and so on).

The AND operator will find records containing all the concepts specified and makes a search more focused or narrower, reducing the size of the results set. In a Population AND Intervention search, the Boolean operator AND is used to find records that contain a Population search term and an Intervention search term. For example, to find records reporting on screening for breast cancer, a search would be structured as follows:

> (breast cancer OR breast neoplasms OR mammary cancer OR mammary carcinoma (and so on)) AND (mammography OR screening OR screen (and so on)).

The NOT operator excludes records from the search. It should generally be avoided, because its use may inadvertently remove relevant records [17, 18]. For example, searching for "(breast AND cancer) NOT (colon AND cancer)" would remove records that are only about colon cancer, but also any records that were about both breast cancer and colon cancer.

When choosing which concepts to combine using Boolean operators, the most specific concept is typically developed and tested first. If only relatively few records are identified, or the review team is willing to screen large numbers of records, a single concept may be adequate. If there are too many records, the next most specific concept may be added via AND to the first concept to keep the number of retrieved records manageable. The impact of adding the second concept should be assessed in terms of the number of relevant records missed and the reasons for missing them. This might lead to the identification of further terms to add to the concepts; to the decision to abandon the second concept and try another concept; or to the conclusion that several different search combinations are necessary. This multi-stranded approach is often required in reviews of diagnostic test accuracy studies and other complex topics [17, 18, 29]. The process continues until the strategy seems to capture most relevant records.

TABLE 3.2   Search syntax.

Option	Description	Examples in the Ovid interface	Examples in the PubMed interface
Truncation	Database-specific symbol that specifies that a word root can be expanded to find word variants	random$ – finds all words beginning with the stem "random" random$3 – finds all word variants (with up to three letters), e.g. "random," "randomly," "randomise," "randomize"	Random* – finds all words beginning with the stem "random" (Note: if truncation is not used in PubMed, the interface will carry out a degree of automatic truncation)
Wildcards	Account for internal spelling variation	"randomi?ed" – identifies "randomised" or "randomized"	Not available
Phrases	Terms must appear next to each other	randomized adj trial "randomized trial"	"randomized trial" (PubMed does not perform adjacency search but uses a phrase index. Phrase searching turns off the automatic term mapping to synonyms and MeSH terms, unless there are zero results in which case term mapping will occur)
Proximity operators	Terms appear near to each other or a maximum distance apart	breast adj3 cancer* – searches for "breast" within three words of the word cancer or within three words of words beginning with the word stem "cancer"	Not available
Explosion of subject headings	Searching a single heading includes all more specific (narrower) subject heading terms	exp Clinical Trial/ – retrieves that heading and all the more specific (narrower) headings such as Controlled Clinical Trial, Randomized Controlled Trial etc.	Clinical Trial [mh] – retrieves that heading and all the more specific (narrower) headings such as Controlled Clinical Trial, Randomized Controlled Trial etc.
Headings without explosion	Searching a single heading finds only that heading	Clinical Trial/	Clinical trial [mh:noexp]

3.4.4   When to Stop Searching

Developing a search is iterative, involving the exploration of trade-offs between sensitivity and precision. It is often difficult to decide objectively when a search is complete. Searchers typically develop "stopping decisions" based on their experience of developing strategies. Researchers have suggested "stopping rules" based on the retrieval of new records: for example, stopping the development process if adding in a series of new terms to a search strategy yields no new relevant records, or precision falls below a certain cut-off point [50]. Stopping might also be appropriate when the removal of terms or concepts results in losing relevant records. Reviews of methods to assist with deciding when to stop developing the search reported few formal evaluations of the approaches [36, 51].

Reviewers need to examine whether a strategy is performing adequately. One simple performance test is to check whether the search finds the publications that are known to be relevant or included in similar reviews [52]. However, this might also signify that the strategy is biased to known studies and might miss other relevant records. Citation searches and reference checking are additional ways to assess performance in finding known and unknown studies. Peer review of searches using the Peer Review of Electronic Search Strategies (PRESS) Checklist [53] should be routine. If some of the PRESS dimensions seem to be missing without adequate explanation or arouse concerns, then the search may not yet be complete. Statistical techniques, such as capture–recapture [54–57] or the relative recall technique [58, 59], can also be used to assess performance.

3.5 CONCLUSIONS

Considerable progress on identifying studies for systematic reviews has been made during the lifetime of this chapter, i.e. over three editions and 25 years. This includes improved access to reports of trials in MEDLINE and Embase and through CENTRAL [6, 9]; improved access to the results of trials before and irrespective of publication [60]; and the establishment of databases providing access to systematic reviews and their included studies. More detailed guidance and standards on conducting and reporting systematic reviews and identifying studies [37–39, 52, 61–64] have become available. New technologies have enabled more objective approaches to building search strategies and designing search filters, such as text mining [65]. Finally, there is greater awareness of the role and value of librarians and information specialists as part of the systematic review team [17, 18, 66–71].

ACKNOWLEDGMENTS

We acknowledge the Cochrane Information Retrieval Methods Group members and others for the various achievements described in this chapter. Concerning CENTRAL, we are grateful to Update Software, the original designers, developers, and publishers of CENTRAL; John Wiley & Sons, the current publishers of CENTRAL; staff, past and present, at the UK Cochrane Centre (now Cochrane UK) and the US Cochrane Center, who contributed records to CENTRAL; the Cochrane Dementia and Cognitive Improvement Group, Metaxis, and York Health Economics Consortium, who continue to build and develop CENTRAL; all Cochrane Trials Search Coordinators/Information Specialists and others who have submitted records for publication in CENTRAL; handsearchers/crowdsource volunteers for screening records to identify reports of trials; all those who contributed in other ways to the building and development of CENTRAL; the funders of the organizations involved in this work; and staff, past and present, of the various organizations that have collaborated with Cochrane with respect to the inclusion of their records in CENTRAL.

REFERENCES

1. Dickersin, K., Scherer, R., and Lefebvre, C. (1995). Identifying relevant studies for systematic reviews. In: *Systematic Reviews* (ed. I. Chalmers and D.G. Altman), 17–36. London: BMJ Publications.

2. Lefebvre, C. and Clarke, M.J. (2001). Identifying randomised trials. In: *Systematic Reviews in Health Care: Meta-Analysis in Context*, 2e (ed. M. Egger, G. Davey Smith and D.G. Altman), 69–86. London: BMJ Books.

3. The Cochrane Controlled Trials Register [updated quarterly]. The Cochrane Library. Oxford: Update Software.

4. Dickersin, K., Manheimer, E., Wieland, S. et al. (2002). Development of the Cochrane Collaboration's CENTRAL Register of Controlled Clinical Trials. *Eval. Health Prof.* 25 (1): 38–64.

5. Egger, M. and Davey Smith, G. (1998). Bias in location and selection of studies. *BMJ* 316 (7124): 61–66.

6. Noel-Storr, A.H., Dooley, G., Wisniewski, S. et al. (2020). Cochrane Centralised Search Service showed high sensitivity identifying randomized controlled trials: a retrospective analysis. *J. Clin. Epidemiol.* 127: 142–150.

7. The Cochrane Central Register of Controlled Trials (CENTRAL) [updated monthly]. The Cochrane Library. Chichester: Wiley-Blackwell.

8. Glanville, J., Bayliss, S., Booth, A. et al. (2008). So many filters, so little time: the development of a search filter appraisal checklist. *J. Med. Libr. Assoc.* 96 (4): 356–361.

9. Lefebvre, C., Glanville, J., Wieland, L.S. et al. (2013). Methodological developments in searching for studies for systematic reviews: past, present and future? *Syst. Rev.* 2: 78.

10. Lefebvre, C., Eisinga, A., McDonald, S. et al. (2008). Enhancing access to reports of clinical trials published world-wide – the contribution of EMBASE records to the Cochrane Central Register of Controlled Trials (CENTRAL) in the Cochrane Library. *Emerg. Themes Epidemiol.* 5: 13.

11. Thomas, J., Noel-Storr, A.H., and Elliott, J.H. (2015). Human and machine effort in Project Transform: how interesting technologies will help us to identify studies reliably, efficiently and at scale. *Cochrane Database Syst. Rev.* 10 (Suppl. 1): 37–41. https://doi.org/10.1002/14651858.CD201501.

12. Glanville, J., Foxlee, R., Wisniewski, S. et al. (2019). Translating the Cochrane EMBASE RCT filter from the Ovid interface to Embase.com: a case study. *Health Inf. Libr. J.* 36 (3): 264–277.

13. Noel-Storr, A., Dooley, G., Elliott, J. et al. (2021). An evaluation of Cochrane crowd found that crowdsourcing produced accurate results in identifying randomized trials. *J. Clin. Epidemiol.* 133: 130–139.

14. McDonald, S. (2002). Improving access to the international coverage of reports of controlled trials in electronic databases: a search of the Australasian Medical Index. *Health Inf. Libr. J.* 19 (1): 14–20.

15. Glanville, J.M., Lefebvre, C., Miles, J.N. et al. (2006). How to identify randomized controlled trials in MEDLINE ten years on. *J. Med. Libr. Assoc.* 94 (2): 130–136.

16. Glanville, J., Dooley, G., Wisniewski, S. et al. (2019). Development of a search filter to identify reports of controlled clinical trials within CINAHL Plus. *Health Inf. Libr. J.* 36 (1): 73–90.

17. Lefebvre, C., Glanville, J., Briscoe, S. et al. (2021). Chapter 4: Searching for and selecting studies. In: *Cochrane Handbook for Systematic Reviews of Interventions* Version 6.2 (updated February 2022) (ed. J.P.T. Higgins, J. Thomas, J. Chandler, et al.). London: Cochrane. https://www.training.cochrane.org/handbook.

18. Lefebvre, C., Glanville, J., Briscoe, S. et al. (2021). Technical supplement to Chapter 4: Searching for and Selecting Studies. In: *Cochrane Handbook for Systematic Reviews of Interventions* Version 6.3 (updated February 2022) (ed. J.P.T. Higgins, J. Thomas, J. Chandler, et al.). London: Cochrane. https://www.training.cochrane.org/handbook.

19. Rada, G., Perez, D., Araya-Quintanilla, F. et al. (2020). Epistemonikos: a comprehensive database of systematic reviews for health decision-making. *BMC Med. Res. Methodol.* 20 (1): 286.

20. Ip, S., Hadar, N., Keefe, S. et al. (2012). A web-based archive of systematic review data. *Syst. Rev.* 1 (1): 15.

21. Lefebvre, C., Glanville, J., Briscoe, S. et al. (2021). Appendix of resources to Chapter 4: Searching for and Selecting Studies. In: *Cochrane Handbook for Systematic Reviews of Interventions* Version 6.3 (updated February 2022) (ed. J.P.T. Higgins, J. Thomas, J. Chandler, et al.). London: Cochrane. https://www.training.cochrane.org/handbook.

22. Page, M.J., Higgins, J.P.T., and Sterne, J.A.C. (2019). Assessing risk of bias due to missing results in a synthesis. In: *Cochrane Handbook for Systematic Reviews of Interventions*, 2e (ed. J.P.T. Higgins, J. Thomas, J. Chandler, et al.), 349–374. Chichester: Wiley.

23. Zarin, D.A., Tse, T., Williams, R.J. et al. (2011). The ClinicalTrials.gov results database: update and key issues. *N. Engl. J. Med.* 364 (9): 852–860.

24. Arber, M., Cikalo, M., Glanville, J. et al. (2013). *Annotated Bibliography of Published Studies Addressing Searching for Unpublished Studies and Obtaining Access to Unpublished Data.* York: York Health Economics Consortium.

25. Isojarvi, J., Wood, H., Lefebvre, C. et al. (2018). Challenges of identifying unpublished data from clinical trials: getting the best out of clinical trials registers and other novel sources. *Res. Synth. Methods* 9 (4): 561–578.

26. Knelangen, M., Hausner, E., Metzendorf, M.-I. et al. (2018). Trial registry searches for randomized controlled trials of new drugs required registry-specific adaptation to achieve adequate sensitivity. *J. Clin. Epidemiol.* 94: 69–75.

27. Glanville, J.M., Duffy, S., McCool, R. et al. (2014). Searching ClinicalTrials.gov and the International Clinical Trials Registry Platform to inform systematic reviews: what are the optimal search approaches? *J. Med. Libr. Assoc.* 102 (3): 177–183.

28. Cooper, C., Court, R., Kotas, E. et al. (2021). A technical review of three clinical trials register resources indicates where improvements to the search interfaces are needed. *Res. Synth. Methods* 12 (3): 384–393.

29. de Vet, H.C.W., Eisinga, A., Riphagen, I.I. et al. (2008). Chapter 7: Searching for studies. In: *Cochrane Handbook for Systematic Reviews of Diagnostic Test Accuracy,* Version 0.4 (updated September 2008). London: Cochrane Collaboration. https://training.cochrane.org/resource/cochrane-handbook-systematic-reviews-diagnostic-test-accuracy.

30. Higgins, J.P.T., Thomas, J., Chandler, J. et al. (ed.) (2019). *Cochrane Handbook for Systematic Reviews of Interventions,* 2e. Chichester: Wiley.

31. Ormstad, S.S. and Isojarvi, J. (2013). Keeping up to date with information retrieval research: Summarized Research in Information Retrieval (SuRe Info). *J. Eur. Assoc. Health Info. Libr.* 9 (2): 17–19.

32. Isojarvi, J. and Glanville, J. (2021). Evidence-based searching for health technology assessment: keeping up to date with SuRe info. *Int. J. Technol. Assess. Health Care* 37 (1): e51.

33. Song, F., Parekh, S., Hooper, L. et al. (2010). Dissemination and publication of research findings: an updated review of related biases. *Health Technol. Assess.* 14 (8): 1–193.

34. Boutron, I., Page, M.J., Higgins, J.P.T. et al. (2019). Chapter 7: considering bias and conflicts of interest among the included studies. In: *Cochrane Handbook for Systematic Reviews of Interventions*, 2e (ed. J.P.T. Higgins, J. Thomas, J. Chandler, et al.), 177–204. Chichester: Wiley.

35. Higgins, J.P.T., Savović, J., Page, M.J. et al. (2019). Chapter 8: assessing risk of bias in a randomized trial. In: *Cochrane Handbook for Systematic Reviews of Interventions*, 2e (ed. J.P.T. Higgins, J. Thomas, J. Chandler, et al.), 205–228. Chichester: Wiley.

36. Arber, M. and Wood, H. (2021). Search strategy development: Summarized Research in Information Retrieval for HTA (SuRe Info). https://sites.google.com/york.ac.uk/sureinfo/home/search-strategy-development.

37. Page, M.J., McKenzie, J.E., Bossuyt, P.M. et al. (2021). The PRISMA 2020 statement: an updated guideline for reporting systematic reviews. *BMJ* 372: n71.

38. Page, M.J., Moher, D., Bossuyt, P.M. et al. (2021). PRISMA 2020 explanation and elaboration: updated guidance and exemplars for reporting systematic reviews. *BMJ* 372: n160.

39. Rethlefsen, M.L., Kirtley, S., Waffenschmidt, S. et al. (2021). PRISMA-S: an extension to the PRISMA statement for reporting literature searches in systematic reviews. *Syst. Rev.* 10 (1): 39.

40. Frandsen, T.F., Bruun Nielsen, M.F., Lindhardt, C.L. et al. (2020). Using the full PICO model as a search tool for systematic reviews resulted in lower recall for some PICO elements. *J. Clin. Epidemiol.* 127: 69–75.

41. Richardson, W.S., Wilson, M.C., Nishikawa, J. et al. (1995). The well-built clinical question: a key to evidence-based decisions. *ACP J. Club* 123 (3): A12–A13.

42. Jenkins, M. (2004). Evaluation of methodological search filters - a review. *Health Inf. Libr. J.* 21 (3): 148–163.

43. Wilczynski, N.L., Lokker, C., McKibbon, K.A. et al. (2016). Limits of search filter development. *J. Med. Libr. Assoc.* 104 (1): 42–46.

44. Arber, M., Glanville, J., Wood, H. et al. (2020). Search filters: Summarized Research in Information Retrieval for HTA (SuRe Info). https://sites.google.com/york.ac.uk/sureinfo/home/search-filters.

45. Glanville, J., Kotas, E., Featherstone, R. et al. (2020). Which are the most sensitive search filters to identify randomized controlled trials in MEDLINE? *J. Med. Libr. Assoc.* 108 (4): 556–563.

46. Petticrew, M. and Roberts, H. (ed.) (2006). *Systematic Reviews in the Social Sciences.* Oxford: Blackwell.

47. Paynter, R.A., Featherstone, R., Stoeger, E. et al. (2021). A prospective comparison of evidence synthesis search strategies developed with and without text-mining tools. *J. Clin. Epidemiol.* 139: 350–360.

48. Hausner, E., Guddat, C., Hermanns, T. et al. (2015). Development of search strategies for systematic reviews: validation showed the noninferiority of the objective approach. *J. Clin. Epidemiol.* 68 (2): 191–199.

49. Paynter, R., Bañez, L, Berliner, E. et al. (2016). EPC Methods: An Exploration of the Use of Text-Mining Software in Systematic Reviews. Research White Paper. Rockville, MD: Agency for Healthcare Research and Quality.

50. Chilcott, J., Brennan, A., Booth, A. et al. (2003). The role of modelling in prioritising and planning clinical trials. *Health Technol. Assess.* 7 (23): 1–125.

51. Booth, A. (2010). How much searching is enough? Comprehensive versus optimal retrieval for technology assessments. *Int. J. Technol. Assess. Health Care* 26 (4): 431–435.

52. EUnetHTA JA3WP6B2-2 Authoring Team (2019). *Process of Information Retrieval for Systematic Reviews and Health Technology Assessments on Clinical Effectiveness. Methodological Guidelines.* Diemen: European network for Health Technology Assessment.

53. McGowan, J., Sampson, M., Salzwedel, D.M. et al. (2016). PRESS Peer Review of Electronic Search Strategies: 2015 guideline statement. *J. Clin. Epidemiol.* 75: 40–46.

54. Spoor, P., Airey, M., Bennett, C. et al. (1996). Use of the capture-recapture technique to evaluate the completeness of systematic literature searches. *BMJ* 313 (7053): 342–343.

55. Kastner, M., Straus, S.E., McKibbon, K.A. et al. (2009). The capture-mark-recapture technique can be used as a stopping rule when searching in systematic reviews. *J. Clin. Epidemiol.* 62 (2): 149–157.

56. Ferrante di Ruffano, L., Davenport, C., Eisinga, A. et al. (2012). A capture-recapture analysis demonstrated that randomized controlled trials evaluating the impact of diagnostic tests on patient outcomes are rare. *J. Clin. Epidemiol.* 65 (3): 282–287.

57. Lane, D., Dykeman, J., Ferri, M. et al. (2013). Capture-mark-recapture as a tool for estimating the number of articles available for systematic reviews in critical care medicine. *J. Crit. Care* 28 (4): 469–475.

58. Sampson, M., Zhang, L., Morrison, A. et al. (2006). An alternative to the hand searching gold standard: validating methodological search filters using relative recall. *BMC Med. Res. Methodol.* 6 (33).

59. Sampson, M. and McGowan, J. (2011). Inquisitio validus Index Medicus: a simple method of validating MEDLINE systematic review searches. *Res. Synth. Methods* 2 (2): 103–109.

60. Zarin, D.A., Tse, T., Williams, R.J. et al. (2017). Update on trial registration 11 years after the ICMJE policy was established. *N. Engl. J. Med.* 376 (4): 383–391.

61. Agency for Healthcare Research and Quality (2014). *Methods Guide for Effectiveness and Comparative Effectiveness Reviews*. Rockville, MD: Agency for Healthcare Research and Quality.

62. Higgins, J.P.T., Lasserson, T., Chandler, J. et al. (2022). *Methodological Expectations of Cochrane Intervention Reviews Version February 2021*. London: Cochrane. https://community.cochrane.org/mecir-manual.

63. Institute of Medicine (US) Committee on Standards for Systematic Reviews of Comparative Effectiveness Research (2011). *Finding What Works in Health Care: Standards for Systematic Reviews* (ed. J. Eden, L. Levit, A. Berg, et al.). Washington, DC: National Academies Press https://doi.org/10.17226/13059.

64. Kugley, S., Wade, A., Thomas, J. et al. (2017). Searching for studies: a guide to information retrieval for Campbell systematic reviews. *Campbell Syst. Rev.* 13: 1–73.

65. O'Mara-Eves, A., Thomas, J., McNaught, J. et al. (2015). Using text mining for study identification in systematic reviews: a systematic review of current approaches. *Syst. Rev.* 4 (1): 5.

66. Li, L., Tian, J., Tian, H. et al. (2014). Network meta-analyses could be improved by searching more sources and by involving a librarian. *J. Clin. Epidemiol.* 67 (9): 1001–1007.

67. Koffel, J.B. (2015). Use of recommended search strategies in systematic reviews and the impact of librarian involvement: a cross-sectional survey of recent authors. *PLoS One* 10 (5): e0125931.

68. Rethlefsen, M.L., Farrell, A.M., Trzasko, L.C.O. et al. (2015). Librarian co-authors correlated with higher quality reported search strategies in general internal medicine systematic reviews. *J. Clin. Epidemiol.* 68 (6): 617–626.

69. Meert, D., Torabi, N., and Costella, J. (2016). Impact of librarians on reporting of the literature searching component of pediatric systematic reviews. *J. Med. Libr. Assoc.* 104 (4): 267–277.

70. Metzendorf, M.-I. (2016). Why medical information specialists should routinely form part of teams producing high quality systematic reviews – a Cochrane perspective. *J. Eur. Assoc. Health Info. Libr.* 12 (6–9).

71. Aamodt, M., Huurdeman, H., and Strømme, H. (2019). Librarian co-authored systematic reviews are associated with lower risk of bias compared to systematic reviews with acknowledgement of librarians or no participation by librarians. *Evid. Based Libr. Inf. Pract. [Internet]* 14 (4): 103–127.

CHAPTER 4

Assessing the Risk of Bias in Randomized Trials

Matthew J. Page, Douglas G. Altman, and Matthias Egger

Methodological characteristics of clinical trials are of obvious relevance to systematic reviewers. If the primary studies are flawed, then the conclusions of a systematic review will be compromised and may be misleading. Following the recommendations of organizations such as Cochrane [1], and the US Institute of Medicine [2], many reviewers formally assess the risk of bias (RoB) (or quality) of the included trials [3]. However, the methods for assessing RoB and its incorporation into systematic reviews remain a matter of ongoing debate [4, 5].

In this chapter, we discuss the concept of *risk of bias* and distinguish it from *quality*. We describe different sources of bias that can occur in randomized trials, and review the empirical evidence underpinning each source. We compare the composite scale and domain-based approaches to RoB assessment. Finally, we outline strategies for incorporating RoB assessments into meta-analysis.

4.1   RISK OF BIAS AND QUALITY

Bias refers to a systematic distortion of the study results or conclusions – in other words, an underestimation or overestimation of the true intervention effect [6]. In some trials bias is trivial, but in others it could be substantial. There is good empirical evidence that, on average, particular flaws in the design, conduct, and analysis of randomized trials are associated with biased intervention effects (see below). However, it is usually

Systematic Reviews in Health Research: Meta-Analysis in Context, Third Edition. Edited by Matthias Egger, Julian P.T. Higgins, and George Davey Smith.
© 2022 John Wiley & Sons Ltd. Published 2022 by John Wiley & Sons Ltd.
Companion website: www.systematic-reviews3.org

impossible to know whether and to what extent methodological flaws have affected the results of a particular trial. For example, lack of participant blinding may result in underestimation of an effect in one study but overestimation in another. Also, the results of a study may in fact be unbiased despite a methodological flaw. For these reasons, it is more appropriate to consider whether a study is at *risk of bias* rather than claiming with certainty that it is biased.

RoB can be distinguished from *quality*. In this context, quality refers to the extent to which study authors conducted their research to the highest possible standards. Some quality standards that have been described in the literature include methods that minimize RoB (e.g. blinding participants), obtaining ethical approval, performing a sample size calculation, and reporting a trial in line with recommended guidelines (e.g. Consolidated Standards of Reporting Trials [CONSORT] 2010 [7]) [1]. The key distinction between RoB and quality is that trialists may have conducted their trial as well as was possible, yet an important RoB remains. For example, the results of a trial comparing physical therapy with surgery for knee osteoarthritis is unlikely to be free of bias due to the inability to blind participants and personnel; however, characterizing such a trial as being of low quality is overly harsh when all other aspects of trial design, conduct, and reporting were performed appropriately. Further, not all markers of trial quality are directly associated with biased intervention effects. In addition, it is important to distinguish the quality of a study from the quality of the report; poor reporting of clinical trials is widespread [8], but a poorly reported study still may have been conducted well.

4.2   THE EVIDENCE BASE FOR RISK OF BIAS

Following a landmark study by Schulz et al. in 1995 [9], researchers have used *meta-epidemiology* to identify which methodological features of randomized trials are associated with biased results [10]. In most meta-epidemiological studies, a collection of meta-analyses is assembled and the individual trials within each meta-analysis are classified into those with or without a particular characteristic. Summary effects from the two sets of trials are then compared. For example, investigators may explore whether estimated treatment effects such as odds ratios systematically differ in trials without double blinding compared with trials with double blinding (Figure 4.1). They may quantify the average bias in trials that lack double blinding by calculating the ratio of odds ratios (ROR), which divides the pooled odds ratio of trials that lack double blinding by the pooled odds ratio of trials with double blinding (ROR = $OR_{with\ flaw}$/$OR_{without\ flaw}$) [12]. An important caveat of such studies is that the assessment of methodological characteristics is often entirely based on what is reported in articles, yet reported methods do not always reflect actual trial conduct. Despite the wide adoption of CONSORT [7], reporting is often still incomplete [8]. Some well-conducted but poorly reported trials will thus be misclassified if quality is assumed to be inadequate unless information to the contrary is provided (the commonly used guilty-until-proved-innocent approach) [13]. Despite this limitation, meta-epidemiology provides important evidence and we refer to the results of such studies throughout this chapter.

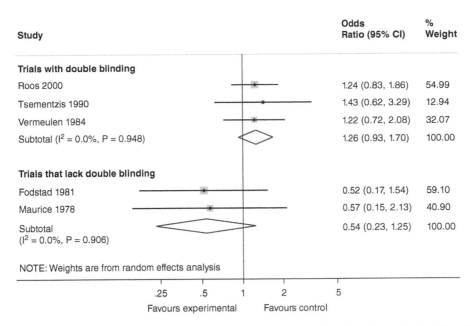

Study	Odds Ratio (95% CI)	% Weight
Trials with double blinding		
Roos 2000	1.24 (0.83, 1.86)	54.99
Tsementzis 1990	1.43 (0.62, 3.29)	12.94
Vermeulen 1984	1.22 (0.72, 2.08)	32.07
Subtotal ($I^2 = 0.0\%$, P = 0.948)	1.26 (0.93, 1.70)	100.00
Trials that lack double blinding		
Fodstad 1981	0.52 (0.17, 1.54)	59.10
Maurice 1978	0.57 (0.15, 2.13)	40.90
Subtotal ($I^2 = 0.0\%$, P = 0.906)	0.54 (0.23, 1.25)	100.00

NOTE: Weights are from random effects analysis

Favours experimental — Favours control

FIGURE 4.1 Example of the use of meta-epidemiology to investigate bias due to lack of double blinding in a meta-analysis of antifibrinolytic treatment versus control for people with aneurysmal subarachnoid hemorrhage [11]. The outcome was hydrocephalus at the end of follow-up, which was reported less often in trials without double blinding than trials with double blinding. In other words, the trials that lacked double blinding overestimated the benefits of antifibrinolytic treatment on this outcome.

4.3 SOURCES OF BIAS IN RANDOMIZED TRIALS

Bias can occur at various stages throughout a randomized trial, from enrollment and allocation to intervention groups, to reporting of the study findings (Figure 4.2). In this section, we describe key sources of bias using the framework that underpins the revised Cochrane RoB tool for randomized trials [14]. We also discuss the methodological features that may safeguard against each source of bias (Table 4.1) and the empirical evidence supporting each feature.

4.3.1 Bias Arising from the Randomization Process

The aim of randomization is to create groups that are comparable with respect to any known or unknown prognostic factors such as age or disease severity. If such factors are not balanced at the start of the trial, they may wholly or partially account for any observed difference in outcomes between intervention groups [15]. The success of randomization depends on two interrelated procedures: *sequence generation* and *allocation concealment*. First, a random allocation sequence must be generated, for example by using a computer algorithm or tables of random numbers [16]. Second, this sequence must be concealed from investigators enrolling participants by, for example, performing randomization centrally at a site remote from trial location, or using sequentially numbered, sealed, opaque envelopes [16].

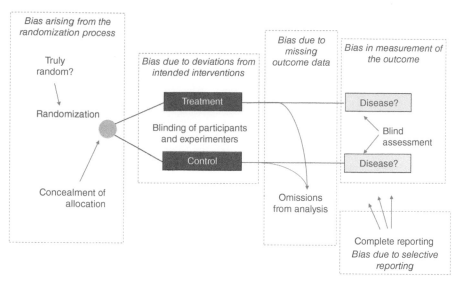

FIGURE 4.2   Sources of bias in randomized trials.

TABLE 4.1   Eligible sources of bias in randomized trials.

Type of bias	Possible methodological features that can lead to bias
Bias arising from the randomization process	Inadequate generation of a random sequence, inadequate allocation concealment, imbalance in baseline characteristics that suggests a problem with randomization
Bias due to deviations from intended interventions	Unblinded participants, unblinded personnel (clinician/treatment provider), unbalanced deviations from intended interventions that arose because of the trial context
Bias due to missing outcome data	Missing/incomplete outcome data (dropouts, losses to follow-up)
Bias in measurement of outcomes	Unblinded outcome assessor
Bias due to selective reporting	Selective reporting of subset of measured outcome domains, or of a subset of outcome measurements or analyses for a particular outcome domain

The randomization process can be subverted in several ways. Awareness of impending assignments, which can occur, for example, when a random number table is openly posted on a bulletin board, can allow selective enrollment of patients based on prognostic factors. Extremely ill patients who would have been assigned to the experimental group, but who are less likely to recover, may be prevented from participating [16]. Or some patients may deliberately be directed to the "appropriate" intervention by delaying their entry into the trial until the desired allocation becomes available [17]. An allocation schedule also may be deciphered by opening sealed assignment envelopes or holding them against a bright light to reveal the contents [17].

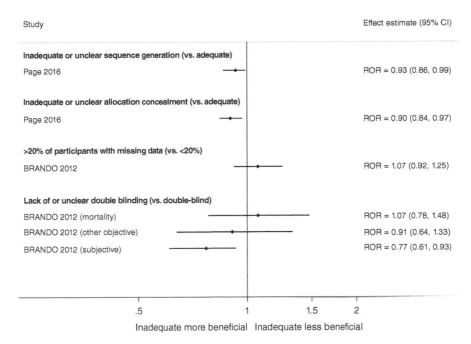

FIGURE 4.3   Results of syntheses of meta-epidemiological studies relating methodological aspects of randomized trials to their effect estimates. CI, confidence interval; ROR, ratio of odds ratios. A ROR <1 denotes a larger intervention effect estimate in trials with an inadequate or unclear (versus adequate) characteristic. Effect estimates for double blinding are subgrouped into mortality, other objective outcomes, and subjective outcomes.

Evidence from a systematic review of meta-epidemiological studies suggests that odds ratios may be exaggerated by 7%, on average, in trials with inadequate or unclear sequence generation (Figure 4.3) [18]. Odds ratios also tend to be exaggerated by 10% on average in trials with inadequate or unclear allocation concealment [18]. These results are similar to those observed in the more recent ROBES study [12].

4.3.2   Bias Due to Deviations from the Intended Interventions

Following assignment to groups, each intervention should be delivered to and received by participants as planned. However, participants may receive additional aspects of care, or intended aspects of care may not be delivered. Bias can arise when there are systematic differences between groups in such deviations from the intended interventions.

Keeping participants, carers, health care providers, and trial personnel unaware of the assigned intervention – a process known as blinding or masking – can reduce the RoB due to deviations from the intended interventions [19]. Steps to achieve blinding include administering a placebo (inactive) drug, or a "sham" device that appears to be functioning, but is actually switched off, to a comparator group [20, 21]. Successful blinding should prevent knowledge of the intervention assignment from influencing receipt of cointerventions other than what is intended, switching from the intended intervention to the alternative intervention, nonadherence to intervention, or failure to implement some or all intervention components as planned [22].

It is not always possible to blind participants, carers, health care providers, and trial personnel. However, absence of blinding need not lead to bias in all instances. If interest is in the effect of *assigning* people to an intervention, which is the focus of an intention-to-treat (ITT) analysis, then absence of blinding is problematic only when it leads to deviations from the intended intervention that arose because of the trial context and are not balanced across groups. Such deviations usually arise due to an expectation of a difference between the experimental intervention and comparator. For example, awareness that trial participants could have been assigned to surgery may make some who were assigned to physical therapy feel unlucky, which could influence them to seek surgery from a different hospital or self-administer a cointervention such as simple analgesics. If all deviations from the intended intervention are consistent with what would occur outside the trial context (for example, participants might stop taking the assigned drug intervention because of its toxicity), there is a low RoB in the estimate of the effect of assignment to intervention [22]. In contrast, if our interest is in the effect of *adhering* to the intervention, then any nonadherence to the intended interventions or imbalances in cointerventions will increase the RoB in the effect [22]. The assessment of possible bias must take the type of question the review aims to answer into account, which may range from efficacy to real-world effectiveness [23].

Evidence of bias due to deviations from intended interventions largely comes from studies exploring the association of *double blinding* with intervention effects. The term "double blinding" is interpreted in different ways [24]. In the BRANDO study, it was defined as blinding of participants and either caregivers or outcome assessors or both. The BRANDO study found that lack of or unclear double blinding in trials with subjective outcomes was associated with a 23% exaggeration of odds ratios, while there was little evidence of such bias in trials of mortality or other objective outcomes (Figure 4.3) [25]. In contrast, the MetaBLIND study found no evidence of an average difference in estimated treatment effect between trials with and without blinded patients or health care providers, which could reflect that blinding is less important than is often believed or meta-epidemiological study limitations, such as residual confounding or imprecision [26].

4.3.3   Bias Due to Missing Outcome Data

The benefits provided by randomization – that is, to balance distributions of known and unknown prognostic factors – are jeopardized when outcome data are missing for some participants. Outcome data can be missing for several reasons, such as when participants are unable to be contacted because they moved without giving notice, or respondents accidentally miss some items in a questionnaire [27]. Also, participants who do not fully adhere to the intended intervention may be excluded from the analysis when, for example, a per-protocol analysis is performed.

Participants whose outcome data are missing are unlikely to be representative of all enrolled participants. Some participants assigned to an experimental intervention may not return for follow-up if they experience an adverse reaction to a treatment, while others might not return if they are in complete remission [28]. Bias can arise when there are systematic differences between groups in the proportions of and reasons for missing outcome data.

To minimize bias due to missing outcome data, outcome data should be obtained from as many randomized participants as possible. Analysis performed according to the ITT principle [29, 30] requires outcomes to be recorded for all randomized participants. Complete outcome data can usually be achieved if the endpoint of interest is mortality from all causes. However, ascertaining other outcomes for all participants is frequently impossible, and most trials that report using an ITT analysis have data missing for some participants [31, 32]. Therefore, having complete data often requires that data for some participants need to be imputed: trialists estimate the missing values and then analyze the known and estimated data [33].

Empirical evidence of bias due to missing outcome data is conflicting [18]. In one meta-epidemiological study, trials using a "modified" ITT analysis had odds ratios that were exaggerated by 20% compared with trials using ITT analysis [34]. Modified ITT analyses do not comply with the ITT principle, but include patients who received at least one dose of the study drug or had at least one assessment [32]. In another study, trials with a dropout rate greater than 20% had odds ratios similar to trials with less than or equal to 20% dropout (Figure 4.3) [25]. In the ROBES study, trials rated at high/unclear RoB due to incomplete outcome data (using version 1 of the Cochrane RoB tool [35]) had similar effect estimates as trials rated at low RoB (ROR 0.98, 95% credible interval 0.92, 1.05) [12]. It would be useful to know whether bias varies according to different amounts of and reasons for missing data, but this has not yet been explored in any meta-epidemiological study.

4.3.4   Bias in Measurement of Outcomes

Procedures for measuring outcomes such as recording events on a case report form should be similar regardless of the group to which participants are assigned. However, problems can occur if assessors are aware of the assigned intervention. For example, participants in an experimental intervention group may be monitored more closely for evidence of symptom reduction than participants receiving the comparator, particularly if assessors have a vested interest in the findings. Also, participants receiving the comparator may exaggerate the severity of their symptoms, especially if they believe they have received an inferior intervention [14].

Blinding assessors to the intervention assignments can reduce the RoB in measurement of outcomes. Such blinding might be achieved by having an independent physician who was not otherwise involved record events or interpret results of a biological test [36]. If the outcome measure is objective, measurement can always be performed by a blinded assessor [19]. However, if the outcome measure is patient reported, blinded assessment is only possible when the participants are unaware of their assigned intervention.

Some studies investigating bias in measurement of outcomes have found that intervention effect estimates were larger in trials with unblinded assessment of subjective outcomes [37–39], although the recent MetaBLIND study found no evidence of such an association [26].

4.3.5   Bias Due to Selective Reporting

Trialists should always provide a complete account of all measured and analyzed outcomes. However, some trialists report data for only a subset of outcomes, depending on the statistical significance, magnitude, or direction of the results [40]. For example, participant deaths may be counted and compared between intervention groups, but trialists present no data because the effect favored the comparator [41]. This selective reporting of results would put a meta-analysis of deaths, which cannot include the nonreported data, at RoB. It is similar to publication bias resulting from an entire study remaining unpublished because of its unfavorable results (see Chapter 5).

In some cases, the intervention effect estimate that is reported in an article has been selected based on the results from multiple measurements or analyses. For example, trialists carry out analyses of change scores and post-intervention scores adjusted for baseline, yet only report analyses that yielded the most favorable effect estimate [42]. Such bias in selection of the reported result typically arises from a desire for findings to be sufficiently noteworthy to merit publication. This type of selective reporting puts effect estimates from individual primary studies at RoB in the same way as the other sources of bias described in this chapter.

Publicly disclosing the prespecified outcomes and analytic methods (for example, in a trial protocol or clinical trials register such as http://ClinicalTrials.gov) has been recommended to help minimize selective reporting [43]. In theory, such prespecification should hold trialists to account to fully report all data, and prevent them from cherry picking the most noteworthy results.

Studies that have compared source documentation such as protocols or register entries from before the start of a trial with the final trial publication have found many discrepancies in the outcomes listed, and in the ways that analyses were planned and conducted [44, 45]. A large study of protocols submitted to a Swiss Ethics Committee found that 7% of protocol-defined primary outcomes and 19% of secondary outcomes were not reported in the corresponding publications [46]. While some of these discrepancies may have been influenced by an attribute of the results such as statistical significance, others may be legitimate, or due to an unintentional omission [41]. Systematic reviewers must try to disentangle such reasons when assessing the RoB due to selective reporting, which makes this one of the most challenging sources of bias to assess.

4.4   APPROACHES TO ASSESSING RISK OF BIAS IN RANDOMIZED TRIALS

Having outlined several important sources of bias that may affect the results of randomized trials, we now consider how systematic reviewers can assess each source in the trials included in their review, and outline the advantages and disadvantages of each.

4.4.1   Composite Scale Approach

Many scales have been developed to assess RoB (or quality). Scales combine information on a range of components into a single numerical score, which may then be used to characterize trials as high or low quality. A search of the literature covering the years up to 1993 identified 25 different quality assessment scales for randomized trials [47], a number that had increased to 94 by the year 2007 [48].

Although composite quality scales may provide a useful overall assessment when comparing populations of trials, there are many problems with their use in individual systematic reviews. Different scales vary considerably in terms of dimensions covered, size, and complexity. Many scales include items for which little evidence exists that they are in fact related to RoB. For example, the widely used Physiotherapy Evidence Database (PEDro) scale assesses whether between-group statistical comparisons or both point measures and measures of variability are reported [49]. Some scales do not cover all of the most important sources of bias in randomized trials (i.e. those that are supported by empirical evidence); the commonly used scale developed by Jadad et al. [50] does not include an item on allocation concealment. Calculating a summary score assumes that each item in a scale deserves equal weight, whereas some features may be more important – that is, more bias inducing – than others. Also, the combination of individual responses into an overall score is meaningful only if all items relate to the same underlying construct. A recent study of the psychometric properties of the PEDro scale showed that it lacked construct validity [51]. Finally, reporting a quality score does not provide a transparent account of the problems identified in a trial.

Unsurprisingly, different scales often reach discordant conclusions. Jüni et al. re-analyzed a meta-analysis of 17 trials comparing low molecular weight heparin to standard heparin for thromboprophylaxis in general surgery patients [52]. Each of 25 different quality assessment scales was used to stratify trials into high or low quality, and the results of stratified analyses differed depending on the scale used. While risk ratios of high-quality trials suggested that low molecular weight heparin was not superior to standard heparin when using certain scales, with other scales the opposite was the case [52]. Further, in a meta-epidemiological study the PEDro scale and Cochrane domain-based approach led to different sets of trials of adequate quality, and different combined treatment estimates from meta-analyses of these trials [53].

4.4.2   Domain-Based Approach

A preferable alternative to the composite scale approach is to judge RoB within separate specified bias domains and to record the information on which each judgment is based: the domain-based approach. This is more transparent to users of a systematic review than a single quality score. The most popular domain-based tool in use is the Cochrane RoB tool for randomized trials [54].

4.4.2.1   Cochrane Risk of Bias tool for Randomized Trials

Originally released in 2008 [55] and revised slightly in 2011 [35], the Cochrane RoB tool provided a systematic way to organize and present the available evidence relating to RoB in randomized trials. The default (and recommended) application was to examine six evidence-based domains: random sequence generation, allocation concealment, blinding of participants and personnel, blinding of outcome assessment, missing outcome data, and selective reporting. Each domain could be judged as being at either low, high, or unclear RoB, and rationale (such as verbatim quotes from the journal article) could be provided to support each judgment. An "other bias" domain was also available to record additional concerns defined by the systematic reviewers. This flexibility inherent in the tool meant different teams implemented it in different ways [56]. An example of how assessments are typically presented in tables and figures is shown in Table 4.2 and Figure 4.4.

TABLE 4.2   Example of a completed Cochrane risk of bias table for a trial comparing physiotherapy to glucocorticoid injection for shoulder pain.

Bias	Reviewers' judgment	Support for judgment
Random sequence generation	Low risk	Quote: "Treatment allocation was according to the study number. Numbers were issued in a predetermined random sequence, in blocks of 10 by general practice, generated by a random number table." Comment: An adequate method was used to generate the allocation sequence
Allocation concealment	Low risk	Quote: "The number corresponded with that on a sealed envelope issued to the patient by the nurse. Participants were instructed not to open the envelope until the nurse had left. The envelope contained information instructing the participant to either make an appointment with one of the trial physiotherapists or to return to their GP for a local steroid injection." Comment: An adequate method was used to conceal the allocation sequence
Blinding of participants and personnel	High risk	Comment: Given the nature of the interventions, participants were not blind to treatment, and may have had different expectations about the benefits of each intervention
Blinding of outcome assessment (self-reported outcomes)	High risk	Comment: Unblinded participants who may have had different expectations about the benefits of the intervention they received self-reported some outcomes
Blinding of outcome assessment (objective outcomes)	Low risk	Quote: "Outcome assessments were performed by the study nurse, who was unaware of the treatment allocation." Comment: Assessor of objective outcomes was likely blinded to the intervention
Incomplete outcome data	Low risk	Quote: "The completion rate of the trial at six months was 95% (196/207) with the following reasons for loss to follow-up: five other medical complications, two personal problems, four could not be contacted/refused visit. Intention to treat analysis was used." Comment: The amount and reasons for dropout are unlikely to have affected the results

TABLE 4.2 (*Continued*)

Bias	Reviewers' judgment	Support for judgment
Selective reporting (reporting bias)	Unclear risk	Comment: Outcome data were fully reported for all outcomes reported in the methods section of the publication, but without a trial protocol it is unclear whether other outcomes were measured but not reported based on the results
Other bias	Low risk	Comment: No other sources of bias were identified

Source: Reproduced from [57]. The source trial is [58].

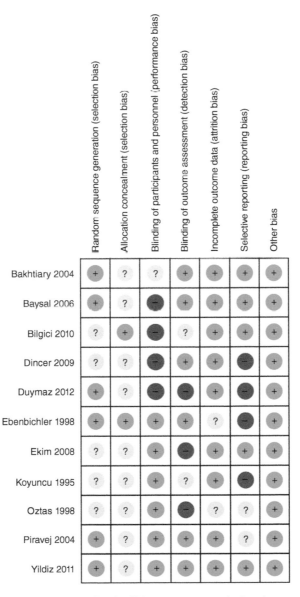

FIGURE 4.4 Example presentation of risk of bias assessments (using the 2011 Cochrane risk of bias tool for randomized trials) for studies in a Cochrane review of therapeutic ultrasound for carpal tunnel syndrome [59]. Review authors' judgments about each risk of bias item presented for each included study.

Use of the RoB tool was made mandatory in Cochrane reviews, and it also became the most commonly used domain-based tool in non-Cochrane reviews of interventions [54, 60]. However, several problems with the tool have been identified. Its inter-rater reliability is modest [61, 62], and some users have found the wording in the guidance confusing [63]. The tool is frequently implemented in ways that are not recommended [64–67], such as merging domains addressing different types of bias into a single domain. Some review authors also consider non-bias-related processes like sample size or industry funding under the other bias domain [56]. Finally, the tool lacks a formal mechanism for reaching an overall RoB judgment.

4.4.2.2 RoB 2

In response to concerns identified in previous evaluations, a revised tool for assessing RoB in randomized trials (RoB 2) was developed. An initial draft of RoB 2 was released in 2016 [68] and a finalized version in 2019 [14]. The RoB 2 tool includes five domains that are broadly consistent with the existing tool, but have different terminology to explain more clearly what each domain addresses (Figure 4.5). These domains are intended to be comprehensive, covering all issues that might lead to a RoB, and for this reason review authors cannot add other domains to the tool. The tool provides signaling questions, which are reasonably factual in nature and whose answers flag the potential for bias. Assessments are directed at a specific trial result, reflecting the fact that a particular methodological feature such as lack of participant blinding may bias results for certain outcomes like patient-reported quality of life but not others, for example all-cause mortality. The tool includes a rule that the overall RoB for the result is driven by the worst judgment across all domains in the tool. Thus, if any domain is assessed

Cochrane Risk of Bias tool (original version)	RoB 2
Random sequence generation (selection bias)	Bias arising from the randomization process
Allocation concealment (selection bias)	
Blinding of participants and personnel (performance bias)	Bias due to deviations from intended interventions
Incomplete outcome data (attrition bias)	Bias due to missing outcome data
Blinding of outcome assessment (detection bias)	Bias in measurement of the outcome
Selective reporting (reporting bias)	Bias in selection of the reported result
Other bias	–
–	Overall bias

FIGURE 4.5 Domains of bias in the initial and revised Cochrane risk of bias tool for randomized trials (RoB 2).

to be at high RoB, then that is the assessment overall. Further, separate templates are available for individually randomized parallel group trials, cluster-randomized parallel group trials, and individually randomized crossover trials.

The revised tool builds on the Risk of Bias In Non-Randomized Studies of Interventions (ROBINS-I) tool [22], described in Chapter 15. Some domains of bias are applicable to both randomized trials and nonrandomized studies of interventions (e.g. bias due to missing outcome data, bias in measurement of the outcome) and so are addressed by both tools. This consistency should facilitate the comparison of RoB across different study designs in systematic reviews that include both randomized and nonrandomized studies of interventions.

4.5   INCORPORATING RISK OF BIAS IN META-ANALYSIS

As noted at the start of this chapter, if there is a high RoB in the primary studies, then the conclusions of a systematic review may be misleading. Accounting for RoB assessments in meta-analysis therefore makes sense. However, surveys of user practice show that while most systematic reviewers routinely assess RoB, they infrequently incorporate those assessments into the meta-analysis [3, 54, 60, 69]. In this section, we outline a number of different approaches that have been proposed for this purpose.

4.5.1   Excluding Studies at High Risk of Bias from the Meta-Analysis

When RoB varies across studies included in a meta-analysis, one option is to restrict the primary meta-analysis to trials rated at low RoB [1]. Selecting this strategy involves a trade-off between bias and precision, because if only a few studies are rated at low RoB the meta-analysis result may be imprecise. Systematic reviewers who restrict their primary analysis in this way are encouraged to perform a sensitivity analysis including all trials to see if the treatment effect changes when trials at high RoB are included [1].

When using this approach, deciding how to categorize trials as low risk or high risk overall requires some consideration. Systematic reviewers could adopt criteria by which the overall RoB is classified as low if all key domains are at low RoB, high if at least one key domain is at high RoB, or some concerns if at least one key domain is rated at some concerns in the absence of high risk. However, such criteria will be unhelpful if none of the included trials is rated at low RoB overall (as is quite common) [54]. Systematic reviewers may therefore consider performing separate sensitivity analyses based on each of the domains of RoB that are considered important in the context of a given meta-analysis [70].

4.5.2   Quality Score as a Weight in Meta-Analysis

An alternative approach is to directly incorporate information on trial quality as weighting factors in the analysis. In standard meta-analysis, effect estimates of individual trials are weighted by the inverse of their variance [71]. The larger the trial, the smaller the variance of the effect estimate and the greater the weight the trial receives in meta-analysis (see Chapter 9 for a discussion of statistical methods). Trial weights can be multiplied by quality scores that increase the weight of trials deemed to be of high quality and decreasing the weight of low-quality trials [5, 40, 72, 73]. A trial with a quality score of 40 out of 100 might thus get the same weight in the analysis as a trial with half the amount of information but a quality score of 80.

Several criticisms have been raised against weighting by quality scores [49, 72, 74–76]. The choice of quality scale will influence the weight of individual trials in an analysis, and the combined effect estimate and its confidence interval therefore depend on the choice of scale. Also, if some of the studies have particularly important methodological flaws, but these have not been picked up by the quality scale, the result of the trial will not be sufficiently down weighted in the meta-analysis [74, 76]. Finally, down weighting does not address bias itself, which is better addressed using adjustment approaches.

4.5.3   Adjusting Results of Trials for Bias

Methods have recently been proposed to adjust the results of trials included in meta-analyses for expected biases. In other words, the effect estimates are adjusted to what they should be if they were unbiased. One method uses the evidence from meta-epidemiological studies to provide empirically based prior information on the degree of bias that can be expected from studies at high RoB. This information is then used to adjust the observed trial effects for expected bias within a Bayesian paradigm [77]. Incorporating uncertainty in the degree of bias leads to additional down weighting of trials at high RoB. This approach relies on the assumption that bias in the present study is similar to the average bias in previous studies with the same methodological flaw. The down weighting can be substantial if the adjustment takes into account both variability of bias across trials and variability of bias across meta-analyses in the meta-epidemiological data, as is commonly recommended, since this variability leads to a high amount of uncertainty in the degree of bias in a new trial [25].

In another approach, trial results are adjusted based on a detailed assessment of the methodological characteristics of each trial and opinions elicited from experts about the degree of bias that is likely to result. Trial-specific, bias-adjusted estimates are then combined using standard meta-analysis models [78]. The disadvantages of this approach are that obtaining expert opinions can be time-consuming, and the opinions are themselves subjective.

Both approaches require the use of specialized statistical techniques with increased complexity and software constraints, and at present are not sufficiently well developed for widespread use.

4.6   CONCLUSIONS

Ample evidence shows that many trials are methodologically weak and that their deficiencies translate into biased findings of systematic reviews. Assessing the RoB in randomized trials and conducting sensitivity analyses based on RoB should therefore be considered routine procedures in meta-analysis. Although composite quality scales may provide a useful overall assessment when comparing populations of trials, such scales should not be used to identify trials of apparent low or high RoB in a given meta-analysis. Rather, the relevant methodological aspects should be assessed individually, using comprehensive, evidence-based tools. These should generally include key sources of bias, including bias arising from the randomization process, bias due to deviations from intended interventions, bias due to missing outcome data, bias in measurement of the outcome, and bias due to selective reporting.

REFERENCES

1. Boutron, I., Page, M.J., and Higgins, J.P.T. (2019). Considering bias and conflicts of interest among the included studies. In: *Cochrane Handbook for Systematic Reviews of Interventions*, 2e (eds. J.P.T. Higgins, J. Thomas, J. Chandler, et al.), 177–204. Chichester: Wiley.

2. IOM (Institute of Medicine) (2011). *Finding What Works in Health Care: Standards for Systematic Reviews*. Washington, DC: National Academies Press.

3. Page, M.J., Shamseer, L., Altman, D.G. et al. (2016). Epidemiology and reporting characteristics of systematic reviews of biomedical research: a cross-sectional study. *PLoS Med.* 13 (5): e1002028.

4. Jüni, P., Altman, D.G., and Egger, M. (2001). Assessing the quality of controlled clinical trials. In: *Systematic Reviews in Health Care: Meta-Analysis in Context*, 2e (eds. M. Egger, G. Davey Smith and D.G. Altman). London: BMJ Books.

5. Jüni, P., Altman, D.G., and Egger, M. (2001). Systematic reviews in health care: assessing the quality of controlled clinical trials. *Br. Med. J.* 323 (7303): 42–46.

6. Whiting, P., Savović, J., Higgins, J.P.T. et al. (2016). ROBIS: a new tool to assess risk of bias in systematic reviews was developed. *J. Clin. Epidemiol.* 69: 225–234.

7. Schulz, K.F., Altman, D.G., and Moher, D. (2010). CONSORT 2010 statement: updated guidelines for reporting parallel group randomised trials. *Br. Med. J.* 340: c332.

8. Dechartres, A., Trinquart, L., Atal, I. et al. (2017). Evolution of poor reporting and inadequate methods over time in 20 920 randomised controlled trials included in Cochrane reviews: research on research study. *Br. Med. J.* 357: j2490.

9. Schulz, K.F., Chalmers, I., Hayes, R.J., and Altman, D.G. (1995). Empirical evidence of bias. Dimensions of methodological quality associated with estimates of treatment effects in controlled trials. *J. Am. Med. Assoc.* 273 (5): 408–412.

10. Sterne, J.A.C., Jüni, P., Schulz, K.F. et al. (2002). Statistical methods for assessing the influence of study characteristics on treatment effects in "meta-epidemiological" research. *Stat. Med.* 21 (11): 1513–1524.

11. Baharoglu, M.I., Germans, M.R., Rinkel, G.J. et al. (2013). Antifibrinolytic therapy for aneurysmal subarachnoid haemorrhage. *Cochrane Database Syst. Rev.* (8): Cd001245.

12. Savović, J., Turner, R.M., Mawdsley, D. et al. (2018). Association between risk-of-bias assessments and results of randomized trials in Cochrane reviews: the ROBES meta-epidemiologic study. *Am. J. Epidemiol.* 187 (5): 1113–1122.

13. Devereaux, P.J., Choi, P.T., El-Dika, S. et al. (2004). An observational study found that authors of randomized controlled trials frequently use concealment of randomization

and blinding, despite the failure to report these methods. *J. Clin. Epidemiol.* 57 (12): 1232–1236.

14. Sterne, J.A.C., Savović, J., Page, M.J. et al. (2019). RoB 2: a revised tool for assessing risk of bias in randomised trials. *Br. Med. J.* 366: l4898.

15. Altman, D.G. and Bland, J.M. (1999). Statistics notes. Treatment allocation in controlled trials: why randomise? *Br. Med. J.* 318 (7192): 1209.

16. Altman, D.G. and Schulz, K.F. (2001). Statistics notes: concealing treatment allocation in randomised trials. *Br. Med. J.* 323 (7310): 446–447.

17. Schulz, K.F. (1995). Subverting randomization in controlled trials. *J. Am. Med. Assoc.* 274 (18): 1456–1458.

18. Page, M.J., Higgins, J.P.T., Clayton, G. et al. (2016). Empirical evidence of study design biases in randomized trials: systematic review of meta-epidemiological studies. *PLoS One* 11 (7): e0159267.

19. Schulz, K.F. and Grimes, D.A. (2002). Blinding in randomised trials: hiding who got what. *Lancet* 359 (9307): 696–700.

20. Boutron, I., Estellat, C., Guittet, L. et al. (2006). Methods of blinding in reports of randomized controlled trials assessing pharmacologic treatments: a systematic review. *PLoS Med.* 3 (10): e425.

21. Boutron, I., Guittet, L., Estellat, C. et al. (2007). Reporting methods of blinding in randomized trials assessing nonpharmacological treatments. *PLoS Med.* 4 (2): e61.

22. Sterne, J.A.C., Hernan, M.A., Reeves, B.C. et al. (2016). ROBINS-I: a tool for assessing risk of bias in non-randomised studies of interventions. *Br. Med. J.* 355: i4919.

23. Egger, M., Moons, K.G.M., Fletcher, C., and GetReal, W. (2016). GetReal: from efficacy in clinical trials to relative effectiveness in the real world. *Res. Synth. Methods* 7 (3): 278–281.

24. Haahr, M.T. and Hróbjartsson, A. (2006). Who is blinded in randomized clinical trials? A study of 200 trials and a survey of authors. *Clin. Trials* 3 (4): 360–365.

25. Savović, J., Jones, H.E., Altman, D.G. et al. (2012). Influence of reported study design characteristics on intervention effect estimates from randomized, controlled trials. *Ann. Intern. Med.* 157 (6): 429–438.

26. Moustgaard, H., Clayton, G.L., Jones, H.E. et al. (2020). Impact of blinding on estimated treatment effects in randomised clinical trials: meta-epidemiological study. *Br. Med. J.* 368: l6802.

27. Akl, E.A., Briel, M., You, J.J. et al. (2012). Potential impact on estimated treatment effects of information lost to follow-up in randomised controlled trials (LOST-IT): systematic review. *Br. Med. J.* 344: e2809.

28. Sackett, D.L. and Gent, M. (1979). Controversy in counting and attributing events in clinical trials. *N. Engl. J. Med.* 301 (26): 1410–1412.

29. Detry, M.A. and Lewis, R.J. (2014). The intention-to-treat principle: how to assess the true effect of choosing a medical treatment. *J. Am. Med. Assoc.* 312 (1): 85–86.

30. Bell, M.L., Fiero, M., Horton, N.J., and Hsu, C.H. (2014). Handling missing data in RCTs; a review of the top medical journals. *BMC Med. Res. Methodol.* 14: 118.

31. Hollis, S. and Campbell, F. (1999). What is meant by intention to treat analysis? Survey of published randomised controlled trials. *Br. Med. J.* 319 (7211): 670–674.

32. Abraha, I. and Montedori, A. (2010). Modified intention to treat reporting in randomised controlled trials: systematic review. *Br. Med. J.* 340: c2697.

33. White, I.R., Horton, N.J., Carpenter, J., and Pocock, S.J. (2011). Strategy for intention to treat analysis in randomised trials with missing outcome data. *Br. Med. J.* 342: d40.

34. Abraha, I., Cherubini, A., Cozzolino, F. et al. (2015). Deviation from intention to treat analysis in randomised trials and treatment effect estimates: meta-epidemiological study. *Br. Med. J.* 350: h2445.

35. Higgins, J.P.T., Altman, D.G., Gøtzsche, P.C. et al. (2011). The Cochrane Collaboration's tool for assessing risk of bias in randomised trials. *Br. Med. J.* 343: d5928.

36. Yordanov, Y., Dechartres, A., Porcher, R. et al. (2015). Avoidable waste of research related to inadequate methods in clinical trials. *Br. Med. J.* 350: h809.

37. Hróbjartsson, A., Thomsen, A.S., Emanuelsson, F. et al. (2012). Observer bias in randomised clinical trials with binary outcomes: systematic review of trials with both blinded and non-blinded outcome assessors. *Br. Med. J.* 344: e1119.

38. Hróbjartsson, A., Thomsen, A.S.S., Emanuelsson, F. et al. (2013). Observer bias in randomized clinical trials with measurement scale outcomes: a systematic review of trials with both blinded and nonblinded assessors. *CMAJ* 185 (4): E201–E211.

39. Hróbjartsson, A., Thomsen, A.S.S., Emanuelsson, F. et al. (2014). Observer bias in randomized clinical trials with time-to-event outcomes: systematic review of trials with both blinded and non-blinded outcome assessors. *Int. J. Epidemiol.* 43 (3): 937–948.

40. Kirkham, J.J., Altman, D.G., Chan, A.-W. et al. (2018). Outcome reporting bias in trials: a methodological approach for assessment and adjustment in systematic reviews. *Br. Med. J.* 362: k3802.

41. Chan, A.W., Hróbjartsson, A., Haahr, M.T. et al. (2004). Empirical evidence for selective reporting of outcomes in randomized trials: comparison of protocols to published articles. *J. Am. Med. Assoc.* 291 (20): 2457–2465.

42. Page, M.J. and Higgins, J.P.T. (2016). Rethinking the assessment of risk of bias due to selective reporting: a cross-sectional study. *Syst. Rev.* 5 (1): 108.

43. Chan, A.W., Song, F., Vickers, A. et al. (2014). Increasing value and reducing waste: addressing inaccessible research. *Lancet* 383 (9913): 257–266.

44. Dwan, K., Altman, D.G., Clarke, M. et al. (2014). Evidence for the selective reporting of analyses and discrepancies in clinical trials: a systematic review of cohort studies of clinical trials. *PLoS Med.* 11 (6): e1001666.

45. Dwan, K., Gamble, C., Williamson, P.R., and Kirkham, J.J. (2013). Systematic review of the empirical evidence of study publication bias and outcome reporting bias - an updated review. *PLoS One* 8 (7): e66844.

46. Redmond, S., von Elm, E., Blumle, A. et al. (2013). Cohort study of trials submitted to ethics committee identified discrepant reporting of outcomes in publications. *J. Clin. Epidemiol.* 66 (12): 1367–1375.

47. Moher, D., Jadad, A.R., Nichol, G. et al. (1995). Assessing the quality of randomized controlled trials: an annotated bibliography of scales and checklists. *Control. Clin. Trials* 16 (1): 62–73.

48. Bai, A., Shukla, V.K., Bak, G., and Wells, G. (2012). *Quality Assessment Tools Project Report*. Ottawa: Canadian Agency for Drugs and Technologies in Health.

49. da Costa, B.R., Hilfiker, R., and Egger, M. (2013). PEDro's bias: summary quality scores should not be used in meta-analysis. *J. Clin. Epidemiol.* 66 (1): 75–77.

50. Jadad, A.R., Moore, R.A., Carroll, D. et al. (1996). Assessing the quality of reports of randomized clinical trials: is blinding necessary? *Control. Clin. Trials* 17 (1): 1–12.

51. Albanese, E., Bütikofer, L., Armijo-Olivo, S. et al. (2020). Construct validity of the Physiotherapy Evidence Database (PEDRo) quality scale for randomized trials: item response theory analyses. *Res. Synth. Methods* 11 (2): 227–236. https://doi.org/10.1002/jrsm.385.

52. Jüni, P., Witschi, A., Bloch, R., and Egger, M. (1999). The hazards of scoring the quality of clinical trials for meta-analysis. *J. Am. Med. Assoc.* 282 (11): 1054–1060.

53. Armijo-Olivo, S., da Costa, B.R., Cummings, G.G. et al. (2015). PEDro or Cochrane to assess the quality of clinical trials? A meta-epidemiological study. *PLoS One* 10 (7): e0132634.

54. Jorgensen, L., Paludan-Muller, A.S., Laursen, D.R. et al. (2016). Evaluation of the Cochrane tool for assessing risk of bias in randomized clinical trials: overview of published comments and analysis of user practice in Cochrane and non-Cochrane reviews. *Syst. Rev.* 5 (1): 80.

55. Higgins, J.P.T., Altman, D.G., and Sterne, J.A.C. (2008). Assessing risk of bias in included studies. In: *Cochrane Handbook for Systematic Reviews of Interventions* (eds. J.P.T. Higgins and S. Green), 187–241. Chichester: Wiley.

56. Babic, A., Pijuk, A., Brázdilová, L. et al. (2019). The judgement of biases included in the category "other bias" in Cochrane systematic reviews of interventions: a systematic survey. *BMC Med. Res. Methodol.* 19 (1): 77.

57. Page, M.J., Green, S., McBain, B. et al. (2016). Manual therapy and exercise for rotator cuff disease. *Cochrane Database Syst. Rev.* (6): CD012224.

58. Hay, E.M., Thomas, E., Paterson, S.M. et al. (2003). A pragmatic randomised controlled trial of local corticosteroid injection and physiotherapy for the treatment of new episodes of unilateral shoulder pain in primary care. *Ann. Rheum. Dis.* 62: 394–399.

59. Page, M.J., O'Connor, D., Pitt, V., and Massy-Westropp, N. (2013). Therapeutic ultrasound for carpal tunnel syndrome. *Cochrane Database Syst. Rev.* 3: CD009601.

60. Hopewell, S., Boutron, I., Altman, D.G., and Ravaud, P. (2013). Incorporation of assessments of risk of bias of primary studies in systematic reviews of randomised trials: a cross-sectional study. *BMJ Open* 3 (8): e003342.

61. Armijo-Olivo, S., Ospina, M., da Costa, B.R. et al. (2014). Poor reliability between Cochrane reviewers and blinded external reviewers when applying the Cochrane risk of bias tool in physical therapy trials. *PLoS One* 9 (5): e96920.

62. Hartling, L., Hamm, M.P., Milne, A. et al. (2013). Testing the risk of bias tool showed low reliability between individual reviewers and across consensus assessments of reviewer pairs. *J. Clin. Epidemiol.* 66 (9): 973–981.

63. Savović, J., Weeks, L., Sterne, J.A.C. et al. (2014). Evaluation of the Cochrane Collaboration's tool for assessing the risk of bias in randomized trials: focus groups, online survey, proposed recommendations and their implementation. *Syst. Rev.* 3: 37.

64. Babic, A., Tokalic, R., Amílcar Silva Cunha, J. et al. (2019). Assessments of attrition bias in Cochrane systematic reviews are highly inconsistent and thus hindering trial comparability. *BMC Med. Res. Methodol.* 19 (1): 76.

65. Barcot, O., Boric, M., Dosenovic, S. et al. (2019). Risk of bias assessments for blinding of participants and personnel in Cochrane reviews were frequently inadequate. *J. Clin. Epidemiol.* 113: 104–113.

66. Barcot, O., Boric, M., Poklepovic Pericic, T. et al. (2019). Risk of bias judgments for random sequence generation in Cochrane systematic reviews were frequently not in line with Cochrane handbook. *BMC Med. Res. Methodol.* 19 (1): 170.

67. Saric, F., Barcot, O., and Puljak, L. (2019). Risk of bias assessments for selective reporting were inadequate in the majority of Cochrane reviews. *J. Clin. Epidemiol.* 112: 53–58.

68. Higgins, J.P.T., Savović, J., Page, M.J., and Sterne, J.A.C., on behalf of the development group for RoB 2.0. (2016) Revised Cochrane risk of bias tool for randomized trials (RoB 2.0, 28 October 2016). Available at www.riskofbias.info. Accessed 21 February 2022.

69. Gerber, S., Tallon, D., Trelle, S. et al. (2007). Bibliographic study showed improving methodology of meta-analyses published in leading journals 1993–2002. *J. Clin. Epidemiol.* 60 (8): 773–780.

70. Dechartres, A., Altman, D.G., Trinquart, L. et al. (2014). Association between analytic strategy and estimates of treatment outcomes in meta-analyses. *J. Am. Med. Assoc.* 312 (6): 623–630.

71. Borenstein, M., Hedges, L.V., Higgins, J.P.T., and Rothstein, H.R. (2009). *Introduction to Meta-Analysis*. Chichester: Wiley.

72. Detsky, A.S., Naylor, C.D., O'Rourke, K. et al. (1992). Incorporating variations in the quality of individual randomized trials into meta-analysis. *J. Clin. Epidemiol.* 45 (3): 255–265.

73. Moher, D., Pham, B., Jones, A. et al. (1998). Does quality of reports of randomised trials affect estimates of intervention efficacy reported in meta-analyses? *Lancet* 352 (9128): 609–613.

74. Greenland, S. and O'Rourke, K. (2001). On the bias produced by quality scores in meta-analysis, and a hierarchical view of proposed solutions. *Biostatistics* 2 (4): 463–471.

75. Herbison, P., Hay-Smith, J., and Gillespie, W.J. (2006). Adjustment of meta-analyses on the basis of quality scores should be abandoned. *J. Clin. Epidemiol.* 59 (12): 1249–1256.

76. Ahn, S. and Becker, B.J. (2011). Incorporating quality scores in meta-analysis. *J. Educ. Behav. Stat.* 36 (5): 555–585.

77. Welton, N.J., Ades, A.E., Carlin, J.B. et al. (2009). Models for potentially biased evidence in meta-analysis using empirically based priors. *J. R. Stat. Soc. A. Stat. Soc.* 172 (1): 119–136.

78. Turner, R.M., Spiegelhalter, D.J., Smith, G.C., and Thompson, S.G. (2009). Bias modelling in evidence synthesis. *J. R. Stat. Soc. Ser. A Stat. Soc.* 172 (1): 21–47.

CHAPTER 5

Investigating and Dealing with Publication Bias and Other Reporting Biases

Matthew J. Page, Jonathan A.C. Sterne, Julian P.T. Higgins, and Matthias Egger

Consider the (fictional) city of Melstol. The council recently called residents to vote on a proposal to ban cheering and clapping at the local football stadium to placate noise-sensitive residents. Passionate campaigning on both sides of the debate led to a record turnout on election day. Officials declared a close victory for the ban, and supporters rejoiced noiselessly with vigorous air punches. However, journalists later discovered that officials had withheld voting forms for 10% of the electorate living in an area that overwhelmingly opposed the measure. A recount including the suppressed votes overturned the original result, to the relief of diehard football fans. Yet all residents remain concerned by the systematic suppression of votes and credibility of the council was dented.

Systematic reviewers seeking to identify all relevant evidence face a similar situation. Study investigators may make decisions about dissemination of their research findings based on P values, or the magnitude or direction of their results. Results that are not available to reviewers may therefore differ systematically from those that are. The phenomenon is widely known as reporting bias, although it might be described more accurately as nonreporting bias [1, 2]. Omission of relevant study results can bias the results of a meta-analysis, putting the credibility of the review in doubt. Reporting biases can also lead to bias in published results, if they are selected for publication from multiple analyses of the same association (described as bias in selection of the reported result [3, 4]). Such bias is addressed by tools to assess risk of bias within studies (see Chapter 4).

In this chapter, we summarize the empirical evidence for various reporting biases that lead to study results being unavailable for inclusion in systematic reviews, with a focus on health research. We describe processes that systematic reviewers can use to minimize the risk of bias due to missing results in a meta-analysis. We also outline different tools, plots, and statistical methods that have been designed for assessing risk of bias due to missing results in meta-analyses.

5.1   THE EVIDENCE BASE FOR REPORTING BIASES IN HEALTH RESEARCH

Basing decisions about publication on P values, or the magnitude or direction of results, has traditionally been referred to as *publication bias*. To study this phenomenon, investigators have drawn samples of clinical studies from research ethics committee listings [5], conference proceedings [6], and regulatory submissions [7], recorded which studies were published in journal articles, and examined the nature of the results in both the published and unpublished studies. These investigations have found that, on average, studies with statistically significant or "positive" results are more likely to be published than null or "negative" studies (Figure 5.1). Such an association has been observed for randomized and nonrandomized studies of interventions [5], diagnostic test accuracy studies [8], prognostic accuracy studies [9], and qualitative studies [10]. Published randomized trials of health interventions also tend to have larger intervention effect estimates on average than unpublished trials [11], which suggests that studies with smaller effects might be considered less worthy of publication.

Research can be disseminated selectively in other ways. Compared with studies with null or negative results, studies with positive results are more likely to be published earlier (time-lag bias) [12–16], reported in multiple journal articles (duplicate or multiple

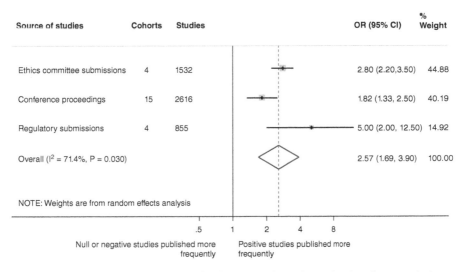

FIGURE 5.1   Random-effects meta-analysis of meta-analyses investigating the association between publication status and the P value, magnitude, or direction of the results. Data for the meta-analysis of studies submitted for research ethics committee approval come from Schmucker et al. [5]. Data for the meta-analysis of randomized trials presented at conferences come from Scherer et al. [6]. Data for the meta-analysis of clinical trials submitted for regulatory approval come from Chan et al. [7].

publication bias) [2, 17], and cited more frequently by others (citation bias) [18], although the magnitudes of the associations vary across clinical areas [12]. When studying pairs of randomized trial reports written by the same authors with one report published in German and the other in English, in 1997 Egger et al. found that the authors were more likely to publish trials in an English-language journal if the results were statistically significant (language bias) [19]. This led to concerns that meta-analyses restricted to studies in English could exaggerate an intervention effect. However, later studies comparing trials published in English with trials published in a language other than English found the opposite direction of bias, with treatment effects slightly smaller in trials published in English than in trials published in another language [11, 20, 21]. A consequence of all these selective dissemination practices (e.g. publication bias, time-lag bias, language bias) is that the subset of studies that are included in systematic reviews may have results that are systematically different from studies that are less readily accessible.

Even when a study report is available, results for some outcomes that were assessed may be missing or incompletely reported because of the P value, or the magnitude or direction of the results (*selective nonreporting bias* or *outcome reporting bias*). Several studies have compared journal article reports of studies with their corresponding protocols [22, 23], trials register entries [24, 25], or documents submitted to regulators [26], and identified frequent nonreporting of results for outcomes that were prespecified. The largest such study compared 227 protocols and amendments with 333 matching articles published between 1990 and 2008 [23] and found that 7% of protocol-defined primary outcomes and 19% of secondary outcomes were not reported. In a more recent analysis, the COMPare study found that results were missing for 42% of outcomes prespecified in 67 trials published between October 2015 and January 2016 in the world's top five general medical journals [27]. Other studies suggest that statistically significant results for beneficial outcomes had higher odds of being completely reported than nonsignificant results [28] (Figure 5.2).

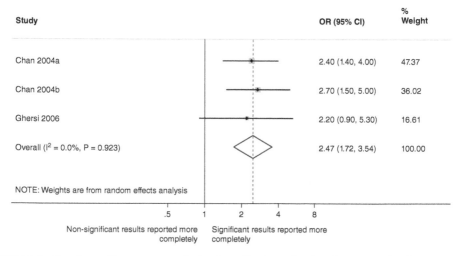

FIGURE 5.2   Random-effects meta-analysis of studies investigating the association between reporting results completely for benefit outcomes and the statistical significance of the results. *Source*: Data come from Chan et al. [22, 29] and Dwan et al. [28].

5.2   APPROACHES TO MINIMIZE RISK OF BIAS DUE TO MISSING RESULTS

Regardless of whether an entire study or a subset of its results is unavailable, the potential consequence for a meta-analysis is bias. In this section, we describe two strategies systematic reviewers can use to minimize the risk of bias due to missing results in a meta-analysis: searching beyond journal articles, and restricting meta-analyses to inception cohorts.

5.2.1   Searching Beyond Journal Articles

As described in Chapter 3, results of health research are available in various sources other than bibliographic databases of published studies like MEDLINE. No single resource gives access to all studies, so systematic reviewers should strive to search multiple sources. These include study registers such as http://ClinicalTrials.gov, databases of conference proceedings, dissertations and other "gray literature" (e.g. unpublished government and institutional reports), and grants databases such as NIH RePORTER [30]. Also, contacting authors or sponsors of studies may yield additional information. For clinical trials of regulated interventions (drugs and devices), reviewers should also consider consulting manufacturer registers such as the Glaxo-SmithKline Study Register, websites of regulatory agencies like the European Medicines Agency, and health technology assessment agencies such as the International Network of Agencies for Health Technology Assessment [30, 31].

Many studies have shown that including results from sources other than journal articles can influence the magnitude or precision of meta-analytic effects [32–35]. For example, Mayo-Wilson et al. found that depending on whether the study data source was a journal article, conference abstract, regulatory document, or individual participant dataset, they were able to produce a meta-analytic result showing that an agent was effective for pain relief in some instances and ineffective in others [36], which shows how valuable it can be to search beyond standard bibliographic databases.

Identifying and using data in sources other than journal articles can present various challenges. For example, search interfaces for trials registers are relatively unsophisticated [31], and there may be long delays between request and receipt of data from regulators or manufacturers [37]. Nevertheless, the task of uncovering such data should be undertaken, especially when the published studies do not report data on key outcomes that are likely to have been measured.

5.2.2   Restricting Meta-Analyses to Inception Cohorts

Study identification is retrospective in most systematic reviews; that is, authors typically search for reports of *completed* studies. However, given the evidence that completed studies with positive results are easier to identify because of the nature of their results, systematic reviews based on completed studies are likely to include a biased subset of all studies conducted. To minimize biased inclusion of studies, systematic reviewers might instead synthesize results of studies that could be identified before their results became known (an inception cohort). For example, different teams of researchers could work together to design and conduct a set of studies addressing the same question, and synthesize the results once all studies are completed (prospective meta-analysis) [38]. Assuming the researchers agreed to include all relevant results in the analysis, there would be no risk of bias due to missing results in the prospective meta-analysis. Few prospective meta-analyses have been conducted, but numbers are increasing: a systematic search for all prospective meta-analyses published up to February 2018 identified 43, almost half of which were published from 2015 onward [39].

Prospective meta-analysis is recommended for high-priority research questions for which limited previous evidence exists and new studies are expected to emerge, and is not suitable in all cases [39]. However, systematic reviewers can generate an inception cohort in other ways, for example by restricting inclusion to prospectively registered (or preregistered) studies addressing the review question [40], or identifying trials from trials registers before results were generated and working together with the trialists to populate the meta-analysis [41]. If all relevant results are available for all prospectively registered studies, there will be no bias due to missing results in a meta-analysis of these studies. If results are unavailable for some of the prospectively registered studies, then authors using this approach will be able to quantify how much evidence is missing, unlike a standard (retrospective) systematic review. However, a limitation of this approach is that the precision of a meta-analysis may be low if there are only a few, small, prospectively registered studies addressing the review question. Restricting a synthesis to an inception cohort may therefore involve a trade-off between bias and precision.

5.3   APPROACHES TO ASSESS RISK OF BIAS DUE TO MISSING RESULTS

Researchers have developed many approaches seeking to assess selective publication or reporting of study results, and the impact this may have on a meta-analysis. A systematic search for scales and checklists designed to help authors make a qualitative judgment about the risk of reporting biases identified 15 tools published up to February 2017 [42]. The tools varied by the type of reporting bias (publication bias or selective nonreporting bias) assessed; the target of assessment (e.g. an individual study or a meta-analysis of studies); and the criteria used to designate a study or meta-analysis as at risk of bias. A systematic search for graphical and statistical approaches designed to detect or adjust for reporting biases identified nearly 100 methods published up to January 2013 [43], and additional methods have been developed since [44]. However, all these approaches have limitations, and few have been validated empirically using examples in which the true amount of missing evidence was known. In the following section, we provide an overview of some of the available methods.

5.3.1   Tools to Assess Selective Nonreporting of Results in The Identified Studies

Various tools have been developed to assess selective nonreporting of results [42]. All emphasize the importance of retrieving the study's protocol, registration record, or statistical analysis plan, so that the planned outcomes and analyses can be compared with those that were reported [42]. If study plans are not available (which is more likely to be the case for older studies, and for nonrandomized studies), an assessment of selective nonreporting is still possible. For example, review authors can check whether any outcomes listed in the Methods section of a report are incompletely reported or have no corresponding results available in the Results section. By "incompletely reported" we mean that the study authors present insufficient data for inclusion of the result in a meta-analysis (for example, stating only that the between-group difference in the number of deaths was not significant, rather than reporting the number of deaths in each group or the risk ratio and 95% confidence interval). Regardless of the study design, users can also gauge the likelihood that a particular outcome of interest was measured, taking into consideration factors such as the clinical importance of the outcome. For example, pain is a defining symptom of shoulder disorders [45], so its absence in a trial report may raise suspicion of selective nonreporting.

An approach commonly used to assess selective nonreporting of results was via one of the domains of the 2011 Cochrane risk of bias tool for randomized trials [46] (introduced in Chapter 4). The tool asks users to judge the risk of selective nonreporting bias in a *study* as either low, unclear, or high, and to provide reasons for their judgment. This approach has limitations [47, 48]. Study-level assessments inform readers which studies the systematic reviewers have concerns about, but not necessarily which results were incompletely reported or missing entirely from those studies. An audit of Cochrane reviews published in 2015 found that in 39% of studies rated at high risk of bias due to selective nonreporting, users of the risk of bias tool failed to specify the particular results that were incompletely reported [48]. Outcome-level assessments, as recommended by the ORBIT (Outcome Reporting Bias In Trials) tool [49], can overcome this problem by displaying which results are unavailable for which studies, and whether the reasons for unavailability give cause for concern.

A limitation of existing tools for assessing selective nonreporting of results is that they do not guide reviewers to assess the risk of bias in meta-analyses that are unable to include the selectively nonreported results. This may explain why only 30% of Cochrane review authors who declared suspicion of selective nonreporting in their included studies acknowledged that the meta-analyses presented in the review were missing results [48]. A new framework that addresses these problems has recently been developed [50].

5.3.2   Qualitative Signals for Additional Missing Results

Some tools for assessing risk of reporting biases guide users to consider various qualitative signals that suggest additional results may be missing from studies that have not been identified [42]. These signals include:

- Sources of unpublished studies (e.g. trials registers) were not consulted.
- Specialized bibliographic databases that are likely to index studies relevant to the review question were not consulted.
- Only English-language studies were eligible, but the review addresses a question frequently investigated in countries speaking a language other than English.
- The research area addressed by the review is fast moving (hence there is a risk of time-lag bias).
- There is prior evidence of reporting bias in the research area addressed by the review.

The presence of one or more of these signals does not prove that additional results are missing from a particular meta-analysis. However, considering them is useful when trying to reach an overall judgment about risk of bias due to missing results, particularly in cases where information on prespecified outcomes and analyses is unavailable for most studies.

5.3.3   Funnel Plots

Funnel plots have long been used to assess the possibility that results are systematically missing from a meta-analysis. However, they should not be considered to be diagnostic of the presence of reporting biases because several other factors influence their appearance [51]. In this section, we describe what funnel plots are and how to interpret them.

First used in educational research and psychology [52], a funnel plot is a simple scatter plot of the intervention effects estimated from individual studies on the x axis against some measure of study size on the y axis, typically the standard error of the effect estimate [53]. The name "funnel plot" is based on the fact that the precision of the estimate of the underlying intervention effect will increase as study sample size increases; effect estimates from small studies will therefore scatter more widely at the bottom of the graph, with the spread narrowing among larger studies. The plot will resemble a symmetric, inverted funnel if there is no bias or between-study heterogeneity, and hence the scatter is due to sampling variation alone (see panel a of Figure 5.3).

Reporting biases are one of several factors that may lead to asymmetry in a funnel plot (Table 5.1). For example, if smaller studies showing no statistically significant effects remain unpublished, then such publication bias will lead to an asymmetric appearance of the funnel plot with a gap in the bottom corner of the graph (see panel b of Figure 5.3). However, studies with less methodological rigor tend to show larger intervention effects [58], so asymmetry also can arise when some smaller studies are at higher risk of bias and therefore produce larger intervention effect estimates (see panel c of Figure 5.3). Therefore, the funnel plot should be seen as a generic means of examining *small-study effects* – the tendency for the smaller studies in a meta-analysis to show larger treatment effects – rather than a tool to diagnose specific types of bias [51, 56].

The studies displayed in a funnel plot may not always estimate the same underlying effect of the same intervention, and such heterogeneity between results may lead to asymmetry in funnel plots if the true intervention effect is larger in the smaller

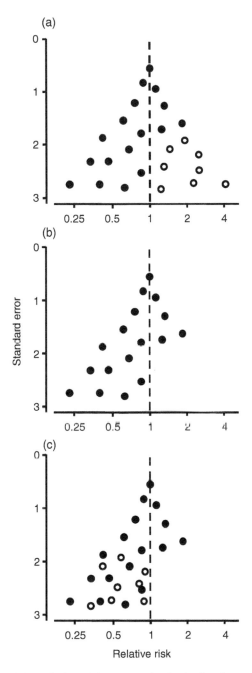

FIGURE 5.3 Hypothetical funnel plots: (a) symmetric plot in the absence of reporting bias (open circles indicate smaller studies showing no statistically significant results); (b) asymmetric plot in the presence of reporting bias (smaller studies showing no statistically significant results are missing); (c) asymmetric plot in the presence of bias due to methodologically flawed smaller studies (open circles indicate small studies using few methodological safeguards, whose results are biased toward larger effects).

TABLE 5.1   Possible sources of asymmetry in funnel plots.

1. Publication bias and other reporting biases
   - Entire study reports, or particular results, of smaller studies are unavailable because of the P value, magnitude, or direction of effect.
2. Poor methodological quality leading to spuriously inflated effects in smaller studies
   - Asymmetry can arise when some smaller studies are of lower methodological quality and produce larger intervention effect estimates.
3. True heterogeneity
   - Substantial benefit may be seen only in patients at high risk for the outcome that is affected by the intervention, and usually these high-risk patients are more likely to be included in small, early studies [54].
   - Some interventions may have been implemented more thoroughly in smaller trials and may therefore have resulted in larger intervention effect estimates [55].
4. Artefactual
   - Some effect estimates are naturally correlated with their standard errors, and this can produce spurious asymmetry in a funnel plot [56, 57]
5. Chance

Source: Adapted from Egger et al. [51].

studies. For example, randomized trials conducted in high-risk patients will tend to be smaller because of the difficulty in recruiting such patients, and because increased event rates mean that smaller sample sizes are required to detect a given effect [54]. Small trials generally are conducted before larger trials are established, and in the intervening years standard, control treatments may have improved, which can reduce the relative efficacy of the experimental treatment. Trialists may have implemented interventions less thoroughly in larger trials, thus explaining the more positive results in smaller trials [55].

Some effect estimates, such as log odds ratios, are naturally correlated with their standard errors. Because of this, a funnel plot that shows no asymmetry when plotted using one effect measure could be asymmetric when plotted using a different one [56]. Finally, it is possible that an asymmetric funnel plot arises merely by chance.

5.3.4   Contour-Enhanced Funnel Plots

An enhancement to the funnel plot includes contour lines corresponding to levels of statistical significance: $P = 0.01, 0.05, 0.1$, etc. [59]. This facilitates inspection of the statistical significance of study effect estimates and whether areas in which studies seem to be missing are related to P values. Such contour-enhanced funnel plots may help systematic reviewers differentiate asymmetry due to reporting biases from bias due to the other factors described in Section 5.3.3.

Consider the funnel plot in Figure 5.4, which represents a meta-analysis of the effect of selective serotonin reuptake inhibitors (SSRIs) versus placebo on treatment response, where a risk ratio greater than 1 indicates benefit of SSRIs [60]. There is a suggestion of missing results in the left-hand side of the plot, where results would be unfavorable to SSRIs, and in the area of statistical nonsignificance, which adds

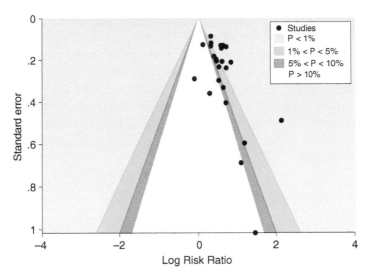

FIGURE 5.4 Contour-enhanced funnel plot for meta-analysis of the effect of selective serotonin reuptake inhibitors (*SSRIs*) versus placebo on treatment response (Clinical Global Impressions Improvement scale [*CGI-I*]) [60]. There is a suggestion of missing results in the left-hand side of the plot, where results would be unfavorable to SSRIs, and in the area of statistical nonsignificance (i.e. the white area where P > 0.10), which adds credence to the possibility that the asymmetry is due to reporting biases.

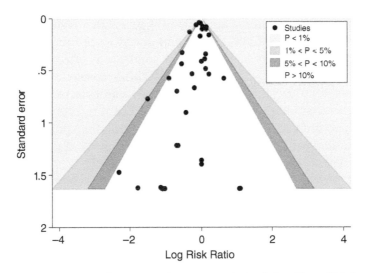

FIGURE 5.5 Contour-enhanced funnel plot for meta-analysis of the effect of higher versus lower intake of long-chain omega-3 fats on all-cause mortality [61]. There is a suggestion of missing results in the right-hand side of the plot, where results would be favorable to lower intake of omega-3, and in the area of statistical nonsignificance (i.e. the white area where P > 0.10). However, given that almost all results in the plot appear in the area of statistical nonsignificance, this reduces the plausibility that reporting bias is the underlying cause of this funnel plot asymmetry.

credence to the possibility that the asymmetry is due to reporting biases. Contrast this with the funnel plot in Figure 5.5, which corresponds to meta-analysis of the effect of higher versus lower intake of long-chain omega-3 fats on all-cause mortality, in which a risk ratio lower than 1 indicates benefit of higher intake [61]. In this case, there is a suggestion of missing results in the right-hand side of the plot, where results would be favorable to lower intake of omega-3, and in the area of statistical nonsignificance. However, given that almost all results in the plot appear in the area of statistical nonsignificance, i.e. both large and small studies finding a beneficial effect of higher or lower intake were nearly all not statistically significant, this reduces the plausibility that reporting bias is the underlying cause of this funnel plot asymmetry.

Funnel plot asymmetry thus may raise the possibility of bias due to missing results, but is not proof of bias. A further concern is that visual interpretation of funnel plots is inherently subjective.

5.3.5   Tests for Funnel Plot Asymmetry

Several statistical tests for funnel plot asymmetry are available. These examine whether the association between estimated intervention effects and a measure of study size or precision is greater than that expected to occur by chance. However, after reviewing the results of simulation studies evaluating test characteristics, and based on theoretical considerations, Sterne et al. advised that tests for funnel plot asymmetry are applicable only in the minority of meta-analyses for which their use is appropriate [56]. For meta-analyses of randomized trials, they suggested that as a rule of thumb, tests for funnel plot asymmetry should be used only when at least 10 trials are included in the meta-analysis. This is because when there are fewer than 10 trials the power of the tests is low. If there is substantial heterogeneity, the minimum number of trials may be substantially more than 10. Sterne et al. also suggested that results of tests for funnel plot asymmetry should be interpreted in the light of visual inspection of the funnel plot. For example, when there is evidence for small-study effects based on the result of an asymmetry test, it may be reasonable to exclude reporting biases as an explanation if there were very few studies with statistically significant results and bias would be expected to favor studies with statistically significant results. These recommendations apply only to meta-analyses of randomized trials, as the performance of tests for funnel plot asymmetry in other contexts (e.g. meta-analyses of prevalence, prognosis, and diagnostic test accuracy studies) is likely to differ [56].

Sterne et al. provided detailed recommendations about which tests to use for meta-analyses of randomized trials of intervention effects measured as mean differences, standardized mean differences, odds ratios, risk ratios, and risk differences [56]. Some tests, including the original and widely used Egger test [51] and Begg and Mazumdar test [62], are not recommended for application to odds ratios and standardized mean differences because of artefactual correlations between the effect size and its standard error [56, 57, 63]. For odds ratios, methods proposed by Harbord et al. [64] and Peters et al. [65] overcome this problem; for standardized mean differences, see methods proposed by Zwetsloot et al. [57] and Pustejovsky et al. [63]. For tests for use in meta-analyses of trials of survival data, see Debray et al. [66].

When a test for funnel plot asymmetry provides evidence of small-study effects, reporting biases should be considered as one of several possible explanations (described in Section 5.3.3), and systematic reviewers should attempt to distinguish the different possible reasons for this. Further information on tests for funnel plot asymmetry can be found in the historical review by Marks-Anglin and Chen [44].

5.3.6   Sensitivity Analyses

Statisticians have proposed several statistical approaches to assess how robust meta-analyses are to various assumptions about the extent and nature of missing results, including trim-and-fill [67], selection models [68], and regression-based adjustment methods [69]. Nearly all are designed to assess robustness to selective publication of studies [70], although some are designed to assess robustness to selective nonreporting of results [71, 72]; none assesses robustness to both sources of bias. Given that it is impossible to know for certain whether reporting biases have influenced the results of a review, or by how much, these methods should be considered only as sensitivity analysis, rather than as a way of ascertaining the "true" meta-analytic effect. Simulation studies have not compared the performance of all proposed methods. However, the available evidence suggests that no single method outperforms others in all scenarios, and thus there is a danger that uncritical application can lead to inappropriate conclusions being drawn [68, 73, 74]. Vevea et al. [70] and Marks-Anglin and Chen [44] summarize the advantages and disadvantages of different methods, indicate circumstances in which each can be used, and describe software available to implement them. Given the complexity of the methods, consultation with a statistician is recommended for their implementation.

5.3.7   Summary of Approaches

We have described several approaches that systematic reviewers can use to assess the risk of reporting biases. These include comparison of prespecified analysis plans with completed reports to detect selective nonreporting of results, consideration of qualitative signals that suggest not all studies were identified, and the use of funnel plots to identify small-study effects, for which reporting bias is one of several causes. Information from approaches such as funnel plots and selection models is more difficult to interpret than from less subjective approaches such as detection of incompletely reported results in studies for which prespecified analysis plans were available. Tools that weigh the various pieces of information gained from each approach to reach an overall judgment of the risk of bias due to missing results in a meta-analysis have recently been proposed. These include the tool for assessing Risk Of Bias due to Missing Evidence (ROB-ME) in pairwise syntheses, available at https://www.riskofbias.info, and its extension for network meta-analysis (ROB-MEN).

5.4   CONCLUSIONS

The evidence that dissemination of research findings can be influenced by the nature of the findings themselves is convincing; and when available results differ systematically from missing results, meta-analyses will be biased. Systematic reviewers should comprehensively search for study reports and consult not only multiple bibliographic databases but trials registers, manufacturers, regulators, and study authors and sponsors. Unless they use prospective approaches to meta-analysis, which can eliminate the potential for bias due to missing results, reviewers should formally assess the risk of bias due to missing results in their review. Several approaches can facilitate such assessment: tools to record selective nonreporting of results, ascertaining qualitative signals that suggest not all studies were identified, and the use of funnel plots to identify small-study effects, one cause of which is reporting bias. Tools that weigh diverse information about the likelihood and nature of missing results in the judgment of the risk of bias in a meta-analysis have recently been proposed and should facilitate appropriate interpretation of results.

REFERENCES

1. Dickersin, K. (1990). The existence of publication bias and risk factors for its occurrence. *J. Am. Med. Assoc.* 263 (10): 1385–1389.

2. Easterbrook, P.J., Berlin, J.A., Gopalan, R., and Matthews, D.R. (1991). Publication bias in clinical research. *Lancet* 337 (8746): 867–872.

3. Sterne, J.A.C., Savović, J., Page, M.J. et al. (2019). RoB 2: a revised tool for assessing risk of bias in randomised trials. *Br. Med. J.* 366: l4898.

4. Sterne, J.A.C., Hernan, M.A., Reeves, B.C. et al. (2016). ROBINS-I: a tool for assessing risk of bias in non-randomised studies of interventions. *Br. Med. J.* 355: i4919.

5. Schmucker, C., Schell, L.K., Portalupi, S. et al. (2014). Extent of non-publication in cohorts of studies approved by research ethics committees or included in trial registries. *PLoS One* 9 (12): e114023.

6. Scherer, R.W., Meerpohl, J.J., Pfeifer, N. et al. (2018). Full publication of results initially presented in abstracts. *Cochrane Database Syst. Rev.* (11): MR000005. https://doi.org/10.1002/14651858.MR000005.pub4.

7. Chan, A.-W., Song, F., Vickers, A. et al. (2014). Increasing value and reducing waste: addressing inaccessible research. *Lancet* 383 (9913): 257–266.

8. Treanor, L., Frank, R.A., Cherpak, L.A. et al. (2020). Publication bias in diagnostic imaging: conference abstracts with positive conclusions are more likely to be published. *Eur. Radiol.* 30 (5): 2964–2972.

9. Vollgraff Heidweiller-Schreurs, C.A., Korevaar, D.A., Mol, B.W.J. et al. (2019). Publication bias may exist among prognostic accuracy studies of middle cerebral artery Doppler ultrasound. *J. Clin. Epidemiol.* 116: 1–8.

10. Petticrew, M., Egan, M., Thomson, H. et al. (2008). Publication bias in qualitative research: what becomes of qualitative research presented at conferences? *J. Epidemiol. Community Health* 62 (6): 552–554.

11. Dechartres, A., Atal, I., Riveros, C. et al. (2018). Association between publication characteristics and treatment effect estimates: a meta-epidemiologic study. *Ann. Intern. Med.* 169 (6): 385–393.

12. Tanner-Smith, E.E. and Polanin, J.R. (2015). A retrospective analysis of dissemination biases in the brief alcohol intervention literature. *Psychol. Addict. Behav.* 29 (1): 49–62.

13. Sune, P., Sune, J.M., and Montoro, J.B. (2013). Positive outcomes influence the rate and time to publication, but not the impact factor of publications of clinical trial results. *PLoS One* 8 (1): e54583.

14. Song, S.Y., Koo, D.H., Jung, S.Y. et al. (2017). The significance of the trial outcome was associated with publication rate and time to publication. *J. Clin. Epidemiol.* 84: 78–84.

15. Khan, N.A., Singh, M., Spencer, H.J., and Torralba, K.D. (2014). Randomized controlled trials of rheumatoid arthritis registered at http://ClinicalTrials.gov: what gets published and when. *Arthritis Rheumatol* 66 (10): 2664–2674.

16. Korevaar, D.A., van Es, N., Zwinderman, A.H. et al. (2016). Time to publication among completed diagnostic accuracy studies: associated with reported accuracy estimates. *BMC Med. Res. Methodol.* 16: 68.

17. Tramer, M.R., Reynolds, D.J., Moore, R.A., and McQuay, H.J. (1997). Impact of covert duplicate publication on meta-analysis: a case study. *Br. Med. J.* 315 (7109): 635–640.

18. Duyx, B., Urlings, M.J.E., Swaen, G.M.H. et al. (2017). Scientific citations favor positive results: a systematic review and meta-analysis. *J. Clin. Epidemiol.* 88: 92–101.

19. Egger, M., Zellweger-Zahner, T., Schneider, M. et al. (1997). Language bias in randomised controlled trials published in English and German. *Lancet* 350 (9074): 326–329.

20. Juni, P., Holenstein, F., Sterne, J. et al. (2002). Direction and impact of language bias in meta-analyses of controlled trials: empirical study. *Int. J. Epidemiol.* 31 (1): 115–123.

21. Egger, M., Juni, P., Bartlett, C. et al. (2003). How important are comprehensive literature searches and the assessment of trial quality in systematic reviews? Empirical study. *Health Technol. Assess.* 7 (1): 1–76.

22. Chan, A.W., Hrobjartsson, A., Haahr, M.T. et al. (2004). Empirical evidence for selective reporting of outcomes in randomized trials: comparison of protocols to published articles. *J. Am. Med. Assoc.* 291 (20): 2457–2465.

23. Redmond, S., von Elm, E., Blumle, A. et al. (2013). Cohort study of trials submitted to ethics committee identified discrepant reporting of outcomes in publications. *J. Clin. Epidemiol.* 66 (12): 1367–1375.

24. Jones, C.W., Keil, L.G., Holland, W.C. et al. (2015). Comparison of registered and published outcomes in randomized controlled trials: a systematic review. *BMC Med.* 13: 282.

25. Korevaar, D.A., Ochodo, E.A., Bossuyt, P.M., and Hooft, L. (2014). Publication and reporting of test accuracy studies registered in http://ClinicalTrials.gov. *Clin. Chem.* 60 (4): 651–659.

26. Jefferson, T., Doshi, P., Boutron, I. et al. (2018). When to include clinical study reports and regulatory documents in systematic reviews. *Br. Med. J. Evid. Based Med.* 23 (6): 210–217.

27. Goldacre, B., Drysdale, H., Dale, A. et al. (2019). COMPare: a prospective cohort study correcting and monitoring 58 misreported trials in real time. *Trials* 20 (1): 118.

28. Dwan, K., Gamble, C., Williamson, P.R., and Kirkham, J.J. (2013). Systematic review of the empirical evidence of study publication bias and outcome reporting bias - an updated review. *PLoS One* 8 (7): e66844.

29. Chan, A.W., Krleža-Jeric, K., Schmid, I., and Altman, D.G. (2004). Outcome reporting bias in randomized trials funded by the Canadian Institutes of Health Research. *Can. Med. Assoc. J.* 171 (7): 735–740.

30. Lefebvre, C., Glanville, J., Briscoe, S. et al. (2019). Searching for and selecting studies. In: *Cochrane Handbook for Systematic Reviews of Interventions* (eds. J.P.T. Higgins, J. Thomas, J. Chandler, et al.), Chapter 4, 67–108. Chichester: Wiley.

31. Isojarvi, J., Wood, H., Lefebvre, C., and Glanville, J. (2018). Challenges of identifying unpublished data from clinical trials: getting the best out of clinical trials registers and other novel sources. *Res. Synth. Methods* 9 (4): 561–578.

32. Baudard, M., Yavchitz, A., Ravaud, P. et al. (2017). Impact of searching clinical trial registries in systematic reviews of pharmaceutical treatments: methodological systematic review and reanalysis of meta-analyses. *Br. Med. J* 356: j448.

33. Hart, B., Lundh, A., and Bero, L. (2012). Effect of reporting bias on meta-analyses of drug trials: reanalysis of meta-analyses. *Br. Med. J* 344: d7202.

34. Schmucker, C.M., Blumle, A., Schell, L.K. et al. (2017). Systematic review finds that study data not published in full text articles have unclear impact on meta-analyses results in medical research. *PLoS One* 12 (4): e0176210.

35. Golder, S., Loke, Y.K., Wright, K., and Norman, G. (2016). Reporting of adverse events in published and unpublished studies of health care interventions: a systematic review. *PLoS Med.* 13 (9): e1002127.

36. Mayo-Wilson, E., Li, T., Fusco, N. et al. (2017). Cherry-picking by trialists and meta-analysts can drive conclusions about intervention efficacy. *J. Clin. Epidemiol.* 91: 95–110.

37. Doshi, P. and Jefferson, T. (2016). Open data 5 years on: a case series of 12 freedom of information requests for regulatory data to the European Medicines Agency. *Trials* 17 (1): 78.

38. Thomas, J., Askie, L.M., Berlin, J.A. et al. (2019). Prospective approaches to accumulating evidence. In: *Cochrane Handbook for Systematic Reviews of Interventions* (eds. J.P.T. Higgins, J. Thomas, J. Chandler, et al.), Chapter 22, 549–568. Chichester: Wiley.

39. Seidler, A.L., Hunter, K.E., Cheyne, S. et al. (2019). A guide to prospective meta-analysis. *Br. Med. J* 367: l5342.

40. Roberts, I., Ker, K., Edwards, P. et al. (2015). The knowledge system underpinning healthcare is not fit for purpose and must change. *Br. Med. J* 350: h2463.

41. Sterne, J.A.C., Murthy, S., Diaz, J.V. et al. (2020). Association between administration of systemic corticosteroids and mortality among critically ill patients with COVID-19: a meta-analysis. *J. Am. Med. Assoc.* 324 (13): 1330–1341.

42. Page, M.J., McKenzie, J.E., and Higgins, J.P.T. (2018). Tools for assessing risk of reporting biases in studies and syntheses of studies: a systematic review. *Br. Med. J Open* 8: e019703.

43. Mueller, K.F., Meerpohl, J.J., Briel, M. et al. (2016). Methods for detecting, quantifying and adjusting for dissemination bias in meta-analysis are described. *J. Clin. Epidemiol.* 80: 25–33.

44. Marks-Anglin, A. and Chen, Y. (2020). A historical review of publication bias. *Res. Synth. Methods* 11 (6): 725–742.

45. Page, M.J., Huang, H., Verhagen, A.P. et al. (2018). Outcome reporting in randomized trials for shoulder disorders: literature review to inform the development of a core outcome set. *Arthritis Care Res. (Hoboken)* 70 (2): 252–259.

46. Higgins, J.P.T., Altman, D.G., Gøtzsche, P.C. et al. (2011). The Cochrane Collaboration's tool for assessing risk of bias in randomised trials. *Br. Med. J* 343: d5928.

47. Sterne, J.A.C. (2013). Why the Cochrane risk of bias tool should not include funding source as a standard item [editorial]. *Cochrane Database Syst. Rev.* (12): ED000076.

48. Page, M.J. and Higgins, J.P.T. (2016). Rethinking the assessment of risk of bias due to selective reporting: a cross-sectional study. *Syst. Rev.* 5 (1): 108.

49. Kirkham, J.J., Altman, D.G., Chan, A.W. et al. (2018). Outcome reporting bias in trials: a methodological approach for assessment and adjustment in systematic reviews. *Br. Med. J* 362: k3802.

50. Page, M.J., Higgins, J.P.T., and Sterne, J.A.C. (2019). Assessing risk of bias due to missing results in a synthesis. In: *Cochrane Handbook for Systematic Reviews of Interventions* (eds. J.P.T. Higgins, J. Thomas, J. Chandler, et al.), Chapter 13, 349–374. Chichester: Wiley.

51. Egger, M., Davey Smith, G., Schneider, M., and Minder, C. (1997). Bias in meta-analysis detected by a simple, graphical test. *Br. Med. J* 315 (7109): 629–634.

52. Light, R.J. and Pillemer, D.B. (1984). *Summing Up: The Science of Reviewing Research.* Cambridge, MA: Harvard University Press.

53. Sterne, J.A.C. and Egger, M. (2001). Funnel plots for detecting bias in meta-analysis: guidelines on choice of axis. *J. Clin. Epidemiol.* 54: 1046–1055.

54. Davey Smith, G. and Egger, M. (1994). Who benefits from medical interventions? Treating low risk patients can be a high risk strategy. *Br. Med. J.* 308: 72–74.

55. Stuck, A.E., Rubenstein, L.Z., and Wieland, D. (1998). Bias in meta-analysis detected by a simple, graphical test. asymmetry detected in funnel plot was probably due to true heterogeneity. *Lett. Br. Med. J.* 316: 469–471.

56. Sterne, J.A.C., Sutton, A.J., Ioannidis, J.P.A. et al. (2011). Recommendations for examining and interpreting funnel plot asymmetry in meta-analyses of randomised controlled trials. *Br. Med. J.* 343: d4002.

57. Zwetsloot, P.-P., Van Der Naald, M., Sena, E.S. et al. (2017). Standardized mean differences cause funnel plot distortion in publication bias assessments. *Elife* 6: e24260.

58. Page, M.J., Higgins, J.P.T., Clayton, G. et al. (2016). Empirical evidence of study design biases in randomized trials: systematic review of meta-epidemiological studies. *PLoS One* 11: 7.

59. Peters, J.L., Sutton, A.J., Jones, D.R. et al. (2008). Contour-enhanced meta-analysis funnel plots help distinguish publication bias from other causes of asymmetry. *J. Clin. Epidemiol.* 61 (10): 991–996.

60. Williams, T., Hattingh, C.J., Kariuki, C.M. et al. (2017). Pharmacotherapy for social anxiety disorder (SAnD). *Cochrane Database Syst. Rev.* (10): CD001206.

61. Abdelhamid, A.S., Brown, T.J., Brainard, J.S. et al. (2018). Omega-3 fatty acids for the primary and secondary prevention of cardiovascular disease. *Cochrane Database Syst. Rev.* (11): CD003177.

62. Begg, C.B. and Mazumdar, M. (1994). Operating characteristics of a rank correlation test for publication bias. *Biometrics* 50 (4): 1088–1101.

63. Pustejovsky, J.E. and Rodgers, M.A. (2019). Testing for funnel plot asymmetry of standardized mean differences. *Res. Synth. Methods* 10 (1): 57–71.

64. Harbord, R.M., Egger, M., and Sterne, J.A.C. (2006). A modified test for small-study effects in meta-analyses of controlled trials with binary endpoints. *Stat. Med.* 25 (20): 3443–3457.

65. Peters, J.L., Sutton, A.J., Jones, D.R. et al. (2006). Comparison of two methods to detect publication bias in meta-analysis. *J. Am. Med. Assoc.* 295 (6): 676–680.

66. Debray, T.P.A., Moons, K.G.M., and Riley, R.D. (2018). Detecting small-study effects and funnel plot asymmetry in meta-analysis of survival data: a comparison of new and existing tests. *Res. Synth. Methods* 9 (1): 41–50.

67. Duval, S. and Tweedie, R. (2000). Trim and fill: a simple funnel-plot-based method of testing and adjusting for publication bias in meta-analysis. *Biometrics* 56 (2): 455–463.

68. McShane, B.B., Bockenholt, U., and Hansen, K.T. (2016). Adjusting for publication bias in meta-analysis: an evaluation of selection methods and some cautionary notes. *Perspect. Psychol. Sci.* 11 (5): 730–749.

69. Moreno, S.G., Sutton, A.J., Turner, E.H. et al. (2009). Novel methods to deal with publication biases: secondary analysis of antidepressant trials in the FDA trial registry database and related journal publications. *Br. Med. J.* 339: b2981.

70. Vevea, J.L., Coburn, K., and Sutton, A. (2019). Publication bias. In: *The Handbook of Research Synthesis and Meta-Analysis* (eds. H. Cooper, L.V. Hedges and J.C. Valentine), 383–430. New York: Russell Sage Foundation.

71. Copas, J., Marson, A., Williamson, P., and Kirkham, J. (2019). Model-based sensitivity analysis for outcome reporting bias in the meta analysis of benefit and harm outcomes. *Stat. Methods Med. Res.* 28 (3): 889–903.

72. Williamson, P.R. and Gamble, C. (2007). Application and investigation of a bound for outcome reporting bias. *Trials* 8: 9.

73. Carter, E.C., Schönbrodt, F.D., Gervais, W.M., and Hilgard, J. (2019). Correcting for bias in psychology: a comparison of meta-analytic methods. *Adv. Methods Pract. Psychol. Sci.* 2 (2): 115–144.

74. Rucker, G., Carpenter, J.R., and Schwarzer, G. (2011). Detecting and adjusting for small-study effects in meta-analysis. *Biomet. J. Biometrische Zeitschrift* 53 (2): 351–368.

CHAPTER 6

Managing People and Data

Eliane Rohner, Julia Bohlius, Bruno R. da Costa, and Sven Trelle

Systematic reviews and meta-analyses are complex projects that require good management of people and data. Because systematic reviews and meta-analyses summarize current evidence, they are time sensitive. If not well managed, a review will likely be out of date when it is finally completed. Nominating a project manager who will develop a project plan and coordinate the review team is thus strongly advised. Review teams often underestimate the time it takes to perform the different steps of a review, outlined in Chapter 2, from formulating a precise review question to interpreting the results and writing up the study. It is therefore important to agree on realistic timelines for the different steps and monitor adherence to these timelines along the project life cycle. Several types of data are collected in a systematic review and meta-analysis. Good data management is crucial for the success of the project. In this chapter, we discuss the composition and coordination of the team undertaking the work and the management and extraction of aggregate data from study reports.

6.1 THE TEAM

6.1.1 Composition and Roles

Systematic reviews and meta-analyses require a multidisciplinary team with expertise both in the clinical or public health question addressed and in methodology, including literature searching (see Chapter 3), risk of bias assessment (see Chapter 4), and statistical methods for meta-analysis (see Chapters 8–14).

Several roles and tasks need to be defined and distributed among the members of a review team (Box 6.1). Depending on skills, experience, and resources available,

Systematic Reviews in Health Research: Meta-Analysis in Context, Third Edition. Edited by Matthias Egger, Julian P.T. Higgins, and George Davey Smith.
© 2022 John Wiley & Sons Ltd. Published 2022 by John Wiley & Sons Ltd.
Companion website: www.systematic-reviews3.org

Box 6.1   Roles and Tasks to be Defined for a Systematic Review Project

Role	Tasks
Project manager/coordinator	• Serves as the backbone of a systematic review/meta-analysis project • Coordinates the team, develops the project plan, manages the project schedule • Ensures efficient communication between the team members
Reviewer	• Develops specific review questions and the review protocol • Screens references for eligibility • Manages screened references to facilitate transparent reporting of the screening process (PRISMA flow diagram, see Chapter 7) • Assesses study quality and extracts data using a standardized data extraction form • Drafts reports
Information specialist	• Develops, runs, and updates systematic literature searches • Supports management of references • Supports reporting of findings from systematic literature searches
Methods expert	• Guides risk of bias assessment of included studies • Supports data extractions and ensures the correct use of statistical methods
Content expert	• Contributes to the development of the review questions and the protocol • Supports the interpretation of the review findings

one team member can take over several roles and tasks. However, two to three team members, at least, are required to conduct a systematic review, since reference screening and data extraction need to be done by two reviewers, ideally independently, and a third reviewer should be consulted if disagreements arise.

Depending on the complexity of the topic and the number of eligible studies, more team members might be necessary. Developing the specific review question and protocol requires input from content and methods experts as well as information specialists. Developing literature search strategies for systematic reviews can be challenging, and advice from information specialists should be sought early on [1]. Information specialists are also increasingly involved in other systematic review tasks such as the formulation of the research question, screening and managing references, and report writing [2]. To develop the data extraction form, input is needed from content experts on outcomes and other data relevant for the health care question under review and from methods experts to define pertinent items for the assessment of study quality. Support from statisticians can be helpful to handle the extraction of incompletely reported data. A statistician should also be involved to ensure the correct use of statistical methods. Finally, the input of all team members, but in particular of the content experts, is required to interpret the review findings appropriately.

6.1.2 Training

Once the tasks have been distributed among the review team members, sufficient time for training should be allocated. Especially for team members not previously involved in systematic reviews and meta-analyses, comprehensive methodological training is essential. The Cochrane webpage (http://training.cochrane.org/) provides online training materials and a list of training events.

6.1.3 Project Management and Coordination

Project management and coordination is a resource-intensive key task in a systematic review [3, 4]. The project manager develops the project plan, coordinates the review team, and oversees the systematic review and meta-analysis as a whole. Together with the team, the project manager should identify all tasks that need to be completed during the life cycle of the systematic review project. Next, the dependencies between different tasks and the timelines and responsibilities should be defined. Ideally, this is done in a dedicated team meeting in which all team members agree on timelines and responsibilities. It is advisable to display the timelines agreed upon in a Gantt chart; that is, a bar chart that visualizes the start and end date of each task. A Gantt chart can be easily produced in Microsoft Excel, for example, and then shared among team members to serve as a reference document. The Gantt chart in Figure 6.1 gives a hypothetical example of how long the different review tasks may last. The timelines may vary substantially depending on the complexity of the subject, the number of references, and eligible studies identified in the literature search, and the number of outcomes to be analyzed.

Tasks	Months											
	1	2	3	4	5	6	7	8	9	10	11	12
Background reading	▓											
Study other reviews	▓											
Specify question	▓											
Pilot literature search	▓	▓										
Write protocol		▓	▓									
Develop data extraction form			▓	▓								
Literature search and screening			▓	▓	▓							
Appraisal of studies					▓	▓	▓					
Data extraction								▓	▓			
Synthesize data										▓	▓	
Report findings										▓	▓	▓

FIGURE 6.1 Gantt chart for planning and visualizing the schedule of a systematic review project.

6.1.4 Communication

Not all team members might work on the review full-time, and team members may be located in different institutions, countries, or continents. To simplify the management of a review with remote team members, entire parts of the review such as literature screening or data extraction and analysis can be delegated to a remote team. Often, no dedicated funding is available for systematic reviews and meta-analyses, and the team members may do the work on a voluntary basis. In this situation, it is even more important for the project manager to keep up the team spirit with clear communication and well-set timelines. Otherwise, discouragement and frustration from unmet targets can lead to prolonged and, in the worst case, abandoned reviews. This book's website (www.systematic-reviews3.org) provides a list of freeware tools that help manage the group and relevant documents. Updating reviews poses a special challenge as, over time, review team members may move on professionally or lose motivation. Good data management is essential to overcome part of the challenge, since it allows new team members to quickly become acquainted with the review history and ensures that adding new data is as straightforward as possible.

6.2 THE DATA

In general, data management for a systematic review follows the same principles that apply to other studies – whether reviewers decide to manage data on paper or electronically. The data management system should be:

- Reliable
  - The system is readily accessible to persons involved, stable, and fit for purpose
- Supportive
  - The system supports (and does not hinder) tasks related to data collection, manipulation, and storage
- Secure
  - Entering or changing data is restricted to authorized users and data are stored securely with regular data back-ups
- Accountable
  - Changes and access to the data are traceable

Fulfilling these requirements helps ensure that the data are accurate, verifiable, and entered efficiently. A data management plan detailing the mechanisms used to handle data should ideally be specified at the protocol stage of the review [5].

6.2.1 Types and Structure of Data in a Systematic Review

Through the different steps of a systematic review and meta-analysis, various forms of data are collected. These include information on the number of references identified through the literature searches, the eligibility assessment of the identified references, factual data extracted from the included studies to address the study questions, and the risk of bias assessment. Review teams may decide to use separate software tools and databases for each step, or use dedicated systematic review software, allowing data collection and management of more than one step [6].

The structure of the data collected in a systematic review is often complex. The primary unit of analysis in a systematic review is usually the component studies. However, data on a particular study may be available from multiple sources, including conference abstracts and presentations, full-text publications, websites, study protocols, clinical study reports, clinical trial registries, or personal communications. A trial protocol, for example, may contain more information on methods, and therefore on the risk of bias, than a journal article. In this situation, reviewers should combine complementary information and document the different sources of data [7]. Discrepancies between sources could be resolved by contacting the authors or by applying prespecified criteria so that, for example, data from full-text publications are given preference over data from conference abstracts. A single report might include data on multiple studies and can therefore contribute several studies eligible for the systematic review and meta-analysis, adding further complexity.

Moreover, the data extracted from studies often reflect different elements, such as the study population or an outcome of interest. The data structure can become yet more complicated if the review team is interested in subgroups of patients, comparisons of several interventions, or outcomes assessed at different points in time. Data can thus be hierarchically nested across levels of a study. It is essential to identify hierarchical structures early on and manage data extraction accordingly. Otherwise, data may be inconsistent, and the analysis difficult or even impossible to conduct. This hierarchical structure also applies to risk of bias assessments that may relate to the study as a whole, to individual comparisons within a study, or to particular results determined by the study population, outcome, or timepoint.

6.2.2   Reference Management and Eligibility Assessment

After the literature searches, the identified references need to be deduplicated, screened, and assessed for eligibility. Each step of the reference screening and eligibility assessment must be documented rigorously to produce the Preferred Reporting Items for Systematic Reviews and Meta-Analyses (PRISMA) flow diagram of the systematic review [8]. Most review teams use general bibliographic software tools such as EndNote, RefWorks, Mendeley, or Zotero for these steps [9]. Each of these bibliographic tools allows for the importing of references from databases and facilitates deduplication of records. However, they differ in terms of cost and general functionality, which includes the documentation of eligibility assessment. For example, in EndNote screening of references may be organized by creating groups of included and excluded references [10]. Apart from general bibliographic software, dedicated software tools for reference screening and eligibility assessment exist [6]. Some of them cover several review steps, whereas others, like the semi-automated online tool Abstrackr [11, 12], focus on reference screening.

Eligibility assessment is a crucial step in a systematic review, since one wants to make sure that no relevant studies are missed. We recommend that at least two reviewers screen references and assess eligibility. Clear inclusion and exclusion criteria must be specified at the protocol stage to reduce subjectivity in decisions [5]. During title and abstract screening, it is usually sufficient to document whether a reference is excluded or should be assessed in more detail. At the full-text stage, however, the reasons for exclusion need to be recorded. It is helpful to define a hierarchy of potential exclusion reasons based on the eligibility criteria, and then use them for classification of the excluded full texts. Reviewers may decide to do the classification directly in the reference manager software or on a separate eligibility form created for this purpose. Independently of the approach used, reviewer disagreements about eligibility should be resolved by discussion or involvement of a third person, and the decision should be documented.

6.2.3   Data Extraction from Component Studies

Data extraction for systematic reviews should be carefully planned, with variables defined at the protocol stage [5]. Upon completion of data extraction, relevant data should be available in electronic form and ready for analysis. As in other studies, systematic review data should be collected using a standardized data extraction form. However, there is an essential difference between data collection in systematic reviews and primary studies. A systematic review is secondary research, and the data used for analysis were generated by others, for different purposes. Therefore, the data available from the eligible studies will often not fit the needs of the review exactly. The required data might need to be calculated from available data or even be approximated, which in turn requires making strong assumptions (see Section 6.2.5). Because these assumptions are often not testable, it is important to be transparent regarding the assumptions made and the derivations or approximations applied.

In general, because the amount of data to extract can quickly become unmanageable, less is often more. An example illustrates the challenge. A review team considered the following aspects as being particularly relevant to their research question:

- Comparison of two interventions (drug X versus placebo).
- Three outcomes of interest (mortality, quality of life, and serious adverse events).
- Results overall and for two subgroups (two different age groups).
- Results at two different timepoints (6 and 12 months after randomization).

This situation, which is not unusual, makes it necessary to extract data for 18 different comparisons of interest for each component study. This number can quickly increase into the hundreds if the systematic review is part of a network meta-analysis (see Chapter 13) where many more interventions are compared.

6.2.3.1   Development and Piloting of Data Extraction Forms

The development of a reliable and valid data extraction form is a crucial task in a systematic review and enough time should be allocated for this step [13–15]. For every systematic review, the data extraction form needs to be carefully tailored to the specific research question. This step is challenging, and it requires in-depth knowledge of the research topic and the relevant literature. A data extraction form usually captures information on study characteristics and the outcomes of interest. It should be designed parsimoniously to ensure that time and resources are not wasted on extracting unnecessary data. Each data item should serve a clear purpose at the data synthesis and presentation stage. The form should be developed with this explicitly in mind. It should begin with an administrative section, including information on the study identifier (e.g. first author's name and publication year), name of data extractor, extraction date, source of information, and publication type. A notes section for queries that need to be discussed within the team may also be useful. This section is usually followed by data items related to study design, characteristics of the study population, and outcomes of interest. Data extraction templates developed by several groups of the Cochrane Collaboration can be downloaded from www.cochrane.org. On this book's website (www.systematic-reviews3.org) we provide further examples of forms for different types of outcomes.

It is important to define explicitly how data should be recorded in the forms. Ideally, the definitions and instructions can be included in the data extraction form itself, but if detailed instructions are required, the forms will become confusing. It may then be helpful to put the data extraction guidelines in a separate document. The more structured the format of the data entry fields, the cleaner the entered data will be. For example, for each data field, the data type (e.g. text, numeric), the format (for dates, dd/mm/yyyy), and the unit of measurement, if applicable, should be defined.

Moreover, outcome data might have been assessed at different times using different methods or instruments (e.g. different rating scales). Sometimes it is also necessary to reference extracted data points with the exact source (report, page, line, or table/graph). The entry of fixed-format or precoded data is generally preferred over free-text fields. However, attention should also be paid to not losing relevant information through overzealous coding. It is therefore advisable to use more rather than fewer categories for a specific data item. If necessary, categories can be collapsed during analysis. Also, if information about a particular variable is unclear or not available, it is vital to record this to distinguish these data from incomplete data extractions.

The development of the data extraction form is an iterative process. It is essential to pilot the data extraction form on a sample of included studies [15, 16]. In our experience, it often takes several revisions of the data extraction form to reach the right balance between collecting all relevant information validly and reliably, and keeping data extraction and analysis efficient by reducing the number of data items collected. Piloting data extraction forms also allows rearrangement of data items to improve the flow of data collection, and the identification of inconsistencies and logical errors. Ideally, different data extractors pilot the form on the same studies. Should the data extractors reach different conclusions for a given data item, the description or definition of that item needs to be clarified. Even after the pilot phase, data extraction forms may still need adaptation. However, any revisions during data extraction should be kept to a minimum, and their implications for previously extracted data must be carefully checked. It might be advisable not to implement changes on an ongoing basis, but instead to wait until several shortcomings have been identified and then implement them all at once. It is sometimes easier to produce a short additional data extraction form for new data items instead of adapting the main data extraction form already in use.

6.2.3.2   Implementation of Data Extraction Forms

Many different data management systems for systematic reviews are in use [17]. Reviewers may decide to manage data extraction on paper first, followed by electronic data entry, or choose electronic data extraction directly. The decision is mainly based on the personal preferences of the review team, but advantages and disadvantages should be considered (Box 6.2).

Paper data extraction forms can be generated, for example, in Microsoft Word. Tick boxes are useful for data items with prespecified categorical response options. Paper forms have the advantage that they readily allow marginal notes and comments.

Box 6.2   Advantages and Disadvantages of Different Data Extraction Methods

Advantages	Disadvantages
Paper-based data extraction forms	
• Easy and cheap to implement	• Separate data entry step needed to obtain variables for analysis
• Allow marginal notes and comments during the extraction process	• Risk of losing data/forms
• No computers needed to do the data extraction	• Handwriting may impair readability
	• Management becomes impractical with a large number of included studies
Electronic data extraction forms	
In general:	In general:
• Combine data extraction and entry	• More rigid than paper forms
• Clear data entry structure may reduce errors	• Require access to a computer and possibly the internet to do the data extraction
• Allow for quality checks with error messages highlighting implausible values	
• Option to store forms on server or cloud with regular back-ups	
• Automatic comparison of data collection forms from two reviewers to identify disagreements	
• Direct data transfer to analysis software such as Stata or R possible	

Advantages	Disadvantages
Electronic data extraction forms	
Generic software:	Generic software:
• Full control over the design of data extraction forms	• Specialized skills needed to develop electronic data extraction form
	• Documentation of the consensus process often not straightforward
Dedicated software tools:	Dedicated software tools:
• Online access facilitates collaboration between reviewers working from different locations	• Costs (for some of the tools)
	• Limited customizability
• Often easy navigation in long forms	• The risk that software tools may be abandoned and no longer available (especially relevant to large, long-lasting review projects that are regularly updated)
• Convenient for inexperienced reviewers as template forms often available that include variables commonly extracted for systematic reviews	
• Additional help files and support may be available	

However, this can also quickly lead to confusing situations at the data entry stage. Therefore, notes should be added cautiously. When using paper forms, the comparison between the data extractions done by two reviewers cannot be automated. One data extraction form usually will be chosen as the main form. If discrepancies occur in data recorded on the other form, they should be resolved by the involvement of a third reviewer. If entries in the main form need to be changed after discussion, this should be documented with a note stating the persons involved and the date.

While paper forms may be an attractive option for reviews with a small number of studies and variables, they tend to become inefficient and unreliable for larger reviews. Electronic forms can be implemented in specialized, dedicated software tools or generic data management software. Generic solutions are developed by the review team using nonspecialized software such as Microsoft Access, LibreOffice Base, FileMaker, and EpiData. Many researchers are familiar with spreadsheet software like Microsoft Excel, which is therefore relatively easy to use. However, spreadsheets do not fulfill the criteria for a data management system described above and quickly become impractical if data for a larger number of studies and variables are extracted. We therefore generally advise against using spreadsheets for data extraction. Relational databases like Microsoft Access or LibreOffice Base are well suited to capture the typical hierarchical data structure in systematic reviews, but setting up these databases requires data management and software expertise.

Dedicated software solutions have been developed specifically for the purpose of data extraction in systematic reviews, and they may also accommodate other phases of the review process, such as literature searches, eligibility assessment, and data synthesis [6]. There are numerous commercial and noncommercial solutions available. The Systematic Review (SR) Toolbox (http://systematicreviewtools.com) allows searching for available tools based on specific criteria such as the review step or cost. Once data have been entered electronically, they are exported in file formats readable by standard analysis software such as Stata or R. Some dedicated software tools also enable direct data synthesis and analysis [6].

6.2.3.3   Data Extraction Process

Extracting data is prone to error [18–20]. Box 6.3 lists the most important pitfalls. Previous reviewing experience reduces the time required to extract data, but does not necessarily improve data accuracy [21]. Therefore, at least two independent reviewers

---

Box 6.3   Common Pitfalls in Data Extraction

Data extraction is one of the most challenging parts of the systematic review process. The following list contains a selection of the most common pitfalls.

Confusing standard deviations and standard errors
- These two statistics are sometimes not explicitly labeled in reports or are misspecified by the authors. Extractors should always check whether a number is reasonable before extraction (standard errors are always smaller than the corresponding standard deviations), record it in the correct data extraction field, and add a note if the statistic had been misspecified.

Performing derivations/calculations by hand and entering these results directly in the extraction form
- Extractors should stick to the rule that extraction and calculations should always be separated. The first step is to extract all relevant data. In a second step, reviewers should do the calculations in a reproducible way using a statistical software package with statistical code that can be checked and made available to others.

Extracting data with insufficient precision
- Extractors should abstain from rounding numbers. Extracting the data as reported is generally the best approach. If only boundary numbers are reported (">X" or "<X") reviewers should document this and consider obtaining more detailed data from the authors.

Incomplete recording of data
- Reviewers should complete as much of the extraction form as possible. For example, when a report provides the mean difference, 95% confidence interval, P value, and the number of patients, then not only the mean difference and confidence interval should be extracted, but all the data to allow consistency checks.

Assuming extraction is a one-off process
- Data extraction is often an iterative process that develops throughout the review. It is frequently necessary to go over extraction forms multiple times. The process and documentation should foresee this, for example by appropriately referencing individual data items, giving detailed descriptions of decisions made, and version control of forms.

should extract data [15]. Data may also be extracted by one reviewer and checked by a second reviewer. However, this approach seems to increase the data extraction error rate [22]. In general, it is advisable to involve both content experts and methodological experts in the data extraction process [15]. Before data extraction can start, all team members should receive training on how to use the data extraction form and how to handle incomplete or missing information. Clear data extraction guidelines need to be included either in the data extraction form or – if they are extensive – an additional document.

6.2.4   Risk of Bias Assessment

Although the primary unit of analysis in a systematic review is typically the component studies, the risk of bias assessment should be directed at individual study results. As discussed in detail elsewhere (Chapter 4), specific methodological features (e.g. lack of participant blinding) may introduce bias for some outcomes (e.g. patient-reported quality of life) but not for others (e.g. all-cause mortality). The Cochrane Collaboration has developed dedicated tools for assessing risk of bias in randomized trials (RoB 2.0) [23] and in non-randomized studies of interventions (ROBINS-I) [24]. Before starting the risk of bias assessment, review authors need to decide which outcomes to focus on. It is not necessary to assess risk of bias for all reported results, but authors should aim to cover the main outcomes of their review. As for the data extraction process in general, two reviewers should independently perform the risk of bias assessment and resolve discrepancies by discussion or involvement of a third reviewer [15]. Risk of bias assessment is prone to subjectivity, and it is essential to ensure transparency and replicability. In addition to the judgment on risk of bias, supporting information to justify the judgment should be extracted, such as quotes from the source publication and their exact location in the source document, as illustrated in Table 6.1.

6.2.5   Derivation or Approximation of Data

Outcome data are not always available in the form required for meta-analysis. However, it may be possible to derive the information of interest either by simple calculation or, with some assumptions, by approximation. Reviewers should be aware of these options in order not to miss relevant information. Whenever calculations and approximations are made, they should be clearly documented. Reviewers might want to use this information at the analysis stage to test the robustness of the assumptions made through sensitivity analyses. The *Cochrane Handbook for Systematic Reviews of Interventions* provides a comprehensive overview of how to convert outcome data into the format required for meta-analysis and how to deal with missing data [15].

6.2.5.1   Continuous Outcomes

For continuous outcomes, the difference in means and the corresponding standard error are usually required for meta-analysis (see Chapters 8 and 9). If standardized mean differences are to be calculated, standard deviations are needed. Should not all required information be provided in the included studies, methods can be used to

TABLE 6.1   Example of a data extraction field for risk of bias assessment.

Study: Trial X 2019	
Allocation sequence	
Generation of allocation sequences as described by the investigator(s)	
Quote 1	"Patients were randomly assigned to . . ."
Source 1	Smith 2020: p. 123, l. 14
Quote 2	"Patients were randomly assigned using computer-generated random lists. Lists were generated . . . in Stata."
Source 2	Meyer 2019: p. 12, l. 10–11
Assessment	
Generation of allocation sequence	Computer-generated lists
Risk of bias	Low risk

derive the missing information. For example, if standard errors or confidence intervals are provided, the standard deviation can be derived. If P, *t*, or *F* values are reported, derivations of standard errors or standard deviations are also possible [25]. Methods exist to approximate means and standard deviations from reported quantiles such as the median. If only the mean difference is available, one may impute the standard deviation from other, similar studies included in the meta-analysis. This book's website (www.systematic-reviews3.org) provides a graph showing the connections between the different statistics.

6.2.5.2   Binary Outcomes

Binary outcomes are easier to handle in meta-analysis than continuous outcomes. Often the number of events of interest and the number of participants are reported, and reviewers can calculate the required effect measure. Alternatively, absolute numbers may be derived from percentages. Difficulties may arise when only an effect measure such as an odds ratio or a risk ratio (see Chapter 8) is reported, but not the number of study participants with and without the events of interest. In this case, the outcome can be included in the meta-analysis only if a measure of uncertainty is available for the effect size. Methods are available to convert or approximate effect measures [26, 27].

6.2.5.3   Time-to-Event Outcomes

Time-to-event outcomes are often meta-analyzed using the inverse-variance method with the hazard ratio as the effect measure. Hazard ratios can also be derived or approximated from available data [28]. If only Kaplan–Meier plots are available, reviewers may be able to reconstruct individual participant data from the graph and calculate the required numbers, as explained below [29].

6.2.5.4   Extracting Data from Graphs

Outcome data of interest are sometimes not reported in text or tables, but only in graphs. For example, a meta-analysis [30] that assessed the effectiveness of nonsteroidal anti-inflammatory drugs for the treatment of pain in osteoarthritis assessed pain as the primary outcome at different follow-up intervals. One of the included studies did not report standard deviations for every pain assessment. Still, a graph showing the development of mean pain over time per group with standard errors was available [31]. The graph was then used to extract the required outcome data for meta-analysis.

Extracting data from graphs is a three-step process. The reviewers need to:

1. Enlarge the graph to ease extraction.
2. Measure and record distances and lengths.
3. Transform the recorded data using the appropriate conversion factor(s).

In the past, step 1 was done using a photocopier, step 2 using a ruler, and step 3 using a hand calculator. Now, digitizing software leads to more accurate extraction [32]. There are several freely available software tools (e.g. the package metaDigitise [33] for R) that support manual and automatic digital extraction of graphical data. When vector-based graphs are available, a PostScript file can be processed, and exact data points can be extracted [34].

Box 6.4 provides a step-by-step guide for reconstructing data from Kaplan–Meier curves.

Box 6.4   Step-by-Step Guide for Reconstructing Data from Kaplan–Meier Curves in R or Stata

What is needed?
- Digitizing software (several solutions available on the internet).
- Stata or R software (with packages ipdfc [35] for Stata and survHE [36] for R).
- Kaplan–Meier graph available in Portable Document Format (*pdf*) or as an image that can be imported into the digitizing software (usually png, jpg, or gif formats).
- Number of persons at risk at the beginning of the study by group.
- Number of events per group *or* number of persons at risk at various timepoints.

Digitizing the curves
1. If needed, copy graphs from a pdf file using a snapshot tool, and save as image in a format that can be imported into the digitizing software.
2. Import the image into digitizing software.
3. View the original image (avoid automatic analysis features as they are usually not reliable enough).

4. Define axis points (see dotted dark gray arrows in Figure 6.2): maximum on the y-axis (usually at 1), origin (0/0), and maximum on the x-axis (usually maximum follow-up).

5. Define symbols and colors for each curve that you want to reconstruct. Ensure that these are easily distinguishable and clearly labeled (light gray crosses and solid/dashed line in Figure 6.2).

6. Mark the lower edge of each identifiable step of the curve using the appropriate label (see as an example the three dashed light gray arrows in Figure 6.2), or the end of the curve in case of no steps at the end.

7. Check the export settings. Ensure that raw data are exported (and not interpolated data).

8. Export and save the data.

9. Manually add a time 0 with a probability of 1 (y-axis data) to each curve data point.

10. Check whether extracted probabilities (y-axis data) decrease over time (x-axis data) and restart if they do not.

Tip: it is usually not necessary to mark every small step of the curve to obtain sufficiently reliable results. Practicing using different curves is, however, strongly recommended.

Reconstructing data

1. Import the data into R or Stata.

2. Reconstruct data by using the Stata package ipdfc [35] or the survHE package in R [36].

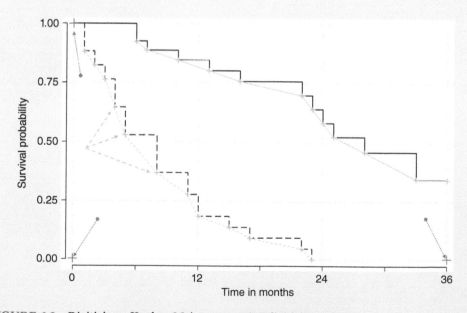

FIGURE 6.2   Digitizing a Kaplan–Meier curve using digitizing software.

3. Reanalyze reconstructed data using the method used in the original report, e.g. standard Cox model.

4. Compare results (e.g. hazard ratio, confidence interval, P value) with published information.

5. Generate Kaplan–Meier curves based on reconstructed data.

6. Save as gif file (with transparent background) or another format that allows for transparent background.

7. Overlay generated Kaplan–Meier curve with the published curve.

8. Redo until quality is sufficient.

6.3 OUTLOOK: AUTOMATION AND DATA SHARING

Automation has the potential to accelerate several steps of a systematic review and meta-analysis (see also Chapters 23 and 24) [37]. Though automation may play a minor role in more creative tasks such as the development of a research question and protocol writing, it can be especially useful for technical tasks such as reference screening, downloading full texts, and data extraction. For example, a machine learning algorithm has been developed to identify randomized controlled trials for Cochrane Reviews [38]. A long-term vision is that a protocol provides the instructions for a systematic review and meta-analysis, and machines can be taught to complete the steps it describes [37]. Indeed, substantial work has been invested in the development of automated or semi-automated tools for different steps of a systematic review. The International Collaboration for the Automation of Systematic Reviews was initiated in 2015 to coordinate the efforts of different groups [39].

Making research data publicly available improves transparency and accelerates scientific discovery [40]. This is why open data access policies are increasingly enforced by funding agencies [41] and scientific journals [42]. To date, data-sharing efforts in health care have focused on clinical trials [40], whereas sharing of data from systematic reviews and meta-analyses has received less attention [43]. However, making data from systematic reviews open access may also yield important benefits. For example, openly available data could be used to replicate or update results, address related research questions, and further develop systematic review and meta-analysis methodologies [43, 44]. Also, these datasets might be useful for training and teaching. To support data sharing of systematic review data, the Agency for Healthcare Research and Quality sponsored the development of the web-based Systematic Review Data Repository [44, 45]. In general, for shared data to be useful, they should follow the FAIR principles; that is, they should be Findable, Accessible, Interoperable, and Reusable [46]. Before sharing their data, review teams need to consider any restrictions that might apply to previously unpublished data obtained through personal communication or from clinical study reports. Thus, the intent to make data publicly available should be discussed early on with the data providers.

REFERENCES

1. Rethlefsen, M.L., Farrell, A.M., Osterhaus Trzasko, L.C., and Brigham, T.J. (2015). Librarian co-authors correlated with higher quality reported search strategies in general internal medicine systematic reviews. *J. Clin. Epidemiol.* 68: 617–626.

2. Spencer, A.J. and Eldredge, J.D. (2018). Roles for librarians in systematic reviews: a scoping review. *J. Med. Libr. Assoc.* 106: 46–56.

3. Baker, P.R.A., Francis, D.P., Hall, B.J. et al. (2010). Managing the production of a Cochrane systematic review. *J. Public Health (Bangkok)* 32: 448–450.

4. Nussbaumer-Streit, B., Ellen, M., Klerings, I. et al. (2021). Resource use during systematic review production varies widely: a scoping review. *J. Clin. Epidemiol.* 139: 287–296.

5. Moher, D. and Shamseer, L. (2015). Preferred reporting items for systematic review and meta-analysis protocols (PRISMA-P) 2015 statement. *Syst. Rev.* 4: 1.

6. Kohl, C., McIntosh, E.J., Unger, S. et al. (2018). Online tools supporting the conduct and reporting of systematic reviews and systematic maps: a case study on CADIMA and review of existing tools. *Environ. Evid.* 7: 1–17.

7. Mayo-Wilson, E., Li, T., Fusco, N., and Dickersin, K. (2018). Practical guidance for using multiple data sources in systematic reviews and meta-analyses (with examples from the MUDS study). *Res. Synth. Methods* 9: 2–12.

8. Moher, D., Liberati, A., Tetzlaff, J., and Altman, D.G. (2009). The PRISMA Group. Preferred reporting items for systematic reviews and meta-analyses: the PRISMA statement. *PLoS Med.* 6: e1000097.

9. Lorenzetti, D.L. and Ghali, W.A. (2013). Reference management software for systematic reviews and meta-analyses: an exploration of usage and usability. *BMC Med. Res. Methodol.* 13: 141.

10. Bramer, W.M., Milic, J., and Mast, F. (2017). Reviewing retrieved references for inclusion in systematic reviews using EndNote. *J. Med. Libr. Assoc.* 105: 84–87.

11. Wallace, B.C., Trikalinos, T.A., Lau, J. et al. (2010). Semi-automated screening of biomedical citations for systematic reviews. *BMC Bioinformatics* 11: 55.

12. Rathbone, J., Hoffmann, T., and Glasziou, P. (2015). Faster title and abstract screening? Evaluating Abstrackr, a semi-automated online screening program for systematic reviewers. *Syst. Rev.* 4: 1–7.

13. Brown, S.A., Upchurch, S.L., and Acton, G.J. (2003). A framework for developing a coding scheme for meta-analysis. *West. J. Nurs. Res.* 25: 205–222.

14. Brown, S.A., Martin, E.E., Garcia, T.J. et al. (2013). Managing complex research datasets using electronic tools: a meta-analysis exemplar. *Comput. Inform. Nurs.* 31: 257–265.

15. Higgins, J., Thomas, J., Chandler, J. et al. (eds.) (2019). *Cochrane Handbook for Systematic Reviews of Interventions*. Chichester: Wiley.

16. Eden, J., Levit, L., Berg, A., and Morton, S. (eds.) (2011). *Finding What Works in Health Care: Standards for Systematic Reviews*. Washington, DC: National Academies Press.

17. Elamin, M.B., Flynn, D.N., Bassler, D. et al. (2009). Choice of data extraction tools for systematic reviews depends on resources and review complexity. *J. Clin. Epidemiol.* 62: 506–510.

18. Mathes, T., Klaßen, P., and Pieper, D. (2017). Frequency of data extraction errors and methods to increase data extraction quality: a methodological review. *BMC Med. Res. Methodol.* 17: 1–8.

19. Jones, A.P., Remmington, T., Williamson, P.R. et al. (2005). High prevalence but low impact of data extraction and reporting errors were found in Cochrane systematic reviews. *J. Clin. Epidemiol.* 58: 741–742.

20. Gotzsche, P.C., Asbjorn, H., Maric, K., and Tendal, B. (2007). Data extraction errors in meta-analyses that use standardized mean differences. *JAMA* 298: 430–437.

21. Horton, J., Vandermeer, B., Hartling, L. et al. (2010). Systematic review data extraction: cross-sectional study showed that experience did not increase accuracy. *J. Clin. Epidemiol.* 63: 289–298.

22. Buscemi, N., Hartling, L., Vandermeer, B. et al. (2006). Single data extraction generated more errors than double data extraction in systematic reviews. *J. Clin. Epidemiol.* 59: 697–703.

23. Sterne, J.A.C., Savović, J., Page, M.J. et al. (2019). RoB 2: a revised tool for assessing risk of bias in randomised trials. *BMJ* 366: l4898.

24. Sterne, J.A., Hernán, M.A., Reeves, B.C. et al. (2016). ROBINS-I: a tool for assessing risk of bias in non-randomised studies of interventions. *BMJ* 355: i4919.

25. Kirkwood, B.R. and Sterne, J.A.C. (2003). *Essential Medical Statistics*, 2e. Malden, MA: Blackwell Science.

26. Wang, Z. (2013). Studies with partial data information. *J. Stat. Softw.* 55: 1–11.

27. Veroniki, A.A., Pavlides, M., Patsopoulos, N.A., and Salanti, G. (2013). Reconstructing 2×2 contingency tables from odds ratios using the Di Pietrantonj method: difficulties, constraints and impact in meta-analysis results. *Res. Synth. Methods* 4: 78–94.

28. Tierney, J.F., Stewart, L.A., Ghersi, D. et al. (2007). Practical methods for incorporating summary time-to-event data into meta-analysis. *Trials* 8: 1–16.

29. Guyot, P., Ades, A.E., MJNM, O., and Welton, N.J. (2012). Enhanced secondary analysis of survival data: reconstructing the data from published Kaplan-Meier survival curves. Additional material, R code. *BMC Med. Res. Methodol.* 12: 1–3.

30. da Costa, B.R., Reichenbach, S., Keller, N. et al. (2017). Effectiveness of non-steroidal anti-inflammatory drugs for the treatment of pain in knee and hip osteoarthritis: a network meta-analysis. *Lancet* 390: e21–e33.

31. Boswell, D.J., Ostergaard, K., Philipson, R.S. et al. (2008). Evaluation of GW406381 for treatment of osteoarthritis of the knee: two randomized, controlled studies. *Medscape J. Med.* 10: 259.

32. Jelicic Kadic, A., Vucic, K., Dosenovic, S. et al. (2016). Extracting data from figures with software was faster, with higher interrater reliability than manual extraction. *J. Clin. Epidemiol.* 74: 119–123.

33. Pick, J., Nakagawa, S., and Noble, D. (2018). metaDigitise: Extract and summarise data from published figures. R package version 1.0.0. https://CRAN.R-project.org/package=metaDigitise (accessed February 22, 2022).

34. Liu, Z., Rich, B., and Hanley, J.A. (2015). Recovering the raw data behind a non-parametric survival curve. *Syst. Rev.* 3: 1–10.

35. Wei, Y. and Royston, P. (2017). Reconstructing time-to-event data from published Kaplan-Meier curves. *Stata J.* 17: 786–802.

36. Baio, G. (2020). survHE: survival analysis for health economic evaluation and cost-effectiveness modeling. *J. Stat. Soft.* 95: 1–47.

37. Tsafnat, G., Glasziou, P., Choong, M.K. et al. (2014). Systematic review automation technologies. *Syst. Rev.* 3: 74.

38. Thomas, J., McDonald, S., Noel-Storr, A. et al. (2021). Machine learning reduced workload with minimal risk of missing studies: development and evaluation of a randomized controlled trial classifier for Cochrane Reviews. *J. Clin. Epidemiol.* 133: 140–151.

39. Beller, E., Clark, J., Tsafnat, G. et al. (2018). Making progress with the automation of systematic reviews : principles of the International Collaboration for the Automation of Systematic Reviews (ICASR). *Syst. Rev.* 7: 1–7.

40. Institute of Medicine (2015). *Sharing Clinical Trial Data*. Washington, DC: The National Academies Press.

41. Walport, M. and Brest, P. (2011). Sharing research data to improve public health. *Lancet* 377: 537–539.

42. Loder, E. and Groves, T. (2015). The BMJ requires data sharing on request for all trials. *BMJ* 350: 9–10.

43. Wolfenden, L., Grimshaw, J., Williams, C.M., and Yoong, S.L. (2016). Time to consider sharing data extracted from trials included in systematic reviews. *Syst. Rev.* 5: 4–6.

44. Ip, S., Hadar, N., Keefe, S. et al. (2012). A Web-based archive of systematic review data. *Syst. Rev.* 1: 1–7.

45. Saldanha, I.J., Smith, B.T., Ntzani, E. et al. (2019). The Systematic Review Data Repository (SRDR): descriptive characteristics of publicly available data and opportunities for research. *Syst. Rev.* 8: 334.

46. Wilkinson, M.D., Dumontier, M., Aalbersberg, I.J.J. et al. (2016). The FAIR guiding principles for scientific data management and stewardship. *Sci. Data* 3: 160018.

CHAPTER 7

Reporting and Appraisal of Systematic Reviews

Larissa Shamseer, Beverley Shea, Brian Hutton, and David Moher

Over the past few decades, systematic reviews have become increasingly central to healthcare decision-making. There has been a corresponding increase in the quantity of reviews being produced. Whereas in 2004, 7 systematic reviews were estimated to be published daily [1], at least 22 were estimated to be published per day in 2016 [2]. This increase in the use of systematic review methods has prompted evolutions in both systematic review methodology and reporting. At the time of publication of the previous edition of this book (c. 2001), guidance was available to guide the reporting of meta-analyses, but not systematic reviews [3, 4]. As systematic reviews (with or without meta-analyses) became more popular than isolated meta-analyses in health research over the past few decades, a reporting guideline specifically for the purpose of reporting of systematic reviews of intervention effectiveness was developed. In 2009, the Preferred Reporting Items for Systematic Reviews and Meta-Analyses (PRISMA) statement [5] and elaboration [6] documents to guide the reporting of systematic reviews of health interventions were first published; these were updated in 2020 [7, 8].

According to the Enhancing the Quality and Transparency Of health Research (EQUATOR) Network, a reporting guideline is a checklist, flow diagram, or explicit text to guide authors in reporting a specific type of research, developed using explicit methodology [9]. At the time of publication of this edition, PRISMA 2020 is the standard for reporting systematic reviews evaluating health care interventions [10]. Reporting guidelines, including PRISMA, extensions of PRISMA, and others mentioned in this chapter, can be found on EQUATOR Network's comprehensive library of reporting guidelines (http://www.equator-network.org/library).

Several other tools have been developed to optimize systematic review reporting. The Methodological Expectations of Cochrane Intervention Reviews (MECIR)

standards [11] and the Methodological Expectations of Campbell Collaboration Intervention Reviews (MECCIR) standards [12] were developed in 2012 and 2016, and cover reporting of Cochrane reviews and Campbell reviews, respectively. Similarly, the National Academy of Medicine (formerly the Institute of Medicine) developed standards for systematic reviews in 2011 [13]. Tools also exist to facilitate quality and methodological appraisal of systematic reviews and are discussed at the end of this chapter.

7.1   CONSEQUENCES OF POOR REPORTING

Systematic reviews are often the primary evidence used to formulate clinical practice guidelines, which are in turn relied on by clinicians, as well as other health system decision-makers and patients, to guide patient care. If they are missing essential information about what was done or what was found (for example, the details and results of outcome measurement), the assumed integrity of evidence-based health care may be compromised.

Systematic reviews can be poorly or incompletely reported in many different ways. Reviews that omit essential methodological details or leave out specific results or outcomes (or portions thereof), and systematic reviews that are never published, are especially problematic. Incompletely reported reviews impede readers' assessment of the appropriateness and trustworthiness of review methods and findings. Additionally, without essential information about review methods, interested parties are unable to replicate review methods for purposes of verification or updating. This may lead to unnecessary redundancy or overlap of reviews, resulting in wasted efforts and resources [1]. When planned outcomes, timepoints, analyses, or entire reviews are not reported or published due to the direction or significance of (summary) effect estimates, this constitutes selective reporting, biasing the evidence base toward favorable outcomes and reviews. Reporting guidelines exist and ought to be used to help ensure that the most accurate, complete, and trustworthy evidence is entering the scholarly record.

7.2   REPORTING SYSTEMATIC REVIEW PROTOCOLS

Documenting a comprehensive protocol is an essential first step in the systematic review process (see Chapter 2). The Preferred Reporting Items for Systematic Reviews and Meta-Analyses extension for protocols (PRISMA-P) provides guidance for documenting planned methods and analyses of systematic reviews in the form of a 17-item checklist [14] and an elaboration document containing explanations and examples for each checklist item [15]. A registry for systematic reviews, PROSPERO (https://www.crd.york.ac.uk/prospero), launched in 2011, provides researchers with a standardized mechanism to document systematic reviews' intentions and methods publicly before they are carried out [16]. PROSPERO has incorporated registration of Cochrane reviews and CAMARADES (Collaborative Approach to Meta-Analysis and Review of Animal Data from Experimental Studies) since November 2013 and December 2017, respectively. Using PRISMA-P to help document review protocols and registering reviews are vital steps to ensuring that review protocols are completely reported and discoverable. This is essential to facilitate the detection of selective reporting within systematic reviews, reduce unintended duplication of efforts (and potentially facilitate collaboration between review groups), and, potentially, encourage the publication of completed, high-quality reviews [2].

7.3   REPORTING SYSTEMATIC REVIEWS

Several tools exist to facilitate and optimize the reporting of completed systematic reviews of various objectives and designs. These are described in this section.

7.3.1   Reviews of Health Interventions

7.3.1.1   The PRISMA Guideline

The PRISMA 2020 guideline supersedes the original PRISMA 2009 guideline [10] as the standard guideline to facilitate optimal reporting of systematic reviews, review updates, and "living" (i.e. continually updated) systematic reviews. It is primarily intended to facilitate reporting of reviews evaluating health care interventions, irrespective of included study designs. It is also applicable to systematic reviews evaluating nonhealth interventions (e.g. behavioral or educational interventions) and those evaluating other objectives (e.g. reviews evaluating etiology, prevalence, or prognosis). It is intended for use in reviews including quantitative studies (including those where qualitative studies are also present). Comprehensive information and resources, such as non-English-language translations and new extensions/applications of PRISMA, can be found on the PRISMA website: http://prisma-statement.org. Reporting guidelines for addressing other types of reviews, including those primarily including qualitative data synthesis, also exist and are listed later in this chapter.

   PRISMA 2020 comprises two publications. The PRISMA 2020 statement presents 27 checklist items that ought to be reported in systematic reviews (PRISMA checklist, Table 7.1), an update to the PRISMA checklist for abstracts, and a flow diagram template for reporting original and updated reviews (Figure 7.1) [7]. (An expanded PRISMA 2020 checklist with additional details is also available as a data supplement in [7].) The PRISMA 2020 explanation and elaboration document contains examples and detailed guidance and evidence for each checklist item [8].

7.3.1.2   The PRISMA Checklist

The PRISMA 2020 checklist consists of a checklist of 27 items, several of which contain subitems. Each item is supported by evidence and published examples in the PRISMA explanation and elaboration document [8]. For example, checklist item 20c, one of the subitems of the "Results of Synthesis" item, recommends providing details about investigations into heterogeneity among included studies. The item, an example of how to report it, and detailed guidance including the importance of reporting it are provided in Box 7.1. Each item also elaborates on the essential elements of reporting referred to by each item, as well as any potential additional elements that it may be helpful to report.

TABLE 7.1 PRISMA 2020 Checklist.

Section and topic	Item #	Checklist item	Location where item is reported
TITLE			
Title	1	Identify the report as a systematic review.	
ABSTRACT			
Abstract	2	See the PRISMA 2020 for Abstracts checklist.	
INTRODUCTION			
Rationale	3	Describe the rationale for the review in the context of existing knowledge.	
Objectives	4	Provide an explicit statement of the objective(s) or question(s) the review addresses.	
METHODS			
Eligibility criteria	5	Specify the inclusion and exclusion criteria for the review and how studies were grouped for the syntheses.	
Information sources	6	Specify all databases, registers, websites, organizations, reference lists, and other sources searched or consulted to identify studies. Specify the date when each source was last searched or consulted.	
Search strategy	7	Present the full search strategies for all databases, registers, and websites, including any filters and limits used.	
Selection process	8	Specify the methods used to decide whether a study met the inclusion criteria of the review, including how many reviewers screened each record and each report retrieved, whether they worked independently, and if applicable, details of automation tools used in the process.	
Data collection process	9	Specify the methods used to collect data from reports, including how many reviewers collected data from each report, whether they worked independently, any processes for obtaining or confirming data from study investigators, and if applicable, details of automation tools used in the process.	
Data items	10a	List and define all outcomes for which data were sought. Specify whether all results that were compatible with each outcome domain in each study were sought (e.g. for all measures, time points, analyses), and if not, the methods used to decide which results to collect.	

TABLE 7.1 *(Continued)*

Section and topic	Item #	Checklist item	Location where item is reported
	10b	List and define all other variables for which data were sought (e.g. participant and intervention characteristics, funding sources). Describe any assumptions made about any missing or unclear information.	
Study risk of bias assessment	11	Specify the methods used to assess risk of bias in the included studies, including details of the tool(s) used, how many reviewers assessed each study and whether they worked independently, and if applicable, details of automation tools used in the process.	
Effect measures	12	Specify for each outcome the effect measure(s) (e.g. risk ratio, mean difference) used in the synthesis or presentation of results.	
Synthesis methods	13a	Describe the processes used to decide which studies were eligible for each synthesis (e.g. tabulating the study intervention characteristics and comparing against the planned groups for each synthesis [item #5]).	
	13b	Describe any methods required to prepare the data for presentation or synthesis, such as handling of missing summary statistics, or data conversions.	
	13c	Describe any methods used to tabulate or visually display results of individual studies and syntheses.	
	13d	Describe any methods used to synthesize results and provide a rationale for the choice(s). If meta-analysis was performed, describe the model(s), method(s) to identify the presence and extent of statistical heterogeneity, and software package(s) used.	
	13e	Describe any methods used to explore possible causes of heterogeneity among study results (e.g. subgroup analysis, meta-regression).	
	13f	Describe any sensitivity analyses conducted to assess robustness of the synthesized results.	
Reporting bias assessment	14	Describe any methods used to assess risk of bias due to missing results in a synthesis (arising from reporting biases).	
Certainty assessment	15	Describe any methods used to assess certainty (or confidence) in the body of evidence for an outcome.	

(Continued)

TABLE 7.1   *(Continued)*

Section and topic	Item #	Checklist item	Location where item is reported
RESULTS			
Study selection	16a	Describe the results of the search and selection process, from the number of records identified in the search to the number of studies included in the review, ideally using a flow diagram.	
	16b	Cite studies that might appear to meet the inclusion criteria, but which were excluded, and explain why they were excluded.	
Study characteristics	17	Cite each included study and present its characteristics.	
Risk of bias in studies	18	Present assessments of risk of bias for each included study.	
Results of individual studies	19	For all outcomes, present, for each study: (a) summary statistics for each group (where appropriate) and (b) an effect estimate and its precision (e.g. confidence/credible interval), ideally using structured tables or plots.	
Results of syntheses	20a	For each synthesis, briefly summarize the characteristics and risk of bias among contributing studies.	
	20b	Present results of all statistical syntheses conducted. If meta-analysis was done, present for each the summary estimate and its precision (e.g. confidence/credible interval) and measures of statistical heterogeneity. If comparing groups, describe the direction of the effect.	
	20c	Present results of all investigations of possible causes of heterogeneity among study results.	
	20d	Present results of all sensitivity analyses conducted to assess the robustness of the synthesized results.	
Reporting biases	21	Present assessments of risk of bias due to missing results (arising from reporting biases) for each synthesis assessed.	
Certainty of evidence	22	Present assessments of certainty (or confidence) in the body of evidence for each outcome assessed.	
DISCUSSION			
Discussion	23a	Provide a general interpretation of the results in the context of other evidence.	
	23b	Discuss any limitations of the evidence included in the review.	

TABLE 7.1   (*Continued*)

Section and topic	Item #	Checklist item	Location where item is reported
	23c	Discuss any limitations of the review processes used.	
	23d	Discuss implications of the results for practice, policy, and future research.	
OTHER INFORMATION			
Registration and protocol	24a	Provide registration information for the review, including register name and registration number, or state that the review was not registered.	
	24b	Indicate where the review protocol can be accessed, or state that a protocol was not prepared.	
	24c	Describe and explain any amendments to information provided at registration or in the protocol.	
Support	25	Describe sources of financial or non-financial support for the review, and the role of the funders or sponsors in the review.	
Competing interests	26	Declare any competing interests of review authors.	
Availability of data, code, and other materials	27	Report which of the following are publicly available and where they can be found: template data collection forms; data extracted from included studies; data used for all analyses; analytic code; any other materials used in the review.	

Source: From [7]. For more information, visit http://www.prisma-statement.org

7.3.1.3   The PRISMA Flow Diagram

PRISMA 2020 also encourages authors to report the flow of studies through sequential stages of the systematic review process (i.e. obtained, excluded, and included) in detail. The PRISMA 2020 flow diagram (Figure 7.1) provides a visual template for doing so. Specifically, within a review, authors are encouraged to report the number of records identified (ideally from each source/database); records remaining after removing duplicates or those deemed ineligible by machine classifiers, and the corresponding number excluded for these reasons; records for which titles and abstracts were screened, and the corresponding number excluded after this process; reports retrieved for full-text screening, and potentially eligible reports that were irretrievable; retrieved reports that did not meet inclusion criteria and the corresponding primary reasons for exclusion

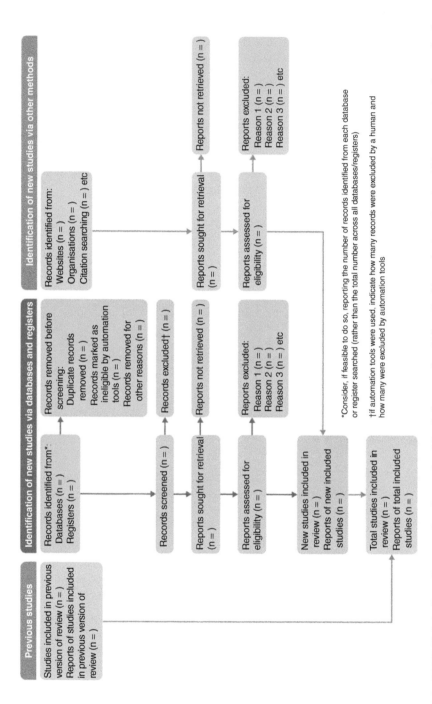

FIGURE 7.1 PRISMA 2020 flow diagram. Gray boxes should only be completed if applicable and otherwise should be removed. A "report" refers to a journal article, preprint, conference abstract, study register entry, clinical study report, dissertation, unpublished manuscript, government report, or any other document providing relevant information. *Source:* From [7].

Box 7.1   Example of a PRISMA Checklist Item

Item 20c. Results of Synthesis: Present results of all investigations of possible causes of heterogeneity among study results

Example: "Among the 4 trials that recruited critically ill patients who were and were not receiving invasive mechanical ventilation at randomization, the association between corticosteroids and lower mortality was less marked in patients receiving invasive mechanical ventilation (ratio of odds ratios (ORs), 4.34 [95% CI, 1.46-12.91]; P = 0.008 based on within-trial estimates combined across trials); however, only 401 patients (120 deaths) contributed to this comparison. . . All trials contributed data according to age group and sex. For the association between corticosteroids and mortality, the OR was 0.69 (95% CI, 0.51-0.93) among 880 patients older than 60 years, the OR was 0.67 (95% CI, 0.48-0.94) among 821 patients aged 60 years or younger (ratio of ORs, 1.02 [95% CI, 0.63-1.65], P = 0.94), the OR was 0.66 (95% CI, 0.51-0.84) among 1215 men, and the OR was 0.66 (95% CI, 0.43-0.99) among 488 women (ratio of ORs, 1.07 [95% CI, 0.58-1.98], P = 0.84)" [17].

Explanation: Presenting results from all investigations of possible causes of heterogeneity among study results is important for users of reviews and for future research. For users, understanding the factors that may, and equally may not, explain variability in the effect estimates may inform decision-making. Similarly, presenting all results is important for designing future studies. For example, the results may help to generate hypotheses about potential modifying factors that can be tested in future studies, or help identify "active" intervention ingredients that might be combined and tested in a future randomized trial. Selective reporting of the results leads to an incomplete representation of the evidence that risks misdirecting decision-making and future research.

Essential elements

- If investigations of possible causes of heterogeneity were conducted:
  - Present results regardless of the statistical significance, magnitude, or direction of effect modification.
  - Identify the studies contributing to each subgroup.
  - Report results with due consideration to the observational nature of the analysis and risk of confounding due to other factors [18, 19].
- If subgroup analysis was conducted, report for each analysis the exact P value for a test for interaction as well as, within each subgroup, the summary estimates, their precision (such as standard error or 95% confidence/credible interval), and measures of heterogeneity. Results from subgroup analyses might usefully be presented graphically (see Fisher et al. [20]).
- If meta-regression was conducted, report for each analysis the exact P value for the regression coefficient and its precision.

- If informal methods (that is, those that do not involve a formal statistical test) were used to investigate heterogeneity – which may arise particularly when the data are not amenable to meta-analysis – describe the results observed. For example, present a table that groups study results by dose or overall risk of bias and comment on any patterns observed [21].

Additional elements

- If subgroup analysis was conducted, consider presenting the estimate for the difference between subgroups and its precision.
- If meta-regression was conducted, consider presenting a meta-regression scatterplot with the study effect estimates plotted against the potential effect modifier [18].

(such as ineligible study design, ineligible population); and the number of studies and reports ultimately included in the review. Where applicable, authors are also encouraged to report the number of ongoing studies and associated reports identified. The PRISMA 2020 flow diagram provides a modifiable template depending on whether the review is an original question or represents an update of a previous review, and depending on whether sources of unindexed literature were searched. A web application to assist in generating a flow diagram can be found at https://www.eshackathon. org/software/PRISMA2020.html.

7.3.1.4 Extensions of the PRISMA Statement

PRISMA has also been modified to provide additional guidance for different scenarios, such as for different types of analyses (e.g. those including network meta-analyses), for different types of data/studies (e.g. individual participant data, diagnostic test accuracy studies), or for specific parts of the review process (e.g. search strategy). Extensions typically incorporate additional checklist items, modify existing items, or expand on certain items, as deemed important through expert consensus and informed by evidence. Each extension is typically accompanied by its own explanatory document containing examples and evidence to support each item. Extensions of PRISMA are summarized in Table 7.2.

7.3.1.5 Synthesizing Review Interventions

Recommendations exist to facilitate considerations related to synthesizing and reporting intervention details in systematic reviews [31]. Eight items are provided for consideration during the planning, conduct, and reporting stages of the review process. These considerations are meant as an aid throughout the review process, so that important and necessary intervention details that need to be reported in a review are planned for and collected/requested during the review (Box 7.2).

TABLE 7.2   Extensions of the PRISMA statement.

PRISMA extension purpose	Description of guidance
Abstracts [7]	Developed based on the premise that readers of published abstracts may never read the full text of a manuscript, instead using only the abstract to identify findings, screen for studies of specific designs, or judge a study's methods. Given the many roles of the abstract, maximizing the structure, transparency, and completeness of information shared in its contents is important. The checklist's primary focus is reviews assessing the relative benefits and harms of interventions.
Acupuncture [22]	Provides guidance for reviews evaluating acupuncture as an intervention. Reporting of such interventions has unique essential elements. This checklist introduces five new subitems and modifies six existing PRISMA items related to title, rationale, eligibility criteria, literature search, data extraction, and study characteristics.
Diagnostic test accuracy studies [23]	Provides reporting guidance for systematic reviews of diagnostic test accuracy (DTA) studies. DTA systematic reviews synthesize data from primary diagnostic studies (i.e. those evaluating the accuracy of one or more index tests against a reference standard), provide estimates of test performance, enable different tests to be compared for accuracy, and facilitate the identification of sources of variability in test accuracy. DTA systematic reviews also provide insight into the ability of medical tests to detect a target condition.
Equity [24]	Provides guidance for equity-based systematic reviews undertaken to help to address avoidable disparities in health. Additional considerations discussed include specification of equity-related questions addressed, methods undertaken specifically to work with data for disadvantaged populations, reporting relevant subgroup analyses, and focused discussion of applicability to disadvantaged populations addressed in the systematic review.
Harms [25]	Developed to facilitate the reporting of harms (or adverse events) as a primary or secondary review outcome. It contains 4 items to complement the original 27-item PRISMA checklist. All PRISMA and PRISMA harms should be reported when the synthesis of harms data is the primary focus of the review, or whether harms are synthesized together with efficacy outcomes.
Individual participant data meta-analyses [26] (see also Chapter 12)	Builds upon the PRISMA statement to address gaps in guidance as it pertains to reporting of systematic reviews that incorporate individual participant data (IPD) within randomized trials as opposed to aggregate study-level data. Considerations for novel items including how IPD data are acquired, checked, and synthesized, how studies without IPD data are managed, considerations for risk of bias appraisal, methods used for the synthesis of the included study data, and modifications to the flow diagram for study selection.

(Continued)

TABLE 7.2   (*Continued*)

PRISMA extension purpose	Description of guidance
Network meta-analysis [27](see also Chapter 13)	Provides guidance for systematic reviews involving a network meta-analysis (NMA). NMA is an extension of traditional meta-analysis allowing the comparison of multiple treatments using direct and indirect evidence (see Chapter 16). There is a need for reviews that use NMA to report details that are not standard components of traditional meta-analyses. This includes rationale for use of NMA, additional details regarding statistical methods, structuring of interventions into a treatment network, techniques to report comparisons of many interventions (and new measures such as treatment rankings), and the extent to which the assumptions of homogeneity, similarity, and consistency are met.
Protocols (PRISMA-P) [14, 15] (see also Chapter 2)	Aimed to facilitate the documentation of protocols for systematic reviews and meta-analyses, the PRISMA-P checklist provides guidance to authors on a minimum set of information that should be included in a review protocol. PRISMA-P is intended to facilitate implementation and replication of review methods, as well as comparisons between protocols and systematic reviews through more complete protocols.
Scoping reviews (PRISMA-ScR) [28]	This 20-item checklist offers guidance for reporting scoping reviews – a type of knowledge synthesis that consists of a systematic approach to map evidence on a topic and identify main concepts, theories, sources, and knowledge gaps.
Literature search [29]	This 16-item checklist (referred to as PRISMA-S) is intended to complement the PRISMA checklist and its extensions by providing general interdisciplinary guidance for ensuring that each essential component of a search is completely reported, such that it could be replicated by others.

Box 7.2   Recommendations for Authors to Improve the Consideration of Interventions When Planning, Conducting, and Reporting Systematic Reviews

Review stage		Consideration
Planning	1	Consider intervention details during question formulation
	2	Describe intervention considerations in the review protocol (following PRISMA-P [15])
Conduct	3	Extract intervention details as part of data extraction
	4	Request missing intervention details
	5	Consider intervention characteristics during statistical analyses and exploration of heterogeneity when appropriate
Reporting	6	Report intervention details in a summary table
	7	Share intervention materials where possible
	8	Describe implications for future research

Source: Adapted from [32].

7.4   REPORTING SYSTEMATIC REVIEWS WITHOUT META-ANALYSES

Meta-analysis in systematic reviews of quantitative studies is not always possible or appropriate (e.g. heterogeneous studies/study characteristics, missing outcome data). About a third of systematic reviews of interventions are estimated not to contain meta-analyses [2]. Such reviews tend to use descriptive text, often referred to as "narrative synthesis," to describe intervention effects, but appear to do so haphazardly [30]. The Synthesis Without Meta-analysis (*SWiM*) guideline, published in 2020, was developed to provide a framework for reporting these studies [21]. SWiM contains nine reporting items, accompanied by explanations and examples. It provides specific guidance for reporting how studies are grouped, synthesis method used (e.g. calculating summary statistics of intervention effect estimates, vote counting based on direction of effect, and combining P values), presentation of data and summary text, and limitations of the synthesis.

7.5   OTHER GUIDANCE FOR REPORTING SYSTEMATIC REVIEWS

7.5.1   Institute of Medicine Standards for Reporting Systematic Reviews

The National Academy of Medicine (formerly the Institute of Medicine) published 21 standards for developing high-quality comparative effectiveness systematic reviews in 2011 [13]. Three of these standards, including 11 substandards, pertain to reporting systematic reviews. These standards are extensively based on PRISMA checklist items, with some additional items to ensure that all steps and judgments required by the preceding standards are reported, and to include a focus on informing the patient and clinical decision-making. For example, a recommendation to include a plain-language summary (following guidance from Cochrane) aims to ensure that research findings are conveyed so that patients can understand and apply them to their personal circumstances.

7.5.2   MECIR and MECCIR Standards

The MECIR standards were developed by consensus within Cochrane and aim to facilitate transparent conduct and reporting of Cochrane intervention reviews. They address six key methodological areas of reviews: (i) scope and question of the review, (ii) review search, (iii) selection of studies and data, (iv) risk of bias, (v) analyzing data and meta-analyses, and (vi) interpreting and presenting results. Some recommendations are indicated as essential/mandatory (e.g. "must do"), while others are highly desirable (e.g. "should do") but not a minimum standard. Several standards relate to the reporting of reviews, including standards for the reporting of Cochrane protocols, new Cochrane reviews, as well as review updates. The Campbell Collaboration, which carries out reviews of social and behavioral interventions including those affecting health policy, adapted the MECIR guidelines to develop MECCIR standards for both conducting and reporting Campbell reviews. Review authors working with these two organizations are expected to follow their respective conduct and reporting standards.

7.6 REPORTING OTHER TYPES OF SYSTEMATIC REVIEWS

Systematic reviews exist that ask questions other than about evaluating interventions, and synthesize nonintervention or nonexperimental studies and data. Several reporting guidelines that have been developed for other review types are described here. An up-to-date listing of reporting guidelines can be found on the EQUATOR Network Library of reporting guidelines at https://www.equator-network.org/library.

7.6.1 Meta-Analyses of Observational Studies

A guideline for reporting meta-analyses of observational studies (MOOSE) was published in 2000, developed using a combination of evidence and consensus-based processes [33]. It provides 35 recommendations pertaining to the reporting of background, search strategy, methods, results, discussion, and conclusion of epidemiological reviews.

7.6.2 Reviews of Experimental Animal Studies

A guideline for reporting systematic reviews of animal experiments was published in 2006 [34]. A more recent set of recommendations for conducting, reporting, and appraising such reviews was published by the CAMARADES group in 2014 [32]. Neither guideline explicitly recommends standards for reporting the 3Rs (i.e. replacement, reduction, and refinement), a widely known set of principles for performing humane animal research [35]. Of systematic reviews of animal research published by 2010, 90% failed to report on any of the 3Rs [35].

7.6.3 Reviews of Qualitative Research

At least four reporting guidelines exist to facilitate the reporting of reviews of qualitative research/data and are listed here for further reference:

- The ENhancing Transparency in Reporting the synthesis of Qualitative research (ENTREQ) guidelines [36].
- The Meta-Ethnography Reporting Guidance (eMERGe) [37].
- Realist And Meta-narrative Evidence Syntheses: Evolving Standards (RAMESES) for realist reviews [38].
- RAMESES for meta-narrative reviews [39].

7.7   OPTIMIZING REPORTING IN PRACTICE

Ideally, authors preparing reports of their systematic reviews for publication should adhere to and report items from the relevant reporting guideline checklist and use flow diagrams to demonstrate the selection and progression of studies throughout a review. In addition, authors can and should follow reporting guidance earlier on in the research process, such as during protocol development (see Chapter 2). Doing so is likely to increase the chances of eventual publication of a systematic review and facilitate transparent reporting of methods and findings.

There is some evidence that systematic reviews published in journals that endorse PRISMA (of which there are over 300) are more completely reported overall [40], [41]. However, direct improvements in review reporting are difficult to track and some users are not using reporting guidelines in the intended manner. For example, journals recommend the use of PRISMA by review authors, but few actually require a completed checklist upon manuscript submission [42]. A systematic review evaluating the effect of reporting guideline endorsement on reporting quality found that systematic reviews were, on average, more completely reported in journals endorsing PRISMA than nonendorsers (mean difference of 0.53 (99% confidence interval [CI] 0.02, 1.03; based on three studies evaluating 143 systematic reviews) [41]. Many studies aiming to evaluate the impact of reporting guidelines, including PRISMA, fail to make meaningful comparisons or use poor study designs from which to draw conclusions about their effects (for example, between journals that endorse vs. do not endorse; in reviews published before or after endorsement in a given journal) [43].

To support authors in complying with reporting guidelines, biomedical journal editors can institute mandatory submission of guideline checklists and peer reviewers could then use them during the editorial decision-making process to make specific recommendations to authors. Widespread use of reporting tools ought to assist in the publication of completely reported systematic reviews.

7.8   APPRAISAL OF SYSTEMATIC REVIEWS

Since systematic reviews are a key tool for informing evidence-based health care, including practice guidelines, readers need to be able to gauge the validity of their findings, which largely hinges on the quality of methods used during the review process. Complete reporting can enable such assessments. Unfortunately, when the reporting of systematic reviews is poor, inadequate, or incomplete, problems with reporting have the potential to be confused with poor methods. Poor reporting of systematic reviews also often limits the strength of evidence practice guidelines can reach.

At least two tools to appraise systematic reviews exist, with slightly different aims. The Risk Of Bias In Systematic reviews (ROBIS) tool evaluates the risk of bias present in the systematic review process [44]. The AMSTAR 2 tool (see below) aims to appraise the methodological quality of systematic reviews [45]. Features of the reliability and validity of both tools are presented in Table 7.3.

TABLE 7.3   Reliability and validity of ROBIS and AMSTAR/AMSTAR 2.

	ROBIS	AMSTAR/AMSTAR 2
Purpose	To facilitate assessment of risk of bias of systematic reviews of most types of research questions, including those evaluating therapy, diagnostic accuracy, prognosis, and etiology	Intended to facilitate critical appraisal of the methodological quality of systematic reviews of health care interventions, including identifying weaknesses in the conduct of the review
Reliability	Interrater reliability (IRR) ranges across questions/domains from $\kappa = 0.03$ to $\kappa = 0.69$ (Fleiss' kappa); varies based on user experience [44]	AMSTAR: • IRR ranges across questions from $\kappa = -0.09$ to $\kappa = 0.76$ (Fleiss' kappa) [44]; $\kappa = 0.38$ to $\kappa = 1.0$ (Cohen's kappa) [44]; $\kappa = 0.41$ to $\kappa = 0.69$ (Cohen's kappa) [46] AMSTAR 2: • $\kappa = 0.32$ to $\kappa = 0.67$ (Cohen's kappa) [46]
Validity	Construct validity strongly correlated with AMSTAR (rs = 0.76, $P < 0.01$) [44]	• High intraclass correlation coefficients (ICC = 0.85, 95% CI 0.65, 0.92) [47] • Construct validity strongly correlated with ROBIS (rs = 0.76, $P < 0.01$) [44]

7.8.1   ROBIS: Risk of Bias in Systematic Reviews

ROBIS facilitates appraisal of the risk of bias related to systematic review methods and conduct [48]. It is intended to be used by experienced users such as clinical guideline developers, authors of overviews of systematic reviews, and review authors looking to assess or avoid bias in their reviews. The tool guides users through a three-phase assessment of systematic reviews [44]:

Phase 1: relevance of the patients/population, interventions, comparators, and outcomes to the review question at hand (i.e. if doing an intervention review).

Phase 2: potential sources of bias in the review, assessed in four domains of the review process: (i) study eligibility, (ii) identification and selection of studies, (iii) data collection and study appraisal, and (iv) synthesis and findings. Phase 2 consists of assessing whether features associated with lower risk of bias are present ("yes," "probably yes," "probably no," "no," and "no information," with "yes" indicating low concerns), and a rating of concern about the domain ("low," "high," or "unclear").

Phase 3: informed by whether concerns in Phase 2 were addressed in the interpretation of findings, users are asked to judge the overall risk of bias of the review.

More information on ROBIS is available at www.bristol.ac.uk/population-health-sciences/projects/robis.

7.8.2   AMSTAR: A MeaSurement Tool to Assess Systematic Reviews

A MeaSurement Tool to Assess systematic Reviews (AMSTAR) is an instrument intended to facilitate critical appraisal of the quality of systematic reviews, originally published in 2007 [49] and updated in 2017 (AMSTAR 2) [45]. AMSTAR 2 provides simple guidance for inexperienced and experienced users for rating the quality of specific methodological elements of published systematic reviews of health care interventions, including randomized controlled trials or nonrandomized studies. The tool comprises 16 items, each of which provides a short single-sentence question with additional guidance on selecting response options (expressed as "yes," "partial yes," and "no"); the resulting assessment provides a broad overall picture of review quality. One recognized limitation of assessing the methodological quality of research, including of systematic reviews, is that it is difficult to distinguish poor methods from poor reporting [50]. More information on AMSTAR is available at https://amstar.ca.

7.9   CONCLUSIONS

Various strategies and tools to improve the reporting of systematic reviews and to facilitate their appraisal exist and continue to evolve. Researchers are encouraged to become familiar with the reporting tools most appropriate to their research and to adhere to their recommendations when preparing reports of systematic review protocols and completed reports. Additionally, reviewers ought to be mindful of employing rigorous and appropriate methods and reporting that will negate any potential biases in the review process.

REFERENCES

1. Moher, D., Tetzlaff, J., Tricco, A.C. et al. (2007). Epidemiology and reporting characteristics of systematic reviews. *PLoS Med.* 4 (3): e78.
2. Page, M.J., Shamseer, L., Altman, D.G. et al. (2016). Epidemiology and reporting characteristics of systematic reviews of biomedical research: a cross-sectional study. *PLoS Med.* 13 (5): e1002028.
3. Moher, D., Cook, D.J.D., Eastwood, S. et al. (1999). Improving the quality of reports of meta-analyses of randomised controlled trials: the QUOROM statement. *Lancet* 354 (9193): 1896–1900.
4. Stroup, D.F., Berlin, J.A., Morton, S.C. et al. (2000). Meta-analysis of observational studies in epidemiology. *JAMA* 283 (15): 2008–2012.
5. Moher, D., Liberati, A., Tetzlaff, J., and Altman, D.G. (2009). Preferred reporting items for systematic reviews and meta-analyses: the PRISMA statement. *BMJ* 339: b2535.
6. Liberati, A., Altman, D.G., Tetzlaff, J. et al. (2009). The PRISMA statement for reporting systematic reviews and meta-analyses of studies that evaluate health care interventions: explanation and elaboration. *PLoS Med.* 6 (7): e1000100.
7. Page, M.J., McKenzie, J.E., Bossuyt, P.M. et al. (2021). The PRISMA 2020 statement: an updated guideline for reporting systematic reviews. *BMJ* 372: n71.

8. Page, M.J., Moher, D., Bossuyt, P.M. et al. (2021). PRISMA 2020 explanation and elaboration: updated guidance and exemplars for reporting systematic reviews. *BMJ* 372: n160.

9. Moher, D., Schulz, K.F., Simera, I., and Altman, D.G. (2010). Guidance for developers of health research reporting guidelines. *PLoS Med.* 7 (2): e1000217.

10. Moher, D., Liberati, A., Tetzlaff, J., and Altman, D.G. (2009). Preferred reporting items for systematic reviews and meta-analyses: the PRISMA statement. *PLoS Med.* 6 (7): e1000097.

11. Higgins, J., Lasserson, T., Chandler, J. et al. (2016). *Methodological Expectations of Cochrane Intervention Reviews (MECIR)*. London: Cochrane. http://community. cochrane.org/mecir-manual (accessed 21 February 2022).

12. Campbell Collaboration (2019). *Methodological Expectations of Campbell Collaboration Intervention Reviews: Reporting Standards*. Oslo: Campbell Collaboration. https://www. campbellcollaboration.org/meccir.html (accessed 21 February 2022).

13. Institute of Medicine (2011). *Finding What Works in Health Care: Standards for Systematic Reviews* (eds. J. Eden, L. Levit, A. Berg and S. Morton). Washington, DC: National Academies Press.

14. Moher, D., Shamseer, L., Clarke, M. et al. (2015). Preferred reporting items for systematic review and meta-analysis protocols (PRISMA-P) 2015 statement. *Syst. Rev.* 4 (1): 1.

15. Shamseer, L., Moher, D., Clarke, M. et al. (2015). Preferred reporting items for systematic review and meta-analysis protocols (PRISMA-P) 2015: elaboration and explanation. *BMJ* 349: g7647.

16. Booth, A., Clarke, M., Dooley, G. et al. (2012). The nuts and bolts of PROSPERO: an international prospective register of systematic reviews. *Syst. Rev.* 1 (2): 2.

17. Sterne, J.A.C., Murthy, S., Diaz, J.V. et al. (2020). Association between administration of systemic corticosteroids and mortality among critically ill patients with COVID-19: a meta-analysis. *JAMA* 324 (13): 1330–1341.

18. Thompson, S.G. and Higgins, J.P.T. (2002). How should meta-regression analyses be undertaken and interpreted? *Stat. Med.* 21 (11): 1559–1573.

19. Schandelmaier, S., Briel, M., Varadhan, R. et al. (2020). Development of the instrument to assess the credibility of effect modification analyses (ICEMAN) in randomized controlled trials and meta-analyses. *CMAJ.* 192 (32): E901–E906.

20. Fisher, D.J., Carpenter, J.R., Morris, T.P. et al. (2017). Meta-analytical methods to identify who benefits most from treatments: daft, deluded, or deft approach? *BMJ* 356: j573.

21. Campbell, M., McKenzie, J.E., Sowden, A. et al. (2020). Synthesis without meta-analysis (SWiM) in systematic reviews: reporting guideline. *BMJ* 368: l6890.

22. Wang, X., Chen, Y., Liu, Y. et al. (2019). Reporting items for systematic reviews and meta-analyses of acupuncture: the PRISMA for acupuncture checklist. *BMC Complement. Altern. Med.* 19: 208.

23. McInnes, M.D.F., Moher, D., Thombs, B.D. et al. (2018). Preferred reporting items for a systematic review and meta-analysis of diagnostic test accuracy studies. *JAMA* 319 (4): 388.

24. Welch, V., Petticrew, M., Tugwell, P. et al. (2012). PRISMA-equity 2012 extension: reporting guidelines for systematic reviews with a focus on health equity. *PLoS Med.* 9 (10): e1001333.

25. Zorzela, L., Loke, Y.K., Ioannidis, J.P. et al. (2016). PRISMA harms checklist: improving harms reporting in systematic reviews. *BMJ* 352: i157.

26. Stewart, L.A., Clarke, M., Rovers, M. et al. (2015). Preferred reporting items for a systematic review and meta-analysis of individual participant data. *JAMA* 313 (16): 1657.

27. Hutton, B., Salanti, G., Caldwell, D.M. et al. (2015). The PRISMA extension statement for reporting of systematic reviews incorporating network meta-analyses of health care interventions: checklist and explanations. *Ann. Intern. Med.* 162 (11): 777–784.

28. Tricco, A.C., Lillie, E., Zarin, W. et al. (2018). PRISMA extension for scoping reviews (PRISMA-ScR): checklist and explanation. *Ann. Intern. Med.* 169: 467–473.

29. Rethlefsen, M.L., Kirtley, S., Waffenschmidt, S. et al. (2021). PRISMA-S: an extension to the PRISMA statement for reporting literature searches in systematic reviews. *Syst. Rev.* 10 (1): 39.

30. Popay, J., Roberts, H., Sowden, A. et al. (2006). Guidance on the conduct of narrative synthesis in systematic reviews. A Product from the ESRC Methods Programme. Version 1. https://www.lancaster.ac.uk/media/lancaster-university/content-assets/documents/fhm/dhr/chir/NSsynthesisguidanceVersion1-April2006.pdf (accessed 21 February 2022).

31. Hoffmann, T.C., Oxman, A.D., Ioannidis, J.P.A. et al. (2017). Enhancing the usability of systematic reviews by improving the consideration and description of interventions. *BMJ* 358: j2998.

32. Sena, E.S., Currie, G.L., McCann, S.K. et al. (2014). Systematic reviews and meta-analysis of preclinical studies: why perform them and how to appraise them critically. *J. Cereb. Blood Flow Metab.* 34 (5): 737–742.

33. Stroup, D.F., Berlin, J.A., Morton, S.C. et al. (2000). Meta-analysis of observational studies in epidemiology: a proposal for reporting. *JAMA* 283 (15): 2008.

34. Peters, J.L., Sutton, A.J., Jones, D.R. et al. (2006 Jan). A systematic review of systematic reviews and meta-analyses of animal experiments with guidelines for reporting. *J. Environ. Sci. Health B.* 41 (7): 1245–1258.

35. Avey, M.T., Fenwick, N., and Griffin, G. (2015). The use of systematic reviews and reporting guidelines to advance the implementation of the 3Rs. *J. Am. Assoc. Lab. Anim. Sci.* 54 (2): 153–162.

36. Tong, A., Flemming, K., McInnes, E. et al. (2012). Enhancing transparency in reporting the synthesis of qualitative research: ENTREQ. *BMC Med. Res. Methodol.* 12 (1): 181.

37. France, E.F., Cunningham, M., Ring, N. et al. (2019). Improving reporting of meta-ethnography: the eMERGe reporting guidance. *BMC Med. Res. Methodol.* 19 (1): 25.

38. Wong, G., Greenhalgh, T., Westhorp, G. et al. (2013). RAMESES publication standards: realist syntheses. *BMC Med.* 11 (1): 21.

39. Wong, G., Greenhalgh, T., Westhorp, G. et al. (2013). RAMESES publication standards: meta-narrative reviews. *BMC Med.* 11 (1): 20.

40. Glasziou, P., Chalmers, I., Altman, D.G. et al. (2010). Taking healthcare interventions from trial to practice. *BMJ* 341: c3852.

41. Stevens, A., Shamseer, L., Weinstein, E. et al. (2014). Relation of completeness of reporting of health research to journals' endorsement of reporting guidelines: systematic review. *BMJ* 348: g3804.

42. Tao, K., Li, X., Zhou, Q. et al. (2011). From QUOROM to PRISMA: a survey of high-impact medical journals' instructions to authors and a review of systematic reviews in anesthesia literature. *PLoS One* 6 (11): e27611.

43. Mannocci, A., Saulle, R., Colamesta, V. et al. (2014). What is the impact of reporting guidelines on public health journals in Europe? The case of STROBE, CONSORT and PRISMA. *J. Public Health (Oxf.)* 23: fdu108.

44. Bühn, S., Mathes, T., Prengel, P. et al. (2017). The risk of bias in systematic reviews tool showed fair reliability and good construct validity. *J. Clin. Epidemiol.* 91: 121–128.

45. Shea, B.J., Reeves, B.C., Wells, G. et al. (2017). AMSTAR 2: a critical appraisal tool for systematic reviews that include randomised or non-randomised studies of healthcare interventions, or both. *BMJ* 358: j4008.

46. Gates, A., Gates, M., Duarte, G. et al. (2018). Evaluation of the reliability, usability, and applicability of AMSTAR, AMSTAR 2, and ROBIS: protocol for a descriptive analytic study. *Syst. Rev.* 7 (1): 85.

47. Shea, B.J., Hamel, C., Wells, G.A. et al. (2009). AMSTAR is a reliable and valid measurement tool to assess the methodological quality of systematic reviews. *J. Clin. Epidemiol.* 62 (10): 1013–1020.

48. Whiting, P., Savović, J., Higgins, J.P.T. et al. (2016). ROBIS: a new tool to assess risk of bias in systematic reviews was developed. *J. Clin. Epidemiol.* 69: 225–234.

49. Shea, B.J., Grimshaw, J.M., Wells, G.A. et al. (2007). Development of AMSTAR: a measurement tool to assess the methodological quality of systematic reviews. *BMC Med. Res. Methodol.* 7 (1): 10.

50. Burda, B.U., Holmer, H.K., and Norris, S.L. (2016). Limitations of A Measurement Tool to Assess Systematic Reviews (AMSTAR) and suggestions for improvement. *Syst. Rev.* 5 (1): 58.

PART II

META-ANALYSIS

CHAPTER 8

Effect Measures

Julian P.T. Higgins, Jonathan J. Deeks, and Douglas G. Altman

An early task in a meta-analysis is the selection of the summary statistic (effect measure) used to describe the observed effect in each study, from which the overall meta-analytical summary can be calculated (see Chapter 9). This chapter considers the choice of a summary statistic from randomized trials. Many of the statistics are also used for observational studies, although analyses of observational studies usually adjust for confounders (see Chapter 15) and so do not use the same computations as we describe here.

The choice of summary statistic depends on the type of outcome data being collected from individual participants. Table 8.1 lists the main types of outcome data and the main measures used to compare outcomes in two arms of a randomized trial. In the chapter, we review the computation and interpretation of these measures, consider their properties, present empirical evidence about their suitability for meta-analysis, and offer guidance on how to choose an appropriate measure for a particular meta-analysis.

8.1 INDIVIDUAL STUDY ESTIMATES OF INTERVENTION EFFECT: BINARY OUTCOMES

Binary data arise when each individual can either experience or not experience a particular outcome. We will refer to experiencing the outcome as the "event." For example, the event may be "death," or "stopped smoking," or "had at least one stroke." The most commonly encountered effect measures used in randomized trials for binary data are:

- Risk ratio (RR) (also called relative risk).
- Odds ratio (OR).

Systematic Reviews in Health Research: Meta-Analysis in Context, Third Edition. Edited by Matthias Egger, Julian P.T. Higgins, and George Davey Smith.
© 2022 John Wiley & Sons Ltd. Published 2022 by John Wiley & Sons Ltd.
Companion website: www.systematic-reviews3.org

TABLE 8.1   Types of data arising from individual participants in a randomized trial.

Data type	Examples	Effect measures commonly used in meta-analysis
Binary	Dead or alive; stop or continue smoking; at least one stroke or no stroke	Odds ratio, risk ratio, risk difference
Simple count	Number of days in hospital; number of strokes	These are often dichotomized and treated as binary data, or may be treated as continuous data
Ordinal scale (few categories)	Level of pain measured as none, mild, moderate, or severe	Odds ratio These may be dichotomized and treated as binary data, or may be treated as continuous data
Ordinal scale (many categories)	Score on Beck Depression Inventory (range 0–63 points)	These are usually treated as continuous data
Continuous	Weight in kg; serum cholesterol in mg/dL; pain measured using a visual analog scale	Mean difference, standardized mean difference, ratio of means
Count per unit time	Number of strokes within a specified length of follow-up	Rate ratio
Time to event (or time observed without experiencing the event)	Time to death (or time observed); time to first stroke (or time observed)	Hazard ratio

- Risk difference (RD) (also called absolute risk reduction, ARR).
- Number needed to treat (NNT).

See Box 8.1 for an explanation of the difference between risk and odds. As events may be desirable rather than undesirable, we would prefer a more neutral term than "risk" (such as probability), but for the sake of convention we use the term "risk" throughout.

Measures of relative effect express the risk of the outcome in one group relative to that in the other. The RR is the ratio of two risks (one for each group), whereas the OR is the ratio of two odds. Note that these relative measures (RR, OR) are sometimes expressed as the percentage reduction in risk or odds. For example, the relative risk reduction is defined as RRR = 100(1 − RR)%. While this representation can help interpretation, it does not affect the choice between different measures: meta-analysis will always be based on the original ratio measures. Summary RRs and ORs estimated from meta-analyses can be converted into relative risk and relative odds reductions in exactly the same way as for individual trials.

Box 8.1   Odds and Risks

In general conversation the phrases "odds" and "risks" are used interchangeably (together with the phrases "chances" and "likelihood"), as if they describe the same quantity. In statistics, however, odds and risks have particular meanings and are calculated in different ways. When the difference between them is ignored, the results of a systematic review may be misinterpreted.

Risk is the concept more familiar to patients and health professionals. Risk describes the probability with which a health outcome (often an adverse event) will occur within a specified period of time. In research, risk is commonly expressed as a decimal number between 0 and 1, although these are occasionally converted into percentages. It is simple to grasp the relationship between a risk and the likely occurrence of events within the time period: in a sample of 100 people the number of events observed will be the risk multiplied by 100. For example, when the risk is 0.1, 10 people out of every 100 will develop the event; when the risk is 0.5, 50 people out of every 100 will develop the event.

Odds is a concept that is more familiar to gamblers than health professionals. The odds is the probability that a particular event will occur divided by the probability that it will not occur, and can be any number from 0 to infinity. In gambling, the odds describe the ratio of the size of the potential winnings to the gambling stake; in health care it is the ratio of the number of people with the event to the number without. It is sometimes expressed as a ratio of two integers. For example, an odds of 0.01 is often written as 1 : 100, odds of 0.33 as 1 : 3, and odds of 3 as 3 : 1. Odds can be converted to risks, and risks to odds, using the formulae

$$\text{risk} = \frac{\text{odds}}{1+\text{odds}}; \text{ odds} = \frac{\text{risk}}{1-\text{risk}}.$$

The practical application of an odds is more complicated than for a risk. The best way to ensure that the interpretation is correct is to convert the odds first into a risk. For example, when the odds are 1:10, or 0.1, one person will have the event for every 10 who do not, and, using the above formula, the risk of the event is 0.1/(1+0.1) = 0.091. In a sample of 100, about 9 individuals will have the event and 91 will not. When the odds are equal to 1, one person will have the event for every one who does not, so in a sample of 100, $100 \times \dfrac{1}{(1+1)} = 50$ will have the event and 50 will not.

The difference between odds and risk is small when the risk is low, as shown in the above example. When events are common, the differences between odds and risks are large. For example, a risk of 0.5 is equivalent to an odds of 1; a risk of 0.9 is equivalent to an odds of 9. Similarly, a ratio of risks (the RR) is similar to a ratio of odds (the OR) when events are rare, but not when events are common (unless the risks in the two groups are very similar), as can be seen in Figure 8.1.

Many epidemiological studies investigate rare events, and here it is common to see the phrases and calculations for risks and odds used interchangeably. However, in randomized controlled trials, event rates are often in the range where risks and odds are very different, and RRs and ORs should not be used interchangeably.

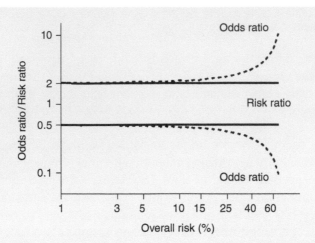

FIGURE 8.1   Risk ratios and odds ratios are similar when the overall risk is small, but get increasingly different as the overall risk increases.

The RD is the difference between the risks in the two groups. This effect measure is often the most natural statistic to use when considering clinical importance, and is often used when carrying out sample size calculations for randomized trials. The RD is sometimes called the ARR. The adjective "absolute" is used here to distinguish this measure from *relative* measures of effect, but it should be recognized that this usage is different from the mathematical usage of "absolute" to mean the size of the effect regardless of the sign. Retaining the sign of the difference is of course vital, as it distinguishes trials that are indicating a beneficial effect from those that are indicating a harmful effect.

8.1.1   Computations

The results of the trial can be presented in a 2×2 table (see Table 8.2), giving the numbers of people who do and do not experience the event in each of the two groups (here called intervention and control). The total number of individuals in the trial is $N_i = n_{1i} + n_{2i}$.

Measures of relative effect (RRs and ORs) are usually combined on the log scale. Hence we give the standard error for the log ratio measure in the following.

The **RR** for each trial is given by

$$\mathrm{RR}_i = \frac{a_i/n_{1i}}{c_i/n_{2i}},$$

the standard error of the log RR being

$$\mathrm{SE}\left[\ln\left(\mathrm{RR}_i\right)\right] = \sqrt{\frac{1}{a_i} - \frac{1}{n_{1i}} + \frac{1}{c_i} - \frac{1}{n_{2i}}},$$

where "ln" denotes logarithms to base e (natural logarithms).

TABLE 8.2 Summary information when outcome is binary.

Study i	Event	No event	Group size
Intervention	a_i	b_i	n_{1i}
Control	c_i	d_i	n_{2i}

The **OR** for each trial is given by

$$OR_i = \frac{a_i d_i}{b_i c_i},$$

the standard error of the log OR being

$$SE\left[\ln\left(OR_i\right)\right] = \sqrt{\frac{1}{a_i} + \frac{1}{b_i} + \frac{1}{c_i} + \frac{1}{d_i}}.$$

Neither the RR nor the OR can be calculated for a trial if no individuals (or all individuals) have the event in one of the groups. In this situation it is customary to add ½ to each cell of the 2×2 table (a_i, b_i, c_i, d_i in Table 8.2). In the case where no individuals have an event in either group (or all individuals have the event in both groups), the trial provides no information about an RR or an OR and should be omitted from the meta-analysis.

The **RD** for each trial is given by

$$RD_i = \frac{a_i}{n_{1i}} - \frac{c_i}{n_{2i}},$$

with standard error

$$SE\left(RD_i\right) = \sqrt{\frac{a_i b_i}{n_{1i}^3} + \frac{c_i d_i}{n_{2i}^3}}.$$

The RD can be calculated for any trial, even when there are no events in either group. The NNT is derived from the RD as

$$NNT = \frac{1}{\left|RD_i\right|}.$$

The vertical bars in the denominator here are directions to *take the absolute (positive) value*. Numbers needed to treat cannot be negative, but it is important to be aware of whether the NNT is a number needed to treat for one person to *benefit*, or a number needed to treat for one person to be *harmed*.

For the **Peto odds ratio** method [1] (see Chapter 9), the individual study ORs are given by

$$OR_i = \exp\left(\frac{a_i - E[a_i]}{v_i}\right),$$

with standard error

$$SE\left[\ln(OR_i)\right] = \sqrt{\frac{1}{v_i}},$$

where $E[a_i] = n_{1i}(a_i + c_i)/N_i$ is the expected number of events in the intervention group if there is no effect of the intervention and

$$v_i = \frac{n_{1i}n_{2i}(a_i + c_i)(b_i + d_i)}{N_i^2(N_i - 1)}$$

the (hypergeometric) variance of a_i.

8.1.2   What is the Event?

Most health care interventions are intended either to reduce the risk of occurrence of an adverse outcome or to increase the chance of a good outcome. These may be seen broadly as prevention and treatment interventions, respectively. All of the effect measures described above apply equally to both types of outcome.

In many situations it is particularly natural to talk about one of the outcome states as being an event. For example, in treatment trials participants are generally ill at the start of the trial, and the event of interest is recovery or cure. In prevention trials participants are well at the beginning of the trial and the event is the onset of disease or death. This distinction is oversimplistic, however, as trials do (and should) investigate both good and bad outcomes. For example, trials of therapy will look at both intended beneficial effects and unintended adverse effects. Because the focus is usually on the intervention group, a trial in which an intervention reduces the occurrence of an adverse outcome will have an OR and RR less than 1, and a negative RD. A trial in which an intervention increases the occurrence of a good outcome will have an OR and RR greater than 1, and a positive RD.

It is also possible to switch events and nonevents and consider instead the proportion of patients *not* recovering or *not* experiencing the event. For meta-analyses using RDs or ORs, the impact of this switch is of no great consequence: the switch simply changes the sign of an RD, while for ORs the new OR is the reciprocal ($1/x$) of the original OR. Similar considerations apply when a trial compares two active treatments, when it might not be clear which should be labeled as the "control" intervention. By contrast, switching the outcome can make a substantial difference for RRs, affecting the effect magnitude, its significance, and the observed heterogeneity across studies. In a meta-analysis, the effect of this reversal cannot be predicted mathematically. An example of the impact the switch can make is given in the case study in Box 8.2.

A simple binary outcome may hide considerable variation in the time from the start of intervention to the event, and many interventions can only aim to delay rather than prevent an event. When interest focuses on the extent to which intervention delays an event, data are best analyzed using methods for the analysis of time-to-event or survival data, the appropriate summary statistic being the hazard ratio (HR; see Section 8.3). Meta-analysis of such studies ideally is based on individual participant data (see Chapter 16), although it may be possible to extract adequate summary information from some papers. The average length of follow-up may vary across trials and could be an important source of heterogeneity in RRs or ORs. Neither the RR nor the OR will be the same as the HR.

8.2 INDIVIDUAL STUDY ESTIMATES OF INTERVENTION EFFECT: CONTINUOUS OUTCOMES

If the outcome is a continuous measure, our analysis options are most flexible if we can obtain the number of participants, the mean response, and standard deviation of responses separately for intervention and control groups (Table 8.3).

The total number of participants in the study is $N_i = n_{1i} + n_{2i}$, and

$$s_i = \sqrt{\frac{(n_{1i} - 1)s_{1i}^2 + (n_{2i} - 1)s_{2i}^2}{N_i - 2}}$$

is the pooled standard deviation of outcomes across the two groups.

The difference in mean responses can be used to compare the two groups when outcome measurements in all trials are made on the same scale. This is usually referred to as the **mean difference** (MD). For a particular study the MD is given by

$$MD_i = m_{1i} - m_{2i},$$

with standard error

$$SE(MD_i) = \sqrt{\frac{s_{1i}^2}{n_{1i}} + \frac{s_{2i}^2}{n_{2i}}}.$$

TABLE 8.3   Summary information when outcome is continuous.

Study i	Mean response	Standard deviation	Group size
Intervention	m_{1i}	s_{1i}	n_{1i}
Control	m_{2i}	s_{2i}	n_{2i}

The MD cannot be used when the trials measure the outcome in a variety of ways, for example if the trials measure depression using different psychometric scales. In this circumstance it is necessary to standardize the results of the trials to a uniform scale before they can be combined.

The **standardized mean difference** (SMD) expresses the difference in mean responses relative to the variability observed in that trial. The method assumes that the differences in standard deviations between trials reflect differences in measurement scales and not real differences in variability between trial populations. This assumption may be problematic in some circumstances, for example where pragmatic and explanatory trials are combined in the same review. For instance, a pragmatic trial with wide patient eligibility criteria might have a large standard deviation, whereas an explanatory trial with narrow patient eligibility criteria might have a small standard deviation. The difference in standard deviations then reflects the different purposes of the trials rather than the use of different measurement scales. The intervention effect can also be difficult to interpret when expressed as an SMD, since it is reported in units of standard deviation rather than in units of any of the measurement scales used in the review.

There are three popular formulations of effect size used in the SMD method. These formulations differ with respect to the standard deviation used in calculations and whether or not a correction for small-sample bias is included. In statistics, small-sample bias arises if there is a difference between the expected value of an estimate given a small sample and the expected value if the sample is very large. Simulations show that the SMD tends to be overestimated with finite samples, although the bias is substantial only if the total sample size is very small (less than 10) [2].

Cohen's d [3] is given by

$$d_i = \frac{m_{1i} - m_{2i}}{s_i},$$

with standard error

$$SE(d_i) = \sqrt{\frac{N_i}{n_{1i}n_{2i}} + \frac{d_i^2}{2(N_i - 2)}}.$$

Hedges' adjusted g [3] is very similar to Cohen's d, but includes an adjustment to correct for the small-sample bias mentioned earlier. It is defined as

$$g_i = \frac{m_{1i} - m_{2i}}{s_i}\left(1 - \frac{3}{4N_i - 9}\right),$$

with approximate standard error

$$SE(g_i) = \sqrt{\frac{N_i}{n_{1i}n_{2i}} + \frac{g_i^2}{2(N_i - 3.94)}}.$$

Finally, **Glass's Δ** [4] takes the standard deviation from the control group as the scaling factor, giving

$$\Delta_i = \frac{m_{1i} - m_{2i}}{s_{2i}},$$

with standard error

$$\text{SE}\left(\Delta_i\right) = \sqrt{\frac{N_i}{n_{1i} n_{2i}} + \frac{\Delta_i^2}{2\left(n_{2i} - 1\right)}}.$$

This method is preferable when the intervention alters the observed variability as well as potentially changing the mean value.

Both the MD and SMD methods assume that the outcome measurements within each trial have a normal distribution. When these distributions are skewed or severely non-normal, the results of these methods may be misleading.

An alternative to both the MD and the SMD is the **ratio of means** (RoM). There are two variants of this. The **ratio of arithmetic means** [5] for each study is given by

$$\text{RoM}_i = \frac{m_{1i}}{m_{2i}},$$

the standard error of the log ratio of arithmetic means being

$$\text{SE}\left[\ln\left(\text{RoM}_i\right)\right] = \sqrt{\frac{s_{1i}^2}{m_{1i}^2 n_{1i}} + \frac{s_{2i}^2}{m_{2i}^2 n_{2i}}}.$$

Alternatively, the **ratio of geometric means** [6] is given by applying the formulae for the MD to the log-transformed data, and exponentiating the result (that is, computing e^{MD}, where MD is computed from means on the log scale). The ratio of geometric means and its confidence interval may be reported directly, especially if the distribution of responses across individuals is skewed. The ratio of geometric means can also be estimated from the data in Table 8.3, with assumptions about the nature of the skewed distribution [6].

8.3 INDIVIDUAL STUDY ESTIMATES OF INTERVENTION EFFECT: TIME-TO-EVENT OUTCOMES

The effect measure most commonly used for time-to-event data is the hazard ratio. The hazard (or hazard rate) is a measure of instantaneous risk. Expressing an intervention effect as an HR involves an assumption that the ratio of hazards is constant over the time period of interest. This assumption is known as the proportional hazards assumption and underlies the most common methods for analyzing time-to-event data, in particular Cox regression (otherwise known as proportional hazards regression). HRs are typically extracted directly from reports of randomized trials rather than computed by reviewers. Often they will be presented as results of a Cox regression analysis. However, several methods are available for approximating the HR, based on other statistics and graphs that might be presented, including Kaplan–Meier curves (which illustrate the survival times of patients in each group of the trial). See Parmar et al., Williamson et al., and Guyot et al. for helpful texts [7–9].

8.4   INDIVIDUAL STUDY ESTIMATES OF INTERVENTION EFFECT: RATES

When the results of a study are reported as a count of events across participants within an intervention group, along with the total amount of follow-up time over which these participants were observed (as in Table 8.4), the two groups may be compared in terms of the *rate* of events. The rate is the number of events divided by the total amount of person-time, and is expressed in relation to the units of observation time. For example, if 80 patients are each followed up for one year and 15 events are observed, the rate is 15 per 80 years of observation time, or 0.19 per person-year. Note that we do not draw a distinction between two participants each having one event and one participant having two events and the other participant having none. Thus, the number of events may exceed the number of individuals, a situation that is not possible with binary data.

The **rate ratio** (RaR) [10] for each study is given by

$$RaR_i = \frac{e_{1i}/t_{1i}}{e_{2i}/t_{2i}},$$

the standard error of the log rate ratio being

$$SE\left[\ln\left(RaR_i\right)\right] = \sqrt{\frac{1}{e_{1i}} + \frac{1}{e_{2i}}}.$$

Note that the number of participants does not feature in the computations. Note also that the choice of time unit (i.e. patient-months, women-years, etc.) is not important, since it is canceled out of the rate ratio and does not feature in the standard error. An adjustment of 0.5 may be added to each count in the case of zero events. Alternative methods of estimating a rate ratio are available, including Poisson regression [11, 12].

The **rate difference** (RaD) [13] for each study is given by

$$RaD_i = \frac{e_{1i}}{t_{1i}} - \frac{e_{2i}}{t_{2i}},$$

TABLE 8.4   Summary information for computing rates.

Study i	Events	Person-time	Group size
Intervention	e_{1i}	t_{1i}	n_{1i}
Control	e_{2i}	t_{2i}	n_{2i}

with standard error

$$\mathrm{SE}\left(\mathrm{RaD}_i\right) = \sqrt{\frac{e_{1i}}{t_{1i}^2} + \frac{e_{2i}}{t_{2i}^2}}.$$

In a randomized trial, rate ratios will often be very similar to RRs obtained after dichotomizing the outcome (for example, into those who did and did not experience at least one event), since the average period of follow-up should be similar in both intervention groups. Rate ratios and RRs will differ, however, if an intervention affects the likelihood of some participants experiencing multiple events.

8.5   INDIVIDUAL STUDY ESTIMATES OF INTERVENTION EFFECT: ORDINAL OUTCOMES

Ordinal outcomes are outcomes that fall into one of several ordered categories. For example, a headache may be categorized as absent, mild, moderate, or severe in intensity. A simple strategy for analyzing ordinal data is to reduce the data to dichotomous data by grouping categories. When there are numerous categories, it is common to assign numeric values to each category and compute means and standard deviations of the scores, analyzing the data as if they were continuous data.

When there is a small number of categories, analyses retaining the ordinal nature of the outcome may give rise to ORs. These are based on models that make particular assumptions about how risks of being in different categories are distributed across the categories and the intervention groups. One popular model is the proportional odds model, which assumes that the intervention effect can be represented by a single OR, where this OR relates to any dichotomization of the outcome into a higher versus a lower category. The ORs are either extracted from trial reports or need to be computed by analyzing the complete dataset. Models and methods are described in detail by Whitehead and Jones [14].

8.6   CRITERIA FOR SELECTION OF A SUMMARY STATISTIC

What are the desirable attributes of a summary statistic (or effect measure) to be used in a meta-analysis? Here we summarize three key criteria to help decide on a suitable statistic to summarize results of a randomized trial.

- **Consistency**: First, we would like the estimated statistic to be applicable across the situations where the trial results will be used. To have this property, estimates of the intervention effect have to be as stable as possible over the various populations from which the trials have been drawn, and to which the intervention will be applied. The more nearly constant the statistic is, the greater the justification for expressing the effect of the intervention as a single summary number [15].
- **Mathematical properties**: Second, the summary statistic must have the mathematical properties required for performing a valid meta-analysis. One of

the most important of these is the availability of a reliable variance estimate. The NNT, for example, does not have a reliable variance estimator and is therefore not a suitable statistic to use in meta-analysis.

- **Ease of interpretation**: Third, a summary statistic should lead to presentation of a summary of the effect of the intervention in a way that helps readers to interpret and apply the results appropriately. "The essence of a good data analysis is the effective communication of clinically relevant findings" [16], so the ability of general readers of a review to understand and make logical decisions based on the reported summary statistic must not be overlooked.

We elaborate on each of these criteria in the three sections that follow. We discuss each with particular reference to the choice of statistic for binary outcome data, where a choice can be particularly difficult to make.

8.6.1   Consistency of Effects Across Studies

A meta-analysis is most useful when the results of the studies are consistent from one to the next. However, a set of trials will often display greater heterogeneity than is expected by chance alone, indicating that a single summary statistic may be an inadequate summary of the intervention effect. Choosing an appropriate summary statistic cannot guarantee consistency of results across studies, but it can sometimes help. Note that we can investigate whether particular study characteristics explain some of the variation either using meta-regression or stratified meta-analysis (see Chapter 10).

In any meta-analysis of binary outcome data, it is likely that there is variation in the underlying risk of the event observed in the control groups across the trials. When this is the case, the RD, RR, and OR cannot all be equally consistent summaries of the trial results. Table 8.5 shows the results of four hypothetical trials, all of which have different control group risks. Trials 2–4 have, respectively, the same OR, the same RR, and the same RD as Trial 1. However, it is clear that when two trials have the same value for one of the measures, they differ on the other two measures. The only situation where this relationship does not hold is when there is no intervention effect. The heterogeneity observed between the trials may thus in part be an artefact of a poor choice of summary statistic, and be reduced or even disappear when an alternative summary statistic is used.

TABLE 8.5   Results of four hypothetical trials with varying control group risks.

Trial	Relation to Trial 1	Intervention group				
		Treatment	Control	OR	RR	RD
1	–	24/100	16/100	**0.60**	**0.67**	**0.08**
2	Same OR	32/100	22/100	**0.60**	0.69	0.10
3	Same RR	42/100	28/100	0.54	**0.67**	0.14
4	Same RD	42/100	34/100	0.71	0.81	**0.08**

8.6.1.1 The L'Abbé Plot

The most common graphical display associated with a meta-analysis is the forest plot (Chapter 2). This plot has a limited ability to help with the question of whether an effect measure is an appropriate summary. A more useful graph here is the L'Abbé plot, in which summary data from the two intervention groups are plotted against each other [17]. Examples are shown in the case studies later in this chapter. The L'Abbé plot is a helpful adjunct to a "standard" meta-analysis. It has several useful features, including the explicit display of the range of variation in responses or response rates in intervention and control groups [18].

The particular value of the L'Abbé plot in deciding on a summary statistic is that it is simple to superimpose contours of constant intervention effect according to each possible measure [19, 20]. The L'Abbé plot for a given set of trials may thus shed light on whether a chosen effect measure is likely to be a good overall summary for a meta-analysis, as illustrated in the case studies in Boxes 8.2 and 8.3.

L'Abbé plots to illustrate contours for RD, RR, and OR are shown in Figure 8.2. The solid lines indicate interventions where the risk is reduced (or the alternative outcome

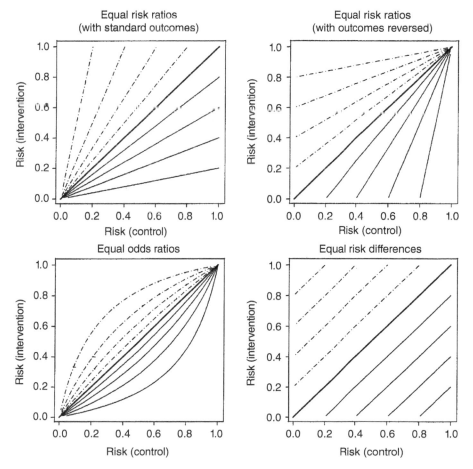

FIGURE 8.2 L'Abbé plots demonstrating constant odds ratios, risk differences, and risk ratios for standard and reversed outcomes.

is increased). The dashed lines indicate interventions where the risk is increased (or the alternative outcome is decreased). In each case, the further the lines are from the diagonal line of no effect, the stronger is the intervention effect. Lines are drawn for RRs and ORs of 0.2, 0.4, 0.6, 0.8, 1, 1.25, 1.67, 2.5 and 5, and for RDs of −0.8 to +0.8 in steps of 0.2. The bold solid line marks the line of no intervention effect (RR = 1, OR = 1, RD = 0).

8.6.1.2   Empirical Evidence of Consistency

A L'Abbé plot is not the only way to assess the consistency of results with the overall summary statistic: it is routine in meta-analysis to evaluate the consistency of results with the summary estimate using tests of homogeneity (see Chapter 7). Rather than visually investigating the appropriateness of different summary statistics, it is possible to undertake the meta-analysis using different measures of intervention effect, and to choose the one that gives the lowest heterogeneity statistic. However, there are problems in this procedure, as the decision is data derived and usually based on very few data points (and thus vulnerable to the play of chance).

An influential empirical investigation assessed the consistency of various different summary statistics across a large sample of meta-analyses [20]. One analysis considered 551 meta-analyses of binary outcomes published from the Cochrane Library. Meta-analyses were performed using RD, RR, and OR methods (described in Chapter 9) on each dataset. The consistency of the results for each meta-analysis was measured using the standard heterogeneity statistic, computing a weighted sum of the squares of the differences between the trial estimates and the overall estimate. The three summary statistics for each analysis were then compared.

Plots of the heterogeneity statistics for comparisons of RR with OR and of RR with RD are given in Figure 8.3. We see from the first plot that there is little difference on average between heterogeneity for ORs and RRs analyses, while from the second plot it is clear that RDs tend to have higher heterogeneity than RRs (more points are below the diagonal line than above it). Even for meta-analyses with high risks in the control group, there was little difference in median heterogeneity scores for the two measures of relative effect [20].

It therefore appears that the RD is likely to be the poorest summary in terms of consistency, while there is little difference between ORs and RRs. However, the findings do not necessarily mean that the RD should never be used. As Figure 8.3 shows, there are meta-analyses that demonstrate less heterogeneity with the RD than the RR. An example of a situation where the RD is the most consistent summary statistic is given in the case study in Box 8.3.

Note that the heterogeneity statistics in the analyses are computed using the standard methods, which use different weights for RR, OR, and RD analyses, although all are considered to approximate to a χ^2 distribution with $k - 1$ degrees of freedom, where k is the number of studies contributing to the meta-analysis.

Similar studies have been performed based on the I^2 statistic rather than the heterogeneity test statistic. These two heterogeneity statistics are equivalent when they are computed from the same meta-analysis, in which case one is a simple transformation of the other. Rhodes et al. examined both binary data and continuous data [21]. Their

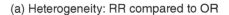

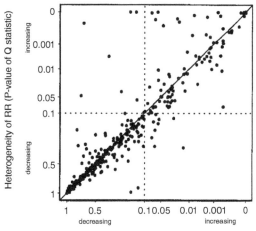

(a) Heterogeneity: RR compared to OR

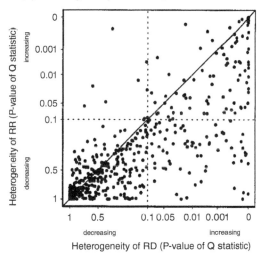

(b) Heterogeneity: RR compared to OR

FIGURE 8.3 Comparison of heterogeneity of the same 551 meta-analyses using risk difference, risk ratio, and odds ratio summary statistics. (a) Heterogeneity: RR compared to OR. (b) Heterogeneity: RR compared to RD.

results are given in Table 8.6; these are summaries of distributions fitted to 3873 meta-analyses of binary outcomes and 5132 meta-analyses of continuous outcomes. Findings for binary data mirror those found by Deeks et al. [20], in that RDs were observed to be less similar across studies than RRs or ORs. For continuous data, no substantial difference was observed between consistency of MDs and consistency of SMDs. These analyses for continuous data were restricted to meta-analyses in which the authors considered the studies to be measuring responses using similar scales, so that use of the MD was appropriate.

TABLE 8.6   Distribution of I^2 statistics for different outcome measures.

Data type	Summary statistic	Median for I^2	Inter-quartile range for I^2
Binary outcome data	Risk ratio	22%	12 to 39%
	Odds ratio	21%	9 to 39%
	Risk difference	41%	24 to 61%
Continuous outcome data	Mean difference	46%	18 to 77%
	Standardized mean difference	40%	15 to 73%

8.6.2   Mathematical Properties

It is important that the chosen summary statistic has the mathematical properties required for performing a valid meta-analysis. A standard meta-analysis is performed as a weighted average of summary statistics across studies, using inverse variances as weights. We therefore need to be able to compute a variance for each study, and we further require that the variance provides an adequate summary of the uncertainty in the summary statistic from each study. The standard meta-analysis method requires that the sampling error in the summary statistic is approximately normally distributed with mean zero. Fulfilling this requirement is the main reason why meta-analyses of relative measures such as the RR and OR are undertaken on the log scale (i.e. they are fundamentally meta-analyses of log RRs and log ORs).

There are mathematical considerations in the choice between summary statistics for binary outcome data. The OR has several mathematical properties that may be advantageous for use as a summary statistic in a meta-analysis. We have already mentioned that the behavior of OR methods does not rely on which of the two outcome states is coded as the event. The OR is also the measure obtained from Peto's approach to the meta-analysis of randomized trials.

The OR has the further advantage over the RR of being "unbounded": this means that it can take values anywhere from 0 to infinity regardless of the underlying risk of the event. On the logarithmic scale, the OR is unbounded in both directions. In contrast, the value of the observed RR is constrained to lie between 0 and $100/p_2$, where p_2 is the risk in the control group. This means that for common events, large values of RR are impossible. For example, when the risk in the control group is 66%, then the observed RR cannot exceed 1.5. This problem only applies for increases in risks, and could be circumvented by considering all trials – whether treatment or prevention – as designed to reduce the risk of a bad outcome. In other words, instead of considering the increase in risk of success, we could consider the decrease in risk of failure.

The RD is also naturally constrained, which may create difficulties when applying results to other patient groups and settings. For example, if a trial or meta-analysis estimates an RD of −10%, then for a group with an initial risk of less than 10% the outcome will have an impossible negative probability. Similar scenarios for increases in risk occur at the other end of the scale. Such problems may arise when the results are applied to patients who have different risks from those of participants in the trial (or meta-analysis).

The NNT does not have a reliable variance estimator and is therefore not a suitable statistic to use in meta-analysis. In most situations the NNT is best obtained by computing an overall RR or OR and applying this to a typical risk of the event without intervention.

For continuous outcomes, all effect measures described here have valid variance estimates. Ratios of means suffer from the same type of constraint as RRs if the measurement scale has a strict upper (or lower) limit. Particular care is needed to avoid using ratio measures when the mean response in either group can be negative.

8.6.3   Issues in Interpretation of Effect Measures

While it is important that results of meta-analyses can be expressed in ways that are readily interpretable, it is not necessary that the summary statistic selected for the meta-analysis is itself easily interpretable. Nevertheless, the better the statistical methods are understood by the reader, the more likely the reader is to understand the results and potentially therefore to accept them.

Among summary statistics for binary outcome data, interpretation of an RR is not difficult, as it describes the multiplication of the risk that occurs with use of the intervention. For example, an RR of 3 implies that the risk with intervention is three times higher than the risk without intervention (or alternatively that intervention increases the risk by $100 \times (RR - 1)\% = 200\%$). Similarly, an RR of 0.25 is interpreted as the risk associated with intervention being one-quarter of that without intervention (or alternatively that intervention decreases risk by $100 \times (RR - 1)\% = 75\%$). Again, the interpretation of the clinical importance of a given RR cannot be made without knowledge of the typical risk in the control group: an RR of 0.75 could correspond to a clinically important reduction in events from 80% to 60%, or a small, less clinically important reduction from 4% to 3%.

ORs, like odds, are more difficult to interpret [22, 23]. ORs describe the multiplication of the odds of the outcome that occur with use of the intervention. To understand what an OR means in terms of changes in numbers of events, it is best to convert it first into an RR in the context of a typical control group risk, as outlined above. Formulae for converting an OR to an RR, and vice versa, are:

$$RR = \frac{OR}{1 - p_2(1 - OR)}; \quad OR = \frac{RR(1 - p_2)}{1 - p_2 RR},$$

where p_2 is the typical control group risk (see the case study in Box 8.2 for an example of the interpretation of an OR).

The nonequivalence of the RR and OR does not indicate that either is wrong; both are entirely valid. Problems may arise, however, if the OR is interpreted directly as an RR [24, 25]. For interventions that increase risk of an event, the OR will be larger than the RR, so the misinterpretation will tend to overestimate the intervention effect, especially when events are common (with, say, risks more than 30%). For interventions that reduce risk, the OR will be smaller than the RR, so that again it overestimates the effect of intervention. This error in interpretation is quite common in published reports of systematic reviews.

The RD is straightforward to interpret. It describes the actual difference in the risk that was observed with intervention; for an individual it describes the estimated change in the probability of experiencing the event. However, the clinical importance of an RD may depend on the underlying risk. For example, an RD of 2% may represent a small, clinically insignificant change from a risk of 58% to 60%, but a proportionally much larger and potentially important change from 1% to 3%. Although there are some grounds to claim that the RD provides more complete information than relative measures [26], it is still important to be aware of the underlying risks and consequences of the events when interpreting an RD.

An RR of 2 will have a much bigger impact on absolute risk if the underlying risk is high than if the underlying risk is small. Several studies have examined whether different ways of expressing numeric results of clinical trial results (such as choice of summary statistics) may influence perceptions about the worth of an intervention. Systematic reviews of the published literature on the effects of information "framing" on the practices of physicians [27] and the preferences of patients [28] have found that expressing intervention effects in terms of an RR (or relative risk reduction) was more likely to elicit use of the intervention than expression of the same results in terms of RDs or numbers needed to treat. These studies cannot assess whether switching summary statistics leads to clinical decisions being more or less rational, only that different decisions are made when the same findings are presented in different ways.

Among summary statistics for continuous outcome data, the SMD is particularly challenging to interpret. It expresses the difference in mean response between the two groups in terms of how many standard deviations apart they are. These standard deviations describe between-participant variability in individual responses. Rules of thumb have been proposed for interpreting SMDs. One particular schema is to interpret 0.2 as representing a small effect, 0.5 a medium effect, and 0.8 a large effect [29]. Variations exist (for example, <0.40 = small, 0.40–0.70 = moderate, >0.70 = large). However, such rules of thumb are not universally applicable. An alternative is to convert the SMD into an unstandardized MD on a particular well-known scale. This requires a typical standard deviation for that scale, which might be obtained from the trials in the meta-analysis or from an external source (such as a large cohort study). The conversion is straightforward: $MD_s = s_s \times SMD$, where MD_s represents the MD on the chosen scale s, and s_s, is a typical standard deviation for responses on that scale. MDs are much easier to interpret. Interpretation is enhanced when there is a good understanding of how large a difference on the scale can be considered to be clinically important.

8.7   CASE STUDIES

Many of the issues mentioned in the preceding sections are illustrated by two case studies: Box 8.2 shows results from a meta-analysis of eradication of *Helicobacter pylori* in non-ulcer dyspepsia, and Box 8.3 shows results from a meta-analysis of trials of vaccines to prevent influenza.

Box 8.2   Case Study: Eradication of *Helicobacter Pylori* in Non-Ulcer Dyspepsia

H. pylori is a bacterium that inhabits the stomach and has been linked to the development of peptic ulcer; eradication of the bacterium with antibiotics is an effective cure for most ulcer disease. *H. pylori* is also considered to have a possible causal role in the development of non-ulcer dyspepsia. A meta-analysis of the five relevant trials reported a small reduction in dyspepsia rates 12 months after eradication, which was just statistically significant [30]. The effect measure used in the published analysis was the RR for remaining dyspeptic 12 months after eradication. This was chosen as it was thought to be the most clinically relevant outcome and had been pre-stated in the review protocol. No alternative effect measures were considered.

Eight alternative meta-analyses are presented in Table 8.7. Results are shown using fixed-effect and random-effects analyses for ORs, RDs, and the two RRs of dyspepsia recovery and remaining dyspeptic. (Estimates of the ORs and RDs of remaining dyspeptic rather than of dyspepsia cure can be determined from the cure results by taking reciprocals and by multiplying by −1, respectively, as explained earlier in the chapter.) In the following we discuss the interpretation of these results, considering random-effects analyses.

The tests of homogeneity clearly indicate that the authors' chosen effect measure, the RR of remaining dyspeptic, is the most consistent estimator across all the trials, with heterogeneity being indicated for the three alternative summary statistics. In fact, the strength of conclusion from the overall estimate crucially depends on this choice of summary statistic: the random-effects analyses for ORs, RDs, and the RR for cure are all not statistically significant at the $P = 0.05$ level. Inspection of the L'Abbé plot in Figure 8.4 also suggests that the pattern of the trial estimates is consistent with the RR for the reversed outcome of remaining dyspeptic, although this is somewhat hard to discern with so few data points. Selection of the RR of remaining dyspeptic on the basis of minimal heterogeneity and maximum statistical significance would be a data-driven decision. Where the interpretation of the analysis so critically depends on the choice of effect measure, it is essential for the effect measure to be pre-stated before the analysis (as was the case in this review), the selection being based on clinical and scientific argument.

TABLE 8.7 Alternative analyses of eradication trials for non-ulcer dyspepsia.

Measure	Effect	95% CI	Test of homogeneity
Odds ratio of cure			
Fixed-effect model	1.31	1.03 to 1.68	Q = 10.8, df = 4, P = 0.03
Random-effects model	1.38	0.90 to 2.11	
Risk difference for cure			
Fixed-effect model	0.05	0.01 to 0.09	Q = 8.3, df = 4, P = 0.08
Random-effects model	0.06	−0.01 to 0.12	
Risk ratio for cure			
Fixed-effect model	1.21	1.02 to 1.43	Q = 12.7, df = 4, P = 0.01
Random-effects model	1.28	0.92 to 1.77	
Risk ratio for remaining dyspeptic			
Fixed-effect model	0.93	0.88 to 0.99	Q = 6.4, df = 4, P = 0.18
Random-effects model	0.92	0.85 to 0.99	

It is also of interest to consider the consistency (or otherwise) of the estimates of treatment benefit across the different analyses. The choice of effect measure can lead to different predictions of benefit. The RR for cure of 1.28 can be interpreted as the chances of recovery increasing by 28% (around one-quarter) with treatment, or that recovery is 1.28 times more likely with treatment. This effect may be important if symptomatic recovery commonly occurs without treatment, but not if it is rare. It is necessary to obtain an estimate of this typical recovery rate, p_2, to gauge the likely impact of the effect in terms of numbers of patients recovering. In the review there was considerable variation of baseline recovery rates between 10% and 50%, as shown in the L'Abbé plot in Figure 8.4. Consider a scenario where the spontaneous recovery rate is 10%: for every 100 people receiving eradication therapy, $100 \times (0.1 \times 1.28) = 13$ will not have dyspeptic symptoms later this year, 10 of whom would have recovered without treatment and 3 due to treatment.

Alternatively, the RD analysis estimated an absolute increase in recovery rates of 0.06, or 6%. This can be interpreted as showing that the chance of recovery increases by 6 percentage points regardless of baseline recovery rates. Thus, for every 100 people treated, 6 will recover as a result of treatment, regardless of how many recover anyway.

The estimate of the OR of 1.38 is interpreted as showing that eradication treatment increases the odds of cure by 38%, or that the odds are 1.4 times higher. To understand the effect that this OR describes, it is necessary first to convert it into an RR. Taking the same spontaneous recovery rate of 10%, the equivalent RR is 1.33, which leads to an estimate of 3 additional people being cured for every 100 treated.

The fourth option differs, in that the event being described is *remaining dyspeptic*. The estimate suggests that the risk of dyspepsia with treatment will be 92% of

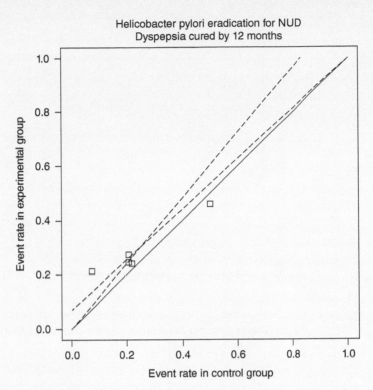

FIGURE 8.4 L'Abbé plot of the results of the five trials of *H. pylori* eradication therapy in the treatment of non-ulcer dyspepsia. The dashed line ascending from point (0,0) corresponds to an RR for dyspepsia cured at 12 months of 1.21 (Mantel–Haenszel fixed-effect estimate; test for heterogeneity: Q = 12.7, df = 4, P = 0.01). The dashed line descending from point (1,1) corresponds to an RR for remaining dyspeptic at 12 months of 0.93 (Mantel–Haenszel fixed-effect estimate; test for heterogeneity: Q = 6.4, df = 4, P = 0.18).

the risk without treatment, or that the risk has decreased by 8%. In terms of numbers of people remaining dyspeptic, this should be considered in the context of the reversed event risk. We estimate the proportion remaining dyspeptic at 12 months to be 0.9 to fit in with the previous scenario. Using this value, for every 100 people receiving eradication therapy, 100 × (0.9 × 0.92) = 83 will still be dyspeptic at the end of follow-up, 7 fewer than would be the case without treatment.

The choice of summary statistic therefore also makes a difference to the estimated benefit of treatment in a particular scenario, the number of people benefiting from treatment varying between 3 and 7 per 100 depending on the chosen summary statistic. These discrepancies are less for projections at typical event risks close to the mean of those observed in the trials. The pattern of predictions of absolute benefit according to placebo response rates for the four effect measures are shown in Figure 8.5.

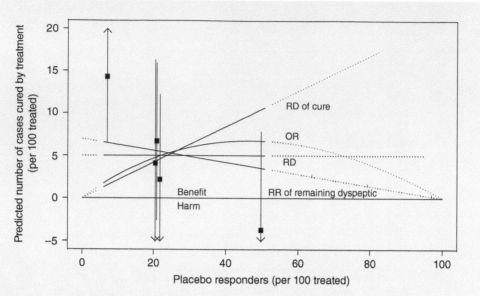

FIGURE 8.5   Predictions of treatment benefit at 6–12 months using *H. pylori* eradication therapy in non-ulcer dyspepsia. Solid lines indicate predictions within the range of the trial data, dotted lines indicate predictions beyond the observed range. The black boxes and vertical lines indicate the point estimates and confidence intervals of the five trials.

Box 8.3   Case Study: Prevention of Influenza Through Vaccination

Only a small proportion of cases of clinical influenza are caused by the influenza A virus, the target of most vaccines that protect against influenza. This means that in clinical trials of influenza vaccines, a large proportion of the cases of clinical influenza would not be prevented even by a totally efficacious vaccine. Also, the proportion of clinical influenza cases unrelated to influenza A fluctuates between trials according to seasonal and geographic variations in other viral infections that cause "flu-like illnesses."

In a systematic review of the efficacy of influenza vaccines [31], it was argued that, in this situation, the RD is the most appropriate summary statistic if the proportion of participants acquiring influenza A cases is more stable than the proportion acquiring other influenza-like viruses across the trials. Inspection of a L'Abbé plot (Figure 8.6) and heterogeneity statistics (Table 8.8) indicates that this is the case. However, strong evidence of heterogeneity is present whichever summary statistic is used. This may in part be explained by the test of homogeneity being powerful enough to detect small variations in intervention effects in reviews with large samples (more than 30 000 participants were included in this review). It may also be explained through variation in the formulation of the vaccine used in the different trials, and to changes in circulating influenza A viral subtypes.

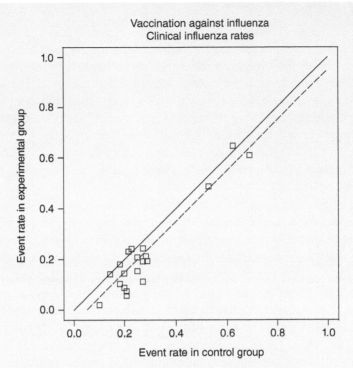

FIGURE 8.6   L'Abbé plot of the results of 20 trials of influenza vaccination in healthy adults. The dashed line indicates the summary RD of −5.1%.

TABLE 8.8   Alternative analyses of influenza vaccination trials.

Measure	Effect	95% CI	Test of homogeneity
Odds ratio for clinical illness			
Random-effects model	0.66	0.53 to 0.81	Q = 84.75, df = 19, P < 0.001
Risk difference for clinical illness			
Random-effects model	−0.051	−0.078 to −0.023	Q = 57.86, df = 19, P < 0.001
Risk ratio for clinical illness			
Random-effects model	0.75	0.65 to 0.86	Q = 86.98, df = 19, P < 0.001

For this situation it does not make clinical sense to reverse the outcome and consider the RR for remaining free of clinical influenza. Such a model would predict the largest absolute benefit of vaccination in a population where risk of influenza-like illness is very low, and no benefit in a population where risk is very high (see the patterns of RRs in Figure 8.6).

8.8   DISCUSSION

The choice of effect measure for a meta-analysis depends first on the type of data, and in particular whether the outcomes measured on individual participants are binary, continuous, time-to-event, ordinal, categorical, or something else. For some types of data, a systematic reviewer has the opportunity to select which measure will be used to compare outcomes between two intervention groups. For binary outcome data, an RR, OR, or RD can be chosen; for continuous outcome data, an MD, an SMD, or an RoM can be chosen. In this chapter we have considered three criteria on which the selection of a measure might be based: consistency across studies, mathematical behavior, and ease of comprehension.

The three effect measures for binary outcome are equally valid measures of the intervention effect for a randomized controlled trial, but each has strengths and limitations. No single measure is uniformly best, so the choice inevitably involves a compromise. The OR has the strongest mathematical properties, but is the hardest to comprehend and to apply in practice. There are many published examples where ORs from meta-analyses have been misinterpreted by authors as if they were RRs [24, 32]. Indeed, Schwartz et al. observed that "odds ratios are bound to be interpreted as risk ratios" [33]. There must always be some concern that routine presentation of the results of systematic reviews as ORs will lead to frequent overestimation of the benefits and harms of interventions when the results are applied in clinical practice.

While there are strong advocates of the OR [34, 35], some statisticians and epidemiologists have argued that the OR is often not the most suitable choice of summary statistic for summarizing the results of randomized trials and systematic reviews [22]. Presentation of RDs or RRs appears on the surface to be more likely to be correctly interpreted than one based on ORs. The RD is the easiest measure to understand, but is the measure least likely to be consistent across a set of trials. Its use is problematic when it is applied to real patients with widely ranging expected risks, because intervention benefit often depends on underlying risk. The RR has some undesirable mathematical properties, but these are a problem only in situations where underlying risks are very high and RRs are much greater than 1. In many situations, the RR may be a reasonable choice as it is relatively easy to comprehend, and our empirical study shows that it is as likely to be as consistent across trials as an OR. However, two opposing RRs are available for any analysis according to whether we focus on the event or the nonevent, and selecting the "wrong" one can dramatically alter the results of the systematic review, as shown in the case study in Box 8.2.

Selection of summary statistics for continuous data is principally determined by whether trials all report the outcome using the same scale. If this is not the case, use of an MD method would be erroneous. However, the SMD method can be used for either circumstance. Differences in results between these two methods can reflect differences in both the intervention effects calculated for each study and the study weights. Interpretation of a weighted MD is easier than that of an SMD, as it is expressed in natural units of measurement rather than standard deviations.

A commonly recommended approach is to use one statistic to analyze the data and to present the results using another. The choice of statistic for analysis might be based on considerations of mathematics and consistency, while an easily interpreted statistic could be used for presentation. This approach might, for example, indicate the use of the OR for analysis, with results converted to an RR or a NNT for presentation (see Box 8.4); or the use of an SMD for analysis, with results converted to an unstandardized MD for presentation (see Section 8.6.3). A difficulty here is that conversions require assumptions about additional quantities (the control group risk in the case of ORs, and the standard deviation on the selected presentation scale for SMDs). These quantities may vary greatly according to the situation to which the results are to be applied. For conversion of ORs, an average value for the control group risk is often estimated from the control groups of the clinical trials, but as trials are rarely designed to provide a valid estimate of this value, this estimate may be inappropriate when applying the results of the review. A better approach might be to choose these external values based on studies other than clinical trials, or on clinical experience.

The impact of the choice of summary statistic can also be considered in sensitivity analyses. Clearly, we would hope that the interpretation of the results would be consistent irrespective of the summary statistic, indicating that the broad qualitative conclusions of the review do not depend on the use of a particular effect measure. However, we have seen that this will not always be the case (see Box 8.2). In some situations,

Box 8.4 Computing Absolute Risks and Number Needed to Treat From A Meta-Analysis

Here we show how to estimate both an absolute risk associated with intervention and the NNT from estimates of RR or OR as summaries of treatment effect from a meta-analysis. The formulae apply similarly to an individual clinical trial. The computations require a typical risk of the event without intervention (or with the control intervention), p_2. This underlying risk might be obtained from the control group of a highly relevant clinical trial or perhaps from a cohort study.

The absolute risk of the event for an individual given the intervention, p_1, can be computed directly from summary ORs or RR according to the following formulae:

$$p_1 = \frac{p_2 \times \mathrm{OR}}{\left(1 - p_2 + p_2 \times \mathrm{OR}\right)}; \quad p_1 = p_2 \times \mathrm{RR},$$

where p_2 is the typical risk of the event without treatment.

The NNT is estimated from a summary RD simply as $\mathrm{NNT} = 1/\mathrm{RD}$. NNT can be computed directly from a summary OR or RR according to the following formulae:

$$\mathrm{NNT} = \frac{1 - p_c\left(1 - \mathrm{OR}\right)}{p_c\left(1 - p_c\right)\left(1 - \mathrm{OR}\right)}; \quad \mathrm{NNT} = \frac{1}{p_c\left(1 - \mathrm{RR}\right)}.$$

As the typical risk increases, the NNT based on a summary RR will decrease. The NNT based on a summary OR, however, will decrease as the risk increases to 50%, and increases thereafter. This pattern for the OR echoes the symmetry in the weights given to the trials in the meta-analysis.

changing the effect measure can have a large effect on the interpretation of the results, especially where the size as well as the direction of the effect are critical.

A priori specification of the effect measure on clinical or scientific grounds undoubtedly seems preferable to a post hoc selection based on comparisons of analyses. But how could such an a priori selection be determined? The choice of a summary statistic can often be viewed as a choice between different mathematical models of the relationship between control group responses and treatment group responses. The underlying patterns for these models are shown in the L'Abbé plots in Figure 8.2 (which show contours of constant effect for each measure) or more clearly in the plot of treatment benefit against control group risks in Box 8.4 (which shows predictions of actual benefit of treatment for the results of the first case study). Significant variation in control group responses between trials must reflect variation in participant characteristics, control group interventions, outcome measures, study quality, or variation in length of follow-up (for example, event risk usually increases with time). If the causes of variation in control group responses between the trials can be identified, and if the shape of the relationship between these and intervention benefit can be hypothesized, it may be possible to choose the summary statistic that most closely fits the predicted patterns of these relationships.

REFERENCES

1. Yusuf, S., Peto, R., Lewis, J. et al. (1985). Beta blockade during and after myocardial infarction: an overview of the randomised trials. *Prog. Cardiovasc. Dis* 27: 335–371.
2. Hedges, L.V. and Olkin, I. (1985). *Statistical Methods for Meta-Analysis*. London: Academic Press.
3. Rosenthal, R. (1994). Parametric measures of effect size. In: *The Handbook of Research Synthesis* (eds. H. Cooper and L.V. Hedges), 231–244. New York: Russell Sage Foundation.
4. Glass, G.V. (1976). Primary, secondary and meta-analysis of research. *Educ. Res.* 5: 3–8.
5. Friedrich, J.O., Adhikari, N.K., and Beyene, J. (2008). The ratio of means method as an alternative to mean differences for analyzing continuous outcome variables in meta-analysis: a simulation study. *BMC Med. Res. Methodol.* 8: 32.
6. Higgins, J.P.T., White, I.R., and Anzures-Cabrera, J. (2008). Meta-analysis of skewed data: combining results reported on log-transformed or raw scales. *Stat. Med.* 27 (29): 6072–6092.
7. Parmar, M.K.B., Torri, V., and Stewart, L. (1998). Extracting summary statistics to perform meta-analyses of the published literature for survival endpoints. *Stat. Med.* 17: 2815–2834.
8. Williamson, P.R., Tudor Smith, C., Hutton, J.L., and Marson, A.G. (2002). Aggregate data meta-analysis with time-to-event outcomes. *Stat. Med.* 21: 3337–3351.
9. Guyot, P., Ades, A.E., Ouwens, M.J., and Welton, N.J. (2012). Enhanced secondary analysis of survival data: reconstructing the data from published Kaplan-Meier survival curves. *BMC Med. Res. Methodol.* 12: 9.
10. Rothman, K.J. and Greenland, S. (1998). *Modern Epidemiology*, 2e. Philadelphia, PA: Lippincott Williams & Wilkins.

11. Spittal, M.J., Pirkis, J., and Gurrin, L.C. (2015). Meta-analysis of incidence rate data in the presence of zero events. *BMC Med. Res. Methodol.* 15: 42.

12. Herbison, P., Robertson, M.C., and McKenzie, J.E. (2015). Do alternative methods for analysing count data produce similar estimates? Implications for meta-analyses. *Syst. Rev.* 4 (1): 163.

13. Hasselblad, V.I.C. and McCrory, D.C. (1995). Meta-analytic tools for medical decision making: a practical guide. *Med. Decis. Making.* 15: 81–96.

14. Whitehead, A. and Jones, N.M.B. (1994). A meta-analysis of clinical trials involving different classifications of response into ordered categories. *Stat. Med.* 13: 2503–2515.

15. Breslow, N.E. and Day, N.E. (1980). Combination of results from a series of 2 x 2 tables; control of confounding. In: *Statistical Methods in Cancer Research, Volume 1: The Analysis of Case-Control Data* (eds. N.E. Breslow and N.E. Day) (IARC Scientific Publications No 32), 136–146. Lyon: International Agency for Health Research on Cancer.

16. Pocock, S.J. (1983). *Clinical Trials: A Practical Approach.* Chichester: Wiley.

17. L'Abbe, K.A., Detsky, A.S., and O'Rourke, K. (1987). Meta-analysis in clinical research. *Ann. Intern. Med.* 107: 224–233.

18. Song, F. (1999). Exploring heterogeneity in meta-analysis: is the L'Abbe plot useful? *J. Clin. Epidemiol.* 52 (8): 725–730.

19. Jimenez, F.J., Guallar, E., and Martinmoreno, J.M. (1997). A graphical display useful for meta-analysis. *Eur. J. Public Health.* 7: 101–105.

20. Deeks, J.J. (2002). Issues in the selection of a summary statistic for meta-analysis of clinical trials with binary outcomes. *Stat. Med.* 21 (11): 1575–1600.

21. Rhodes, K.M., Turner, R.M., and Higgins, J.P.T. (2015). Empirical evidence about inconsistency among studies in a pair-wise meta-analysis. *Res. Synth. Methods* 7 (4): 346–370.

22. Sinclair, J.C. and Bracken, M.B. (1994). Clinically useful measures of effect in binary analyses of randomized trials. *J. Clin. Epidemiol.* 47: 881–889.

23. Sackett, D.L., Deeks, J.J., and Altman, D.G. (1996). Down with odds ratios! *Evid. Based Med.* 1 (6): 164–166.

24. Deeks, J. (1998). When can odds ratios mislead? Odds ratios should be used only in case-control studies and logistic regression analyses. *BMJ.* 317 (7166): 1155–1156. author reply 6-7.

25. Knol, M.J., Duijnhoven, R.G., Grobbee, D.E. et al. (2011). Potential misinterpretation of treatment effects due to use of odds ratios and logistic regression in randomized controlled trials. *PLoS One* 6 (6): e21248.

26. Laupacis, A., Sackett, D.L., and Roberts, R.S. (1988). An assessment of clinically useful measures of the consequences of treatment. *New Engl. J. Med.* 318: 1728–1733.

27. McGettigan, P., Sly, K., O'Connell, D. et al. (1999). The effects of information framing on the practices of physicians. *J. Gen. Intern. Med.* 14 (10): 633–642.

28. Moxey, A., O'Connell, D., McGettigan, P., and Henry, D. (2003). Describing treatment effects to patients. *J. Gen. Intern. Med.* 18 (11): 948–959.

29. Cohen, J. (1988). *Statistical Power Analysis for the Behavioral Sciences*, 2e. Mahwah, NJ: Erlbaum.

30. Moayyedi, P., Soo, S., Deeks, J. et al. (2000). Systematic review and economic evaluation of Helicobacter pylori eradication treatment for non-ulcer dyspepsia. Dyspepsia review group. *BMJ.* 321 (7262): 659–664.

31. Demicheli, V., Rivetti, D., Deeks, J.J., and Jefferson, T.O. (2000). Vaccines for preventing influenza in healthy adults. *Cochrane Database Syst. Rev.* **2**: CD001269. https://doi.org/10.1002/14651858.CD001269.

32. Altman, D.G., Deeks, J.J., and Sackett, D.L. (1998). Odds ratios should be avoided when events are common. *BMJ* 317 (7168): 1318.

33. Schwartz, L.M., Woloshin, S., and Welch, H.G. (1999). Misunderstandings about the effects of race and sex on physicians' referrals for cardiac catheterization. *N. Engl. J. Med.* 341 (4): 279–283. discussion 286-7.

34. Senn, S. and Walter, S. (1998). Odds ratios revisited. *Evid. Based Med.* 3: 71.

35. Cook, T.D. (2002). Up with odds ratios! A case for odds ratios when outcomes are common. *Acad. Emerg. Med.* 9 (12): 1430–1434.

CHAPTER 9

Combining Results Using Meta-Analysis

Jonathan J. Deeks, Richard D. Riley, and Julian P.T. Higgins

In this chapter we consider the general principles of meta-analysis, and introduce the most commonly used methods for performing meta-analysis. We shall focus on meta-analysis of randomized trials evaluating the effects of an intervention, but much the same principles apply to other comparative studies, notably case–control and cohort studies evaluating risk factors. An important first step in a systematic review of controlled trials is the thoughtful consideration of whether it is appropriate to combine all (or perhaps some) of the trials in a meta-analysis, to yield an overall statistic (together with its confidence interval) that summarizes the effect of the intervention of interest. Decisions regarding the "combinability" of results should largely be driven by consideration of the similarity of the trials (in terms of participants, experimental and comparator interventions, and outcomes), but statistical investigation of the degree of variation between individual trial results, which is known as heterogeneity, can also contribute.

9.1 META-ANALYSIS

9.1.1 General Principles

Meta-analysis usually involves a two-stage process. In the first stage a summary statistic is calculated for each trial to be included in the meta-analysis. The summary statistics describe the observed intervention effect, and are usually risk ratios, odds ratios or risk differences for binary outcome data, differences in means or standardized differences in means for continuous outcome data, or hazard ratios for survival (time-to-event) data. In the second stage, the overall estimate of the intervention effect is calculated as a weighted average of these

Systematic Reviews in Health Research: Meta-Analysis in Context, Third Edition. Edited by Matthias Egger, Julian P.T. Higgins, and George Davey Smith.
© 2022 John Wiley & Sons Ltd. Published 2022 by John Wiley & Sons Ltd.
Companion website: www.systematic-reviews3.org

summary statistics. The weights are trial specific, and are chosen to reflect the amount of information that each trial contains. In practice the weight for a trial is often the inverse of the variance (the square of the standard error) of the trial's summary statistic, which relates closely to sample size (and number of events for binary or time-to-event data). The precision (confidence interval) and statistical strength of evidence (e.g. P value) for an overall estimate are also calculated. The most commonly used methods of meta-analysis follow these basic principles. There are, however, some other aspects that vary between alternative methods, as described in this chapter.

In a meta-analysis we do not combine the data from all of the trials as if they were from a single large trial. Such an approach is inappropriate for several reasons and can give misleading results, especially when the number of participants in each group is not balanced within trials [1].

9.1.2   Heterogeneity

An important component of systematic reviews is to investigate the consistency of the intervention effects across the individual trials. As trials will not have been conducted according to a common protocol, there will usually be some variation between the trials in trial characteristics, such as the participants, clinical settings, concomitant care, methods of delivery of the intervention, and measurement of outcomes. While some divergence of trial results from the overall estimate is always expected purely by chance, the effectiveness of an intervention may also vary according to trial characteristics. Such variation in effectiveness is known as heterogeneity, and it will increase the variability of the observed trial results. Consistency of trial results across a variety of circumstances provides important and powerful corroboration of the generalization of the effect of the intervention, so that a greater degree of certainty can be placed on its application to wider clinical practice.

The possibility of excess variability (heterogeneity) between the results of the different trials may be examined by a statistical test of homogeneity (often described as a test for heterogeneity). If the test result yields a small P value, the between-trial variability is more than expected by chance alone, and it can be concluded that the intervention has a variable effect. However, if the test of homogeneity is inconclusive (the P value is large), the possibility of a Type II (false-negative) error must always be considered, because the test has low power to detect excess variation, especially when there are not many trials. Partly because the test has limited usefulness in this situation, it is preferable to focus on the magnitude of heterogeneity (often denoted by τ^2, also known as the between-trial variance), which if greater than zero suggests there is between-trial variability in the size of the effect. This variation can be incorporated into the analysis using a random-effects model (see below). One may additionally consider the magnitude of heterogeneity *relative* to the variability of trial results themselves, for example using the I^2 statistic, to determine the potential impact of heterogeneity on the meta-analysis. Fuller details on these methods are given later in the chapter.

Where the amount of heterogeneity is deemed considerable, the meta-analyst ought to consider an investigation of reasons for the differences between trial results (see Chapter 10), and if the differences cannot be explained, may even consider not undertaking a meta-analysis at all. Meta-analysis of the studies in subgroups and statistical methods of meta-regression (see Chapter 10) can be used to examine potential associations between trial characteristics and the estimated intervention effect.

9.1.3   Summary Statistics for Intervention Effects

A meta-analysis of randomized trials is performed for a specific summary statistic. For example, if the outcome for each individual within each trial is binary, then the standard options for a summary statistic are the odds ratio, the risk ratio, and the risk difference. If the outcome is continuous, then the usual choices are the difference in mean response (often called the mean difference) and the standardized difference in mean response (often called the standardized mean difference or SMD, and known in some fields as the "effect size"). For time-to-event data, the hazard ratio is the usual measure for comparing survival between the two intervention groups. These summary statistics are described in more detail in Chapter 8. In most circumstances we combine log-transformed values of ratio measures (odds ratios, risk ratios, and hazard ratios), because the sampling distribution for these measures is symmetric only on the log scale. Heterogeneity may be larger for one summary statistic than for another. For instance, if odds ratios are similar across trials but baseline risks differ substantially, then risk differences would be expected to very markedly across trials, producing greater heterogeneity than on the odds ratio scale (see Chapter 8).

9.2   FORMULAE FOR DERIVING A SUMMARY ESTIMATE OF THE INTERVENTION EFFECT BY COMBINING TRIAL RESULTS (META-ANALYSIS)

We first describe a general class of meta-analysis methods that combine individual trial summary statistics. Each summary statistic is an estimate of the intervention effect for a particular metric, such as a standardized mean difference. We denote the summary statistic generically by $\hat{\theta}_i$, with each given a weight w_i that is related to $SE\left(\hat{\theta}_i\right)$, where SE denotes the standard error. All the methods described are available in the Stata, R, or Comprehensive Meta-Analysis routines described in Chapters 25–27.

9.2.1   Fixed-Effect and Random-Effects Methods

One approach to meta-analysis is to assume that there is a single true intervention effect common to all trials; in other words, the intervention effect is **fixed** at the same value for each trial. The differences between trial results are therefore due solely to the play of chance, which relates to the sample size of each trial. This approach has often been described as a **fixed-effect meta-analysis**. although some refer to it (perhaps more appropriately) as a common-effect or equal-effects meta-analysis. The estimate from a fixed-effect meta-analysis provides the best estimate of this single intervention effect.

In a **random-effects meta-analysis** the intervention effects for the individual trials are assumed to vary around some average value. The summary estimate from the meta-analysis provides the best estimate of this average intervention effect. Usually the intervention effects in the different trials are assumed to have a normal distribution with between-trial variance τ^2. In essence, the test of homogeneity tests whether τ^2 is zero. The smaller the value of τ^2, the more similar are the fixed-effect and random-effects analyses in terms of the summary intervention effect and its interpretation.

Peto describes his method for obtaining a summary odds ratio (described below) as assumption free [2], arguing that it does not assume that all the trials are estimating the same intervention effect. Although alternative interpretations of the fixed-effect meta-analysis result are available [3], in the current chapter we adopt the conventional assumption that, in a fixed-effect meta-analysis, the same intervention effect is assumed for every trial. We also interpret the Peto method in the same way.

There has been historical debate over when to use fixed-effect or random-effects models. Many recommend using random-effects models when heterogeneity is expected. Given that random-effects estimates and fixed-effect estimates are usually very similar when there is little or no heterogeneity, they consider it reasonable to use random-effects models in most circumstances so that any heterogeneity is incorporated into the analysis if it is present. However, random-effects models have limitations when data and events are sparse, when fixed-effect models may be preferred, and may be very misleading if trial findings are related to their sample sizes (sometimes described as the presence of "small-study effects"), as discussed later.

9.2.2 Fixed-Effect Meta-Analysis using the Inverse-Variance Method

Inverse-variance methods may be used to combine summary statistics for binary, continuous, time-to-event, and other types of outcome data. In the general formula below, the estimated summary statistic, denoted by $\hat{\theta}_i$, could for example be the log odds ratio, log risk ratio, log hazard ratio, risk difference, difference in means, or standardized difference in means from the ith trial.

The summary statistics are combined to give an overall summary estimate by calculating a **weighted average** of the estimates from the individual trials:

$$\hat{\theta}_{IV} = \frac{\sum w_i \hat{\theta}_i}{\sum w_i}.$$

The summation notation indicates summation across the i trials included in the analysis. In a fixed-effect meta-analysis, the weights (w_i) are the reciprocal of the variances (or squared standard errors):

$$w_i = \frac{1}{\left[SE\left(\hat{\theta}_i\right) \right]^2}.$$

Thus larger trials, which have smaller standard errors, are given more weight than smaller trials, which have larger standard errors. This choice of weight minimizes the uncertainty in the summary estimate, $\hat{\theta}_{IV}$. For binary outcome data, where one or more cells in the 2×2 table is zero, both the summary statistic $\hat{\theta}_i$ and its standard error $SE\left(\hat{\theta}_i\right)$ may be undefined due to divide-by-zero errors. Where this occurs a small quantity, typically 0.5, is added to each cell in the 2×2 table before the computations are undertaken, though other options are available [4].

The standard error of $\hat{\theta}_{IV}$ is given by

$$SE\left(\hat{\theta}_{IV}\right) = \frac{1}{\sqrt{\sum w_i}}.$$

The heterogeneity test statistic is given by [5]

$$Q = \sum w_i \left(\hat{\theta}_i - \hat{\theta}_{IV}\right)^2.$$

For a formal test of homogeneity, the statistic Q will follow approximately a χ^2 distribution on $k-1$ degrees of freedom, under the null hypothesis that the true intervention effect is the same for all trials. However, as previously mentioned, it is better to focus on the absolute magnitude of heterogeneity (τ^2, see below) and its magnitude relative to the variation within each trial (the $SE\left(\hat{\theta}_i\right)$). The latter can be summarized by the I^2 statistic, which is given by

$$I^2 = 100\% \times \frac{\left(Q - \left(k-1\right)\right)}{Q},$$

where k is the number of trials in the meta-analysis [6, 7]. I^2 measures the percentage of variability in intervention effect estimates that is due to between-trial heterogeneity rather than chance. A common mistake is to interpret I^2 as a measure of the (absolute) amount of heterogeneity. The value of I^2 should not be used on its own to decide between a fixed-effect or random-effects meta-analysis [8]; it simply quantifies the potential *impact* of heterogeneity on the summary estimate. If I^2 is close to 0% then the impact of heterogeneity is small, whereas an I^2 closer to 100% indicates it may be substantial.

The strength of the inverse-variance approach is its wide applicability. It can be used to combine any type of estimate where standard errors are available. Thus it also can be used for estimates of a wide variety of measures, including standardized mortality ratios, risk and prognostic factor effects, and prevalence; and from many types of study, including crossover trials, cluster-randomized trials, and observational studies. It is also possible to use this method when arm-specific summary data (such as 2×2 tables for binary outcomes) cannot be obtained for each study, but intervention effects and confidence intervals are available, such as when intervention effects have been adjusted for design or prognostic variables.

When applying the inverse-variance method to meta-analyses of binary outcomes, it is important to remember that different choices of summary statistic will affect the relative weights that are assigned to different trials. For a trial with a given sample size, it will be given the highest weight in a meta-analysis if using the risk ratio scale when the absolute risks of the event in the two groups are both high (near 100%), and the lowest weight when they are both low (near 0). In a meta-analysis of odds ratios, the trial will be given the highest weight when both absolute risks are near to 50%. For a meta-analysis of risk differences, the pattern is the opposite to that for odds ratios: the trial will have the highest weight when the absolute risks are both low (near 0%) or high (near 100%) [9].

9.2.3 Mantel–Haenszel Methods for Binary Outcomes

When binary outcome data are sparse, both in terms of event risks being low and trials being small, the estimates of the standard errors of the intervention effects that are used in the inverse-variance methods may be poor. Mantel–Haenszel methods are an alternative weighting scheme for conducting a fixed-effect meta-analysis for binary outcome data, which have been shown to be more robust when data are sparse and may therefore be preferable to the inverse-variance method in that situation. In other situations they give similar estimates to the inverse-variance method. They are available only for binary outcomes.

For each trial, the summary statistic from each trial $\hat{\theta}_i$ is given weight w_i in the analysis, where w_i is defined below. The summary estimate of effect, $\hat{\theta}_{MH}$, is given by

$$\hat{\theta}_{MH} = \frac{\Sigma w_i \hat{\theta}_i}{\Sigma w_i}.$$

Unlike with inverse-variance methods, relative effect measures are combined on their natural scale, although their standard errors (and confidence intervals) are still computed on the log scale.

We will use the same notation for the data as in Chapter 8, summarized in Table 9.1. This gives the numbers of people who do or do not experience the event in each of the two groups (here called intervention and control).

For combining **odds ratios**, each trial's OR is given weight [10, 11]

$$w_i = \frac{b_i c_i}{N_i}.$$

Thus the summary estimate can be expressed as

$$\hat{\theta}_{MH} = OR_{MH} = \frac{\Sigma \left(a_i d_i / N_i \right)}{\Sigma \left(b_i c_i / N_i \right)}.$$

This illustrates that adjustments for zero events are not required to compute the summary Mantel–Haenszel estimate, although in practice several software routines have introduced them to ensure that the odds ratio, $\hat{\theta}_i$, is defined for each trial (including **metan** in Stata, and Review Manager).

The logarithm of OR_{MH} has standard error given by [12]

$$SE\left[\ln\left(OR_{MH} \right) \right] = \sqrt{\frac{1}{2}\left(\frac{E}{R^2} + \frac{F+G}{R \times S} + \frac{H}{S^2} \right)},$$

TABLE 9.1 Summary information when outcome is binary.

Trial i	Event	No event	Group size
Intervention	a_i	b_i	n_{1i}
Control	c_i	d_i	n_{2i}
Total			N_i

where

$$R = \sum \frac{a_i d_i}{N_i}; \quad S = \sum \frac{b_i c_i}{N_i};$$

$$E = \sum \frac{(a_i + d_i) a_i d_i}{N_i^2}; \quad F = \sum \frac{(a_i + d_i) b_i c_i}{N_i^2};$$

$$G = \sum \frac{(b_i + c_i) a_i d_i}{N_i^2}; \quad H = \sum \frac{(b_i + c_i) b_i c_i}{N_i^2}.$$

For combining **risk ratios**, each trial's RR is given weight [13]

$$w_i = \frac{c_i n_{1i}}{N_i},$$

and the logarithm of RR_{MH} has standard error given by

$$SE\left[\ln\left(RR_{MH}\right)\right] = \sqrt{\frac{P}{R \times S}},$$

where

$$P = \sum \frac{\left(n_{1i} n_{2i} \left(a_i + c_i\right) - a_i c_i N_i\right)}{N_i^2}; \quad R = \sum \frac{a_i n_{2i}}{N_i}; \quad S = \sum \frac{c_i n_{1i}}{N_i}.$$

For **risk differences**, each trial's RD has the weight [13]

$$w_i = \frac{n_{1i} n_{2i}}{N_i},$$

and RD_{MH} has standard error given by

$$SE\left(RD_{MH}\right) = \sqrt{\frac{J}{K^2}},$$

where

$$J = \sum \frac{a_i b_i n_{2i}^3 + c_i d_i n_{1i}^3}{n_{1i} n_{2i} N_i^2}; \quad K = \sum \frac{n_{1i} n_{2i}}{N_i}.$$

However, the test of homogeneity is based upon the inverse-variance weights and not the Mantel–Haenszel weights, and computed using log-transformed estimates for ratio measures. The heterogeneity statistic is given by

$$Q = \sum w_i \left(\ln\left(\hat{\theta}_i\right) - \ln\left(\hat{\theta}_{MH}\right)\right)^2$$

where $\hat{\theta}_{MH}$ is the summary odds ratio (OR_{MH}), or risk ratio (RR_{MH}), or

$$Q = \sum w_i \left(\hat{\theta}_i - \hat{\theta}_{MH}\right)^2$$

where $\hat{\theta}_{MH}$ is the summary risk difference (RD_{MH}). Zero-cell corrections are required when $\hat{\theta}_i$ is not estimable.

9.2.4   Peto's Odds Ratio Method

An alternative to the Mantel–Haenszel methods is a method due to Peto (sometimes attributed to Yusuf, or to Yusuf and Peto) [2]. This is again a fixed-effect approach to meta-analysis. The overall odds ratio is given by

$$OR_{Peto} = \exp\left(\frac{\sum w_i \ln\left(OR_i\right)}{\sum w_i}\right),$$

where the odds ratio for each individual study OR_i is calculated using the approximate Peto method described in Chapter 8, and the weight w_i is equal to the hypergeometric variance of the event count in the intervention group, v_i. The summation notation indicates summation of the trials included in the analysis.

The logarithm of the overall odds ratio has standard error

$$SE\left[\ln\left(OR_{Peto}\right)\right] = \frac{1}{\sqrt{\sum v_i}}.$$

The heterogeneity statistic is given by

$$Q = \sum v_i \left(\ln\left(OR_i\right) - \ln\left(OR_{Peto}\right)\right)^2.$$

The approximation upon which Peto's method relies has been shown to fail when intervention effects are very large, and when the size of the arms of the trials is seriously unbalanced [14]. Severe imbalance with, for example, four times as many participants in one group than the other is possible, but rare in randomized trials. In other circumstances, including when event rates are very low, the method performs well [15]. Unlike the inverse-variance and Mantel–Haenszel methods, corrections for zero-cell counts are not necessary for either the summary OR or its standard error.

9.2.5   Extending the Peto Method for Combining Time-to-Event Data

Meta-analysis for time-to-event outcomes can be performed either by computing hazard ratios for each trial and combining them using the inverse-variance method above, or by exploiting a link between the log-rank test statistic and the Peto method, as follows.

For each trial, the calculation of a log-rank statistic involves dividing the follow-up period into a series of discrete time intervals. For each interval the number of events observed in the treated group O_{ij}, the number of events that would be expected in the intervention group under the null hypothesis E_{ij} and its variance v_{ij}, are calculated [16]. The expected count and its variance are computed taking into account the number still at risk of the event within each time period. The log-rank test for the ith trial is computed from $\sum O_{ij}$, $\sum E_{ij}$ and $\sum v_{ij}$ summed over all the time periods, j.

Following the same format as the Peto odds ratio method, an estimate of the hazard ratio in each trial is given by [16]

$$HR_i = \exp\left(\frac{\sum O_{ij} - \sum E_{ij}}{\sum v_{ij}}\right),$$

with standard error

$$SE\left[\ln\left(HR_i\right)\right] = \frac{1}{\sqrt{\sum v_{ij}}}.$$

Note that the summation notation here indicates summation of the j time period intervals, and is computed separately for each trial.

The summary estimate of the hazard ratio is given by the weighted average of the log hazard ratios

$$HR_{Peto} = \exp\left(\frac{\sum w_i \ln\left(HR_i\right)}{\sum w_i}\right),$$

where the summation is now over the i trials again, and the weights w_i are equal to the variances computed from the trials, $\sum v_{ij}$.

The logarithm of the overall hazard ratio has standard error

$$SE\left[\ln\left(HR_{Peto}\right)\right] = \frac{1}{\sqrt{\sum w_i}}.$$

Computation of the components of the log-rank statistic $\sum O_{ij}$, $\sum E_{ij}$, and $\sum v_{ij}$ is straightforward if individual participant data (IPD) are available. However, the method has been noted to suffer from bias in some situations [17]. Methods have been proposed for indirectly estimating the log hazard ratio and its variance from graphical and numeric summaries commonly published in reports of randomized controlled trials [18–21].

9.2.6 Random-Effects Meta-Analysis using the Inverse-Variance Method

Under the random-effects model, the assumption of a single, fixed (common) intervention effect is relaxed, and the true intervention effects are considered to vary across trials. Conventionally, the θ_i are assumed to follow a normal distribution with a mean θ and variance τ^2. A simple estimate of τ^2, after DerSimonian and Laird [5], is given by

$$\hat{\tau}^2 = \frac{Q - (k-1)}{\sum w_i - \frac{\sum w_i^2}{\sum w_i}},$$

where Q is the heterogeneity statistic, with $\hat{\tau}^2$ set to zero if $Q < k-1$, and the w_i are calculated as in the inverse-variance method. The value of Q is typically obtained by the formula shown within the inverse-variance method section, although the formula based on the Mantel–Haenszel approach is also an option (and has been implemented as the default in some software, such as **metan** in Stata and Review Manager). Again, for odds ratios, risk ratios, and hazard ratios, the intervention effect is considered on the logarithmic scale.

When deriving the summary effect estimate for the random-effects inverse-variance approach, each trial's intervention effect is given weight

$$w_i' = \frac{1}{\left[\text{SE}\left(\hat{\theta}_i\right)\right]^2 + \hat{\tau}^2}.$$

The summary estimate is given by

$$\hat{\theta}_{\text{DL}} = \frac{\sum w_i' \hat{\theta}_i}{\sum w_i'},$$

with standard error

$$\text{SE}\left(\hat{\theta}_{\text{DL}}\right) = \frac{1}{\sqrt{\sum w_i'}}.$$

Note that when $\tau^2 = 0$, i.e. where the heterogeneity statistic Q is smaller than its degrees of freedom $(k-1)$, the weights reduce to those given by the fixed-effect inverse-variance method.

If the estimate of τ^2 is greater than zero, then the weights in random-effects models ($w_i' = 1/\left(\left[\text{SE}\left(\hat{\theta}_i\right)\right]^2 + \hat{\tau}^2\right)$) will be smaller and more similar to each other than the weights in fixed-effect models ($w_i = 1/\left[\text{SE}\left(\hat{\theta}_i\right)\right]^2$). This means that summary estimates from random-effects meta-analyses have larger standard errors (the confidence intervals will be wider) than fixed-effect analyses [22], since the variance of the summary effect is the inverse of the sum of the weights, which are smaller when the estimate of τ^2 is greater than zero. It also means that random-effects models give relatively more weight to smaller trials than the fixed-effect model, which will alter the summary estimate if there is a relationship between trial findings and sample size. This may not always be desirable (see Chapter 5).

The random-effects inverse-variance method has the same wide applicability as the fixed-effect inverse-variance method, and can be used to combine any type of estimates, provided standard errors are available.

9.2.7   Other Random-Effects Meta-Analysis Methods

There are many other competing approaches for the estimation of τ^2, most of which are computationally more complex than the DerSimonian and Laird method, but can be readily obtained with modern software such as Stata, R, or Comprehensive Meta-Analysis (see Chapters 25–27). At least 16 different estimators are available [23]. Re-analysis across many meta-analyses using several of these methods found that meta-analysis conclusions can differ depending on which is used [24]. However, an estimate using restricted maximum likelihood (REML) has been recommended based on an extensive simulation study [25]. We provide one example of a re-analysis using different approaches in Box 9.1. Regardless of the chosen method, the estimated τ^2 is used to obtain the trial weights, $w_i' = 1 / \left(\left[\mathrm{SE}\left(\hat{\theta}_i\right) \right]^2 + \hat{\tau}^2 \right)$, and then the summary effect and standard error computed as outlined above. Whichever estimate of τ^2 is used in the inverse-variance approach, it will be accompanied by substantial uncertainty when the number of studies is small.

Box 9.1   Consideration of Different Estimation Methods for Random-Effects Models

Cornell et al. illustrate how the choice of estimation method and confidence interval can lead to different conclusions (Figure 9.1) [26]. The methods that account for uncertainty in the between-trial variance (profile likelihood, Hartung–Knapp, and Bayesian) all lead to wider 95% confidence intervals than the DerSimonian and Laird approach with standard confidence interval derivation.

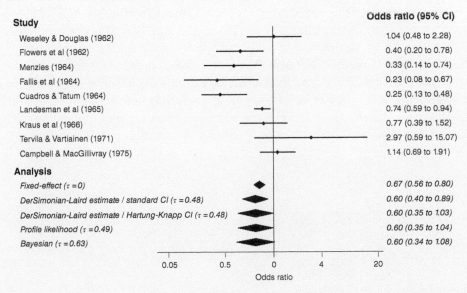

FIGURE 9.1   Summary meta-analysis results for a meta-analysis of the effect of diuretics on preeclampsia, as taken from Cornell et al. [26].

9.3　CONFIDENCE INTERVAL FOR OVERALL EFFECT

The standard $100(1-\alpha)\%$ confidence interval for the overall estimate $\hat{\theta}$ is given by

$$\hat{\theta} - \left(z_{1-\alpha/2} \times \mathrm{SE}\left(\hat{\theta}\right) \right) \quad \text{to} \quad \hat{\theta} + \left(z_{1-\alpha/2} \times \mathrm{SE}\left(\hat{\theta}\right) \right),$$

where $\hat{\theta}$ is the log odds ratio, log risk ratio, log hazard ratio, risk difference, mean difference, or standardized mean difference, and z is the standard normal deviate. For example, if $\alpha = 0.05$, then $z_{1-\alpha/2} = 1.96$ and the standard 95% confidence interval is given by

$$\hat{\theta} - \left(1.96 \times \mathrm{SE}\left(\hat{\theta}\right) \right) \quad \text{to} \quad \hat{\theta} + \left(1.96 \times \mathrm{SE}\left(\hat{\theta}\right) \right).$$

Confidence intervals for log odds ratios, log risk ratios, and log hazard ratios are exponentiated to provide confidence intervals for the summary odds ratio, risk ratio, or hazard ratio, respectively.

There are growing calls to replace this standard confidence interval with methods that more fully account for the uncertainty in the within-trial weights [26]. When deriving the summary estimate, the estimated weights are assumed to be known. However, the weights in a fixed-effect meta-analysis and both components of the weights in a random-effects meta-analysis ($\mathrm{SE}\left(\hat{\theta}_i\right)$ and $\hat{\tau}^2$) are in fact estimates that may have considerable uncertainty. Thus, the concern is that the standard approach produces confidence intervals that are too narrow, leading to conclusions that are too precise. Hartung and Knapp (and independently Sidik and Jonkman) propose an alternative confidence interval for random-effects meta-analyses, which uses a modified estimate of $\mathrm{SE}\left(\hat{\theta}\right)$ and replaces $z_{1-\alpha/2}$ with $t_{k-1,1-\alpha/2}$, the value from a t-distribution with degrees of freedom equal to the number of trials (k) minus one [27, 28]. The method is the default approach in the **metareg** Stata module (see Chapter 25), and simulation studies suggest this method performs very well unless there are few trials with very unequal sample sizes [29]. Other options include profile likelihood estimation [30] and Bayesian methods. The latter can incorporate prior information from other sources. Empirical prior distributions for τ^2 have been proposed for different outcome types across various disease fields, based on previous meta-analyses in Cochrane [31, 32] (see Box 9.2).

9.4　TEST STATISTIC FOR OVERALL EFFECT

A standard test statistic for the overall intervention effect is derived as

$$Z = \frac{\hat{\theta}}{\mathrm{SE}\left(\hat{\theta}\right)},$$

Box 9.2   Bayesian Meta-Analysis

Bayesian meta-analysis provides an alternative to the specific methods described in more detail in this chapter. In a Bayesian meta-analysis, the combined results of the studies are combined with a *prior distribution*, producing a *posterior distribution* for the quantities of interest. In a simple Bayesian fixed-effect meta-analysis, the prior distribution describes an a priori belief about the magnitude of the underlying effect. In a simple Bayesian random-effects meta-analysis, the prior distribution describes a priori beliefs about the mean and variability of effects across studies. The prior distribution may be derived from data external to the meta-analysis, or from expert opinions. It influences the analysis such that the main results of the meta-analysis (extracted from the posterior distribution) reflect a combination of the information in the prior distribution and the information in the data.

Usually the prior belief about the magnitude of the effect size is specified to be that of ignorance, with a flat prior distribution that does not favor any particular effect size over another. However, notable gains in precision can be obtained by using informative prior distributions for the amount of between-study heterogeneity in a random-effects meta-analysis [31]. This is particularly the case for meta-analyses of clinical trials, since empirical distribution for the typical amount of heterogeneity have been derived based on many thousands of historical meta-analyses. The impact of using such prior distribution is greatest when there are very few trials in the meta-analysis, since in this situation the between-study heterogeneity is estimated very poorly based on the trials alone.

There are further advantages of taking a Bayesian approach. One is that they offer great flexibility to model the data more meaningfully, for example by allowing different studies to be analyzed in different ways, and easily facilitating the clustering of studies, for example by drug classes. The flexibility arises because Bayesian meta-analyses are typically implemented using bespoke code within a simulation approach to analysis (specifically, Markov chain Monte Carlo methods). A further advantage, argued by many, is that inferences more naturally follow intuition: Bayesian analyses focus on our uncertainty about the underlying effects, treating the data as fixed, rather than our uncertainty about the data, treating the underlying effects as fixed. Result are expressed using *credible intervals* and direct probabilities, rather than using confidence intervals and P values.

where the odds ratio, risk ratio, or hazard ratio is again considered on the log scale. Under the null hypothesis that there is no intervention effect, Z will follow approximately a standard normal distribution. However, as for the derivation of confidence intervals, other test statistics that account for uncertainty may be preferred [33].

Note that the interpretation of the test of overall effect differs between fixed-effect and random-effects analyses. For the fixed-effect model it tests the hypothesis that there is no effect of the intervention, while for the random-effects model it tests the hypothesis that the average effect of the intervention is zero.

9.5   PREDICTION INTERVAL FOR THE INTERVENTION EFFECT IN A NEW TRIAL

The overall summary from a fixed-effect meta-analysis estimates the assumed *fixed* (or *common*) effect of the intervention. For a random-effects analysis, the overall summary estimates the *average* effect rather than a *fixed* effect, an important difference that is often overlooked. When interpreting the overall summary for a random-effects analysis, it is important to describe the expected *variability* as well as the average effect of the intervention, to be able to help predict, for example, what might be observed in a new trial, or when the intervention is applied in a different setting. Assuming that the trials included in the meta-analysis provide a representative sample of intervention effects and that intervention effects are normally distributed between trials, a prediction interval can be computed for the effect of the intervention in further trials or settings. A prediction interval is approximately found by [34, 35]

$$\hat{\theta} - t_{k-2}\sqrt{\hat{\tau}^2 + \left[SE\left(\hat{\theta}\right)\right]^2} \text{ to } \hat{\theta} + t_{k-2}\sqrt{\hat{\tau}^2 + \left[SE\left(\hat{\theta}\right)\right]^2},$$

Box 9.3   Interpretation of Summary Results from Random-Effects Models

Figure 9.2 presents two hypothetical meta-analyses (Example 1 and Example 2), taken from Riley et al. [35]. In each meta-analysis, intervention effect estimates are computed and synthesized from 10 hypothetical trials. Each trial provides an unbiased estimate of the intervention effect expressed as a standardized mean difference. Assume that negative intervention effects indicate benefit. The two meta-analyses give identical summary intervention effect estimates of −0.33 with a standard 95% confidence interval of −0.48 to −0.18. Both are computed using a DerSimonian and Laird random-effects model. However, visual inspection of the forest plots makes it clear that there is substantially more between-trial variation in Example 2 than in Example 1. So why do the analyses give the same result, and is it appropriate that they do?

The reason for the discrepancy is that two factors are impacting on the width of the confidence interval. The first is the sizes of the trials. The trials are generally larger in Example 2 and have narrower confidence intervals. The effect of the larger trials is to give the meta-analysis more precision and give the diamond at the bottom a narrower confidence interval. The second factor is the amount of heterogeneity. This is much larger in Example 2. The effect of this heterogeneity is to give the meta-analysis less precision and give the diamond at the bottom a wider confidence interval. The examples were constructed so that the effects of these two factors cancel out, such that the summary estimates in both examples have the same precision. However, the width of the confidence interval in Example 2 does not describe the amount of heterogeneity across the trials. The confidence interval reflects only uncertainty in the location of the average intervention effect.

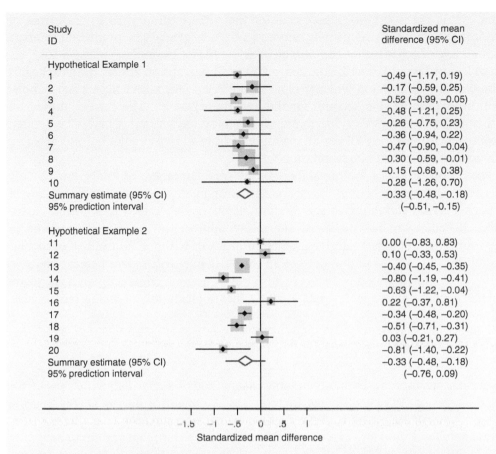

FIGURE 9.2 Forest plots of two distinct hypothetical meta-analyses that give the same summary estimate (center of the diamond) and 95% confidence interval (width of the diamond). Example 1 is a random-effects meta-analysis with smaller trials with little heterogeneity. Example 2 is a random-effects meta-analysis with larger trials with greater heterogeneity. N.B. The center of each square gives an individual trial estimate of intervention effect, and the horizontal line gives its 95% confidence interval; the size of the square is proportional to the weight of the trial in the meta-analysis.

Adding prediction intervals helps reveal the difference in interpretation for these two meta-analyses. In Figure 9.2, the prediction interval for the first forest plot is essentially the same as the confidence interval for the average effect, because there is no discernible heterogeneity across the trials (the slight difference arises because the prediction interval is computed using a t-distribution whereas the confidence interval is computed using a normal distribution). However, the 95% prediction interval for the second forest plot is much wider than the confidence interval: −0.76 to 0.09. Although most of this interval is below zero, indicating that the intervention will be beneficial in the majority of settings, the interval overlaps zero and so in some settings the intervention effect may be small or even slightly harmful. This finding was masked when just focusing on the average effect estimate and its confidence interval.

where t_{k-2} is the $100(1-\alpha/2)$ percentile of the t-distribution with $k-2$ degrees of freedom. The value of α is usually chosen as 0.05, to give a 95% prediction interval, although use of other values can also be considered (for example, quoting a 50% prediction interval would describe the central 50% of intervention effects, akin to the box in the center of a box and whisker plot). A t-distribution, rather than a normal distribution, is used to help account for the uncertainty of $\hat{\tau}^2$. The correct number of degrees of freedom for this t-distribution is complex, and the value of $k-2$ will often be approximate. See Box 9.3 for an example of how adding prediction intervals to a meta-analysis helps with interpretation.

Prediction intervals for meta-analyses of small numbers of trials can be very wide, and may not be helpful. They are also strongly dependent on the accuracy of the between-trial variability in the random-effects model following a normal distribution. Recent work has proposed alternative approaches, using bootstrapping or nonparametric methods, to derive prediction intervals without assuming a particular distribution [36, 37]. Note that prediction intervals may encompass heterogeneity in intervention effects caused by biases in addition to genuine clinical differences, so are most useful clinically when the meta-analysis does not include trials at high risk of bias.

9.6   META-ANALYSIS WITH INDIVIDUAL PARTICIPANT DATA

The same basic approaches and meta-analysis methods described above are useful for meta-analyses of IPD [38, 39] (see Chapter 12). A benefit of having IPD is that the meta-analyst calculates the summary tables or statistics for each trial directly from the raw data, and therefore can ensure that all data are complete and up to date, that the same inclusion/exclusion criteria are used, that the outcome definitions are harmonized, and that the same method of analysis is used for all trials. A key advantage of having IPD is that the meta-analysis can address participant-level characteristics. Thus, summary statistics can be calculated that are adjusted for prognostic factors, or for specific groups of participants, enabling subgroup analyses to be produced and differences between them quantified.

9.7   ADDITIONAL ANALYSES

Additional analyses undertaken after the main meta-analysis investigate *influence*, *robustness*, and *bias*. Influence and robustness can be assessed in sensitivity analyses by repeating the meta-analysis on subsets of the original dataset (see Chapter 2 for an example). The influence of each trial can be estimated by deleting each in turn from the analysis and noting the degree to which the size and uncertainty of the intervention effect change. Other sensitivity analyses can assess robustness to uncertainties and assumptions. Examples include implementing different statistical models and estimation methods (for example, different methods for estimating heterogeneity variances); removing or adding sets of trials (such as those at higher risk of bias); and changing the data for individual trials (for example, by using different methods to impute missing data, or when it is not clear which result should be extracted from a trial report). Methods for investigating between-trial bias, including publication bias, are described in Chapter 5.

9.8   SOME PRACTICAL ISSUES

Although it is desirable to include trial results according to intention-to-treat principles, this is not always possible given the data provided in published reports. Reports commonly omit participants who do not comply, receive the wrong intervention, or drop out of the trial. All of these individuals can easily be included in intention-to-treat analyses if follow-up data are available, and it is most important that they are included if the reasons for exclusion relate to the intervention that they received (such as dropouts due to side effects and poor tolerability of the intervention). Occasionally full details of the outcomes of those excluded during the trial may be mentioned in the text of the report, or IPD may be available, but in many situations assumptions must be made regarding their fate. By using sensitivity analysis based on plausible assumptions about the missing values, it is possible to assess the influence of these excluded cases on the final results [40, 41]; see Chapter 11. The issue is more problematic for continuous outcomes, where there is a continuum of possible scenarios for every excluded participant.

Other problems can occur when trials have no events in one or both arms [4, 15]. In these many of the methods described in this chapter require the addition of a small quantity (usually 0.5) to the cell counts to avoid division by zero errors. Many software implementations of these methods automatically add this correction to all cell counts regardless of whether it is strictly needed. When both groups have event rates of zero (there being no events in either arm), then the trial contains no information about an odds ratio or a risk ratio, and such trials must be excluded from the analysis unless assumptions are made about the absolute risk of the event (for example, Kuss has proposed alternative methods [42]). The risk difference in such situations is zero, so the trials will still contribute to an analysis of risk differences. However, for all effect measures, both inverse-variance and Mantel–Haenszel methods perform poorly when event rates are very low, underestimating intervention effects and overestimating P values [15]. Peto's odds ratio method has been observed to produce more accurate estimates of the intervention effects and their confidence intervals, providing the sample sizes of the arms in the trials are not severely unbalanced.

9.9   DISCUSSION

We have outlined a variety of standard methods for combining results from several trials in a systematic review. There are three aspects of choosing the right method for a particular meta-analysis: identifying the data type (binary, continuous, time to event, etc.), choosing an appropriate summary statistic, and selecting a method for combining the summary statistics across trials. These are summarized in Box 9.4. Although we have discussed meta-analysis in the context of clinical trials, the methods apply equally for meta-analysis of observational and other experimental studies.

Box 9.4 Considerations in Choosing a Method of Meta-Analysis

Choice of summary statistic depends upon

(a) the type of data being analyzed (e.g. binary, continuous, time-to-event)

(b) the consistency of estimates of the intervention effect across trials and subgroups

(c) the ease of interpretation of the summary statistic

Choice of weighting method depends upon

(a) the reliability of the method when sample sizes are small

(b) the reliability of the method if events are very rare

(c) the degree of imbalance in allocation ratios in the trials

Consideration of heterogeneity can affect

(a) whether a meta-analysis should be considered, depending on the similarity of trial characteristics

(b) whether an overall summary can have a sensible meaning, depending on the degree of disagreement observed between the trial results

(c) whether a random-effects method is used to account for between-trial variation

(d) whether the impact of other factors on the intervention effect can be investigated using stratified analyses and methods of meta-regression

A key decision is whether the meta-analysis will use a fixed-effect or random-effects model. For fixed-effect analyses of binary outcome measures, it is important to be aware of circumstances in which Mantel–Haenszel, inverse-variance, and Peto methods give erroneous results. Inverse-variance methods have poor properties when most trials are small (or events are few) and are rarely preferable to Mantel–Haenszel methods for a fixed-effect meta-analysis. Both Mantel–Haenszel and inverse-variance methods have poor properties when event rates are very low, and Peto's method can be misleading when intervention effects are large, and when there are severely unequal numbers of participants in intervention and control groups in some or all of the trials [17]. Some of these points are illustrated in the case studies discussed in Boxes 9.5 and 9.6.

The interpretation of summary results is different for fixed-effect and random-effects models. The former provides the best estimate of an assumed common (fixed) summary effect, whereas the latter provides an estimate of the average summary effect from a distribution of possible intervention effects. This distinction is not well recognized in the literature. The derivation of prediction intervals following a random-effects analysis can help illustrate the heterogeneity around the summary estimate more clearly, though the interval may often be very wide. It is important to note that none of the analyses described can compensate for publication bias (see Chapter 5), nor can they account for bias introduced through poor trial design and execution.

Box 9.5   Case study: Support from Caregivers during Childbirth

Descriptive studies of women's childbirth experiences have suggested that women appreciate advice and information from their caregivers, comfort measures and other forms of tangible assistance to cope with labor, and the continuous presence of a sympathetic person. A systematic review included trials that evaluated the effects of intrapartum support from caregivers on a variety of childbirth outcomes, medical as well as psychosocial [43]. One outcome included in the review was the use of epidural anesthesia during delivery. Nine trials reported this outcome, five from North America, two from Europe, and one each from Central America and South America. In four of the six trials husbands, partners, or other family members were also usually present. The person providing the support intervention was variously described in the trials as a midwife, nurse, *monitrice,* and a *doula.* The results of the nine trials are given in Table 9.2.

TABLE 9.2   Rates of use of epidural anesthesia in trials of caregiver support.

Trial	Caregiver present Epidurals/N	Standard care Epidurals/N
Kennell 1991 (USA)	47/212	94/200
Bréart 1992 (Belgium)	55/133	62/131
Bréart 1992 (France)	281/652	319/666
Gagnon 1997 (Canada)	139/209	142/204
Langer 1998 (Mexico)	295/335	302/346
Torres 1999 (Chile)	202/217	195/218
Hodnett 2002 (Canada)	2349/3454	2436/3461
Campbell 2006 (USA)	247/291	260/295
McGrath 2008 (USA)	145/224	149/196

Ten alternative methods have been described in this chapter that can be used to perform a meta-analysis of these data. The results are shown in Table 9.3, with the standard method used to derive confidence intervals and P values.

There are some notable patterns in the results in Table 9.3. First, there is substantial agreement between Peto, Mantel–Haenszel, and fixed-effect inverse-variance methods for odds ratios. For risk ratio meta-analyses, the differences in the trial weights between the methods can be high when event rates are high, as is the case for many trials in this analysis. For example, the largest trial (Hodnett 2002) is given very different weights (48.5% in the inverse-variance, 61.4% in the Mantel–Haenszel, and 17.1% in the random-effects analyses) which has led to differences in the meta-analytical findings. (Meta-analysis of risk ratios of *not* having an epidural – switching the definition of the event – would give similar weights to each trial, since event rates would be low.)

Second, there are substantial differences between intervention effects expressed as odds ratios and risk ratios. Considering the Mantel–Haenszel results, the reduction in the odds of having an epidural with additional caregiver support is 16% ($100 \times [1-0.84]$), while the relative risk reduction is 5% ($100 \times (1-0.95)$), only around one-third the size. Where events are common, odds and risks are very different, and care must be taken in a meta-analysis of odds ratios to ensure that a reader of the review is not misled into believing that benefits of intervention are larger than is truly the case [32].

Between-trial heterogeneity is present, and tests of homogeneity have small P values for all summary statistics (OR, RR, and RD), with values for I^2 of 72.1, 80.8, and 77.7%, respectively. As a result, the confidence intervals for the random-effects estimates are wider than those calculated from fixed-effect models. The estimates of the benefit of intervention also increase, as the random-effects model attributes proportionally greater weight to the smallest trials, which in this example report larger relative benefits of intervention.

The 95% prediction intervals provide ranges that reflect the heterogeneity across trials. In each case, the prediction interval indicates that the effect of intervention in a subsequent, similar trial will not necessarily indicate benefit.

TABLE 9.3 Results of meta-analyses of epidural rates from trials of caregiver support.

Method	Estimate of effect (95% CI)	Statistical evidence of effect	Statistical evidence of heterogeneity
Odds ratio			
Peto	0.84 (0.77,0.91)	Z = 4.19, P < 0.0001	$\chi_8^2 = 29.1$, P < 0.001
Mantel–Haenszel	0.84 (0.77, 0.91)	Z = 4.19, P < 0.0001	$\chi_8^2 = 28.7$, P < 0.001
Inverse variance (fixed effect)	0.84 (0.76, 0.91)	Z = 4.13, P < 0.0001	$\chi_8^2 = 28.7$, P < 0.001; $I^2 = 72.1\%$
Inverse variance (random effects[a])	0.78 (0.63, 0.96)	Z = 2.35, P = 0.019	
	95% prediction interval: (0.40, 1.49)		
Risk ratio of receiving epidural			
Mantel–Haenszel	0.95 (0.93, 0.97)	Z = 4.19, P < 0.0001	$\chi_8^2 = 41.7$, P < 0.001
Inverse variance (fixed effect)	0.97 (0.95, 0.99)	Z = 2.60, P < 0.009	$\chi_8^2 = 37.3$, P < 0.001; $I^2 = 80.8\%$
Inverse variance (random effects[a])	0.93 (0.88, 0.99)	Z = 2.16, P = 0.03	
	95% prediction interval: (0.77, 1.14)		
Risk difference			
Mantel–Haenszel	−0.035 (−0.052, −0.019)	Z = 4.20, P < 0.0001	$\chi_8^2 = 36.6$, P < 0.001
Inverse variance (fixed effect)	−0.029 (−0.045, −0.013)	Z = 3.59, P < 0.0001	$\chi_8^2 = 35.9$, P < 0.001; $I^2 = 77.7\%$
Inverse variance (random effects[a])	−0.048 (−0.088, −0.007)	Z = 2.32, P = 0.02	
	95% prediction interval: (0.18, 0.08)		

[a] Random-effects meta-analyses use the DerSimonian and Laird estimate of between-study variance.

Box 9.6   Case study: Effect of Reduced Dietary Sodium on Blood Pressure

Restricting the intake of salt in the diet has been proposed as a method of lowering blood pressure, in both hypertensives and people with normal blood pressure. A 1996 systematic review of randomized trials included 56 trials comparing salt-lowering diets with control diets [44]. Only trials that assessed salt reduction through measurement of sodium excretion were included. Hypertensive participants were recruited for 28 of the trials; the other 28 recruited normotensive participants; 41 trials used a crossover design, while 15 used a parallel-group design.

The focus of interest in these trials is the difference in mean blood pressure (both diastolic and systolic) between the salt-reducing diet and the control diet. As all measurements are in the same units (mmHg), the difference in means can be used directly as a summary statistic in the meta-analysis. The trials estimated this difference in mean blood pressure in four different ways:

- In a parallel-group trial, as the difference in mean final blood pressure between those receiving the salt-lowering and the control diets.
- In a parallel-group trial, as the difference in mean change in blood pressure while on the diets, between those on the salt-lowering diet and those on the control diet.
- In a crossover trial, as the mean within-person difference between final blood pressure at the end of the salt-lowering diet and at the end of the control diet.
- In a crossover trial, as the mean within-person difference in the change in blood pressure while on the salt-lowering diet compared with the control diet.

Results from these four different designs all estimate the same summary measure. However, it is likely that trials using within-person changes are more efficient than those using final values, and that those with crossover designs are more efficient than those with parallel groups. These differences are encapsulated in the standard errors of the estimates in differences in mean blood pressure between the two diets, provided appropriate consideration is given to the within-person pairing of the data for change scores and crossover trials in the analysis of those trials. As the standard inverse-variance approach to combining trials uses weights inversely proportional to the square of these standard errors, it copes naturally with data of these different formats, so that the trials are given appropriate weights according to the relative efficiency of their designs.

The authors of the review reported that they had used a variety of techniques to estimate these standard errors, as they were not always available in the original reports. If necessary, standard errors can be derived directly from standard deviations, confidence intervals, t values, and exact P values. However, when paired data (both for change scores and for crossover trials) are used, it is occasionally necessary to make an assumption about the within-participant correlation between two timepoints if the analysis presented mistakenly ignores the pairings. Similarly, when results are reported simply either as significant or nonsignificant, particular P values must be assumed from which the standard errors can be derived. Such problems are common in meta-analyses of continuous data, due to the use of inappropriate analyses and the poor standard of presentation commonly encountered in published trial reports.

Meta-analyses were undertaken separately for the trials in normotensive and hypertensive groups, and for systolic and diastolic blood pressure. The results are given in Table 9.4, with standard methods used to derive confidence intervals and P values.

The analysis shows reductions of around 5–6 mmHg in systolic blood pressure in hypertensive participants, with a smaller reduction in diastolic blood pressure. The size of the reductions observed in normotensive participants was much smaller, the differences between the hypertensive and normotensive subgroups being convincing for both systolic ($Z = 4.12 : P < 0.0001$) and diastolic ($Z = 5.61 : P < 0.0001$) measurements. The confidence intervals for the random-effects analyses for all reductions are much wider than those of the fixed-effect analyses, reflecting the significant heterogeneity detected in all analyses (as indicated by the I^2 statistics). The prediction intervals indicate that the range of possible intervention effects is wide, particularly in the hypertension trials. The authors investigated this further using methods of meta-regression (see Chapter 10) and showed that the heterogeneity between trials could in part be explained by a relationship by the reduction in salt intake achieved in each trial.

On the basis of these analyses, the authors concluded that salt-lowering diets may have some worthwhile impact on blood pressure for hypertensive people but not for normotensive people, contrary to current recommendations for universal dietary salt reduction.

TABLE 9.4   Impact of salt-lowering diets on systolic and diastolic blood pressure.

Method	Estimated difference in blood pressure reduction (95% CI) (diet-control) (mmHg)	Statistical evidence of effect	Statistical evidence of heterogeneity
Normotensive trials			
Systolic			
Inverse variance (fixed effect)	−1.2 (−1.6, −0.8)	$Z = 6.4, P < 0.001$	$\chi^2_{27} = 75.1, P < 0.001$
Inverse variance (random effects[a])	−1.7 (−2.4, −0.9)	$Z = 4.3, P < 0.001$	$I^2 = 64.0\%$
	95% prediction interval	(−4.6, 1.3)	
Diastolic			
Inverse variance (fixed effect)	−0.7 (−1.0, −0.3)	$Z = 3.4, P = 0.001$	$\chi^2_{27} = 56.1, P = 0.001$

TABLE 9.4 *(Continued)*

Method	Estimated difference in blood pressure reduction (95% CI) (diet-control) (mmHg)	Statistical evidence of effect	Statistical evidence of heterogeneity
Inverse variance (random effects)	−0.5 (−1.2, 0.2)	$Z = 1.50$, $P = 0.13$	$I^2 = 55.1\%$
	95% prediction interval	(−2.9, 1.9)	
	Hypertensive trials		
Systolic			
Inverse variance (fixed effect)	−5.4 (−6.3, −4.5)	$Z = 12.0$, $P < 0.001$	$\chi^2_{27} = 99.2$, $P < 0.001$
Inverse variance (random effects)	−5.9 (−7.8, −4.1)	$Z = 6.4$, $P < 0.001$	$I^2 = 72.8\%$
	95% prediction interval	(−14.2, 2.3)	
Diastolic			
Inverse variance (fixed effect)	−3.5 (−4.0, −2.9)	$Z = 11.6$, $P < 0.001$	$\chi^2_{27} = 57.3$, $P = 0.001$
Inverse variance (random effects)	−3.8 (−4.8, −2.9)	$Z = 8.0$, $P < 0.001$	$I^2 = 52.9\%$
	95% prediction interval	(−7.5, −0.2)	

[a] Random-effects meta-analyses use the DerSimonian and Laird estimate of between-study variance.

ACKNOWLEDGMENTS

We are grateful to Julian Midgley for allowing us access to the data on which the second case study is based.

REFERENCES

1. Deeks, J.J. (1998). *Systematic reviews of published evidence: miracles or minefields? Ann. Oncol.* 9: 703–709.
2. Yusuf, S., Peto, R., Lewis, J. et al. (1985). *Beta blockade during and after myocardial infarction: an overview of the randomised trials. Prog. Cardiovasc. Dis.* 27: 335–371.
3. Rice, K., Higgins, J.P.T., and Lumley, T. (2018). *A re-evaluation of fixed effect(s) meta-analysis. J. R. Stat. Soc. Ser. A Stat. Soc.* 181 (1): 205–227.
4. Sweeting, M.J., Sutton, A.J., and Lambert, P.C. (2004). *What to add to nothing? Use and avoidance of continuity corrections in meta-analysis of sparse data. Stat. Med.* 23 (9): 1351–1375.

5. DerSimonian, R. and Laird, N. (1986). *Meta-analysis in clinical trials. Control. Clin. Trials* 7: 177–188.

6. Higgins, J.P.T. and Thompson, S.G. (2002). *Quantifying heterogeneity in a meta-analysis. Stat. Med.* 21 (11): 1539–1558.

7. Higgins, J.P.T., Thompson, S.G., Deeks, J.J. et al. (2003). *Measuring inconsistency in meta-analysis. BMJ* 327: 557–560.

8. Rucker, G., Schwarzer, G., Carpenter, J.R. et al. (2008). *Undue reliance on I(2) in assessing heterogeneity may mislead. BMC Med. Res. Methodol.* 8: 79.

9. Deeks, J.J. (2002). *Issues in the selection of a summary statistic for meta-analysis of clinical trials with binary outcomes. Stat. Med.* 21 (11): 1575–1600.

10. Mantel, N. and Haenszel, W. (1959). *Statistical aspects of the analysis of data from retrospective studies of disease. J. Natl. Cancer Inst.* 22: 719–748.

11. Breslow, N.E. and Day, N.E. (1980). *Combination of results from a series of 2 x 2 tables; control of confounding.* In: *Statistical Methods in Cancer Research, Volume 1: The Analysis of Case-Control Data* (IARC Scientific Publications No. 32) (eds. N.E. Breslow and N.E. Day), 136–146. Lyon: International Agency for Health Research on Cancer.

12. Robins, J., Greenland, S., and Breslow, N.E. (1986). *A general estimator for the variance of the Mantel-Haenszel odds ratio. Am. J. Epidemiol.* 124 (5): 719–723.

13. Greenland, S. and Robins, J.M. (1985). *Estimation of a common effect parameter from sparse follow-up data. Biometrics* 41 (1): 55–68.

14. Greenland, S. and Salvan, A. (1990). *Bias in the one-step method for pooling study results. Stat. Med.* 9: 247–252.

15. Bradburn, M.J., Deeks, J.J., Berlin, J.A. et al. (2006). *Much ado about nothing: a comparison of the performance of meta-analytical methods with rare events. Stat. Med.* 26 (1): 53–77.

16. Simmonds, M.C., Tierney, J., Bowden, J. et al. (2011). *Meta-analysis of time-to-event data: a comparison of two-stage methods. Res. Synth. Methods* 2 (3): 139–149.

17. Bowden, J., Tierney, J.F., Simmonds, M. et al. (2011). *Individual patient data meta-analysis of time-to-event outcomes: one-stage versus two-stage approaches for estimating the hazard ratio under a random effects model. Res. Synth. Methods* 2 (3): 150–162.

18. Parmar, M.K.B., Torri, V., and Stewart, L. (1998). *Extracting summary statistics to perform meta-analyses of the published literature for survival endpoints. Stat. Med.* 17: 2815–2834.

19. Tierney, J.F., Steward, L.A., Ghersi, D. et al. (2007). *Practical methods for incorporating summary time-to-event data into meta-analysis. Trials* 8: 16.

20. Guyot, P., Ades, A.E., Ouwens, M.J. et al. (2012). *Enhanced secondary analysis of survival data: reconstructing the data from published Kaplan-Meier survival curves. BMC Med. Res. Methodol.* 12: 9.

21. Wei, Y. and Royston, P. (2017). *Reconstructing time-to-event data from published Kaplan-Meier curves. Stata Journal* 17 (4): 786–802.

22. Berlin, J.A., Laird, N.M., Sacks, H.S. et al. (1989). *A comparison of statistical methods for combining event rates from clinical trials. Stat. Med.* 8: 141–151.

23. Veroniki, A.A., Jackson, D., Viechtbauer, W. et al. (2016). *Methods to estimate the between-study variance and its uncertainty in meta-analysis. Res. Synth. Methods* 7 (1): 55–79.

24. Langan, D., Higgins, J.P.T., and Simmonds, M. (2015). *An empirical comparison of heterogeneity variance estimators in 12 894 meta-analyses. Res. Synth. Methods* 6 (2): 195–205.

25. Langan, D., Higgins, J.P.T., Jackson, D. et al. (2019). *A comparison of heterogeneity variance estimators in simulated random-effects meta-analyses. Res. Synth. Methods* 10 (1): 83–98.

26. Cornell, J.E., Mulrow, C.D., Localio, R. et al. (2014). *Random-effects meta-analysis of inconsistent effects: a time for change. Ann. Intern. Med.* 160 (4): 267–270.

27. Hartung, J. and Knapp, G. (2001). *A refined method for the meta-analysis of controlled clinical trials with binary outcome. Stat. Med.* 20: 3875–3889.

28. Sidik, K. and Jonkman, J.N. (2002). *A simple confidence interval for meta-analysis. Stat. Med.* 21 (21): 3153–3159.

29. IntHout, J., Ioannidis, J.P., and Borm, G.F. (2014). *The Hartung-Knapp-Sidik-Jonkman method for random effects meta-analysis is straightforward and considerably outperforms the standard DerSimonian-Laird method. BMC Med. Res. Methodol.* 14: 25.

30. Hardy, R.J. and Thompson, S.G. (1996). *A likelihood approach to meta-analysis with random effects. Stat. Med.* 15: 619–629.

31. Turner, R.M., Davey, J., Clarke, M.J. et al. (2012). *Predicting the extent of heterogeneity in meta-analysis, using empirical data from the Cochrane Database of Systematic Reviews. Int. J. Epidemiol.* 41 (3): 818–827.

32. Rhodes, K.M., Turner, R.M., and Higgins, J.P.T. (2015). *Predictive distributions were developed for the extent of heterogeneity in meta-analyses of continuous outcome data. J. Clin. Epidemiol.* 68 (1): 52–60.

33. Hartung, J. and Knapp, G. (2001). *On tests of the overall treatment effect in meta-analysis with normally distributed responses. Stat. Med.* 20: 1771–1782.

34. Higgins, J.P.T., Thompson, S.G., and Spiegelhalter, D.J. (2009). *A re-evaluation of random-effects meta-analysis. J. R. Stat. Soc. Ser. A Stat Soc* 172 (1): 137–159.

35. Riley, R.D., Higgins, J.P.T., and Deeks, J.J. (2011). *Interpretation of random effects meta-analyses. BMJ* 342: d549.

36. Wang, C.C. and Lee, W.C. (2019). *A simple method to estimate prediction intervals and predictive distributions: summarizing meta-analyses beyond means and confidence intervals. Res. Synth. Methods* 10 (2): 255–266.

37. Nagashima, K., Noma, H., and Furukawa, T.A. (2019). *Prediction intervals for random-effects meta-analysis: a confidence distribution approach. Stat. Methods Med. Res.* 28 (6): 1689–1702.

38. Riley, R.D., Lambert, P.C., and Abo-Zaid, G. (2010). *Meta-analysis of individual participant data: rationale, conduct, and reporting. BMJ* 340: c221.

39. Tierney, J.F., Vale, C., Riley, R. et al. (2015). *Individual Participant Data (IPD) meta-analyses of randomised controlled trials: guidance on their use. PLoS Med.* 12 (7): e1001855.

40. Higgins, J.P.T., White, I.R., and Wood, A.M. (2008). *Imputation methods for missing outcome data in meta-analysis of clinical trials. Clin. Trials* 5 (3): 225–239.

41. Mavridis, D., White, I.R., Higgins, J.P.T. et al. (2015). *Allowing for uncertainty due to missing continuous outcome data in pairwise and network meta-analysis. Stat. Med.* 34 (5): 721–741.

42. Kuss, O. (2015). *Statistical methods for meta-analyses including information from studies without any events-add nothing to nothing and succeed nevertheless*. Stat. Med. 34 (7): 1097–1116.

43. Bohren, M.A., Hofmeyr, G.J., Sakala, C. et al. (2017). *Continuous support for women during childbirth*. Cochrane Database Syst. Rev. **7**: CD003766. https://doi.org/10.1002/14651858.CD003766.pub6.

44. Midgley, J.P., Matthew, A.G., Greenwood, C.M.T. et al. (1996). *Effect of reduced dietary sodium on blood pressure: a meta-analysis of randomized controlled trials*. JAMA 275: 1590–1597.

CHAPTER 10

Exploring Heterogeneity

Julian P.T. Higgins and Tianjing Li

The ultimate purpose of a systematic review is often considered to be the production of an overall effect estimate, obtained by combining results across studies in a meta-analysis. In reality, studies brought together in a systematic review are likely to vary in terms of where, when, why, and how they were undertaken. A meta-analysis cannot, therefore, be interpreted in quite the same way as an individual study. For example, a particular clinical trial investigating the effectiveness of face masks in reducing the spread of influenza viruses might compare surgical masks with no masks, given to parents of sick children at schools during a flu season, using a particular selection of outcome measures. The purpose of a meta-analysis may be broader: for example, to estimate the extent to which using facial barriers of any kind reduces the transmission of a range of respiratory viruses during an outbreak. Meta-analyses almost invariably ask broader questions than do individual studies so that they can gain from the increased precision and greater generalizability that ensue (see Chapter 1).

The inevitable differences between studies brought together within a systematic review can pose problems in interpreting the overall effect. Consider, for example, the meta-analysis of randomized trials of intrapartum support from caregivers during childbirth [1], introduced as a case study in Chapter 9 and illustrated in Figure 10.1. As the review authors noted, the trials were conducted "under widely disparate hospital conditions, regulations and routines," and individuals providing the support "varied in their experience, qualifications and relationships to the laboring women." Furthermore, a critical evaluation of trials revealed differences in the risk of bias in their results (see Chapter 4), with variation in whether outcome assessors were blinded and in the extent of missing outcome data. In the presence of such heterogeneity, to whom would the results of the overall synthesis apply? Meta-analyses are often criticized for mixing apples and oranges, sometimes with good justification. The key to a convincing meta-analysis is to articulate a meaningful underlying question that is adequately addressed

Systematic Reviews in Health Research: Meta-Analysis in Context, Third Edition. Edited by Matthias Egger, Julian P.T. Higgins, and George Davey Smith.
Companion website: www.systematic-reviews3.org

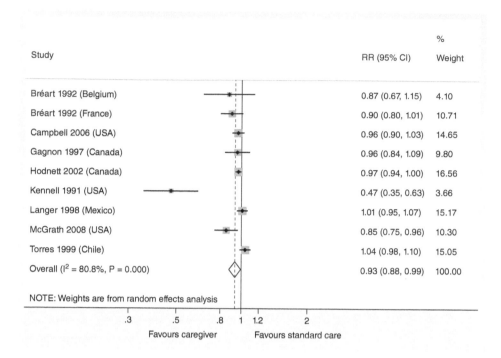

FIGURE 10.1   Meta-analysis of trials comparing the effect of caregiver support with standard care during childbirth on epidural anesthesia use. CI, confidence interval.

by all of the included studies (see Chapter 2). For example, it may be meaningful to ask a question about fruit, in which case mixing apples and oranges, as well as pears and bananas, may be a useful thing to do. Unless a meaningful question exists, the emphasis should be on understanding the differences across the studies.

In this chapter, we explore some of the methods available for exploring heterogeneity in a meta-analysis. These methods should be regarded as central tools, although their implementation needs care to avoid misleading interpretation of their results in practice. The main two approaches are (i) to group the studies into subsets and compare the overall effects across these subsets, an analysis known as *subgroup analysis*; and (ii) to explore the gradient of effects across studies according to one or more numeric study features, an analysis known as *meta-regression*. We also highlight how gathering individual participant data (IPD) from each study provides a stronger basis for exploring how effects vary according to participant characteristics such as age and disease severity, a topic taken forward in Chapter 12.

10.1   CLINICAL, METHODOLOGICAL, AND STATISTICAL VARIABILITY ACROSS STUDIES

It can be helpful to distinguish between three types of variability across studies. The first is variation in the research questions being asked by the different studies, such as the participant groups, the interventions or exposures of interest, and how outcomes or endpoints were defined and measured. The term *clinical diversity* (or sometimes *clinical heterogeneity*) has been used for this type of variability. In the context of a meta-analysis of clinical trials, it relates to variation in the PICOs – Population(s), Intervention(s), Comparator(s), Outcome(s) – of the included studies (see Chapter 2). The second type of variability is in *how* the studies were undertaken. This type of variability includes differences in the study design, e.g. randomized trial versus case–control study, and the conduct of the study, e.g. whether or not outcomes (or exposures) were assessed without knowledge of intervention (or case/control) status. Further, it covers variability in how the data were analyzed (e.g. making different assumptions about missing data). We refer to this as *methodological diversity* (or *methodological heterogeneity*); it refers to different biases operating in different studies.

Clinical and methodological diversity is expected in any meta-analysis. Therefore, it is not surprising to observe that the results of the studies are incompatible with each other. We refer to this third type of variability as *statistical heterogeneity*. Statistical heterogeneity (often abbreviated hereafter to heterogeneity) is due to clinical or methodological diversity across the studies, although the actual causes within these categories may be unknown. Importantly, it is often impossible to determine whether clinical or methodological diversity is the main cause. Both are likely to be present: a re-analysis of 117 meta-analyses of clinical trials estimated that a median of 37% (95% confidence interval 0–71%) of statistical heterogeneity could be explained by bias regarding generation and concealment of the allocation sequence and masking of participants and trial personnel, rather than clinical diversity [2]. Note that clinical and methodological diversity among the studies will not *necessarily* lead to heterogeneity. Heterogeneity only arises when these factors influence the magnitudes of effects estimated by the studies. Nevertheless, it is unusual for no factors to influence the magnitude of an effect unless the intervention or exposure is ineffective or unimportant. Even then, it is likely that methodological diversity will be present, since the different studies may be prone to different biases.

To assess whether (statistical) heterogeneity is present, the imprecision in estimating the effect size from each study, as graphically expressed by the confidence intervals in a forest plot such as Figure 10.1, has to be taken into account. Visual inspection of the forest plot is a convenient first step in identifying heterogeneity. Such inspection should focus on whether there is greater variation between the study results than would be expected by the play of chance. This situation will manifest itself in confidence intervals that do not overlap with each other. As might be surmised from inspection of Figure 10.1, a statistical test for heterogeneity yields a small P value ($\chi^2_8 = 41.7$, $P < 0.001$), with an I^2 statistic of 80.8% (see Chapter 9). This is driven largely by the Kennell study, which stands out with a risk ratio much smaller than all the other studies. The cause of this discrepancy is not clear.

The evidence for statistical heterogeneity is strong among the trials of caregiver support. However, in many meta-analyses such statistical evidence is lacking: the test for heterogeneity fails to reject the null hypothesis (of homogeneity), and the I^2 statistic takes a small value or even 0%. Yet this cannot be interpreted as evidence of homogeneity (that is, total consistency) of the results of all the studies included. A statistically nonsignificant test result should not be interpreted as conclusive evidence in favor of the null hypothesis of homogeneity. Tests of homogeneity have low power when there are few studies in a meta-analysis (as is often the case) and thus may fail to detect genuine heterogeneity [3]. Similarly, I^2 values typically come with substantial uncertainty, and a point value of 0% may be observed in the presence of heterogeneity [4].

It may be tempting to ignore the problems of clinical and methodological diversity when interpreting the results of a meta-analysis if clear evidence of statistical heterogeneity is lacking. However, it is more important to examine the extent and sources of statistical heterogeneity than to look for evidence of its existence. Indeed, some have argued that testing for heterogeneity is largely irrelevant because the studies in any meta-analysis will always be clinically or methodologically diverse [5]. The extent of heterogeneity in a meta-analysis may be measured by estimating the standard deviation (or its square, the variance) of underlying effect sizes across studies. This quantity is often called tau (τ, with variance τ^2) in the meta-analysis literature and is discussed in more detail in Chapter 9.

10.2   REAL AND SPURIOUS HETEROGENEITY

An essential aspect of a meta-analysis should be to consider how the specific differences between studies might impact their results. In a meta-analysis of thrombolysis trials in the acute phase of myocardial infarction, a classic example, the survival benefit was shown to be greater when there was less delay between onset of symptoms and treatment [6]. Quantifying this relation was influential in drawing up policy recommendations for the use of thrombolysis in routine clinical practice. Whereas a key aim of a meta-analysis may be to estimate the average effect seen in studies asking a similar underlying question, plans should be made when writing the meta-analysis protocol for a careful investigation of potential sources of heterogeneity (see Chapter 2).

When faced with heterogeneity, it is important to pause, explore, and identify reasons for it. It can be present for spurious reasons. Data extraction errors are not uncommon. For instance, the direction of effect may accidentally be reversed for a study, or a standard error may be mistaken for a standard deviation, leading to a very narrow confidence interval and a spurious impression of heterogeneity. Thus, it is always wise to check the data, particularly for outlying studies (see Chapter 6). The impact of outlying studies, if found to be error free, can be evaluated by conducting sensitivity analyses with and without them. However, excluding discrepant studies post hoc, solely based on their results without a sound justification, can introduce bias.

Heterogeneity may be present because of the choice of effect measure. Risk differences are unlikely to give consistent estimates of intervention effects. When the risks in the comparison group vary substantially, homogeneous risk ratios or odds ratios will induce heterogeneous risk difference and vice versa. For example, a meta-analysis found that blood pressure–lowering treatment leads to a similar reduction in the risk of cardiovascular events irrespective of baseline cardiovascular risk, but absolute risk reductions, of course, were much larger for those with higher baseline risks [7]. It is crucial always to recognize that heterogeneity observed in a meta-analysis is specific to the choice of effect measure or summary statistic. Ideally, a summary statistic for meta-analysis should be specified in advance (see Chapter 8).

In the following sections of this chapter, we describe subgroup analysis and meta-regression as two useful approaches to understanding the causes of heterogeneity. If the results are considerably different, particularly if the direction of effect is inconsistent, calculating an average effect may be misleading. If attempts to explain heterogeneity are unsuccessful, a standard option is to perform a random-effects meta-analysis to allow for the unexplained variation in effects across studies (see Chapter 9). Note that a random-effects meta-analysis is not a remedy for heterogeneity; it is intended primarily for incorporating heterogeneity that cannot be explained. Further, we should keep in mind that the confidence interval from a random-effects meta-analysis describes uncertainty in the location of the mean of systematically different effects among studies; it does not describe the degree of heterogeneity among them. In contrast, the prediction interval, also covered in Chapter 9, captures the impact of heterogeneity. The prediction interval can be interpreted as a summary of the spread of underlying effects in the studies included in the random-effects meta-analysis, providing there are sufficient studies for the interval to be reasonably accurate.

10.3   SUBGROUP ANALYSIS: DIVIDING THE EVIDENCE INTO SUBSETS

The direction and magnitude of an average effect from a meta-analysis of clinical trials help guide broad clinical practice and policy decisions. Its usefulness depends on the assumption that participants included in the contributing studies represent the people about whom decisions are being made. However, physicians are used to managing patients according to their specific characteristics [8]. It is implausible to assume that the effect of a given treatment is identical across different groups of patients, such as the young and the elderly, or those with mild or severe disease. Therefore, it may seem reasonable to base treatment decisions on the trials that included participants with similar characteristics to the patient under consideration, rather than on the totality of the evidence provided by a meta-analysis.

Decisions based on subgroup analyses are often misleading, however. Consider, for example, the story of the physician in Germany being confronted by the meta-analysis of long-term beta-blockade following myocardial infarction that was presented in Chapter 2. While there was a robust beneficial effect in the overall analysis, in the only large trial recruiting a substantial proportion of German patients, the European Infarction Study (EIS) [9], there was, if anything, a detrimental effect of using beta-blockers. Should the physician prescribe beta-blockers to German post-infarct patients? Common sense would suggest that being German does not prevent a patient from obtaining benefits from beta-blockade. Thus, the best estimate of the outcome for German patients may actually come through essentially discounting the trial carried out in German patients and borrowing information from trials carried out in non-German patients. This may seem paradoxical. Indeed, the statistical expression of this phenomenon is known as Stein's paradox [10] (see Box 10.1).

Box 10.1   Stein's Paradox

Applying the findings from meta-analyses to clinical practice often means that results from a particular trial are disregarded in favor of the overall intervention effect estimate, assuming that the contradictory study results reflect the game of chance. However, even if we assume that the effect in the patients included in a particular study truly differs, the overall estimate may provide the best effect estimate for that patient group, a manifestation of Stein's paradox [10]. In 1955, Charles Stein of Stanford University showed that it is generally better to esti- mate a quantity by also considering the results of related surveys rather than solely focusing on one particular study. His method can be used to show that the regional prevalence of a disease is more accurately estimated, on average, when the results of studies done in other parts of the country are considered. This may seem paradoxical: why should the Oxford data affect what we believe to apply to Bristol? The central principle of Stein's method is to "shrink" the individual data points to the grand mean, i.e. to the average of all the studies. If the Oxford survey gives a higher prevalence than the UK as a whole, then the estimate for Oxford is reduced. Conversely, if the Bristol survey gives a lower prevalence, the figure for Bristol is increased. The amount of such shrinkage depends on the precision of the observed value: an extreme result from a small study is more likely to be due to chance than is a similar result from a large study. A deviant data point measured inaccurately will therefore be shrunk more than an outlier measured with precision. In the case of the beta-blockers trials in myocardial infarction discussed in the main text, the EIS results, which account for only 6.5% of the weight in the meta-analysis, would shrink a long way toward the overall estimate of a beneficial effect of beta-blockade [11].

Deciding whether to be guided by overall effects or by the results for a particular group of study participants is not just a problem created by meta-analysis; it also applies to the interpretation of individual clinical trials [12]. Trialists often spend more time on discussing the results seen within subgroups of patients included in the trial than on the overall results. Yet frequently, the findings of these subgroup analyses fail to be con- firmed by later research. The various trials of beta-blockade after myocardial infarction yielded several subgroup findings with apparent clinical significance [13]. Treatment was said to be beneficial in patients under 65, but harmful in older patients; or only beneficial in patients with anterior myocardial infarction. These findings received no support when examined in subsequent studies [13] or a formal pooling project [14]. This is not surprising: if an overall treatment effect is statistically significant at the 5% level ($P < 0.05$) and the patients are divided at random into two groups, then there is a 1 in 3 chance that the treatment effect will be large and statistically highly significant in one, but small and nonsignificant in the other group [15]. Which subgroup apparently benefits from an intervention is thus often a chance phenomenon, inundating the literature with contradictory findings from subgroup analyses and wrongly inducing clinicians to withhold treatments from some patients [8, 16].

10.3.1   Between-Study and Within-Study Subgroups

In a subgroup analysis, the evidence in a meta-analysis is stratified (or grouped) according to a particular feature or characteristic, and a separate meta-analysis is car- ried out within each subgroup. One option is simply to divide the studies into subsets of studies. This is the only option if the characteristic is genuinely at the study level, e.g. the length of follow-up or the risk of bias. The approach can also be used when the characteristics vary within studies, for example by subgrouping studies according to the average age of participants (see also Section 10.5.2).

Often there are too few trials, or differences in the average characteristics of participants in the trials are too small to subgroup at the level of the study. It may then be possible to consider strata within the trials (e.g. male versus female, or those with or without existing disease). Thus, in a meta-analysis, subgroup analysis may be of subgroups of studies or participants, across or within studies.

10.3.2   Investigating Within-Study Variability through Meta-Analysis

Subgrouping participants within studies requires that data are available for each participant subgroup separately (e.g. men and women), although such data are often lacking in practice. Comparisons of subgroups within studies are common when IPD are collected (see Chapter 12). An IPD meta-analysis of trials of corticosteroids for patients with COVID-19 is shown in Figure 10.2 [17]. In this collaborative meta-analysis, the trialists provided summary data separately for each participant subgroup, allowing consistent stratification by each characteristic. The left-hand side of the plot gives the effect estimate for the subgroups of participants receiving and not receiving invasive mechanical ventilation when they were randomized in each trial, along with meta-analyses for each subgroup. Note that some trials include only patients receiving invasive mechanical ventilation. The right-hand side of the plot shows the preferable way to investigate participant-level characteristics, which is to estimate subgroup differences within studies

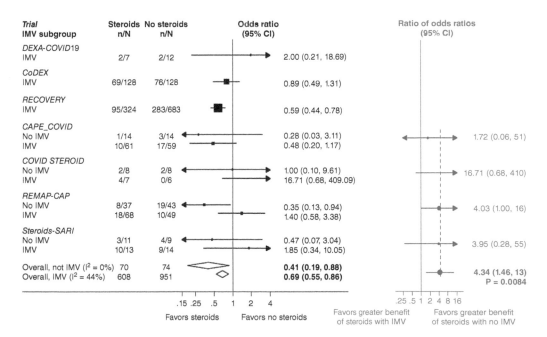

FIGURE 10.2   Within-study subgroup analyses examining the effect of corticosteroids on 28-day mortality in patients critically ill with COVID-19, stratified by whether or not patients received invasive mechanical ventilation (IMV) at the time of randomization. CI, confidence interval; n, deaths; N, total. Source: Redrawn using data from [17].

and combine these across studies, rather than to combine across studies within each subgroup and then take the difference. These issues are further discussed in Chapter 12.

Differences in effects between different subgroups of participants reflect effect modification by the subgrouping characteristic, or interaction between that characteristic and the intervention, on the scale of the effect metric used to perform the analysis. As an aside, we note an alternative approach to detecting effect modification, which has been attracting attention in the meta-analysis literature. It is a meta-analysis based on the outcome's variances rather than the central values [18]. If an intervention interacts with participant characteristics, some participants will see larger impacts on their outcome than others. In a trial comparing the intervention with no intervention, this effect modification will manifest as an increased variability (or variance) of the outcome in the intervention group compared with the control group. Conversely, if an intervention does not interact with participant characteristics, the variances are expected to be similar. Estimating the difference or ratio of variances between the two groups from each trial, and undertaking a meta-analysis of these differences, therefore provides a way to detect effect modification. In one application of this approach across 52 trials of antipsychotic medications for schizophrenia, the variance ratio was 0.97 (95% confidence interval 0.95–0.99) [19]. This small *reduction* in variance was taken as evidence against arguments that patients vary substantially in their response to antipsychotics [19].

10.3.3   Examining Differences between Subgroups

When subgroup analyses are based on subsets of studies, the overall summaries calculated for each subgroup can be inspected for evidence of whether effects vary across the subgroups, which would suggest that the stratifying characteristic is an important source of heterogeneity and so is associated with the magnitude of effect. An inference that the treatment effect differs between two or more subsets of the studies may be based on a formal statistical test. There are several methods to do this. If there are only two subsets, yielding estimates $\hat{\theta}_A$ and $\hat{\theta}_B$ with standard errors $SE\left(\hat{\theta}_A\right)$ and $SE\left(\hat{\theta}_R\right)$, respectively, the statistical evidence for a difference between the two subsets can be examined by considering the Z statistic:

$$Z = \frac{\hat{\theta}_A - \hat{\theta}_B}{\sqrt{\left[SE\left(\hat{\theta}_A\right)\right]^2 + \left[SE\left(\hat{\theta}_B\right)\right]^2}}$$

The Z statistic is then compared with critical values of the normal distribution.

An alternative approach, which can be used regardless of the number of subsets, is to apply the standard test for heterogeneity (see Chapter 9) to examine the evidence for variability across the subsets of studies rather than across individual studies. The meta-analytic result for each subgroup takes the place of the result of each individual study. The test statistic is then compared with critical values of the χ^2 distribution with $S - 1$ degrees of freedom, where S is the number of subgroups.

In a meta-analysis of clinical trials, the stratifying factor is often the type of intervention. For example, a systematic review may include placebo-controlled trials of several drugs, all for the same condition. A meta-analysis may then be stratified by drug, providing an estimate of the intervention effect for each drug separately. Here a test of differences between subgroups effectively involves making indirect comparisons of the effects of the different drugs. A better way to undertake such analyses is network meta-analysis, as discussed in Chapter 13.

10.4   META-REGRESSION

Subgroup analysis is used when studies are grouped into a few categories according to a particular study characteristic. Meta-regression generalizes this idea and can also be used when the characteristic is a continuous measure. Meta-regression is much like standard linear regression. Variation in a response variable (or dependent variable, or outcome variable) is to be explained by one or more predictor variables (variously called covariates, moderators, explanatory variables, or independent variables). In a meta-regression, the response variable is the underlying effect size specific to each study measured as, for example, a mean difference or a (logarithmically transformed) odds ratio. The predictor variables are study features expressed as numeric or categorical variables. Thus, the meta-regression seeks to explain variation in effect sizes (i.e. heterogeneity) according to key study characteristics.

Berkey and colleagues introduced meta-regression methods in 1995, illustrating them using studies of the effectiveness of the Bacillus Calmette–Guérin (BCG) vaccine against tuberculosis from different parts of the world [20]. There was reason to believe that the vaccine might be less effective in warmer climates. Using each study location's latitude (i.e. its distance from the equator) as a surrogate for climate, we can depict the relationship in a scatter plot, as illustrated in Figure 10.3. The X-axis represents the predictor variable (i.e. latitude of the study) and the Y-axis the effect estimate of the vaccine efficacy (i.e. log risk ratio). The regression coefficient obtained from the meta-regression analysis describes how the response variable changes with a one-unit increase in the continuous predictor variable. In the BCG vaccine example, the coefficient for latitude is −0.029, which means that every 1° of latitude corresponds to a decrease of 0.029 unit in log risk ratio (or multiplication by 0.971 of the risk ratio). The confidence interval around the regression coefficient can be used to evaluate whether there is a robust relationship between the (transformed) model's performance and the predictor variable. The analysis of the BCG vaccine trials has become a textbook example of meta-regression, because it provides a compelling case of variability in effects being well explained by a single predictor variable. In practice, meta-regression analyses are often less clean, with study-level predictor variables failing to provide good explanations of heterogeneity and several potential predictors competing for such a role.

10.4.1   Meta-Regression: Technicalities

For the same reasons that simple meta-analyses use weighted averages, meta-regression analyses should be based on weighted regression. Also, in common with simple meta-analyses, meta-regression can be performed under either a fixed-effect model or a random-effects model (see Chapter 9). However, in most cases the latter is much to be

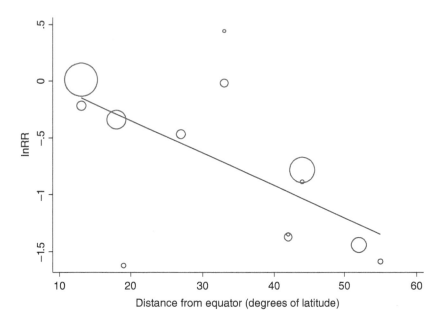

FIGURE 10.3   Meta-regression analysis using latitude to explain variation in log risk ratio of Bacillus Calmette–Guérin vaccine efficacy among 13 randomized trials. lnRR, log risk ratio. In the regression model, the absolute latitude is centered at the mean 33.4615. Source: Based on [19].

preferred. Simulation studies have shown that fixed-effect meta-regression analyses have a considerably greater risk of false-positive findings regarding the impact of the predictor variable(s) [21]. Furthermore, if heterogeneity is present among studies in a meta-analysis, it is usually considered unlikely that the specific predictor variables included in the model will account for it entirely. Therefore, meta-regression analyses are generally undertaken using a random-effects model.

In a random-effects meta-regression, the variance of each effect estimate has two components: the within-study variance (which is specific to the study) and the residual among-studies variance (which is common to all studies in the meta-analysis). The within-study variance is the same as that used in standard meta-analysis. For example, in the case of log odds ratios, the within-study variance is simply estimated as the sum of the reciprocal cell counts in the 2×2 table for that study (see Chapter 8). The among-studies variance represents the residual heterogeneity of effects; that is, the variability between true effects across studies not explained by the predictor variable. Specifically, it refers to the distribution of effects for studies with the same predictor variable(s) value.

To be explicit, consider the analysis presented in Figure 10.4. It shows the results of nine clinical trials of aerobic exercise interventions to reduce pain in people with knee osteoarthritis. The interest here is in examining whether the effectiveness of the exercise intervention depends on the number of supervised exercise sessions, a study-level predictor variable. We index the trials by $i = 1, \ldots, 9$. For the ith trial, we denote the observed standardized mean difference (SMD) in the pain score by y_i, its estimated within-trial variance by v_i, and the number of sessions by x_i. The linear regression of the SMD in pain score on the number of sessions can be expressed as $y_i = \alpha + \beta x_i$. We are not forcing the regression through the origin, and α represents the intercept of the regression line.

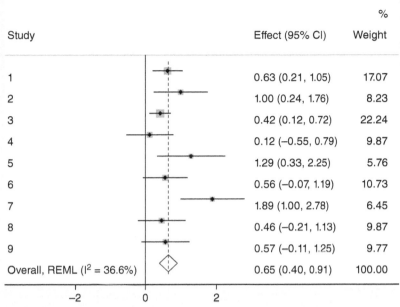

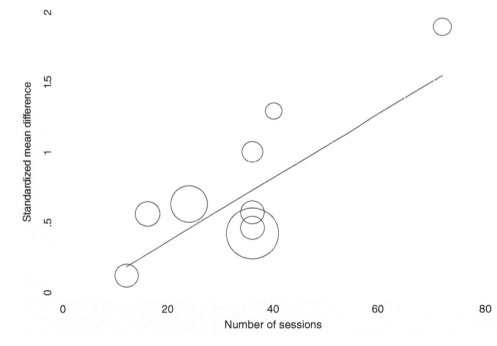

FIGURE 10.4   Meta-regression analysis using the number of sessions to explain variation in the standardized mean differences (SMD) in pain scores among nine randomized trials of aerobic exercise interventions in people with knee osteoarthritis. CI, confidence interval; REML, restricted maximum likelihood.

TABLE 10.1   Meta-regression results using the number of sessions to explain variation in standardized mean differences (SMD) in pain scores among nine randomized trials of aerobic exercise interventions in people with knee osteoarthritis.

Coefficient	Estimate	95% confidence interval[a]	P value[a]
Intercept, α	−0.087	−0.799–0.626	0.78
Impact of an additional session, β	0.023	0.002–0.043	0.04

Heterogeneity statistics

Residual among-studies variance[b] ($\tau^2_{unexplained}$): 0.028
   I^2 (residual): 10.9%
Adjusted R^2: 45.2%

[a] Using Hartung–Knapp adjustment.
[b] Restricted maximum likelihood estimate.

The purpose of the analysis is to provide estimates of α and β, together with their confidence intervals. The meta-regression analysis yields the results in Table 10.1. The interpretation of the β coefficient is as follows: for every 1 unit increase in supervised exercise session (i.e. for each additional session), there is a 0.023 unit increase in the SMD for pain. The 95% confidence interval for this improvement ranges from 0.002 to 0.043.

The weights for the regression are equal to $1/\left(v_i + \hat{\tau}^2\right)$, where $\hat{\tau}^2 = 0.028$ is the estimated residual heterogeneity variance. There are several ways of estimating τ^2. The restricted maximum likelihood (REML) estimate is often recommended [22, 23] and is used here. An intuitive interpretation of the estimate of τ^2 is not straightforward. However, we can consider its meaning for a particular prediction from the model. Consider the predicted SMD for pain in a trial running 20 sessions, which is estimated as $-0.087 + 0.023 \times 20 = 0.37$. Given the heterogeneity between studies expressed by τ^2, the 95% range of true SMDs for different studies is approximately $-0.087 + 0.023 \times 20 \pm 1.96 \times \sqrt{0.028}$; that is, from 0.05 to 0.70.

Programs to carry out such random-effects weighted regression analyses are available in various software packages, including Stata, R, and Comprehensive Meta-analysis (see Chapters 25–27). Note that these analyses are not the same as the usual weighted regression where weights are inversely proportional to the variances. In addition, assumptions of linearity of predictor variable effects or normality of the residual variation between trial results can be difficult to assess in practice [24].

10.4.2   Subgroup Analysis Is a Special Case of Meta-Regression

Subgroup analyses in which studies are grouped into subsets can be formulated as a meta-regression. To perform such a subgroup analysis as a meta-regression, $S-1$ dummy variables are created to indicate membership of the S subgroups in the standard manner used in multiple regression. The coefficients estimated for each of these dummy variables provide an estimate of the differences between the overall effect in the respective subgroup compared with the reference subgroup (which has no dummy variable). If the subgroup categories are ordered, then meta-regression may be used to test for a trend by denoting group membership by a single variable indicating the ranked order of each subgroup.

10.4.3   Proportion of Variance Explained

A useful question is how much the between-study heterogeneity is reduced by taking into account the predictor variable(s). In meta-regression (and subgroup analysis formulated as meta-regression), we can define a statistic R^2 (sometimes referred to as "adjusted R^2") as the proportion of total heterogeneity variance explained by predictor variables. The total variance is the variance estimated in a standard meta-analysis that ignores the predictor variables; we shall call this τ^2_{total} here. The R^2 statistic is defined as:

$$R^2 = \frac{\tau^2_{explained}}{\tau^2_{total}}$$

or, equivalently,

$$R^2 = 1 - \left(\frac{\tau^2_{unexplained}}{\tau^2_{total}} \right),$$

where $\tau^2_{unexplained}$ is the variance that remains after accounting for the impact of the predictor variable(s) in the meta-regression model (referred to as τ^2 in Section 10.4.1). Using the knee osteoarthritis example, the τ^2_{total} for the full set of studies turns out to be 0.051 (using REML), and $\tau^2_{unexplained}$ after running the meta-regression was 0.028. So

$$R^2 = 1 - \left(\frac{0.028}{0.051} \right) = 0.45.$$

The interpretation is that the number of exercise sessions explains approximately 45% of the between-studies variance. In general, R^2 ranges from 0 to 1 (or 0 to 100%) and describes the percent reduction in true variance, analogous to the R^2 index used in regression analyses of primary studies.

10.4.4   Extensions to Meta-Regression

Imaginative coding of predictor variables in meta-regression can make efficient use of meta-analytic evidence to answer novel questions, particularly about the effects of interventions. An example is provided by a meta-analysis addressing the impact of drinking-water sanitation on childhood diarrheal disease in low- and middle-income settings [25]. Several water supply characteristics were examined: whether or not the water source was treated by chlorine, solar, or filters; and levels and quality of piped water supply into the premises. Each of these characteristics was represented by a predictor in a meta-regression model. The specific intervention in each study could then be coded as a combination of the predictors. The meta-regression model enabled indirect estimation of sanitation approaches that had not been directly observed, following the ideas of network meta-analysis (Chapter 13). This approach is increasingly popular to examine complex interventions [26] and is sometimes known as component network meta-analysis. In a meta-analysis addressing psychological preparation for surgery, this approach allowed the authors to derive estimates of the effects of the individual components of the psychological interventions, even when delivered in combination [27]. These models can further explore whether the component effects are additive or whether there are interactions between them [28, 29].

10.5   PRACTICAL PROBLEMS IN THE EXPLORATION OF HETEROGENEITY

10.5.1   Correlated Predictor Variables and Causal Conclusions

Associations between study characteristics and study results are observational and are subject to confounding. Study-level confounding occurs when an association observed between a study characteristic and the effect size arises not because one causes the other, but because a third study characteristic is a common cause of variation in both the characteristic of interest and the effect size. For example, drug trials and diet trials may have different degrees of success in lowering cholesterol. However, this may be due to differences in baseline cholesterol levels rather than due to the type of intervention. In practice, it can be challenging to tell which aspect of a study (e.g. type of intervention, baseline characteristics, risk of bias) is the cause of any difference in effect estimates.

A related problem arises from the correlation between study characteristics. For example, in a meta-regression analysis of total mortality outcomes of cholesterol-lowering trials, various factors appeared to influence the outcome: greater cholesterol reduction led to greater benefit; trials including participants at a higher level of coronary heart disease risk showed larger mortality reductions; and the fibrate drugs led to less benefit than other interventions [30, 31]. These findings were difficult to interpret since the variables included were strongly correlated: the fibrate trials recruited lower-risk participants, and fibrates lowered cholesterol less than statins. In this situation, all the problems of performing multivariable analyses with correlated predictor variables are introduced [32].

10.5.2   Aggregating Participant-Level Predictor Variables at the Study Level

Subgroup analysis or meta-regression that uses averages of participant characteristics in each study (such as the average age of all the participants) can give misleading results. It is tempting to interpret the relationship between average age and effect size as if it applies to individual participants. This may, however, not be the case because of *aggregation bias* (sometimes called the "ecological fallacy") [33]. Aggregation bias can arise when aggregate data for a group are used to make inferences about individuals. For example, suppose that all studies had the same average age. In that case, any age dependence of an intervention effect will be missed, yielding a coefficient of zero in the regression analysis and the impression that age might not be important.

Evidence about the modifying effect of a participant-level characteristic is most robust when the characteristic varies substantially within studies, and the individual (within-study) data are available to the meta-analyst. Study characteristics that vary between studies only can be assessed at the study level and are more prone to confounding by other study-level factors.

10.5.3   Spurious Findings and Undetected Associations

Subgroup analysis and meta-regression can readily generate spurious findings, particularly when there are few studies [21]. Suppose two studies produce estimates with nonoverlapping confidence intervals. Then any factor that differs between studies will be strongly related to the "heterogeneity" between the studies, and hence a potential explanation of it. Many of the explanations will not be biologically or clinically plausible. We could, for example, take the star sign of the first author. The likelihood of a false-positive result is greatest when there are few studies and substantial heterogeneity. In such situations, a permutation may be considered instead of the standard parametric test [34].

False associations are also more likely when many predictor variables are included. Indeed, performing multiple analyses is a major concern for spurious findings. The rule of thumb that 10 or 20 observations should be available per predictor variable should be observed. The numbers indicated by these rules of thumb may not be sufficient if the predictor variables are unevenly distributed across studies, for example if most of the studies are very similar in their characteristics or most of the variation is observed in a small proportion of them. If more than one or two characteristics are included in the model, adjustments for multiplicity might be considered. Different techniques are available, including correction of P values, testing all candidate characteristics simultaneously, or using shrinkage estimators [35, 36]. More importantly, only a few scientifically justified characteristics should be selected for subgroup analysis or meta-regression. The credibility of a result is strengthened when such factors and their direction of effect are hypothesized a priori.

10.5.4   Statistical Artefacts when Investigating Small-Study Effects and Underlying Risk

Two particular sources of heterogeneity can lead to statistical problems when investigated without due care. The first is study size. Small-study effects (see Chapter 5) refer to the phenomenon that smaller studies show different, often more beneficial, effects of interventions than larger studies. A common method of investigating small-study effects is to examine the relationship between the effect estimates and their precisions, for example expressed as standard errors. This is the basis of the Egger test, which is widely used [37]. In principle, small-study effects will lead to the situation where larger effect estimates are associated with larger standard errors. Unfortunately, in some situations an artefactual correlation is present between effect estimates and their standard errors, simply because they are computed from the same data and not because of any genuine small-study effects [38]. This issue led to the development of other tests for small-study effects, as discussed in Chapter 5 (Section 5.4.5).

Similar problems occur when examining the association between intervention effects and baseline risk. If the baseline risk is measured by the risks observed in the control groups of trials and a meta-regression, e.g. of the log odds ratios on the risks of the control groups, is performed, then a spurious association will emerge because both are calculated from the same 2×2 table. Specifically, a trial that observes a higher control group risk by chance alone will also observe a smaller odds ratio due to the same chance phenomenon. Similarly, a trial that observes a lower control group risk by chance alone will also observe a larger odds ratio. This will result in the impression of an association between the odds ratios and the baseline risks across trials, but drawing such an inference would be a spurious finding due to this statistical artefact [39, 40].

10.6   CLOSING REMARKS

Sources of heterogeneity in meta-analysis should always be investigated. In some types of meta-analysis, the focus is almost exclusively on understanding heterogeneity, with relatively little interest in overall average effects (see also Chapter 19). However, attempting to explore possible reasons for heterogeneity can come with overinterpretation, because such investigations are often inspired, at least to some extent, by looking at the results at hand. Moreover, apparent heterogeneity may be due to chance and searching for its causes would then be misleading. The problem is akin to that of subgroup analyses within an individual clinical trial. However, the degree of clinical and methodological diversity across different studies is greater than within individual studies and represents a more serious problem.

Guidelines for deciding whether to believe results from investigating heterogeneity depend on, for example, the magnitude and strength of evidence for the differences identified, the extent to which the potential sources of heterogeneity have been specified in advance, and indirect evidence and biological considerations that support the investigation [41, 42]. The risk of overinterpretation is greatest when there are many differences between studies, but only a few studies are available. There may be several alternative explanations for statistical heterogeneity in such situations, and ideas about sources of heterogeneity can be considered only as hypotheses for evaluation in future studies.

ACKNOWLEDGMENTS

This chapter draws on material from chapters by Simon G. Thompson ("Why and how sources of heterogeneity should be investigated"), George Davey Smith and Matthias Egger ("Going beyond the grand mean: subgroup analyses in meta-analysis of randomized controlled trials"), and Jonathan J. Deeks, Douglas G. Altman, and Michael

J. Bradburn ("Statistical methods for examining heterogeneity and combining results from several studies in meta-analysis") published in the second edition of this book.

REFERENCES

1. Bohren, M.A., Hofmeyr, G.J., Sakala, C. et al. (2017). Continuous support for women during childbirth. *Cochrane Database Syst. Rev.* 7 (7): CD003766. https://doi.org/10.1002/14651858.CD003766.pub6.

2. Rhodes, K.M., Turner, R.M., Savovic, J. et al. (2018). Between-trial heterogeneity in meta-analyses may be partially explained by reported design characteristics. *J. Clin. Epidemiol.* 95: 45–54.

3. Hedges, L.V. and Pigott, T.D. (2001). The power of statistical tests in meta-analysis. *Psychol. Methods* 6: 203–217.

4. Higgins, J.P.T. and Thompson, S.G. (2002). Quantifying heterogeneity in a meta-analysis. *Stat. Med.* 21: 1539–1558.

5. Higgins, J.P.T., Thompson, S.G., Deeks, J.J., and Altman, D.G. (2003). Measuring inconsistency in meta-analysis. *BMJ* 327: 557–560.

6. Boersma, E., Maas, A.C., Deckers, J.W., and Simoons, M.L. (1996). Early thrombolytic treatment in acute myocardial infarction: reappraisal of the golden hour. *Lancet* 348: 771–775.

7. Blood Pressure Lowering Treatment Trialists C (2014). Blood pressure-lowering treatment based on cardiovascular risk: a meta-analysis of individual patient data. *Lancet* 384: 591–598.

8. Davey Smith, G. and Egger, M. (1998). Incommunicable knowledge? Interpreting and applying the results of clinical trials and meta-analyses [see comments]. *J. Clin. Epidemiol.* 51: 289–295.

9. (1984). European Infarction Study (E.I.S.). A secondary prevention study with slow release oxprenolol after myocardial infarction: morbidity and mortality. *Eur. Heart J.* 5: 189–202.

10. Efron, B. and Morris, C. (1977). Stein's paradox in statistics. *Sci. Am.* 236: 119–127.

11. Stijnen, T. and Van Houwelingen, J.C. (1990). Empirical Bayes methods in clinical trials meta-analysis. *Biom. J.* 32: 335–346.

12. Oxman, A.D. and Guyatt, G.H. (1992). A consumer's guide to subgroup analyses. *Ann. Intern. Med.* 116: 78–84.

13. Yusuf, S., Wittes, J., Probstfield, J., and Tyroler, H.A. (1991). Analysis and interpretation of treatment effects in subgroups of patients in randomized clinical trials. *J. Am. Med. Assoc.* 266: 93–98.

14. (1988). The Beta-Blocker Pooling Project (BBPP): subgroup findings from randomized trials in post infarction patients. The Beta-Blocker Pooling Project Research Group. *Eur. Heart J.* 9: 8–16.

15. Ingelfinger, J.A., Mosteller, F., Thibodeau, L.A., and Ware, J.H. (1994). *Biostatistics in Clinical Medicine*. New York: McGraw-Hill.

16. Buyse, M.E. (1989). Analysis of clinical trial outcomes: some comments on subgroup analyses. *Control. Clin. Trials* 10: 187S–194S.

17. WHO Rapid Evidence Appraisal for COVID-19 Therapies Working Group, Sterne, J.A.C., Murthy, S. et al. (2020). Association between administration of systemic corticosteroids and mortality among critically ill patients with COVID-19: a meta-analysis. *JAMA* 324: 1330–1341.

18. Mills, H.L., Higgins, J.P.T., Morris, R.W. et al. (2021). Detecting heterogeneity of intervention effects using analysis and meta-analysis of differences in variance between trial arms. *Epidemiology* **32** (6): 846–854.

19. Winkelbeiner, S., Leucht, S., Kane, J.M., and Homan, P. (2019). Evaluation of differences in individual treatment response in schizophrenia spectrum disorders: a meta-analysis. *JAMA Psychiatry* 76: 1063–1073.

20. Berkey, C.S., Hoaglin, D.C., Mosteller, F., and Colditz, G.A. (1995). A random-effects regression model for meta-analysis. *Stat. Med.* 14: 395–411.

21. Higgins, J.P.T. and Thompson, S.G. (2004). Controlling the risk of spurious findings from meta-regression. *Stat. Med.* 23: 1663–1682.

22. Thompson, S.G. and Sharp, S.J. (1999). Explaining heterogeneity in meta-analysis: a comparison of methods. *Stat. Med.* 18: 2693–2708.

23. Langan, D., Higgins, J.P.T., Jackson, D. et al. (2019). A comparison of heterogeneity variance estimators in simulated random-effects meta-analyses. *Res. Synth. Methods* 10: 83–98.

24. Hardy, R.J. and Thompson, S.G. (1998). Detecting and describing heterogeneity in meta-analysis. *Stat. Med.* 17: 841–856.

25. Wolf, J., Hunter, P.R., Freeman, M.C. et al. (2018). Impact of drinking water, sanitation and handwashing with soap on childhood diarrhoeal disease: updated meta-analysis and meta-regression. *Tropical Med. Int. Health* 23: 508–525.

26. Higgins, J.P.T., López-López, J.A., Becker, B.J. et al. (2018). Synthesising quantitative evidence in systematic reviews of complex health interventions. *BMJ Glob. Health* 4: e000858.

27. Freeman, S.C., Scott, N.W., Powell, R. et al. (2018). Component network meta-analysis identifies the most effective components of psychological preparation for adults undergoing surgery under general anesthesia. *J. Clin. Epidemiol.* 98: 105–116.

28. Welton, N.J., Caldwell, D.M., Adamopoulos, E., and Vedhara, K. (2009). Mixed treatment comparison meta-analysis of complex interventions: psychological interventions in coronary heart disease. *Am. J. Epidemiol.* 169: 1158–1165.

29. Caldwell, D.M. and Welton, N.J. (2016). Approaches for synthesising complex mental health interventions in meta-analysis. *Evid. Based Ment. Health* 19: 16–21.

30. Holme, I. (1996). Relationship between total mortality and cholesterol reduction as found by meta-regression analysis of randomized cholesterol- lowering trials. *Control. Clin. Trials* 17: 13–22.

31. Davey Smith, G. (1997). Low blood cholesterol and non-atherosclerotic disease mortality: where do we stand? *Eur. Heart J.* 18: 6–9.

32. Davey Smith, G. and Phillips, A.N. (1992). Confounding in epidemiological studies: why "independent" effects may not be all they seem. *BMJ* 305: 757–759.

33. Piantadosi, S., Byar, D.P., and Green, S.B. (1988). The ecological fallacy. *Am. J. Epidemiol.* 127: 893–904.

34. Higgins, J., Thompson, S., Deeks, J., and Altman, D. (2002). Statistical heterogeneity in systematic reviews of clinical trials: a critical appraisal of guidelines and practice. *J. Health Serv. Res. Policy* 7: 51–61.

35. Bender, R., Bunce, C., Clarke, M. et al. (2008). Attention should be given to multiplicity issues in systematic reviews. *J. Clin. Epidemiol.* 61: 857–865.

36. Efthimiou, O. and White, I.R. (2020). The dark side of the force: multiplicity issues in network meta-analysis and how to address them. *Res. Synth. Methods* 11: 105–122.

37. Egger, M., Davey Smith, G., Schneider, M., and Minder, C. (1997). Bias in meta-analysis detected by a simple, graphical test. *BMJ* 315: 629–634.

38. Irwig, L., Macaskill, P., Berry, G., and Glasziou, P. (1998). Bias in meta-analysis detected by a simple, graphical test. Graphical test is itself biased [letter; comment]. *BMJ* 316: 470.

39. Thompson, S.G., Smith, T.C., and Sharp, S.J. (1997). Investigating underlying risk as a source of heterogeneity in meta-analysis. *Stat. Med.* 16: 2741–2758.

40. Sharp, S.J. and Thompson, S.G. (2000). Analysing the relationship between treatment benefit and underlying risk in meta-analysis: comparison and development of approaches. *Stat. Med.* 19: 3251–3274.

41. Deeks, J.J., Higgins, J.P.T., and Altman, D.G. (2019). Analysing data and undertaking meta-analyses. In: *Cochrane Handbook for Systematic Reviews of Interventions* (ed. J.P.T. Higgins, J. Thomas, J. Chandler, et al.), 241–284. Chichester: Wiley.

42. Schandelmaier, S., Briel, M., Varadhan, R. et al. (2020). Development of the instrument to assess the credibility of effect modification analyses (ICEMAN) in randomized controlled trials and meta-analyses. *CMAJ* 192: E901–E906.

CHAPTER 11

Dealing with Missing Outcome Data in Meta-Analysis

Ian R. White and Dimitris Mavridis

This chapter addresses the inclusion of studies with incomplete outcome data in a meta-analysis. Missing data are not only a threat to the validity of the analysis of a single study [1], they can threaten the validity of a meta-analysis. Yet more attention is often paid to missing data in the analysis of single studies than in meta-analysis. This chapter explores what we may know about missing data, describes the analysis options in single studies, discusses the methods available in meta-analysis, and makes suggestions for practice with a primary focus on aggregate data meta-analysis. A modified version of this chapter was previously published [2].

This chapter does not address meta-analyses in which entire studies are missing, or studies within which particular outcomes are unreported. These issues are addressed in Chapter 5. Throughout this chapter, the term *missing data* refers only to missing outcome data. We discuss the consequences of missing data for randomized controlled trials (RCTs) without adjustment for baseline covariates. The methods discussed here could equally be used in an observational study such as a genetic study in which adjustment for confounders is unnecessary.

11.1 ANALYSIS OF A SINGLE STUDY WITH MISSING DATA

An RCT sets the standard for testing the efficacy of an intervention. Randomizing with high numbers tends toward equal distribution of prognostic factors across arms, so that we have confidence that any systematic difference in outcome can be attributed

Systematic Reviews in Health Research: Meta-Analysis in Context, Third Edition. Edited by Matthias Egger, Julian P.T. Higgins, and George Davey Smith.
© 2022 John Wiley & Sons Ltd. Published 2022 by John Wiley & Sons Ltd.
Companion website: www.systematic-reviews3.org

to the intervention. But participants can, for example, drop out, and under certain circumstances missing data may introduce bias and yield misleading conclusions. The problem is well recognized and many methods have been suggested to account for missing data in RCTs [3–6].

The intention to treat (ITT) principle requires all participants in an RCT to be included in the analysis in the arm to which they were randomized, to preserve randomization and avoid bias introduced by dropout and protocol deviations [7]. However, there is no consensus on how to perform ITT analysis when outcomes are missing [8]. Some argue that the ITT principle requires missing values be imputed using methods such as last observation carried forward (LOCF) or multiple imputation [9].

From a statistical perspective, any analysis of a study with missing data makes an assumption about the missing data. A principled approach starts by considering what assumption is plausible and chooses a suitable primary analysis [10]. The validity of the analysis rests on the plausibility of its assumptions, not on whether or not missing values were imputed. Sensitivity analyses are then needed to explore how robust the results are to plausible deviations from the assumption in the primary analysis. These ideas lead to an ITT analysis strategy, which emphasizes the inclusion of all randomized participants in sensitivity analyses [11].

Assumptions about missing data are often described using Rubin's framework [12]. Data are missing completely at random (MCAR) if missing data have the same distribution as observed data. For example, blood pressure data are likely to be MCAR if they are missing due to breakdown of an automatic sphygmomanometer [5]. Data are missing at random (MAR) if missing data have the same distribution as observed data, conditional on other variables included in the analysis. For example, blood pressure data are likely to be MAR if age, but no other factor, predicts blood pressure measurement. Finally, if data are not MAR then they are missing not at random (MNAR) or informatively missing (IM). For example, blood pressure data are likely to be MNAR if, within age groups, the outcomes for participants who dropped out might be worse than those for participants with observed outcomes. However, other assumptions are possible: for example, the assumption underlying an LOCF analysis is that missing values do not differ on average from last observed values, which does not fit neatly into the MCAR/MAR/MNAR framework.

In practice, the starting point of an analysis is usually to ignore missing data in an available case analysis (ACA), also called a complete case analysis. This assumes that data are MAR. If instead the data are MNAR, then ACA risks bias in the intervention effect, especially if dropout rates vary between arms [13].

Several approaches have been suggested to handle missing data in clinical trials. Some of the most popular methods are summarized in Table 11.1.

11.2   META-ANALYSIS WITH MISSING DATA

Inappropriate analysis with missing data in RCTs leads to biased meta-analytic estimates. The meta-analyst therefore faces four tasks.

TABLE 11.1   Methods for handling missing outcome data in clinical trials.

Method	Description	Assumptions about missing outcome data	Use in meta-analysis
Available case analysis	Ignores missing participants	MAR	Common starting point in AD and IPD meta-analysis
Single imputation methods for binary data			
Impute failure	Imputes missing values as failures	Always failures	Possible starting point in AD and IPD meta-analysis (e.g. smoking cessation trials)
Worst-(best-) case scenario	Imputes failures in the treatment arm and successes in the control (or vice versa)	Always failures or always successes depending on arm	Extreme assumption in AD and IPD meta-analysis that may be useful in sensitivity analysis
Single imputation methods for all data			
Last observation carried forward	Imputes missing values with the participants' last observation	The missing value for a participant has the same mean as the last observed value	Often used in trial reports, and hence also in AD meta-analysis; can be avoided in IPD meta-analysis. Usually an unrealistic assumption; can underestimate uncertainty [14]
Single imputation	Imputes missing values, usually borrowing information from observed outcomes (not necessarily from the same arm or study)	Missing values equal a pre-specified value without uncertainty	Does not take uncertainty in the imputed values into account
Methods that take uncertainty into account			
Multiple imputation	Builds a model to predict missing outcome from the participants' observed outcome, and adds appropriate random error [15]	MAR	Useful in IPD meta-analysis but rarely used with AD
Likelihood methods	Fits a model to the observed data	MAR	Useful in IPD meta-analysis but rarely used with AD
	Fits a model to the observed data and the probability of being missing	MNAR	Hard to implement but potentially useful in IPD meta-analysis

TABLE 11.1   (*Continued*)

Method	Description	Assumptions about missing outcome data	Use in meta-analysis
Pattern mixture model	Builds a model for the outcome conditional on whether it is missing or not and a model for the missingness mechanism [13]	Addresses departures from the MAR assumption (MNAR)	Useful in AD and IPD meta-analysis. The relation between missing and observed outcomes can be informed by expert opinion or by a sensitivity analysis

AD, aggregate data; IPD, individual participant data; MAR, missing at random; MNAR, missing not at random.

11.2.1   Understand the Extent of Missing Data in Each Included Study

Standard data extraction yields the number of individuals analyzed in each arm with summary statistics (count, or mean and standard deviation). To allow for missing data, we also need to know at least the number of study participants with missing data in each arm. The CONSORT statement expects reporting of the number of participants who were randomly assigned, and the number of participants in each arm included in each analysis [16]. This is usually available from the participant flow diagram (CONSORT diagram), which should report the number lost to follow-up. It is also usually available in results tables, where the numbers analyzed should be reported. Surveys have shown that 95% of trials in major medical journals report some missing outcome data [17] and 94% of palliative care trials report the number of participants not included in the primary outcome analysis [18]. Systematic reviews have lower rates of reporting numbers of participants with missing data: 47% of Cochrane reviews and 7% of non-Cochrane reviews [19].

When possible, the number of missing values in each arm should be broken down by the reasons why the data are missing: for example, the number of missing values that were due to loss to follow-up and the number that were due to disillusioned patients withdrawing from a trial (which are likely to be MNAR with worse outcomes than those observed). The meta-analyst needs to define a classification of reasons to make results comparable between studies. If the outcome in the review is a trial's secondary outcome, it may be necessary to use reasons reported for the trial's primary outcome, which are likely to be better reported.

As an example, we use a meta-analysis of studies comparing haloperidol with placebo in the treatment of schizophrenia [20]. The outcome is coded as success or failure on the basis of clinical improvement. Information about missing values was extracted and analyzed by Higgins and colleagues [21], and reproduced in Table 11.2. Two studies have particularly large numbers of missing values; this may be because other studies imputed missing outcomes without reporting their numbers. Table 11.2 also tabulates reasons for missing data using codes explained below.

TABLE 11.2 Haloperidol meta-analysis: main results and reasons for missing data. In some cases, reasons refer to a different outcome.

First author	Year	Main results data						Reasons for missing data							
		Haloperidol arm			Placebo arm			Haloperidol arm				Placebo arm			
		Successes	Failures	Missing	Successes	Failures	Missing	ICA-0	ICA-1	ICA-p_c	ICA-p	ICA-0	ICA-1	ICA-p_c	ICA-p
Arvanitis	1997	25	25	2	18	33	0	17	0	17	0	30	0	5	0
Beasley	1996	29	18	22	20	14	34	19	0	15	5	32	0	13	1
Bechelli	1983	12	17	1	2	28	1	0	0	0	1	0	0	0	1
Borison	1992	3	9	0	0	12	0	0	0	0	0	0	0	0	0
Chouinard	1993	10	11	0	3	19	0	11	0	2	0	10	0	6	0
Durost	1964	11	8	0	1	14	0	0	0	0	0	0	0	0	0
Garry	1962	7	18	1	4	21	1	0	0	1	0	0	0	1	0
Howard	1974	8	9	0	3	10	0	0	0	0	0	0	0	0	0
Marder	1994	19	45	2	14	50	2	25	0	0	13	41	0	0	4
Nishikawa	1982	1	9	0	0	10	0	0	0	0	0	0	0	0	0
Nishikawa	1984	11	23	3	0	13	0		0	0		0	0	0	0
Reschke	1974	20	9	0	2	9	0	0	0	0	2	6	0	0	0
Selman	1976	17	1	11	7	4	18	4	0	0	7	8	0	0	10
Serafetinides	1972	4	10	0	0	13	1	0	0	0	0	1	0	0	0
Simpson	1967	2	14	0	0	7	1	0	0	0	0		0	0	
Spencer	1992	11	1	0	1	11	0	0	0	0	0	0	0	0	0
Vichaiya	1971	9	20	1	0	29	1	0	0	0	1	0	0	0	1

Abbreviations are explained in Section 11.3.

11.2.2   Understand How the Missing Data were Handled in Each Published Report

The quality of published analyses can be hard to judge: studies typically report results from ACA or from some simple imputation method, but reporting of methods used can be poor. For example, in 2000 only 34% of studies in PubMed reported the handling of attrition [22], but by 2013 methods could be classified in 100% of trials in major medical journals [17].

Errors can arise by misunderstanding how data were handled. For example, a meta-analysis of the effectiveness of brief interventions targeting excessive drinkers in general practice set out to regard missing values as failures (thus giving a lower bound to the success rate) [23], but was overzealous: one study's reported results included all participants, with missing values imputed as failures, but the reviewers took this study as reporting only available cases and applied a further correction [24].

11.2.3   Evaluate the Risk of Bias Due to Missing Data in Each Published Report

Participants in a focus group reported that the risk of bias due to incomplete outcome data was more difficult to assess than other biases [25]. The Cochrane Risk of Bias tool includes risk of bias due to missing data [26]. The original version of the Cochrane tool asked assessors to describe the completeness of outcome data for each outcome, the numbers in each intervention arm (compared with total randomized participants), and the reasons for attrition or exclusions. The revised version of the tool asks assessors to think specifically about whether a missing outcome is likely to depend on its true value [26]. See Chapter 4 for more details.

11.2.4   Perform Alternative Analyses Exploring the Impact of the Missing Data under Different Assumptions

This is the main focus of this chapter. Valid statistical methods are needed to account for missing outcome data in meta-analysis, and several methods have been suggested [27]. As well as correcting for bias in individual studies and inflating the standard error of the pooled estimate to allow for uncertainty about missing data, we also aim to change the weights assigned to studies to reflect which studies are more uncertain. Studies with high missing rates should be penalized relatively more when pooled in a meta-analysis because their effect estimates are more likely to be biased (under MNAR).

The primary analysis is commonly an ACA; a sensitivity analysis is then needed to explore the impact of departures from the MAR assumption implied in an ACA on the point estimate and its standard error. The methods we propose are primarily intended to be used in such a sensitivity analysis. However, in a meta-analysis in which bias from missing data is a serious concern, the methods proposed could form a primary analysis.

In this chapter, we assume we have access only to aggregate data (AD), so we cannot use all the methods presented in Table 11.1 (e.g. multiple imputation). If we have individual participant data (IPD), suitable methods from Table 11.1 can be used to analyze each study, as we note below; the methods in this chapter would be less appropriate for primary analysis, but would be useful in sensitivity analysis.

Among 140 systematic reviews in mental health published in the Cochrane Database of Systematic Reviews since 2009, only 27 (19%) reported a sensitivity analysis [28]. In those 27 reviews, 14 considered a best/worst-case scenario and 13 of these did that only for the experimental arm. In 109 (78%) of the 140 reviews, missing data were imputed using LOCF in at least one study.

The best/worst-case scenarios are typically used as sensitivity analyses, but may produce unrealistic results in practice, especially if missing rates are high. Gamble and Hollis suggested that the discrepancy between best- and worst-case scenarios should be used to inform the down weighting of studies with more missing data [29]. However, because best- and worst-case scenarios are implausible in most meta-analyses, their method is unrealistically conservative. Methods based on single imputation such as imputing the worst observed mean have also been suggested for meta-analysis of continuous outcomes [30].

We next describe two improvements on the above methods. In Section 11.3, we use data on reasons for missing data to improve our analysis. In Section 11.4, we specify the magnitude of plausible departures from the MAR assumption.

11.3   METHOD 1: USING REASONS FOR MISSING DATA AND SIMPLE ASSUMPTIONS

Our first approach requires data on the distribution of reasons for missing data in at least some studies. The methods described here were proposed for meta-analyses with binary outcomes [21]. If reasons for missing data are unreported in some studies, then they can be imputed by the within-arm average across other studies.

The key idea is to consider the individuals in each reason group within each arm, and to impute the missing data by making specific assumptions about the missing data mechanism (an imputed case analysis, ICA). These specific assumptions could involve imputing failures (ICA-0), imputing successes (ICA-1), imputing the control arm proportion (ICA-p_c), and imputing the arm-specific proportion (ICA-p) [21]. In the haloperidol meta-analysis in Table 11.2, ICA-0 was used for reasons such as lack of therapeutic benefit, and ICA-1 for positive response. ICA-p_c was used for adverse events because patients with adverse events would withdraw from treatment and therefore might be expected to perform like untreated patients; this implicitly assumed that patients withdrawing from treatment did not differ in any other way from those remaining on treatment. Finally, ICA-p was used for reasons such as loss to follow-up, which could plausibly be considered to be MAR. Once imputations have been done, care is needed to obtain correct standard errors. It would be wrong to treat the imputed data as real data, since this would deflate standard errors and give too much weight to studies with missing data as well as overestimate the certainty of the results [21].

This approach is broad and equally applicable to AD or to IPD, subject only to what is known about reasons for missing data. For example, it includes best- and worst-case analyses (by setting ICA-1 in the treatment arm and ICA-0 in controls, and vice versa). A further extension is given in Section 11.4.

11.4   METHOD 2: QUANTIFYING DEPARTURES FROM MAR

The method in Section 11.3 only allows a limited range of assumptions within each reason group. Now we expand the range of assumptions by quantifying departures from MAR. We do not require data on reasons for missing data, although these can be used later.

Prior beliefs about missing data are expressed using an *informative missingness parameter* (IMP), which relates the mean outcome in the missing data to that in the observed data for each arm of each trial and expresses the degree of departure from the MAR assumption. The IMP is unknown and cannot be informed by the data; ideally, expert (clinical) opinion is used to elicit information about likely values of the IMP. These prior beliefs are then incorporated into the analysis in a two-stage approach [31]. At the first stage, we compute study-specific effect estimates and their standard errors adjusted for the prior beliefs about the missing data. At the second stage, the adjusted estimates are combined in a standard meta-analysis.

With binary outcome data, a suitable IMP is the ratio of the odds of the outcome among participants with missing outcomes to the odds of the outcome among observed participants, and is referred to as the *informative missingness odds ratio* (IMOR) [22]. The IMOR approach incorporates the best/worst-case scenarios as special cases, but allows less extreme assumptions. An IMOR of 2 in a beneficial outcome states that the odds of success in the missing participants are double the odds in the observed participants because, for example, participants left the study due to early response. An IMOR of 0.5 states that the odds in the missing participants are half the odds in the observed participants because, for example, participants lacking improvement left the study. Suppose we have 100 participants randomized in an arm, 40 of whom recovered, 20 of whom did not (odds in observed = 40/20), and there are 40 who did not provide any outcome data. Suppose that an expert believes that only 10 of the 40 unobserved participants would have recovered (odds in missing = 10/30). Then the expert's estimate of the IMOR is the ratio of the odds in missing to the odds in observed, and equals 1/6.

With continuous outcomes, the IMP compares the mean in missing participants to the mean in the observed participants [32]. It may be defined as the *informative missingness difference of means* (IMDoM) or the *informative missingness ratio of means* (IMRoM). An IMDoM of 1 states that the mean value in the missing participants exceeds the mean value of the observed participants by 1 unit. An IMRoM of 1.5 states that the mean value in the missing participants is 1.5 times the mean value in the observed participants. The IMDoM or IMRoM can be elicited by giving an expert the mean value in the observed data and asking for the mean value in the missing data.

In practice, experts should express a range of plausible values of the IMP. These may be used in a sensitivity analysis. For example, if the plausible range of the IMP is from −2 to 2, then the meta-analysis could be performed with the IMP assumed to be −2 in all arms of all studies, and then repeated with −1, 0, 1, and 2. Alternatively, the range of plausible values of the IMP may be viewed as a prior belief distribution specified by a mean IMP and a standard deviation. For example, the IMP above could be taken as normally distributed with mean 0 and standard deviation 1 (so that the expert is 95% sure that the true IMP is within the plausible range).

In this approach, a nonzero mean IMP tends to shift the point estimates, while uncertainty about the IMP (expressed through its standard deviation) tends to increase the study-specific standard errors, with two consequences: studies with fewer missing data tend to receive greater weight, and the standard error of the pooled estimate tends to increase. An important extension of the method allows the IMP to differ across treatment arms [13, 31].

The method has been extended for network meta-analysis models for both dichotomous and continuous outcomes [32, 33]. The methods of Sections 11.3 and 11.4 can be combined so that one category of reasons is imputed with a specified IMP. In principle, a distribution of IMPs could be used for each reason group, but this is not currently available in statistical software. IPD would facilitate more complex analyses, perhaps using multiple imputation with MNAR mechanisms [34]. Alternative fully Bayesian approaches have been proposed [35, 36].

11.5　TWO WORKED EXAMPLES

11.5.1　Haloperidol Meta-Analysis

These data with a binary outcome (clinical improvement) were introduced in Section 11.2 and are listed in Table 11.2. We consider fixed-effect meta-analyses for the risk ratio (RR; see Chapter 9).

We present four possible ways of handling the missing data out of a wide possible range. First, an ACA would be the standard choice. However, in this mental health setting, missing values are likely to show less improvement than observed values. A second analysis therefore imputes all missing values as failures (ICA-0). Because the outcome here is clinical improvement, this may be considered to be an LOCF analysis. However, the truth about the missing data is likely to lie between ACA and ICA-0. In our third analysis, we express this by using the reasons for missing data given in Table 11.2. Finally, our fourth analysis expresses uncertainty about the missing data by using a plausible distribution for the IMOR (Figure 11.1) in which the IMOR lies between 0.5 and 1 with probability 2/3.

Figure 11.2 shows the results of the four analyses. We first look at the study-specific estimates listed under RR (95% confidence interval) for the Beasley and Selman studies, which have substantial amounts of missing data, and more missing data in the placebo arm (Table 11.2). Compared with the ACA analysis, the ICA-0 analysis tends to impute more failures in the placebo arm and therefore gives larger estimated risk ratios for these studies. The confidence intervals widen because uncertainty for the risk ratio increases with lower risk, outweighing the benefit of increased sample size; for other measures such as the odds ratio, the confidence interval would narrow. The analysis using reasons imputes some but not all missing values as failures and therefore gives smaller increases in the estimated risk ratios and confidence interval widths. The analysis using IMORs imputes the missing values as slightly more likely to be failures than does the ACA analysis, and slightly increases the estimated risk ratios, while the added uncertainty widens the confidence intervals. For the other 15 studies, all four analyses give similar estimates.

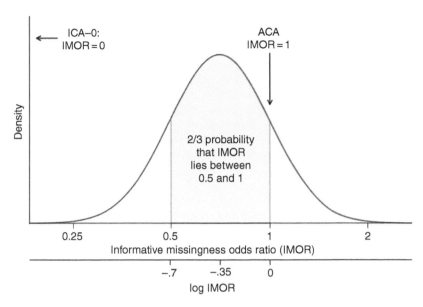

FIGURE 11.1   Plausible distribution for the informative missingness odds ratio (IMOR) in the haloperidol meta-analysis. ACA, available case analysis; ICA-0, imputed case analysis imputing failures.

The changes in confidence interval width reduce the weight given to the Beasley study from 31% in the ACA analysis to 25–27% in the other analyses, and similarly reduce the weight for the Selman study from 19% to 10–16%. The reduction in weight given to the Beasley study is important, because this study has a lower risk ratio than other studies. The meta-analysis results in Figure 11.2 therefore show that the pooled estimate increases from 1.57 in the ACA analysis to 1.68–1.90 in the other analyses, with corresponding increases in confidence interval width.

11.5.2   Mirtazapine Meta-Analysis

Our second example comprises eight studies comparing the effectiveness of mirtazapine and placebo in patients with major depression [37]. The continuous outcome is the change in depression symptoms measured on a standardized rating scale. For both mirtazapine and placebo arms, we have the mean change, standard deviation, and numbers of patients with observed and missing data (Table 11.3). We synthesize the mean differences using a random-effects model.

We present two of the possible ways to handle the missing data. ACA is the starting point in the analysis. As an alternative, we use a plausible distribution for the IMDoM, in which the IMDoM is considered to lie between −3 and 3 with 95% probability (Figure 11.3). This implies that the mean value of IMDoM is zero. We do not believe that data are MAR, but we do believe that departures from MAR are equally likely in both directions.

Figure 11.4 shows the results. Both methods give the same point estimate for the individual studies because the IMDoM distribution in the MNAR analysis is centered at zero (its value in the MAR analysis). Study-specific confidence intervals are wider for MNAR than MAR analyses by 5–10% in most studies, but by 23% in the fifth study (MIR 003-021), which has a larger proportion of missing data (Table 11.3).

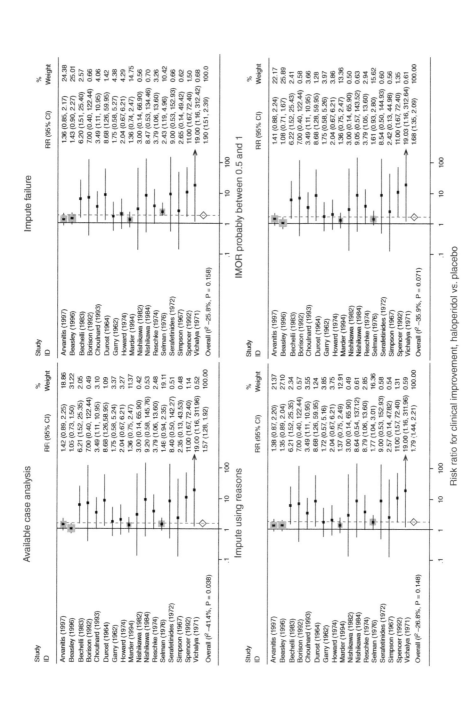

FIGURE 11.2 Haloperidol meta-analysis under four different assumptions about the missing data. CI, confidence interval; RR, risk ratio.

TABLE 11.3   Mirtazapine meta-analysis: mean change in depression scores, standard deviations (SDs), and numbers of observed and missing outcomes for the mirtazapine and placebo arms.

Study	Mirtazapine arm				Placebo arm			
	Mean	SD	Observed	Missing	Mean	SD	Observed	Missing
Claghorn 1995	−14.5	8.8	26	19	−11.4	10.2	19	26
MIR 003–003	−14.0	7.3	27	18	−11.5	8.3	24	21
MIR 003–008	−12.6	8.0	23	37	−11.4	8.0	17	13
MIR 003–020	−13.0	9.0	23	21	−6.2	6.5	24	19
MIR 003–021	−13.8	5.9	22	28	−17.4	5.3	21	29
MIR 003–024	−15.7	6.7	30	20	−11.1	9.9	27	23
MIR 84023a	−14.2	7.6	35	25	−11.9	8.6	33	24
MIR 84023b	−14.7	8.4	51	13	−11.8	8.3	48	18

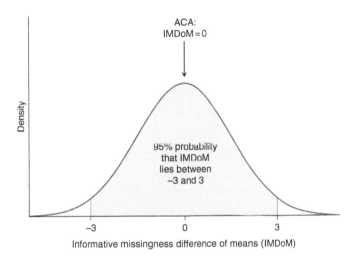

FIGURE 11.3   Plausible distribution for the informative missingness difference of means (IMDoM) in the mirtazapine meta-analysis. ACA, available case analysis.

The MNAR analysis therefore assigns slightly smaller weight to MIR 003-021. Since this is the only study favoring placebo, the summary estimate shifts slightly toward mirtazapine and the heterogeneity variance declines, which is reflected in the decreased I^2 value and the narrower confidence interval about the summary estimate. Although the differences are not large, the MAR assumption gives a marginally non-significant result, whereas the MNAR assumption gives a marginally significant result in favor of mirtazapine.

All these analyses may be performed using our software for Stata, available from the Statistical Software Components (SSC) archive. For binary outcomes, the

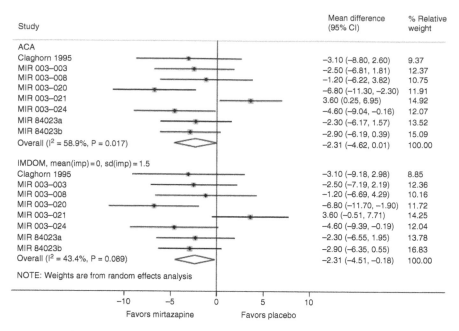

FIGURE 11.4 Mirtazapine meta-analysis under two different assumptions about the missing data. CI, confidence interval.

IMOR approach and the approach using reasons are implemented in the `metamiss` command [38]. For continuous outcomes, the IMDoM and IMRoM approaches are implemented in the `metamiss2` command [39].

11.6 RECOMMENDATIONS

Trial investigators should report the numbers of missing participants and results even if they go on to impute missing data, and they should collect and report the reasons for dropout by trial arm.

Reviewers should consider the possibility of missing outcome data when planning a systematic review and plan to extract data about numbers of missing values and reasons why data are missing.

Reviewers should be alert to the possibility that missing values have already been imputed, and when conducting a systematic review should aim to extract the unimputed data so that alternative imputation approaches can be used.

When performing a meta-analysis, a simple analysis such as ACA or ICA-0 will often be used as a main analysis, but the more sophisticated methods described above form important sensitivity analyses [21]. These should involve one or more analyses that make plausible assumptions about the missing data. The sensitivity analyses are typically specified after the systematic review so that the nature of the trials can inform the plausible assumptions. With large amounts of missing data, results can be adjusted in so many ways that it would be difficult to know which estimates to believe. Thus, it is sensible to define the relevant sensitivity analyses a priori in order to avoid the risk of data dredging. For example, if rich data on reasons are available, then imputation strategies should be defined for each reported reason. Alternatively, background knowledge should be used to specify a plausible range of IMORs and thus to define an uncertainty approach. More suggestions for the uncertainty approach are given by White et al. [31].

Further research is needed in developing questionnaires to elicit values of the IMOR, IMDoM, or IMRoM [40]; in developing statistical methods allowing reason-specific IMPs with uncertainty; and in developing methods for using reasons for missing data with continuous outcomes.

Supporting Research Grants

IW was supported by the Medical Research Council Unit Programme number MC_UU_12023/21. DM is funded by the European Union's Horizon 2020 COMPAR-EU project (No 754936).

REFERENCES

1. National Research Council (2010). *The Prevention and Treatment of Missing Data in Clinical Trials*. Washington, DC: National Academies Press.

2. Mavridis, D. and White, I.R. (2019). Dealing with missing outcome data in meta-analysis. *Res. Synth. Methods* 11 (1): 2–13.

3. Little, R.J., D'Agostino, R., Cohen, M.L. et al. (2012). The prevention and treatment of missing data in clinical trials. *N. Engl. J. Med.* 367 (14): 1355–1360.

4. Molenberghs, G. and Kenward, M.G. (2007). *Missing Data in Clinical Studies*. Chichester: Wiley.

5. Sterne, J.A.C., White, I.R., Carlin, J.B. et al. (2009). Multiple imputation for missing data in epidemiological and clinical research: potential and pitfalls. *BMJ* 338: b2393.

6. Carpenter, J.R. and Kenward, M.G. (2007). *Missing Data in Randomised Controlled Trials—a Practical Guide*. Birmingham: Health Technology Assessment Methodology Programme. https://researchonline.lshtm.ac.uk/id/eprint/4018500 (accessed February 21, 2022).

7. Higgins, J.P.T., Deeks, J.J., and Altman, D.G. (2008). Special topics in statistics. In: *Cochrane Handbook for Systematic Reviews of Interventions* (eds. J. Higgins and S. Green), 481–529. Chichester: Wiley.

8. Hollis, S. and Campbell, F. (1999). What is meant by intention to treat analysis? Survey of published randomised controlled trials. *BMJ* 319 (7211): 670–674.

9. Elobeid, M.A., Padilla, M.A., McVie, T. et al. (2009). Missing data in randomized clinical trials for weight loss: scope of the problem, state of the field, and performance of statistical methods. *PLoS One* 4 (8): e6624.

10. Kenward, M.G., Goetghebeur, E.J.T., and Molenberghs, G. (2001). Sensitivity analysis for incomplete categorical data. *Stat. Model.* 1 (1): 31–48.

11. White, I.R., Horton, N.J., Carpenter, J., and Pocock, S.J. (2011). Strategy for intention to treat analysis in randomised trials with missing outcome data. *BMJ* 342: d40.

12. Little, R.J.A. and Rubin, D.B. (2002). *Statistical Analysis with Missing Data*. Chichester: Wiley.

13. White, I.R., Carpenter, J., Evans, S., and Schroter, S. (2007). Eliciting and using expert opinions about dropout bias in randomized controlled trials. *Clin. Trials* 4 (2): 125–139.

14. Leucht, S., Engel, R.R., Bauml, J., and Davis, J.M. (2006). Is the superior efficacy of new generation antipsychotics an artifact of LOCF? *Schizophr. Bull.* 33 (1): 183–191.

15. White, I.R., Royston, P., and Wood, A.M. (2011). Multiple imputation using chained equations: issues and guidance for practice. *Stat. Med.* 30 (4): 377–399.

16. Schulz, K.F., Altman, D.G., and Moher, D. (2010). CONSORT 2010 statement: updated guidelines for reporting parallel group randomised trials. *BMJ* 340: c332.

17. Bell, M., Fiero, M., Horton, N., and Hsu, C.-H. (2014). Handling missing data in RCTs; a review of the top medical journals. *BMC Med. Res. Methodol.* 14 (1): 118.

18. Hussain, J.A., Bland, M., Langan, D. et al. (2017). Quality of missing data reporting and handling in palliative care trials demonstrates that further development of the CONSORT missing data reporting guidance is required: a systematic review. *J. Clin. Epidemiol.* 88: 81–91.

19. Akl, E.A., Shawwa, K., Kahale, L.A. et al. (2015). Reporting missing participant data in randomised trials: systematic survey of the methodological literature and a proposed guide. *BMJ Open* 5 (12): e008431.

20. Adams, C.E., Bergman, H., Irving, C.B., and Lawrie, S. (2013). Haloperidol versus placebo for schizophrenia. In: *Cochrane Database of Systematic Reviews*, no. 11 (ed. C.E. Adams), CD003082. Chichester: Wiley.

21. Higgins, J.P.T., White, I.R., and Wood, A.M. (2008). Imputation methods for missing outcome data in meta-analysis of clinical trials. *Clin. Trials* 5 (3): 225–239.

22. Chan, A.-W. and Altman, D.G. (2005). Epidemiology and reporting of randomised trials published in PubMed journals. *Lancet* 365 (9465): 1159–1162.

23. Beich, A., Thorsen, T., and Rollnick, S. (2003). Screening in brief intervention trials targeting excessive drinkers in general practice: systematic review and meta-analysis. *BMJ* 327 (7414): 536–542.

24. White, I.R. (2003). Intention-to-treat analysis was over-zealous—but this does not affect findings. *BMJ* 327: 7414.

25. Savović, J., Weeks, L., Sterne, J.A.C. et al. (2014). Evaluation of the Cochrane Collaboration's tool for assessing the risk of bias in randomized trials: focus groups, online survey, proposed recommendations and their implementation. *Syst. Rev.* 3 (1): 1–12.

26. Sterne, J.A.C., Savović, J., Page, M.J. et al. (2019). ROB 2: a revised tool for assessing risk of bias in randomised trials. *BMJ* 366: l4898.

27. Mavridis, D., Chaimani, A., Efthimiou, O. et al. (2014). Addressing missing outcome data in meta-analysis. *Evid. Based Ment. Health* 17 (3): 85–89.

28. Spineli, L.M., Pandis, N., and Salanti, G. (2015). Reporting and handling missing outcome data in mental health: a systematic review of Cochrane systematic reviews and meta-analyses. *Res. Synth. Methods* 6 (2): 175–187.

29. Gamble, C. and Hollis, S. (2005). Uncertainty method improved on best–worst case analysis in a binary meta-analysis. *J. Clin. Epidemiol.* 58 (6): 579–588.

30. Ebrahim, S., Akl, E.A., Mustafa, R.A. et al. (2013). Addressing continuous data for participants excluded from trial analysis: a guide for systematic reviewers. *J. Clin. Epidemiol.* 66 (9): 1014–1021.

31. White, I.R., Higgins, J.P.T., and Wood, A.M. (2008). Allowing for uncertainty due to missing data in meta-analysis—part 1: two-stage methods. *Stat. Med.* 27 (5): 711–727.

32. Mavridis, D., White, I.R., Higgins, J.P.T. et al. (2015). Allowing for uncertainty due to missing continuous outcome data in pairwise and network meta-analysis. *Stat. Med.* 34 (5): 721–741.

33. Spineli, L.M., Higgins, J.P.T., Cipriani, A. et al. (2013). Evaluating the impact of imputations for missing participant outcome data in a network meta-analysis. *Clin. Trials* 10 (3): 378–388.

34. Leacy, F.P., Floyd, S., Yates, T.A., and White, I.R. (2017). Analyses of sensitivity to the missing-at-random assumption using multiple imputation with delta adjustment: application to a tuberculosis/HIV prevalence survey with incomplete HIV-status data. *Am. J. Epidemiol.* 185: 304–315.

35. White, I.R., Welton, N.J., Wood, A.M. et al. (2008). Allowing for uncertainty due to missing data in meta-analysis—part 2: hierarchical models. *Stat. Med.* 27 (5): 728–745.

36. Turner, N.L., Dias, S., Ades, A.E., and Welton, N.J. (2015). A Bayesian framework to account for uncertainty due to missing binary outcome data in pairwise meta-analysis. *Stat. Med.* 34 (12): 2062–2080.

37. Cipriani, A., Furukawa, T.A., Salanti, G. et al. (2015). Comparative efficacy and acceptability of 21 antidepressant drugs for the acute treatment of adults with major depressive disorder: a systematic review and network meta-analysis. *Lancet* 391 (10128): 1357–1366.

38. White, I.R. and Higgins, J.P.T. (2009). Meta-analysis with missing data. *Stata J.* 9: 57–69.

39. Chaimani, A., Mavridis, D., Higgins, J. et al. (2018). Allowing for informative missingness in aggregate data meta-analysis with continuous or binary outcomes: extensions to metamiss. *Stata J.* 18 (3): 716–740.

40. White, I.R. (2015). Sensitivity analysis: the elicitation and use of expert opinion. In: *Handbook of Missing Data Methodology* (eds. G. Molenberghs, G. Fitzmaurice, M.G. Kenward, et al.), 471–489. London: Chapman and Hall.

CHAPTER 12

Individual Participant Data Meta-Analysis

Mark C. Simmonds and Lesley A. Stewart

Most systematic reviews analyze summary data from published reports of primary studies, extracting effect estimates and combining them across studies. An alternative and increasingly used approach (Figure 12.1) is to seek original datasets for each eligible study and base meta-analysis on the assembled individual participant data (IPD). IPD meta-analyses have been done in many health care fields, although reviews of oncology and cardiovascular medicine predominate [1]. While most IPD analyses are of randomized trials, the approach is gaining popularity for meta-analyses of observational evidence.

IPD meta-analyses offer many advantages over meta-analyses based on summary data, such as the opportunity to mitigate publication and outcome reporting bias [1] and perform more sophisticated analyses, including of participant-level associations, for example to investigate potential effect modifiers. IPD meta-analysis projects are, however, more complex, time-consuming, and resource-intensive, and require greater expertise than standard systematic reviews with meta-analysis of aggregate data. Thus, before embarking on an IPD meta-analysis project, careful consideration needs to be given as to whether an IPD meta-analysis is necessary to address the research question posed and whether it is likely to be feasible. Benefits and challenges of IPD meta-analyses are listed in Box 12.1 and are discussed briefly in the following section.

This chapter provides an outline of IPD meta-analysis processes and overview of the main statistical approaches that can be taken. A more detailed account of the design, planning, conduct, analysis, and reporting of IPD meta-analysis projects can be found in the book edited by Riley, Tierney, and Stewart [2].

Systematic Reviews in Health Research: Meta-Analysis in Context, Third Edition. Edited by Matthias Egger, Julian P.T. Higgins, and George Davey Smith.
© 2022 John Wiley & Sons Ltd. Published 2022 by John Wiley & Sons Ltd.
Companion website: www.systematic-reviews3.org

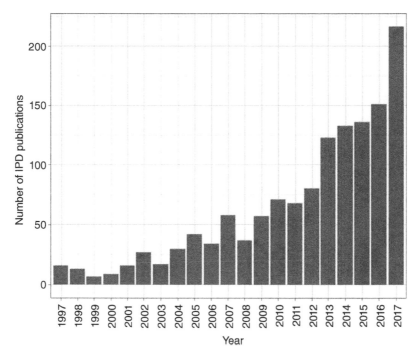

FIGURE 12.1 Popularity of individual participant data (IPD) meta-analyses over time.

Box 12.1 Benefits and Disadvantages of Systematic Reviews Using Individual Participant Data (IPD)

Benefits of collecting IPD

- Supply of additional or updated data
- Improve overall follow-up
- Include previously excluded or missing participants
- Analyze outcomes not reported in publications
- Data can be checked and corrected

Benefits of analyzing IPD

- Analyze on the basis of allocated intervention
- Enable consistent adjustment for key confounding variables
- Analyze participant subgroups
- Analyze by time to event
- Greater choice of analysis methods

Benefits of collaborating with primary investigators in the conduct of the review

- Better identification of studies
- More balanced interpretation of the results of the review

- Wider endorsement
- Increased possibilities for dissemination of the results of the review
- Better clarification of the implications for future research
- Possibilities for collaboration in future research

Possible disadvantages of IPD reviews

- May take longer and cost more
- Review team needs wider range of skills
- Data management is more complicated
- Statistical analysis may be more complex
- IPD may not be available from all relevant studies

12.1   ADVANTAGES AND CHALLENGES OF COLLECTING INDIVIDUAL PARTICIPANT DATA

12.1.1   Access to Additional Outcome Data

A particular benefit of the IPD approach is that data not presented in publications can be collected and analyzed. This may include data from unpublished studies, unpublished long-term follow-up data, and outcomes or timepoints not reported in publications, as well as data not reported in a suitable format for meta-analysis. It may also be possible to obtain data from participants who were excluded from the original study analyses. These additional data can help to reduce the impact of publication and reporting biases.

12.1.2   Data in a Consistent and Usable Format

An important obstacle to undertaking meta-analyses using published data is that results are often presented in different ways: one study might report a risk ratio, another only an odds ratio, and a third only that a comparison was not statistically significant. Access to the participant-level data would allow any of these results to be computed from each study. Similarly, if an outcome measure has been defined using different cutpoints across the studies, or by taking different components of a measurement scale, or by combining outcomes into different composite outcomes, then IPD may enable the original data to be re-coded to a common measurement scale.

Time-to-event outcome data cannot conveniently be summarized using simple statistics like counts or means from each group. Results may be presented in several ways, including Kaplan–Meier curves, statistics from log-rank tests, and effect estimates from proportional hazards models. Although various methods are available for extracting consistent results and converting approximately between them, the results of such different analyses cannot be easily combined in a meta-analysis [3–5]. Thus obtaining and analyzing IPD can be particularly useful for reviews with important time-to-event outcomes.

12.1.3   More Choice of Analysis Options

Provision of IPD enables standardization of data, and results may be combined across studies in ways they otherwise could not. IPD enable re-analysis of the data to include updated results, to perform intention-to-treat analysis, to analyze time-to-event data, and to correct flawed original study analyses. Access to IPD also permits much more flexible and powerful analyses than are possible using summary data, such as application of methods to account for missing outcome data (see also Chapter 11).

12.1.4   Ability to Examine Individual-Level Characteristics

IPD datasets will generally contain demographic information such as age, sex, health condition, previous health care, and possibly socioeconomic variables for each participant. This allows investigation of how such participant-level covariates might affect the impact of the intervention, exposure, or test under investigation. This ability to answer research questions about individual-level effect modification in ways that are typically not possible from aggregate data is a key advantage of IPD meta-analysis, and is often the main scientific reason for seeking IPD.

For all the above reasons and more, an IPD meta-analysis is taken to be the gold standard for meta-analysis [6, 7].

12.1.5   Challenges in Using Individual Participant Data

Despite the advantages, using IPD in meta-analysis poses challenges. IPD meta-analysis is strongly dependent on the availability of data from the studies, which will usually require study investigators to share their data. IPD may not be available for all studies, either because authors do not share data or because the data are no longer available. Considerable effort is be needed to manage and prepare IPD for analysis. The quantity of data is often large, and data may be provided in very different formats. Statistical analysis of IPD is also generally more complex than a conventional meta-analysis.

An IPD review generally takes longer, is more costly, and is more complex than a review of published results. Before embarking on an IPD review, reviewers should therefore consider whether the advantages of an IPD approach outlined here outweigh the extra effort required, particularly if the review question could be answered reliably using data from publications, perhaps supplemented by requesting additional data from authors [8].

12.2   PERFORMING A SYSTEMATIC REVIEW USING INDIVIDUAL PARTICIPANT DATA

12.2.1   Planning the Review and Identifying Studies

The rationale for a systematic review using IPD is the same as that for any systematic review, and many of the processes are similar. Differences occur mainly with respect to obtaining and managing data and in the type of analyses that can be done.

It is particularly important to write a protocol for an IPD review, given the added complexity and potential to conduct multiple analyses and selectively report those that produce favorable results. The protocol is also a valuable communication tool that can be used to explain the proposed project to primary study investigators as an aid to obtaining the data and building collaboration.

As with any systematic review, an early step will be to identify all the studies relevant to the review following the methods discussed elsewhere in this book (see Chapter 3). Searches for gray literature may be particularly useful in identifying studies that have not been published, from which IPD could be sought. Searching trial registries may identify both unpublished studies and ongoing trials for which data may become available, as might clinical trial data repositories. Primary study investigators help identify additional studies, particularly regarding unpublished studies that they have completed or know of. Any available published material for potentially eligible studies should be obtained to confirm eligibility and help understand and check the individual-level dataset, and for data extraction should IPD be unavailable.

A series of additional preparatory steps is usually required for IPD meta-analysis projects. Although full ethics approval may not be required for the IPD review, this should be investigated and clarified. This is important, since confirmation of ethical clearance may be needed before study investigators can gain approval from local ethics committees, institutional review boards, or managers to release IPD. Data protection and security regulations should also be checked to ensure compliance. Formal data-sharing agreements are used increasingly and having these ready as part of negotiating collaboration and provision of data is advisable, as is having prepared a detailed data dictionary that sets out the participant-level data items that the review seeks to collect. Most IPD reviews will require dedicated funding and a research team with appropriate skills and experience will need to be in place [9].

12.2.2   Obtaining Individual Participant Data

Careful consideration should be given to whether the review should be performed in collaboration with primary study investigators. A collaboration can yield substantial benefits and may also be the only means by which some investigators will release their IPD. Under this model, collaborators may be assured that their data are being stored and used appropriately (through the protocol and data use agreements), have some input to design through commenting on the protocol, and gain academic credit through group-authored publications. Such involvement, particularly if a dedicated meeting is held at which results are shared, can facilitate more nuanced interpretation of findings, improve knowledge mobilization, and afford greater credibility among the wider target audience. Often, collaborators will be able to provide material such as trial protocols or adverse event report forms. Collaborations forged through an IPD review may be long-lasting and can facilitate updating the review, instigating new reviews, as well as in some cases leading to planning new clinical trials. However, independence of the central research team undertaking the meta-analysis is important in safeguarding against design and analysis being influenced by primary investigators, who are likely to know the studies and data well, in ways that shape findings to reflect their own views. This may be particularly important in controversial areas.

An alternative, or complement, to obtaining IPD directly from trial investigators is to access IPD through one of the growing number of data-sharing platforms or repositories. Although this may have potential to save time in obtaining IPD, at present the process of gaining approval to access data can be lengthy, and may not save time compared with contacting trial investigators directly [10, 11].

IPD may be medically or commercially sensitive, and this must be considered when obtaining and handling the data for the review. In general, data should be requested to be supplied without names or identifying numbers. A data-sharing agreement that sets out the details of safe data storage and ensures that the limited number of researchers with access to the data will refrain from any attempt to re-identify individuals may be helpful.

12.2.3   Checking and Cleaning the Data

Once data are obtained they will generally need to be harmonized, since different studies will provide data in different formats and will have coded their data differently. Although trial investigators are often willing to re-code data to a specified meta-analysis format, it is likely that considerable data manipulation and transformation will be needed to convert the data received into a consistent format across all studies ready for the meta-analysis. Discussion with the study authors is usually necessary to clarify any areas of uncertainty around what the data contain and how they are coded. Data should also be checked to identify any omissions and possible errors. This could include checking for simple coding errors, checking clinical plausibility of the data, and comparing data with publications.

IPD may usefully contribute to, and supplement, investigations of study quality or risk of bias. For example, whether randomization was adequate in a clinical trial may be checked by examining the distributions of age, sex, and other basic participant characteristics across intervention arms of the trial. Randomization patterns such as dates of allocation of participants to each group may also be informative [12].

12.3   METHODS FOR META-ANALYSIS WITH INDIVIDUAL PARTICIPANT DATA

There are two broad statistical approaches to performing a meta-analysis using IPD. The first follows the strategy of a meta-analysis of aggregate data: each study is analyzed separately to produce a summary effect estimate and these summary effect estimates are then combined using standard meta-analysis techniques. This is the *two-stage* approach. The second approach is to analyze all the IPD in a single analysis using a statistical model that recognizes that the data come from independent studies. This is the *one-stage* approach. We discuss methods for the two approaches separately, focusing initially on estimation of a single overall effect such as a treatment effect across multiple randomized trials.

12.3.1   Two-Stage Approaches for Overall Effect

In the two-stage approach to IPD meta-analysis, the meta-analysis is performed in two distinct parts. In the first stage, data from each study are analyzed separately to obtain estimates of effect and estimates of uncertainty in these estimates. For example, for dichotomous outcome data (e.g. death) in randomized controlled trials, the risk ratio or odds ratio and its 95% confidence interval (on a logarithmic scale) might be calculated. For continuously distributed outcomes (e.g. blood pressure), the mean difference or standardized mean difference between arms and its standard error might be computed.

In the second stage, the effect estimates are combined in a meta-analysis. Any of the standard meta-analytic techniques discussed in Chapter 9 could be used. For a fixed-effect meta-analysis, the standard inverse-variance weighted average may be used. For binary data, alternative methods such as the Mantel–Haenszel approach or Peto method may be used. For a random-effects meta-analysis, the DerSimonian–Laird approach may be used [13].

An advantage of the two-stage approach is that any meta-analysis method used in standard analyses of published data may be used for IPD analysis, including assessment of heterogeneity using Cochran's Q test or the I^2 statistic to measure inconsistency in results [14]. Furthermore, combining effect estimates based on IPD with effect estimates obtained from study reports is straightforward. Forest plots of the results for each study along with the meta-analytic summary may also be presented. Since meta-analysis methods in a two-stage approach are common to IPD and aggregate data meta-analysis, and have been covered in other chapters, we do not discuss them in detail here.

12.3.1.1   Example: The PARIS Review (Part 1)

The Perinatal Antiplatelet Review of International Studies (PARIS) review was a collaborative systematic review and IPD meta-analysis of 31 randomized, placebo-controlled trials investigating the use of antiplatelets to prevent pre-eclampsia and associated outcomes in pregnancy [15]. The use of IPD afforded a number of benefits, among them a consistent definition of pre-eclampsia across the IPD (in contrast to publications that had used a variety of definitions). IPD were included from unpublished trials and provided updated or more complete data from some of the trials. The IPD also contained results for more outcomes than had been reported in publications, and allowed a range of subgroup analyses to explore whether some women and their infants benefited more from antiplatelets than others.

The meta-analysis used a two-stage approach. For the primary outcome of pre-eclampsia, the numbers of women with and without pre-eclampsia in both antiplatelet and placebo arms of each trial were determined and combined in the same way as if they had been extracted directly from publications. Figure 12.2 shows a forest plot of the results of the 24 trials that provided data on pre-eclampsia, with the summary odds ratio from a random-effects meta-analysis; the use of aspirin led to a modest but statistically significant reduction in pre-eclampsia with an odds ratio of 0.85. There is little apparent heterogeneity: the I^2 value of 29% indicates that only one-quarter of the variation in point estimates is due to heterogeneity rather than within-study random errors [16].

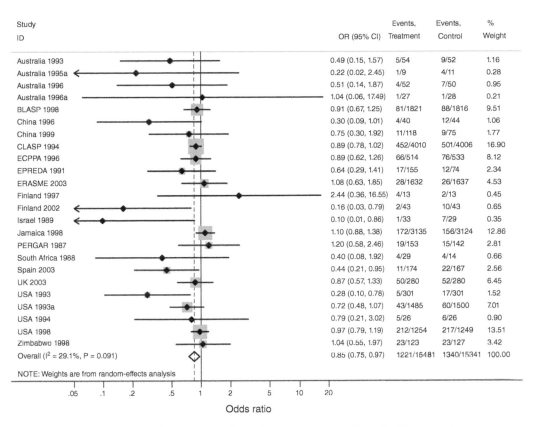

FIGURE 12.2   Forest plot of the impact of aspirin on pre-eclampsia in the PARIS review. CI, confidence interval; OR, odds ratio.

12.3.2   One-Stage Approaches for Overall Effect

The one-stage approach to IPD meta-analysis consists of fitting a single statistical model to all data from all studies simultaneously. The approach is much like analyzing one large study, except that allowance must be made for interstudy differences. Any suitable model may be used, but generalized linear modes are most common in practice. For a meta-analysis of randomized controlled trials, a suitable generalized linear model would include terms for the treatment effect and indicator variables for each study. Assumptions must be made for each parameter across studies. Each parameter may be assumed to be unrelated across studies, equal in every study, or randomly distributed across studies

Parameters representing baseline levels of the outcome across studies (e.g. underlying risks of the event) might reasonably be assumed to be unrelated across studies, replicating the assumptions involved in a standard meta-analysis and ensuring that between-individual comparisons across groups are made only within studies and not across studies. However, alternative model structures are possible, which may have model convergence and stability benefits [17].

The treatment effect is typically assumed to be either equal across studies (a fixed-effect meta-analysis) or randomly distributed across studies (a random-effects meta-analysis). When random effects are included, the model is a generalized linear mixed model and the variance of treatment effects across studies represents the amount of heterogeneity in the treatment effect.

Detailed discussions are available for one-stage meta-analysis of IPD for continuous outcomes using linear regression models [18], dichotomous event data using logistic regression models [19], and ordered categorical data using a proportional odds models [20]; for count data, Poisson regression might be used. One-stage models for time-to-event data are discussed in Section 12.3.3.

12.3.2.1 Example: The PARIS Review (Part 2)

A re-analysis of the PARIS IPD meta-analysis compared one-stage and two-stage approaches to the impact of antiplatelet use on risk of pre-eclampsia [16]. For the one-stage model, a fixed-effect model was fitted using a logistic regression model to estimate the odds ratio for the benefit of antiplatelets. A random-effects logistic regression model was also fitted to the same data. A summary of the results from the four models is given in Table 12.1. The results of the one-stage and two-stage approaches are very similar. The only difference is that the one-stage approach observed no heterogeneity (so that fixed- and random-effects models have the same results). This is an artifact of using heterogeneity estimation methods that differ in the two analyses: two-stage analyses used the DerSimonian–Laird estimator, while the one-stage analysis used a restricted maximum likelihood approach.

12.3.3 Time-to-Event Analysis

Many IPD meta-analyses have been performed on time-to-event outcomes using survival analysis techniques [21]. Survival analysis relies on knowing the timing of each event, not just how many events occurred in each group. As we have mentioned, the data required for these analyses are not generally available in publications, which means that there are considerable advantages of collecting IPD.

Both two-stage and one-stage approaches to meta-analysis of survival data are possible. A commonly used two-stage approach is to perform a log-rank test within each study. Briefly, this consists of calculating the difference between the observed and expected numbers of events along with its variance at a set of times, usually each

TABLE 12.1 Results of one- and two-stage analyses of PARIS review.

Method	Odds ratio for effect of aspirin	95% confidence interval	Heterogeneity (τ^2)
Two-stage fixed-effects	0.887	0.817 to 0.963	$I^2 = 29\%$
Two-stage random-effects	0.849	0.745 to 0.976	$\tau^2 = 0.021$; $I^2 = 29\%$
One-stage fixed-effect	0.886	0.816 to 0.963	–
One-stage random-effects	0.886	0.816 to 0.963	$\tau^2 = 0$

event time. These values are then summed across times to obtain an estimate of the log hazard ratio and its variance. This approach is discussed in detail by Simmonds et al. [22]. The log hazard ratios from each trial are combined in an inverse-variance meta-analysis, using either a fixed-effect or a random-effects approach. Alternatively, the hazard ratio in each trial may be estimated by fitting a Cox proportional hazards model [22] or a parametric survival model such as a Weibull model [23].

The most commonly recommended one-stage approach for survival analysis is to fit a random-effects Cox proportional hazards model [24, 25]. Stratification of the analysis by study is achieved by allowing a separate baseline hazard for each study. Alternatively, a Weibull model or other parametric survival model could be used in a one-stage approach, again stratifying by study and allowing the treatment effect to be equal or randomly varying across studies.

12.3.3.1 Example: Chemotherapy for Non-Small Cell Lung Cancer

An IPD meta-analysis of trials of preoperative chemotherapy for non-small cell lung cancer included 15 trials and 2385 patients [26]. An IPD approach was taken because the original publications did not present sufficient data to be able to meta-analyze hazard ratios for overall survival, and because it enabled subgroup analyses. A two-stage approach was used. Within each trial, the log-rank expected number of events and its variance were used to estimate the hazard ratio for the effect of preoperative radiotherapy on overall survival. Hazard ratios were then combined across trials using both fixed- and random-effects meta-analyses. The result of this meta-analysis is shown in Figure 12.3.

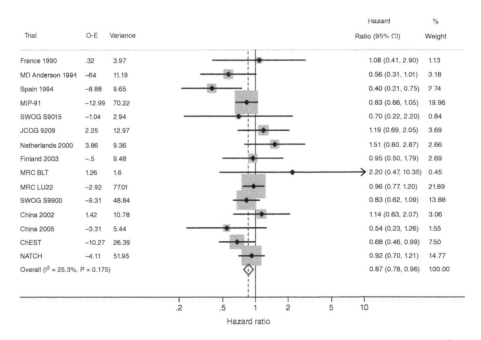

FIGURE 12.3 Results of the two-stage individual participant data (IPD) meta-analysis of non-small cell lung cancer trials. CI, confidence interval; E, expected; O, observed.

12.4   GOING BEYOND ESTIMATING THE SUMMARY EFFECT

The IPD meta-analysis methods described so far have estimated overall effects such as an overall odds ratio for the effect of treatment versus control on a particular outcome. Most IPD analyses aim to do more than this and investigate the situations in which treatment effects are larger or smaller. Further analyses may therefore investigate how characteristics such as participant age or drug dose modify the effectiveness of a treatment. Investigating whether particular types of people benefit more or less from an intervention is important in "precision medicine" [27]. IPD are particularly useful for this, because data on individual-level covariates are generally not available from publications. When investigating the effect of covariates, it is helpful to distinguish between two categories of covariate:

- *Study-level* covariates are the same for all participants within a study, but vary across studies; common examples are intended drug dosage or treatment duration.
- *Participant-level* covariates vary across participants within each study, for example age or sex.

The nature of a covariate affects the choice of analysis. Some covariates may fall between these categories. For example, if we are interested in different subtypes of a disease, some studies may be restricted to only one disease type, while others include participants with a range of disease types.

The methods for investigating the effect of covariates in an IPD meta-analysis differ for one-stage and two-stage approaches.

12.4.1   Two-Stage Approaches for Investigating Covariates

The simplest two-stage method for investigating the effect of a covariate is subgroup analysis. For study-level covariates, this consists of estimating the treatment effect in each study, dividing the studies into subsets according to the value of the covariate in each study, and then performing separate meta-analyses for each subset of studies using standard meta-analysis methods (see Chapter 10). Continuously distributed study-level covariates may be investigated using meta-regression, in which the effect estimates from the studies are regressed against the study-level value of the covariate [28]. Meta-regression has been found to be prone to bias and lacks statistical power, so it should be used with caution [29].

For individual-level covariates such as treatment effects in men versus women, we might calculate a treatment effect separately within each subgroup of individuals. For example, we might estimate the treatment effect among only men and the treatment effect among only women separately for each study, then undertake a meta-analysis across studies using the results for men and, similarly, a meta-analysis across studies from the results for women [29]. A preferable alternative is to focus on the interaction between treatment and the covariate [29–31]. The analysis of each study then targets estimation of this interaction term rather than estimation of the treatment effect, and these estimated interaction terms are combined across studies in the meta-analysis [29]. One disadvantage of this approach is that it is currently unclear how to incorporate studies that do not have variability in the covariate of interest. For example, if the interaction term of interest is between treatment and sex, then a study of only women may be difficult to include in the analysis.

12.4.2   One-Stage Approaches for Investigating Covariates

Investigating the effect of a covariate in a one-stage analysis requires adding interaction terms between treatment and covariate to the one-stage random-effects regression models discussed in Section 12.3.2 for estimation of overall effect. As for other parameters in the model, there is the option of assuming that these interaction terms are equal in every study, unrelated across studies, or randomly distributed across studies. This model can be used for both individual- and study-level covariates, and for continuous or dichotomous covariates. For example, if the covariate is the dose of the drug, then the interaction term would quantify the dose–response relationship. If the covariate is sex, then the interaction term would give the difference in treatment effect between men and women. This model may also be extended to consider multiple covariates in the same model.

12.4.2.1   Example: The PARIS Review (Part 3)

The original analysis of the PARIS data considered several possible factors that might modify the effectiveness of aspirin to reduce pre-eclampsia. In a re-analysis of the impact of diabetes, hypertension, age, and gestational age on the effectiveness of aspirin in the PARIS review, two-stage and one-stage models were used to investigate the interactions between antiplatelet use and each of the four covariates. The results for both approaches, which are similar, are given in Table 12.2.

12.5   INDIVIDUAL PARTICIPANT DATA META-ANALYSIS OF OBSERVATIONAL STUDIES

The examples cited so far in this chapter have all been analyses of randomized trials. The use of IPD is growing in importance in meta-analyses of observational studies in health care, such as cohort and case–control studies. Because of the lack of randomization in observational data, adjustments for potentially confounding factors are usually important to avoid biased results. Unfortunately, publications may not present suitably adjusted results, or the choice of adjustments may vary across studies. We also may be interested in the effects of multiple covariates on an outcome, not just a single treatment, and details of such multivariate analyses are rarely presented in publications. Obtaining the IPD can solve both these problems by allowing the reviewer to fit fully adjusted multivariate models (see also Chapters 17 and 18).

As with analyses of randomized trials, both one- and two-stage approaches may be implemented with observational IPD. The models and methods are similar, although the treatment factor would be replaced with one or more covariates of interest. In a two-stage approach, we may again fit a suitably adjusted linear, logistic, or other model of the effect of the covariate(s) on the specified outcome within each study, and then combine the results of each analysis (typically expressed as a mean change, odds ratio, hazard ratio, or similar) in a standard meta-analysis. A one-stage analysis would fit a similar adjusted regression model to all data from all studies simultaneously.

TABLE 12.2 Results of one- and two-stage analyses of the effect of covariates in the PARIS review.

Covariate	Category	Two-stage analysis		One-stage analysis		
		Odds ratio (95% CI)	P value for difference	Odds ratio (95% CI)	Interaction odds ratio (95% CI)	P value for interaction
Diabetes	With	0.72 (0.49 to 1.04)	0.38	0.74 (0.50 to 1.11)	0.82 (0.57 to 1.20)	0.32
	Without	0.86 (0.74 to 0.99)		0.90 (0.83 to 0.99)		
Hypertension	With	0.90 (0.69 to 1.17)	0.62	0.96 (0.75 to 1.23)	1.10 (0.90 to 1.35)	0.35
	Without	0.83 (0.71 to 0.98)		0.87 (0.79 to 0.96)		
Gestational age	<20 weeks	0.85 (0.73 to 0.98)	0.54	0.89[a] (0.82 to 0.96)	1.004[b] (0.99 to 1.02)	0.55
	≥20 weeks	0.91 (0.76 to 1.09)				
Maternal age	Under 20	0.99 (0.79 to 1.24)	0.19	0.89[a] (0.81 to 0.97)	1.001[b] (0.99 to 1.01)	0.92
	20–35	0.81 (0.70 to 0.95)				
	Over 35	1.03 (0.79 to 1.33)				

[a] Odds ratio of effect at average gestational/maternal age.
[b] Odds ratio per week/year increase in gestational/maternal age.
CI, confidence interval.

In either a one- or a two-stage approach, we need to consider whether to incorporate the same or different adjustment factors within each study, and whether to assume that the effects of each covariate are unrelated across studies, equal in every study (as in a fixed-effect meta-analysis), or randomly distributed across studies (a random-effects meta-analysis). These choices may depend on the nature of the topic and the availability of data.

IPD methods may in principle be used in any meta-analysis. For example, estimates of sensitivity and specificity in a meta-analysis evaluating the accuracy of a diagnostic test could be calculated from IPD and then combined using the methods described in Chapter 16.

12.5.1   Example: Aortic Pulse Wave Velocity and Cardiovascular Disease

An IPD meta-analysis sought to determine the association between aortic pulse wave velocity (aPWV) and later cardiovascular disease [32]. The review obtained IPD from 16 prospective cohort studies. The primary outcome was the incidence of any cardiovascular event. A two-stage analysis was used. Within each included study, the time-to-event data for cardiovascular events were used to fit Cox proportional hazards models to determine the hazard ratio of cardiovascular events per standard deviation increase in aPWV. Such Cox models could only be fitted using IPD. Another advantage of using IPD was that the Cox model could be adjusted for key covariates such as age and sex consistently in every study. Hazard ratio estimates for each study were then combined in a random-effects meta-analysis to estimate the overall effect of aPWV and present a forest plot (see Figure 12.4).

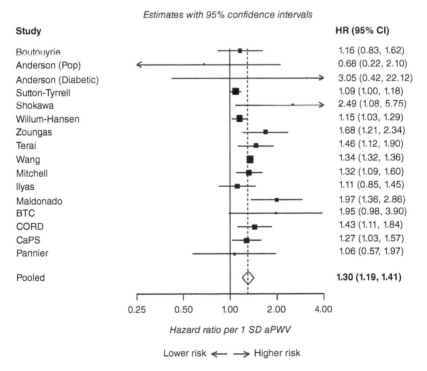

FIGURE 12.4   Results of the individual participant data (IPD) meta-analysis for aortic pulse wave velocity (aPWV) and cardiovascular disease. CI, confidence interval; HR, hazard ratio; SD, standard deviation.

12.6   COMBINING INDIVIDUAL PARTICIPANT DATA WITH PUBLISHED DATA

An obvious possibility in an IPD meta-analysis is that IPD are not available from all of the studies from which they are sought. Study authors may not be willing or able to provide data, or the data may no longer be available. Missing studies will lead to lower precision (wider confidence intervals) and possibly bias if, for example, data are made available only from studies with favorable results (sometimes called "availability bias"). To overcome these problems, a meta-analysis that combines the IPD with published results from studies from which IPD were not obtained will often be necessary.

In a two-stage approach, combining IPD with published data is straightforward. Provided suitable estimates of effect are presented in publications, these may be combined in a meta-analysis with similar estimates derived from the IPD from each study for which they are available [33]. It is possible that the results in the publications are from different types of analyses to those performed on the IPD. For example, analyses using IPD may be adjusted for potential confounding factors, but a publication may only present unadjusted results. Careful consideration should then be given to whether it is appropriate to combine the IPD with published data, and to what assumptions must be made to justify this. A sensitivity analysis to compare the results from combining published data and IPD with the original results from IPD alone may be desirable. If there are important differences, further exploration and explanation are required.

It is usually more difficult to incorporate published data into analyses of the effect of individual-level covariates, since data will generally not be available from publications. Sophisticated one-stage approaches, which combine a one-stage model of the IPD with an analysis of the published data, have been proposed but are more complicated to perform [34].

12.7   REPORTING FINDINGS

Guidance on academic reporting of an IPD systematic review is available in the PRISMA-IPD statement, which expands on the existing PRISMA statement for reporting of systematic reviews and meta-analyses specifically to reviews containing IPD [35].Using a range of tailored outputs and approaches to dissemination will help reach the various audiences who may be interested in IPD review findings [36].

12.8   CONCLUSION

A systematic review based on IPD has many advantages over a systematic review of published aggregate (or summary) data. These advantages include more complete data-sets, and the possibility of carrying out more detailed and flexible analyses and investigating the impact of individual-level covariates. But an IPD meta-analysis requires access to the original data from each study, and greater expertise, time, and resources. Obtaining IPD can be time-consuming or difficult and usually requires close collaboration with study authors. However, given increasing pressure to make data from clinical trials available for re-analysis, access to IPD may become easier.

Statistical methods for a meta-analysis using IPD fall into two categories. Two-stage methods based on standard meta-analysis techniques are more familiar, but one-stage models offer greater flexibility. An IPD review can include both approaches; a two-stage approach may be used for the main outcomes to produce forest plots and a one-stage method can yield more detailed analyses of possible causes of heterogeneity. In general, the two approaches would be expected to produce similar results when estimating an overall effect, but are more likely to differ when estimating the impact of covariates.

Given the complexity of performing a review based on IPD and the additional time, expertise, and resource that they require, early consideration of whether IPD will reward the extra effort of obtaining them is necessary. IPD reviews may be most useful when important results have not been published, or when many participants have been excluded from published results. IPD can be particularly worthwhile for outcomes that are poorly reported, or reported in ways that are not amenable to meta-analysis such as adverse events, long-term outcomes, and time-to-event outcomes. Often an IPD approach is the only way to discern clinically significant differences between subgroups of individuals. The IPD approach thus aligns well with the increasingly prominent goals of precision medicine.

REFERENCES

1. Simmonds, M., Stewart, G., and Stewart, L. (2015). A decade of individual participant data meta-analyses: a review of current practice. *Contemp. Clin. Trials* 45 (Pt A): 76–83.

2. Riley, R.D., Tierney, J.F., and Stewart, L.A. (eds.) (2021). *Individual Participant Data Meta-Analysis: A Handbook for Healthcare Research*. Chichester: Wiley.

3. Parmar, M.K., Torri, V., and Stewart, L. (1998). Extracting summary statistics to perform meta-analyses of the published literature for survival endpoints. *Stat. Med.* 17 (24): 2815–2834.

4. Guyot, P., Ades, A.E., Ouwens, M.J.N.M., and Welton, N.J. (2012). Enhanced secondary analysis of survival data: reconstructing the data from published Kaplan-Meier survival curves. *BMC Med. Res. Methodol.* 12.

5. Williamson, P.R., Smith, C.T., Hutton, J.L., and Marson, A.G. (2002). Aggregate data meta-analysis with time-to-event outcomes. *Stat. Med.* 21 (22): 3337–3351.

6. Stewart, L.A. and Tierney, J.F. (2002). To IPD or not to IPD? *Eval. Health Prof.* 25: 76–97.

7. Stewart, L.A. and Parmar, M.K.B. (1993). Meta-analysis of the literature or of individual patient data: is there a difference? *Lancet* 341: 418–422.

8. Tierney, J.F., Riley, R.D., Tudor Smith, C. et al. (2021). Rationale for embarking on an IPD meta-analysis project. In: *Individual Participant Data Meta-Analysis: A Handbook for Healthcare Research* (eds. R.D. Riley, J.F. Tierney and L.A. Stewart), 9–20. Chichester: Wiley.

9. Stewart, L.A., Riley, R.D., and Tierney, J.F. (2021). Planning and initiating an IPD meta-analysis project. In: *Individual Participant Data Meta-Analysis: A Handbook for Healthcare Research* (eds. R.D. Riley, J.F. Tierney and L.A. Stewart), 21–44. Chichester: Wiley.

10. Veroniki, A.A., Ashoor, H.M., Le, S.P.C. et al. (2019). Retrieval of individual patient data depended on study characteristics: a randomized controlled trial. *J. Clin. Epidemiol.* 113: 176–188.

11. Nevitt, S.J., Marson, A.G., Davie, B. et al. (2017). Exploring changes over time and characteristics associated with data retrieval across individual participant data meta-analyses: systematic review. *BMJ* 357: j1390.

12. Tierney, J.F., Riley, R.D., Rydzewska, L.H.M., and Stewart, L.A. (2021). Running an IPD meta-analysis project: from developing the protocol to preparing data for meta-analysis. In: *Individual Participant Data Meta-Analysis: A Handbook for Healthcare Research* (eds. R.D. Riley, J.F. Tierney and L.A. Stewart), 45–80. Chichester: Wiley.

13. DerSimonian, R. and Laird, N. (1986). Meta-analysis in clinical trials. *Control. Clin. Trials* 7 (3): 177–188.

14. Higgins, J.P.T., Thompson, S.G., Deeks, J.J., and Altman, D.G. (2003). Measuring inconsistency in meta-analyses. *Br. Med. J.* 327 (7414): 557–560.

15. Askie, L.M., Duley, L., Henderson-Smart, D.J. et al. (2007). Antiplatelet agents for prevention of pre-eclampsia: a meta-analysis of individual patient data. *Lancet* 369 (9575): 1791–1798.

16. Stewart, G.B., Altman, D.G., Askie, L.M. et al. (2012). Statistical analysis of individual participant data meta-analyses: a comparison of methods and recommendations for practice. *PLoS One* 7 (10): e46042.

17. Jackson, D., Law, M., Stijnen, T. et al. (2018). A comparison of seven random-effects models for meta-analyses that estimate the summary odds ratio. *Stat. Med.* 37 (7): 1059–1085.

18. Higgins, J.P.T., Whitehead, A., Turner, R.M. et al. (2001). Meta-analysis of continuous outcome data from individual patients. *Stat. Med.* 20 (15): 2219–2241.

19. Turner, R.M., Omar, R.Z., Yang, M. et al. (2000). A multilevel model framework for meta-analysis of clinical trials with binary outcomes. *Stat. Med.* 19 (24): 3417–3432.

20. Whitehead, A., Omar, R.Z., Higgins, J.P.T. et al. (2001). Meta-analysis of ordinal outcomes using individual patient data. *Stat. Med.* 20 (15): 2243–2260.

21. Simmonds, M.C., Higgins, J.P.T., Stewart, L.A. et al. (2005). Meta-analysis of individual patient data from randomized trials: a review of methods used in practice. *Clin. Trials* 2 (3): 209–217.

22. Simmonds, M.C., Tierney, J., Bowden, J., and Higgins, J.P.T. (2011). Meta-analysis of time-to-event data: a comparison of two-stage methods. *Res. Synth. Methods* 2 (3): 139–149.

23. Crowther, M.J., Look, M.P., and Riley, R.D. (2014). Multilevel mixed effects parametric survival models using adaptive Gauss-Hermite quadrature with application to recurrent events and individual participant data meta-analysis. *Stat. Med.* 33 (22): 3844–3858.

24. Therneau, T.M., Grambsch, P.M., and Pankratz, V.S. (2003). Penalized survival models and frailty. *J. Comput. Graph. Stat.* 12 (1): 156–175.

25. Simmonds, M.C., Higgins, J.P.T., and Stewart, L.A. (2013). Random-effects meta-analysis of time-to-event data using the expectation-maximisation algorithm and shrinkage estimators. *Res. Synth. Methods* 4 (2): 144–155.

26. NSCLC Meta-analysis Collaborative Group (2014). Preoperative chemotherapy for non-small-cell lung cancer: a systematic review and meta-analysis of individual participant data. *Lancet* 383 (9928): 1561–1571.

27. Collins, F.S. and Varmus, H. (2015). A new initiative on precision medicine. *N. Engl. J. Med.* 372 (9): 793–795.

28. Thompson, S.G. and Higgins, J.P.T. (2002). How should meta-regression analyses be undertaken and interpreted? *Stat. Med.* 21 (11): 1559–1573.

29. Simmonds, M.C. and Higgins, J.P.T. (2007). Covariate heterogeneity in meta-analysis: criteria for deciding between meta-regression and individual patient data. *Stat. Med.* 26 (15): 2982–2999.

30. Thompson, S.G. and Higgins, J.P.T. (2005). Can meta-analysis help target interventions at individuals most likely to benefit? *Lancet* 365: 341–346.

31. Fisher, D.J., Carpenter, J.R., Morris, T.P. et al. (2017). Meta-analytical methods to identify who benefits most from treatments: daft, deluded, or deft approach? *BMJ* 356: j573.

32. Ben-Shlomo, Y., Spears, M., Boustred, C. et al. (2014). Aortic pulse wave velocity improves cardiovascular event prediction: an individual participant meta-analysis of prospective observational data from 17,635 subjects. *J. Am. Coll. Cardiol.* 63 (7): 636–646.

33. Riley, R.D., Simmonds, M.C., and Look, M.P. (2007). Evidence synthesis combining individual patient data and aggregate data: a systematic review identified current practice and possible methods. *J. Clin. Epidemiol.* 60 (5): 431–439.

34. Riley, R.D., Lambert, P.C., Staessen, J.A. et al. (2008). Meta-analysis of continuous outcomes combining individual patient data and aggregate data. *Stat. Med.* 27 (11): 1870–1893.

35. Stewart, L.A., Clarke, M., Rovers, M. et al. (2015). Preferred reporting items for systematic review and meta-analyses of individual participant data: the PRISMA-IPD statement. *JAMA* 313 (16): 1657–1665.

36. Stewart, L.A., Riley, R.D., and Tierney, J.F. (2021). Reporting and dissemination of IPD meta-analyses. In: *Individual Participant Data Meta-Analysis: A Handbook for Healthcare Research* (eds. R.D. Riley, J.F. Tierney and L.A. Stewart), 253–270. Chichester: Wiley.

CHAPTER 13

Network Meta-Analysis

Georgia Salanti and Julian P.T. Higgins

Evaluation of the role of any health intervention in clinical and public health practice requires consideration of alternative options for intervention. However, the meta-analysis methods described in Chapters 9 and 10 address only pairwise comparison of two interventions. **Network meta-analysis** provides a methodology for analyzing trials that compare three or more interventions [1–6]. For example, there are eight different percutaneous coronary interventions for the treatment of in-stent restenosis [7]. Various clinical trials have compared two or more of these interventions. Connections between the different interventions included in the trials may be viewed as forming a network of evidence, as illustrated in Figure 13.1. A network meta-analysis is a statistical synthesis of evidence across such a network, with the aim of determining which of the available interventions work better for the condition of interest, and it has become increasingly popular in recent years [4, 8–14]. A growing literature highlights its advantages and limitations [15–28] and explores its properties in empirical investigations [29–33] and simulation studies [9, 32, 34]. A glossary of terms commonly used in network meta-analysis is available from Cochrane (http://methods.cochrane.org/cmi/glossary).

13.1 INDIRECT COMPARISON AND TRANSITIVITY

A key concept underlying network meta-analysis is that of indirect comparison. Suppose we are interested in the relative effect of an intervention compared with another intervention, but no trials are available that have compared them directly. This is the case for bare metal stents versus everolimus-eluting stents in the network in

Systematic Reviews in Health Research: Meta-Analysis in Context, Third Edition. Edited by Matthias Egger, Julian P.T. Higgins, and George Davey Smith.
© 2022 John Wiley & Sons Ltd. Published 2022 by John Wiley & Sons Ltd.
Companion website: www.systematic-reviews3.org

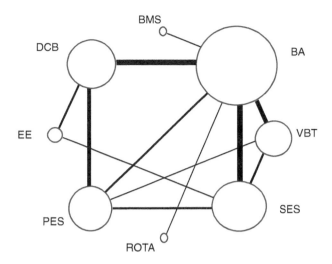

FIGURE 13.1   Complex evidence network of 26 trials comparing percutaneous coronary interventions in the treatment of in-stent restenosis. Nodes represent the different interventions and edges direct comparisons. The size of a node reflects the number of study arms assigned to the corresponding intervention, and the thickness of an edge reflects the number of studies of the corresponding direct comparison. BA, balloon angioplasty; BMS, bare metal stents; DCB, drug-coated balloons; EE, everolimus-eluting stents; PES, paclitaxel-eluting stents; ROTA, rotablation; SES, sirolimus-eluting stents; VBT, vascular brachytherapy. *Source*: Adapted from [7].

Figure 13.1 [7]. A comparison of these two interventions may be made using studies involving bare metal stents and different studies involving everolimus-eluting stents. Such a comparison is indirect because it is not derived from a direct, within-study comparison of the interventions.

A naive comparison of patient outcomes after an intervention (say, A) observed in one trial with patient outcomes after another intervention (B) observed in another trial is likely to be misleading, since results are confounded by other differences between the two trials. A more appropriate indirect comparison can be made if both studies additionally include patients receiving a common reference intervention (C). The difference between A and B may then be estimated by using the difference between A and C from one trial and the difference between B and C from the other trial. This approach to deriving indirect evidence is referred to as **adjusted indirect comparison** and lies at the heart of a network meta-analysis. The confounding present in the naive indirect comparison is reduced by adjusting for outcomes with intervention C.

The argument that A can be compared with B via C reflects an assumption of **transitivity** [35]. Indirect comparisons via the transitivity assumption are observational evidence even when they are based on randomized trials of A versus C and B versus C. Although participants are randomized within trials, interventions A and B have not been randomized against each other. The adjustment achieved through the common comparator intervention, C, adjusts for differences in baseline risk, or levels of a continuous outcome measure, across trials. However, it does not account for differences in effect modifiers, i.e. in characteristics that are associated with the magnitude of intervention effect. Effect modifiers may be related to the characteristics of patients included in a study such as their age, gender, or prevalence of comorbidities, or to study and intervention characteristics such as the inherent risk of bias (see also Chapter 4) or the intensity or delivery mode of an intervention. Effect modifiers are the sources of heterogeneity in a standard meta-analysis, but become potential sources of confounding in an indirect comparison. The validity of the indirect comparison relies on the A versus B studies being similar, on average, to the A versus C studies in all effect modifiers [9, 22, 30].

Transitivity can be violated under various scenarios [22, 35]. The nature of intervention C may differ between the A versus C and the B versus C trials, for example with regard to administration or dose, or the A versus C trials may have been done in populations that differed from those in the B versus C trials. For example, in a network of four interventions for preventing dental caries (toothpaste, rinse, varnish, and gel compared with placebo), it was found that the toothpaste studies were on average carried out much earlier than the other studies. Among other factors, both the quality of trials and the burden of dental disease have improved substantially over time, which might lead to violation of the transitivity assumption and an exaggeration of the relative effect of toothpaste [36].

Transitivity is an untestable assumption because it is impossible to identify and evaluate the comparability of the studies with respect to all possible effect modifiers whether measured or unmeasured. Nevertheless, comparability of suspected effect modifiers can increase confidence in the transitivity assumption.

13.2   INDIRECT AND DIRECT EVIDENCE

Sometimes both direct and indirect evidence are available for a particular comparison. In the example of the treatments of in-stent restenosis (Figure 13.1), 28 pairwise comparisons are possible between the eight active treatments (note that if the number of treatments is T, then the number of possible pairwise comparisons is $T(T-1)/2$). For 10 comparisons, both direct and indirect evidence is available; for two comparisons only direct evidence is available; and for the remaining 16 comparisons only indirect evidence is available.

Figure 13.2 presents a network of trials evaluating unfractionated heparin (UFH), low molecular weight heparin (LMWH), and an inactive control group or placebo in nonsurgical hospitalized patients at risk of venous thromboembolism [37]. Direct and indirect evidence exists for five out of six comparisons, but only indirect evidence was available for the comparison of greatest interest to the investigators: UFH given twice a day (bid) versus three times a day (tid). For this comparison, the authors used indirect evidence via either a control group (no intervention) or LMWH based on 13 trials [37]. In contrast, the comparison of UFH bid or UFH tid with LMWH can be estimated directly or indirectly via control. If transitivity holds and each set of studies is similar with regard to effect modifiers, then the direct and indirect sources of evidence are regarded as estimating the same underlying effect. They can then be combined statistically as described in Box 13.1.

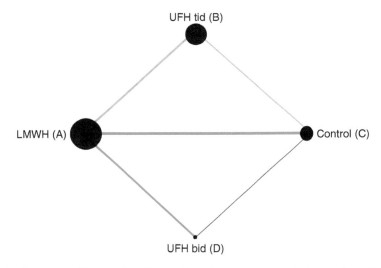

FIGURE 13.2 Network with two closed loops: low-dose unfractionated heparin (UFH) given twice a day (bid) versus three times a day (tid) and low molecular weight heparin (LMWH) to prevent thrombotic complications in nonsurgical hospitalized patients. The colors of the edges represent the risk of bias in the studies comparing pairs of interventions (red = high, yellow = moderate, green = low risk of bias). *Source*: Adapted from [37].

Box 13.1   The Statistics of Indirect Comparisons

The statistical manifestation of transitivity is called **consistency** and can be written mathematically by the **consistency assumption**

$$\mu_{AB} = \mu_{AC} - \mu_{BC} \tag{13.1}$$

where μ_{XY} denotes the average effect of any intervention X versus Y measured on a linear scale such as a mean difference, log odds ratio, or risk difference. Consider a network of trials of tyrosine-kinase inhibitors in the treatment of chronic myeloid leukemia (Figure 13.3) [38].

Let us suppose we undertake a meta-analysis of the nilotinib (A) versus imatinib (C) trials and a meta-analysis of the dasatinib (B) versus imatinib (C) trials, and denote the results as m_{AC}^d and m_{BC}^d, respectively, where d denotes that these are based on direct (head-to-head) trials of the treatments. Either a fixed-effect or a random-effects meta-analysis can be used. An indirect estimate of the nilotinib versus dacatinib difference – that is, of μ_{AB} in Eq. 13.1 – is obtained via the intermediate comparator, imatinib, as

$$m_{AB}^i = m_{AC}^d - m_{BC}^d \tag{13.2}$$

where the i denotes that the estimate is based on an indirect comparison. The variance of the indirect estimate is obtained simply by adding the variances of m_{AC}^d and m_{BC}^d.

Now suppose we have the example of the network presented in Figure 13.2. An indirect estimate for the comparison LMWH (A) versus UFH tid (B) via control

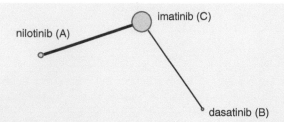

FIGURE 13.3   Network of trials of tyrosine-kinase inhibitors in the treatment of chronic myeloid leukemia.

(C) can be derived as described above. However, there is direct evidence for the LMWH versus UFH tid comparison, yielding a meta-analysis result m^d_{AB}. Under the assumption of consistency, we assume this is also an estimate of μ_{AB} in Eq. 13.1. Thus the indirect and direct estimates are considered to be estimating the same underlying intervention effect. They can therefore be combined using fixed-effect meta-analysis, i.e. using a weighted average with weights w^d_{AB} and w^i_{AB} equal to the respective inverse variances of the estimates m^d_{AB} and m^i_{AB}. Specifically, we obtain

$$m^{mixed}_{AB} = \frac{w^d_{AB} m^d_{AB} + w^i_{AB} m^i_{AB}}{w^d_{AB} + w^i_{AB}} \qquad (13.3)$$

as a further estimate of μ_{AB} in Eq. 13.1, where the term "mixed" refers to the fact that the estimate is based on a mixture of direct and indirect evidence.

It is of interest to examine whether the direct and the indirect estimates of μ_{AB} are statistically similar so that their combination is justified. The discrepancy, or **inconsistency**, between them is obtained simply as

$$\text{Inconsistency} = m^d_{AB} - m^i_{AB} \qquad (13.4)$$

The variance of this discrepancy is obtained by adding together the variances of m^d_{AB} and m^i_{AB}. This simple procedure is known as a "loop-based" evaluation of inconsistency in the context of a network meta-analysis.

Network meta-analyses are built on the same reasoning as the formulae presented in this box. However, they use more sophisticated methods to obtain direct, indirect, or mixed estimates, and measures of discrepancy, simultaneously for all intervention comparisons across the network.

Indirect evidence about two interventions may be produced via more than one route. For example, the comparison of LMWH versus UFH tid in Figure 13.2 has three sources of evidence: direct, indirect via control, and indirect via UFH bid and control. With multiple routes and multiple intervention comparisons, the network of evidence becomes complex and the simple statistical approach described in Box 13.1 becomes inefficient for estimating all effects.

13.3   NETWORK PLOTS OF INTERVENTIONS

Network plots such as those in Figures 13.1 and 13.2 provide a useful visual representation of the evidence base. Nodes in these plots represent the interventions and edges
represent the available direct comparisons. Three important aspects of the evidence
can be examined using such plots.

1. **Network structure**. Plots facilitate understanding of the data structure. For
   each comparison, evidence may come only from direct evidence, only from
   indirect evidence, or from a mixture of direct and indirect evidence. A mixture
   of evidence happens if (and only if) the comparison is part of a **closed loop**,
   which is a closed polygon in the network plot. In a **star network** all evidence is
   either direct or indirect, and there are no closed loops. Figure 13.4 shows a star
   network of four antiepileptic drugs for the treatment of refractory seizures [39].
   Figure 13.5, in contrast, shows a complex network of trials of new-generation
   antidepressants, which includes many direct comparisons between competing
   drugs [40]. Figures 13.1–13.5 were produced using the netgraph command in
   the network package in R [41]. Such plots can also be produced using the net-
   work_plot command from the network_graphs package in Stata [42].
2. **Properties of the evidence**. Typically, the size of a node reflects the number of participants assigned to the corresponding intervention, and the thickness of an edge
   reflects the number of studies of the corresponding direct comparison. Nodes and
   edges may alternatively (or additionally) be given attributes to represent potential
   effect modifiers, facilitating the detection of an uneven distribution of effect modifiers across comparisons [43]. For example, in Figure 13.2 the risk of bias averaged
   over the studies examining the same direct comparison is shown in different colors.
3. **Network connectedness**. The network plot facilitates examination of whether
   the evidence is fully connected. A network is connected when there is a path

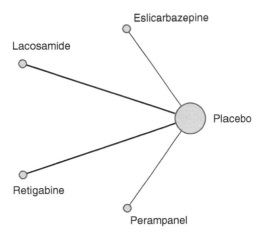

FIGURE 13.4   Star network of trials of antiepileptic drugs for the treatment of refractory seizures.
All active drugs have been compared with placebo, but no direct evidence is available between
active drugs. It is thus impossible to test the consistency assumption by statistical means as there
are no closed loops of evidence. *Source*: Adapted from [39].

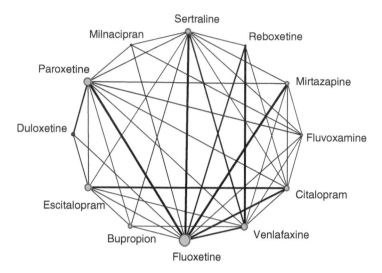

FIGURE 13.5   Complex network of trials of 12 new-generation antidepressants that includes many direct comparisons between competing drugs. The assumption of consistency can be tested in several closed loops and in the entire network. *Source*: Adapted from [40].

from each intervention to any other intervention in the plot. This means that every intervention can be compared with any other intervention either directly or via intermediate comparators. Network meta-analysis requires a connected network and investigation of the network plot for disconnected elements should precede any analysis.

13.4   SYSTEMATIC REVIEWS UNDERLYING NETWORK META-ANALYSIS

Systematic reviews underlying network meta-analyses follow the same general principles as those described earlier in this volume. Some special considerations are listed in Table 13.1. Guidance is available for writing protocols for systematic reviews that plan to synthesize the data using network meta-analysis [45]. Protocols should address issues that relate to the network of interventions to be compared, evaluation of assumptions, statistical methods to be employed, and methods for ranking the competing interventions.

Eligibility criteria for interventions and populations will need to be chosen so that they maximize the plausibility of transitivity. A helpful way to think about this is to require that all competing interventions are **jointly randomizable** for the population considered [22]. Interventions are jointly randomizable for the population if we can imagine a single multi-arm trial comparing all interventions of interest in the eligible participants. This avoids the inclusion of interventions in the network that are not indicated for the same condition. For example, interventions aimed at preventing an infection should not be included in a network with interventions aimed at treating its symptoms, because they will be studied in different populations.

Guidance is also available for reporting network meta-analyses in an extended PRISMA (Preferred Reporting Items for Systematic reviews and Meta-Analyses)

TABLE 13.1 Special considerations in a systematic review and network meta-analysis compared with the traditional process for pairwise comparisons.

Steps of a systematic review	Considerations for a network meta-analysis
1. Specifying the review question and eligibility criteria	Justify how the question would benefit from network meta-analysis Define the interventions in the network and which comparisons are of primary and secondary interest
2. Identifying studies	Search should be broad enough to capture interventions of interest
3. Collecting data and assessing risk of bias	Collect information on potential effect modifiers that may violate the assumption of transitivity
4. Planning the synthesis	Evaluate the network structure Evaluate transitivity
5. Undertaking the statistical synthesis	Conduct pairwise meta-analyses in addition to network meta-analyses Use statistical models appropriate for network meta-analysis Evaluate inconsistency Summarize results for all intervention comparisons, using appropriate numeric or graphical tools such as league tables If intervention hierarchy is of interest, use appropriate ranking statistics, such as SUCRA or mean ranks
6. Interpreting results and drawing conclusions	Carefully interpret results, especially intervention hierarchy Interpret results in context of outcomes examined Evaluate the confidence in network meta-analysis results using the CINeMA framework [44].
7. Reporting findings	Follow the PRISMA extension for network meta-analysis

PRISMA, Preferred Reporting Items for Systematic reviews and Meta-Analyses; SUCRA, surface under the cumulative ranking curve.

statement [46]. This emphasizes the need for detail on how the interventions were structured into a network, description of the statistical methods employed, attention to how to report comparisons of many interventions (including measures such as intervention rankings), and the extent to which the required assumptions could be demonstrated to be met.

13.5 SYNTHESIS OF DATA

Network meta-analyses can be implemented using different yet equivalent statistical approaches, briefly described here. Key to all approaches are the **consistency assumptions** (see Box 13.1), which describe the mathematical connections between the underlying average effect sizes for the various intervention comparisons. In the network of trials of heparins for the prevention of thrombotic complications [37] shown in Figure 13.2, six comparisons are possible. However, of these six possible comparisons only three are independent, while the remaining three can be written as functions of the first three using consistency assumptions. We call the three independent comparisons the **basic comparisons** and the derived comparisons the **functional comparisons**. The number of basic comparisons in a network meta-analysis is equal to the number of interventions minus one. Which comparisons are chosen as basic is unimportant provided that all interventions are represented in at least one basic comparison.

13.5.1   Assumptions About Heterogeneity

Network meta-analysis may take a fixed-effects or a random-effects approach to allow for between-study differences within each comparison. Under the random-effects model, studies of the same comparison are assumed to estimate different yet related intervention effects (see Chapter 9). The vast majority of network meta-analyses make the assumption that all pairwise comparisons have the same amount of heterogeneity. For example, in a simple A versus B versus C network, it is assumed that AB studies have the same heterogeneity as AC and BC studies. This is computationally convenient and reduces heterogeneity estimation problems when few studies are available for some of the comparisons. However, the assumption of equal heterogeneity variances needs to be justified in the context of the clinical setting. Empirical studies indicate that the amount of heterogeneity depends on the nature of the outcome and the types of interventions being compared; heterogeneity is in general higher when nonpharmacological interventions are studied and when the outcome is subjective [47, 48]. If the assumption is unlikely to hold, more complex models are available in which heterogeneity is allowed to differ according to the interventions being compared [49]. For example, we might assume two heterogeneity parameters allowing variability in all placebo-controlled studies to differ from variability in active versus active drug studies (for an example see [50]).

The assumption of equal heterogeneity parameters across all comparisons can lead to apparently paradoxical situations: estimates from network meta-analysis may end up being less precise than estimates from pairwise meta-analysis. For example, assume that AB studies have no heterogeneity ($\tau^2 = 0$, see Chapter 9). When analyzed within an A versus B versus C network where AC and BC studies have important heterogeneity, this heterogeneity is propagated to the AB studies and the estimate for AB will have larger confidence intervals compared with those obtained by a pairwise meta-analysis of AB studies alone.

13.5.2   Statistical Methods

Three mathematically equivalent ways to implement network meta-analysis are meta-regression, multivariate meta-analysis, and hierarchical modeling. In **meta-regression** the basic comparisons are treated as different dummy variables to be included as covariates in a regression model, although careful coding of the model is required to implement the consistency assumptions (see Box 13.2). If a network

Box 13.2   Implementing Network Meta-Analysis Using Meta-Regression

Networks in which all studies compare two interventions can be analyzed using standard meta-regression (see Chapter 10). In the example of the star network of antiepileptic drugs (Figure 13.4), consider four dummy variables defined by the four basic comparisons of each active intervention (eslicarbazepine, lacosamide, retigabine, perampanel; abbreviated as their first letter) versus a placebo control (abbreviated as C): I_{iEC}, I_{iLC}, I_{iRC}, I_{iPC}, where the index i refers to the study. If the ith study provides data on a basic comparison, say E versus C, then $I_{iEC} = 1$ and the other three dummy variables are zero; if the study compares R and C, then $I_{iRC} = 1$ and the other three are zero, and so on.

Denoting with y_i the estimate of the relative intervention effect in study i, network meta-analysis can be fitted as a random-effects meta-regression without an intercept

$$y_i = \mu_{EC} I_{iEC} + \mu_{LC} I_{iLC} + \mu_{RC} I_{iRC} + \mu_{PC} I_{iPC} + \delta_i + \varepsilon_i$$

The δ_i terms are random effects across studies within a comparison, with variance equal to the heterogeneity variance, and the ε_i terms represent random error within studies, with variances estimated from the data.

The estimated regression coefficients corresponding to each of the four dummy covariates are the network meta-analysis estimates for the respective comparisons. The analysis would also provide tests of significance and confidence intervals for the four estimated relative intervention effects. To obtain network meta-analysis estimates for the other comparisons (the functional comparisons), we simply employ the consistency equations – for instance, $m_{ER} = m_{RC} - m_{EC}$.

In this example, there are no head-to-head comparisons and all studies address one of the basic comparisons (i.e. an active intervention against C). If we had a study with a functional comparison, then the consistency assumptions need to be used to work out the values for the four dummies. For instance, if we had a study that compares E versus L, we would have $I_{iEC} = 1$, $I_{iLC} = -1$ and all other dummies zero in line with the consistency Eq. 13.1 in Box 13.1.

includes multi-arm studies, then these studies provide data for more than one comparison and thus contribute more than one effect size. Effect sizes belonging to the same study are correlated, and this needs to be taken into account. Salanti and colleagues provide further details [51].

Multivariate meta-analysis views the basic comparisons as if they were different study outcomes. For the simple A versus B versus C network, we consider two outcomes of interest, AB and AC. An A versus B study reports on the first outcome; an A versus C study reports on the second outcome, while an A versus B versus C study reports on both outcomes. This framework requires a reformatting of the data such that the results of each study are expressed in terms of the basic comparisons alone. In practice this may involve a procedure known as data augmentation, in which a very small amount of data is imputed to create a complete dataset for all basic comparisons (irrespective of whether they have been investigated in each study). This allows the analysis to work, but the information imputed is so little that it does not affect the final results. In the example above, because a B versus C study contributes neither an A versus B comparison nor an A versus C comparison, very small amounts of data for these comparisons are generated (for example, by imputing data for 0.001 patients in the A arm so that A versus B and A versus C comparisons are possible but with near-zero weight). For further details, see White and colleagues [52]. Once the study data are set up so that each study reports on at least one basic comparison, standard multivariate meta-analysis techniques are employed to synthesize the data [53, 54]. The network meta-analysis estimates for all other comparisons are obtained by computing them from results for the basic comparisons.

Hierarchical models implement a random-effects model by considering two levels of variation. At the first level, the observed data are used to estimate the underlying or true study-specific intervention effects for each study. At the second level, these underlying effects are combined for each pairwise comparison under constraints that ensure the transitivity assumption holds. Hierarchical models fitted in a Bayesian framework are the most popular approach so far to network meta-analysis [8, 12]; details can be found in Lu and Ades, and in Salanti and colleagues [3, 51]. Bayesian implementations tend to produce slightly wider confidence intervals (more strictly, these are credible intervals) because, unlike standard implementations of frequentist methods, they allow for full uncertainty in all unknown quantities.

The results from network meta-analysis of trials of heparins for the prevention of thrombotic complications [37] (Figure 13.2) are summarized in Table 13.2. These were obtained using a multivariate meta-analysis approach fitted in Stata using the `mvmeta` command from the `network` package [55] and assuming that all comparisons share the same heterogeneity parameter. We can see from the width of the confidence intervals that most of the evidence comes from studies comparing active interventions versus control. The precision of all comparisons is improved with network meta-analysis compared with pairwise meta-analyses.

13.6   INTRANSITIVITY AND INCONSISTENCY

When transitivity holds, estimates from direct and indirect comparisons are expected to be in agreement (within the margins of random error and heterogeneity). If clinical or methodological study characteristics that are effect modifiers differ across intervention comparisons, then transitivity will not hold. This can be seen in the data as **inconsistency**: estimates from direct and indirect comparisons differ. Several statistical methods are available to detect inconsistency [11, 22, 35, 56, 57]. These methods can be broadly classified into local approaches and global approaches. **Local approaches** detect whether a particular part of the network is inconsistent. They include a loop-based approach [43, 58], the node-splitting approach [59], and the

TABLE 13.2 Results from network meta-analysis and pairwise meta-analysis for the network of interventions to prevent thrombolitic complications presented in Figure 13.2. The overall odds ratio (OR) for efficacy and a 95% confidence interval (CI) are presented. Control describes an inactive control group or placebo.

	Network meta-analysis		For comparison: pairwise meta-analyses		
	OR	95% CI	OR	95% CI	Statistical note
UFH tid vs. Control	0.46	(0.30–0.69)	0.17	(0.05–0.59)	Basic comparison, directly estimated by the network meta-analysis
LMWH vs. Control	0.39	(0.29–0.52)	0.46	(0.34–0.62)	Basic comparison, directly estimated by the network meta-analysis
UFH bid vs. Control	0.32	(0.13–0.76)	0.10	(0.01–0.79)	Basic comparison, directly estimated by the network meta-analysis
UFH tid vs. UFH bid	1.45	(0.59–3.57)	–	–	Functional comparison, computed from the basic comparisons
UFH tid vs. LMWH	1.18	(0.86–1.61)	1.27	(0.37–2.36)	Functional comparison, computed from the basic comparisons
UFH bid vs. LMWH	1.23	(0.53–2.86)	1.06	(0.42–2.70)	Functional comparison, computed from the basic comparisons

net-heat matrix [60]. Perhaps the most useful of these is the node-splitting approach. Confusingly named in relation to a network plot, this takes each edge in the network plot and separates the evidence into the direct (pairwise) comparison represented by this edge and the indirect comparison obtained by synthesizing all the rest of the network. **Global approaches** evaluate whether the network is consistent as a whole, and test whether all potential sources of local inconsistency are simultaneously zero. They can be implemented by comparing results under a consistency assumption with results under either a model that allows the inconsistencies to vary freely (a fixed-effects inconsistency model) or a constrained model (a random-effects inconsistency model). Global tests might be referred to as tests of "design-by-treatment interaction" [41, 60–62].

In the network meta-analysis of trials of heparins for the prevention of thrombotic complications, local inconsistency (using a loop-based approach) can be estimated by comparing the direct and indirect intervention effects within each of the two closed loops of evidence, ABC and ADC. For instance, the indirect odds ratio (OR) of UFH tid versus LMWH via control is 0.37, obtained as 0.17/0.46 from Table 13.2, while the direct OR is 1.27. A statistical test for the discrepancy between the two ORs gives P = 0.07. Following a similar approach, the other closed loop gives P = 0.17. Given the low power of the test and the small number of studies, there are concerns about inconsistency in the loop formed by UFH tid, LMWH, and control. The global test for this network suggests the presence of inconsistency in the whole network (P = 0.03). These findings warrant further investigation of the inconsistency to explain why different sources of evidence yield different conclusions, possibly by accounting for differences in effect modification.

Empirical evidence has shown that about 9% of closed loops of evidence (networks consisting of three interventions) and about 13% of whole networks show inconsistency [34, 56]. Because tests for inconsistency have low power [34, 63], the proportion of networks in which inconsistency is present is likely to be higher than this. Moreover, different assumptions and different ways of estimating the heterogeneity variance can influence detection of inconsistency [63]. Consequently, test results should be interpreted with caution and the absence of statistically significant inconsistency should not be taken as proof of consistency, particularly for networks with few studies or large heterogeneity. To overcome some of the limitations of statistical tests, I^2 measures analogous to those for pairwise meta-analysis (see Chapter 9) have been developed for network meta-analysis [62].

When inconsistency is present, efforts should be made to explain the disagreement between direct and indirect evidence, for example by using network meta-regression techniques to account for differences in study characteristics [36, 64]. When no explanation is found, investigators may use models that accommodate inconsistency in the network meta-analysis by adding extra variability to account for the disagreement between the various sources of evidence [3, 52, 62]. However, such models should be used only if the amount of unexplained inconsistency is small in relation to the variation in mean effect sizes across comparisons.

13.7 RANKING INTERVENTIONS

The estimated relative intervention effects for all comparisons are the typical output from a network meta-analysis. Prediction intervals on top of the confidence intervals, as described in Chapter 9, can also be presented to convey the magnitude of heterogeneity [65]. These comparison-level effects can, however, make it difficult to determine whether there is evidence for the superiority of one intervention over other interventions. Estimating a hierarchy of the competing interventions involves calculating ranking probabilities (the probability that an intervention is at a specific rank) based on the distributions of intervention effects [18, 35].

Rankograms are a graphical way to present both ranking probabilities and their uncertainty [66]. A rankogram is a plot of the probabilities that an intervention takes each of the possible ranks. A cumulative rankogram presents the cumulative versions of these probabilities. The surface under the cumulative ranking curve (SUCRA, a transformation of the mean rank) and the median rank are numerical summaries of a rankogram and can be used to provide a hierarchy of the interventions [66]. They can also be useful in comparing results from different analyses, for example different meta-regression models.

Figure 13.6 shows the rankograms from the network meta-analysis of the example on antidepressants presented in Figure 13.5. For the studied outcome (improvement

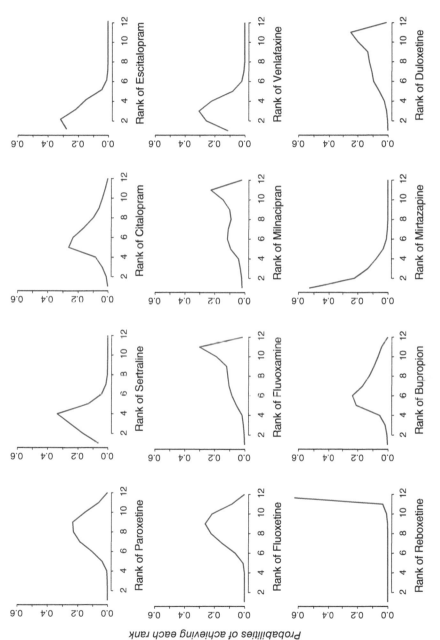

FIGURE 13.6 Rankograms from network of trials of 12 new-generation antidepressants for improvement in symptoms. The horizontal axis shows the 12 possible ranks and the vertical axis the probability of each rank. *Source*: Adapted from [40].

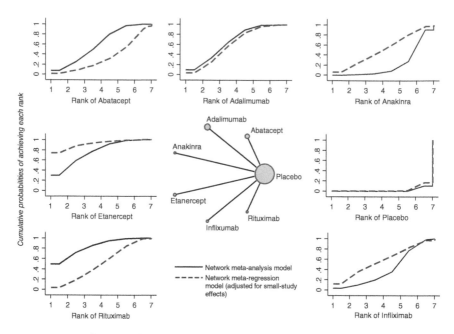

FIGURE 13.7   Cumulative ranking for six biologics for rheumatoid arthritis with respect to improvement in ACR50. The horizontal axis shows the six possible ranks and the vertical axis the cumulative probability for each intervention to be among the best x options, where x ranges from 1 to 7. Solid lines are cumulative ranking probabilities estimated from network meta-analysis. Dashed lines are cumulative ranking probabilities estimated from network meta-regression, adjusting for small-study effects. *Source*: Adapted from [67].

in depression symptoms) mirtazapine and escitalopram have a higher probability of being among the best two interventions, whereas reboxetine has a high probability of ranking as the least effective.

Figure 13.7 shows a network that compares the effectiveness of six biologics in patients with rheumatoid arthritis [67]. Small-study effects where the smaller studies show larger intervention effects than the larger studies were examined in the data (see also Chapter 5). Figure 13.7 shows cumulative rankings from a re-analysis of these data in which intervention effects were adjusted for small-study effects in network meta-regression analysis.

13.8   CONCLUSIONS

Network meta-analyses allow the simultaneous synthesis of multiple clinical trials making different comparisons from among a specific set of alternative interventions. Network meta-analyses play an increasingly important role in evidence-based health care, generalizing the traditional meta-analysis method to facilitate selection of those intervention options that have the most favorable trade-off between benefit and harm. Network meta-analyses are built on the notion of adjusted indirect comparisons, exploiting mathematical connections between the different pairwise comparisons of interventions in the network. The assumptions underlying network analyses require careful examination, however. It is important to ensure that the studies contributing evidence to the different intervention comparisons in the network are sufficiently similar in all important characteristics.

Practical Exercises and Further Resources

Further resources on network meta-analysis are listed on our website at www.systematic-reviews3.org.

Visit our website for practical exercises relevant to this chapter.

REFERENCES

1. Caldwell, D.M., Ades, A.E., and Higgins, J.P.T. (2005). Simultaneous comparison of multiple treatments: combining direct and indirect evidence. *BMJ* 331 (7521): 897–900.
2. Higgins, J.P.T. and Whitehead, A. (1996). Borrowing strength from external trials in a meta-analysis. *Stat. Med.* 15 (24): 2733–2749.
3. Lu, G. and Ades, A.E. (2004). Combination of direct and indirect evidence in mixed treatment comparisons. *Stat. Med.* 23 (20): 3105–3124.
4. Coleman, C.I., Phung, O.J., Cappelleri, J.C. et al. (2012). *Use of Mixed Treatment Comparison in Systematic Reviews*. Prepared by the university of Connecticut/Harford Hospital Evidence-Based Practice Center under Contract No. 290-2007-10067-I. Publication No. 12-EHC119-EF. Rockville, MD: Agency for Healthcare Research and Quality.
5. Lumley, T. (2002). Network meta-analysis for indirect treatment comparisons. *Stat. Med.* 21 (16): 2313–2324.
6. Nikolakopoulou, A., White, I.R., Salanti, G. (2020). *Network Meta-Analysis*. In: Handbook of Meta-Analysis (pp. 187–218). New York: Chapman and Hall/CRC. https://doi.org/10.1201/9781315119403.
7. Siontis, G.C.M., Stefanini, G.G., Mavridis, D. et al. (2015). Percutaneous coronary interventional strategies for treatment of in-stent restenosis: a network meta-analysis. *Lancet* 386 (9994): 655–664.
8. Nikolakopoulou, A., Chaimani, A., Veroniki, A.A. et al. (2014). Characteristics of networks of interventions: a description of a database of 186 published networks. *PLoS One* 9 (1): e86754.
9. Glenny, A.M., Altman, D.G., Song, F. et al. (2005). Indirect comparisons of competing interventions. *Health Technol. Assess.* 9 (1366-5278 (Print)): 1–iv.
10. D'Ascenzo, F. and Biondi-Zoccai, G. (2014). Network meta-analyses: the "White Whale" for cardiovascular specialists. *J. Cardiothorac. Vasc. Anesth.* 28 (1): 169–173.
11. Donegan, S., Williamson, P., Gamble, C., and Tudur-Smith, C. (2010). Indirect comparisons: a review of reporting and methodological quality. *PLoS One* 5 (1932-6203): e11054.
12. Sobieraj, D.M., Cappelleri, J.C., Baker, W.L. et al. (2013). Methods used to conduct and report Bayesian mixed treatment comparisons published in the medical literature: a systematic review. *BMJ Open* 3: 2044–6055.

13. Petropoulou, M., Nikolakopoulou, A., Veroniki, A.-A. et al. (2017). Bibliographic study showed improving statistical methodology of network meta-analyses published between 1999 and 2015. *J. Clin. Epidemiol.* 82: 20–28.

14. Zarin, W., Veroniki, A.A., Nincic, V. et al. (2017). Characteristics and knowledge synthesis approach for 456 network meta-analyses: a scoping review. *BMC Med.* 15 (1): 3.

15. Cooper, N.J., Peters, J., Lai, M.C. et al. (2011). How valuable are multiple treatment comparison methods in evidence-based health-care evaluation? *Value Health* 14 (2): 371–380.

16. Cucherat, M., and Izard, V. (2009). Summary report: Indirect comparisons: methods and validity. Saint-Denis La Plaine: Haute Autorité de Santé. https://www.has-sante.fr/plugins/ModuleXitiKLEE/types/FileDocument/doXiti.jsp?id=c_1027686 (accessed 21 February 2022).

17. EUnetHTA – European Network for Health Technology Assessment (2015). Comparators and comparisons: Direct and indirect comparisons. Amended JA1 Guideline. https://www.eunethta.eu/wp-content/uploads/2018/01/Comparators-Comparisons-Direct-and-indirect-comparisons_Amended-JA1-Guideline_Final-Nov-2015.pdf (accessed 22 February 2022).

18. Jansen, J.P., Fleurence, R., Devine, B. et al. (2011). Interpreting indirect treatment comparisons and network meta-analysis for health-care decision making: report of the ISPOR task force on indirect treatment comparisons good research practices: part 1. *Value Health* 14 (4): 417–428.

19. Jansen, J.P., Crawford, B., Bergman, G., and Stam, W. (2008). Bayesian meta-analysis of multiple treatment comparisons: an introduction to mixed treatment comparisons. *Value Health* 11 (5): 956–964.

20. Malone, D.C. (2007). Using indirect comparisons in pharmacoeconomic studies – time for implementation. *Clin. Ther.* 29: 2454–2455.

21. Naci, H. and Fleurence, R. (2011). Using indirect evidence to determine the comparative effectiveness of prescription drugs: do benefits outweight risks? *Health Outcomes Res. Med.* 2 (4): 241–249.

22. Salanti, G. (2012). Indirect and mixed-treatment comparison, network, or multiple-treatments meta-analysis: many names, many benefits, many concerns for the next generation evidence synthesis tool. *Res. Synth. Methods* 3 (2): 80–97.

23. Sutton, A., Ades, A.E., Cooper, N., and Abrams, K. (2008). Use of indirect and mixed treatment comparisons for technology assessment. *Pharmacoeconomics* 26 (9): 753–767.

24. Welton, N.J., Sutton, A.J., Cooper, N. et al. (2012). Mixed and indirect treatment comparisons. In: *Evidence Synthesis for Decision Making in Healthcare* (eds. N.J. Welton, A.J. Sutton, N. Cooper, et al.). New York: Wiley.

25. Hoaglin, D.C., Hawkins, N., Jansen, J.P. et al. (2011). Conducting indirect-treatment-comparison and network-meta-analysis studies: report of the ISPOR task force on indirect treatment comparisons good research practices: part 2. *Value Health* 14: 429–437.

26. Cipriani, A., Barbui, C., Rizzo, C., and Salanti, G. (2012). What is a multiple treatments meta-analysis? *Epidemiol. Psychiatr. Sci.* 21: 151–153.

27. Sutton, A.J., Cooper, N.J., and Jones, D.R. (2009). Evidence synthesis as the key to more coherent and efficient research. *BMC Med. Res. Methodol.* 9: 29.

28. Nikolakopoulou, A., Mavridis, D., Furukawa, T.A. et al. (2018). Living network meta-analysis compared with pairwise meta-analysis in comparative effectiveness research: empirical study. *BMJ* 360: k585.

29. O'Regan, C., Ghement, I., Eyawo, O. et al. (2009). Incorporating multiple interventions in meta-analysis: an evaluation of the mixed treatment comparison with the adjusted indirect comparison. *Trials* 10: 86.

30. Song, F., Altman, D.G., Glenny, A.M., and Deeks, J.J. (2003). Validity of indirect comparison for estimating efficacy of competing interventions: empirical evidence from published meta-analyses. *BMJ* 326: 472.

31. Song, F., Harvey, I., and Lilford, R. (2008). Adjusted indirect comparison may be less biased than direct comparison for evaluating new pharmaceutical interventions. *J. Clin. Epidemiol.* 61 (5): 455–463.

32. Jonas, D.E., Wilkins, T.M., Bangdiwala, S. et al. (2013; Publication No. 13-EHC039-EF). *Findings of Bayesian Mixed Treatment Comparison Meta-Analysis: Comparison and Exploration Using Real-Word Trial Data and Simulation.* Rockville, MD: AHRQ: Agency for Healthcare Research and Quality.

33. Madan, J., Stevenson, M.D., Cooper, K.L. et al. (2011). Consistency between direct and indirect trial evidence: is direct evidence always more reliable? *Value Health* 14: 953–960.

34. Song, F., Clark, A., Bachmann, M.O., and Maas, J. (2012). Simulation evaluation of statistical properties of methods for indirect and mixed treatment comparisons. *BMC Med. Res. Methodol.* 12 (1): 138.

35. Cipriani, A., Higgins, J.P.T., Geddes, J.R., and Salanti, G. (2013). Conceptual and technical challenges in network meta-analysis. *Ann. Intern. Med.* 159 (2): 130–137.

36. Salanti, G., Marinho, V., and Higgins, J.P.T. (2009). A case study of multiple-treatments meta-analysis demonstrates that covariates should be considered. *J. Clin. Epidemiol.* 62 (8): 857–864.

37. Phung, O.J., Kahn, S.R., Cook, D.J., and Murad, M.H. (2011). Dosing frequency of unfractionated heparin thromboprophylaxis: a meta-analysis. *Chest J.* 140 (2): 374–381.

38. Mealing, S., Barcena, L., Hawkins, N. et al. (2013). The relative efficacy of imatinib, dasatinib and nilotinib for newly diagnosed chronic myeloid leukemia: a systematic review and network meta-analysis. *Exp. Hematol. Oncol.* 2: 5.

39. Khan, N., Shah, D., Tongbram, V. et al. (2013). The efficacy and tolerability of perampanel and other recently approved anti-epileptic drugs for the treatment of refractory partial onset seizure: a systematic review and Bayesian network meta-analysis. *Curr. Med. Res. Opin.* 29 (8): 1001–1013.

40. Cipriani, A., Furukawa, T.A., Salanti, G. et al. (2009). Comparative efficacy and acceptability of 12 new-generation antidepressants: a multiple-treatments meta-analysis. *Lancet* 373 (9665): 746–758.

41. Rucker, G., and Schwarzer, G. (2021). netmeta: An R package for network meta-analysis. https://cran.r-project.org/web/packages/netmeta/netmeta.pdf (accessed 8 September 2021).

42. Chaimani, A. and Salanti, G. (2015). Visualizing assumptions and results in network meta-analysis: the network graphs package. *Stata J.* 15 (4): 905–950.

43. Chaimani, A., Higgins, J.P.T., Mavridis, D. et al. (2013). Graphical tools for network meta-analysis in STATA. *PLoS One* 8 (10): e76654.

44. Nikolakopoulou, A., Higgins, J.P.T., Papakonstantinou, T. et al. (2020). CINeMA: An approach for assessing confidence in the results of a network meta-analysis. *PLoS Med.* 17(4): e1003082.

45. Chaimani, A., Caldwell, D.M., Li, T. et al. (2017). Additional considerations are required when preparing a protocol for a systematic review with multiple interventions. *J. Clin. Epidemiol.* 83: 65–74.

46. Hutton, B., Salanti, G., Chaimani, A. et al. (2014). The quality of reporting methods and results in network meta-analyses: an overview of reviews and suggestions for improvement. *PLoS One* 9 (3): e92508.

47. Turner, R.M., Davey, J., Clarke, M.J. et al. (2012). Predicting the extent of heterogeneity in meta-analysis, using empirical data from the Cochrane database of systematic reviews. *Int. J. Epidemiol.* 41 (3): 818–827.

48. Rhodes, K.M., Turner, R.M., and Higgins, J.P.T. (2016). Empirical evidence about inconsistency among studies in a pair-wise meta-analysis. *Res. Synth. Methods* 7 (4): 346–370.

49. Lu, G. and Ades, A. (2009). Modeling between-trial variance structure in mixed treatment comparisons. *Biostatistics* 7 (4): 346–370.

50. Cipriani, A., Furukawa, T.A., Salanti, G. et al. (2018). Comparative efficacy and acceptability of 21 antidepressant drugs for the acute treatment of adults with major depressive disorder: a systematic review and network meta-analysis. *Lancet* 391 (10128): 1357–1366.

51. Salanti, G., Higgins, J.P.T., Ades, A.E., and Ioannidis, J.P.A. (2008). Evaluation of networks of randomized trials. *Stat. Methods Med. Res.* 17 (3): 279–301.

52. White, I.R., Barrett, J.K., Jackson, D., and Higgins, J.P.T. (2012). Consistency and inconsistency in network meta-analysis: model estimation using multivariate meta-regression. *Res. Synth. Methods* 3 (2): 111–125.

53. Mavridis, D. and Salanti, G. (2013). A practical introduction to multivariate meta-analysis. *Stat. Methods Med. Res.* 22 (2): 133–158.

54. Jackson, D., Riley, R., and White, I.R. (2011). Multivariate meta-analysis: potential and promise. *Stat. Med.* 30 (20): 2481–2498.

55. White, I.R. (2015). Network meta-analysis. *Stata Journal* 15 (4): 951–985.

56. Veroniki, A.A., Vasiliadis, H.S., Higgins, J.P.T., and Salanti, G. (2013). Evaluation of inconsistency in networks of interventions. *Int. J. Epidemiol.* 42 (1): 332–345.

57. Dias, S., Welton, N.J., Sutton, A.J. et al. (2013). Evidence synthesis for decision making 4: inconsistency in networks of evidence based on randomized controlled trials. *Med. Decis. Making* 33 (5): 641–656.

58. Bucher, H.C., Guyatt, G.H., Griffith, L.E., and Walter, S.D. (1997). The results of direct and indirect treatment comparisons in meta-analysis of randomized controlled trials. *J. Clin. Epidemiol.* 50 (6): 683–691.

59. Dias, S., Welton, N.J., Caldwell, D.M., and Ades, A.E. (2010). Checking consistency in mixed treatment comparison meta-analysis. *Stat. Med.* 29: 932–944.

60. Krahn, U., Binder, H., and Konig, J. (2013). A graphical tool for locating inconsistency in network meta-analyses. *BMC Med. Res. Methodol.* 13: 35.

61. Higgins, J.P.T., Jackson, D., Barrett, J.K. et al. (2012). Consistency and insconsistency in network meta-analysis: concepts and models for multi-arm studies. *Res. Synth. Methods* 3 (2): 98–110.

62. Jackson, D., Barrett, J.K., Rice, S. et al. (2014). A design-by-treatment interaction model for network meta-analysis with random inconsistency effects. *Stat. Med.* 33 (21): 3639–3654.

63. Veroniki, A.A., Mavridis, D., Higgins, J.P.T., and Salanti, G. (2014). Characteristics of a loop of evidence that affect detection and estimation of inconsistency: a simulation study. *BMC Med. Res. Methodol.* 14 (1): 106.

64. Cooper, N.J., Sutton, A.J., Morris, D. et al. (2009). Addressing between-study heterogeneity and inconsistency in mixed treatment comparisons: application to stroke prevention treatments in individuals with non-rheumatic atrial fibrillation. *Stat. Med.* 28: 1861–1881.

65. Riley, R.D., Higgins, J.P.T., and Deeks, J.J. (2011). Interpretation of random effects meta-analyses. *BMJ* 342: d549.

66. Salanti, G., Ades, A.E., and Ioannidis, J.P.A. (2011). Graphical methods and numerical summaries for presenting results from multiple-treatment meta-analysis: an overview and tutorial. *J. Clin. Epidemiol.* 64: 163–171.

67. Singh, J.A., Christensen, R., Wells, G.A. et al. (2009). A network meta-analysis of randomized controlled trials of biologics for rheumatoid arthritis: a Cochrane overview. *CMAJ* 181 (11): 787–796.

CHAPTER 14

Dose–Response Meta-Analysis

Nicola Orsini, Susanna C. Larsson, and Georgia Salanti

Dose–response relationships are of great interest in epidemiology and medicine. They are important in the context of etiological, public health, and clinical questions. Recent examples include the relationship between dietary fiber intake and coronary heart disease; markers of immune activation/inflammation and non-Hodgkin lymphoma; and body mass index and COVID-19 mortality [1–3]. The existence of a dose–response mechanism between a presumed cause and the occurrence of an outcome is one of the nine criteria famously proposed by Bradford Hill that should be considered "before deciding that the most likely interpretation of it is causation" [4].

A strategy for meta-analytical assessment of the effect of quantitative predictors and outcomes in observational studies with individual participant data has been recently proposed [5]. The main focus of this chapter is a two-stage dose–response meta-analysis based on summarized data. Studies comparing outcomes at different levels of exposure or different doses of an intervention are often reduced to a table of contrasts relative to a chosen referent [6]. When summarizing these published sets of contrasts, it is quite common to focus on the highest versus lowest contrast, and to synthesize these effect sizes across multiple studies using standard meta-analytic models. An example in nutritional epidemiology is processed meat consumption in relation to mortality risk [7]. This approach is straightforward and easy to implement. It avoids any assumptions about the shape of the relationship between the different levels of exposure and the outcome. However, it does not use all the information contained in the data. Also, the size of the effect may differ across studies, depending on the definition used for the highest and lowest exposure category, thus introducing heterogeneity (see also Chapters 9 and 10) [8].

Systematic Reviews in Health Research: Meta-Analysis in Context, Third Edition. Edited by Matthias Egger, Julian P.T. Higgins, and George Davey Smith.
© 2022 John Wiley & Sons Ltd. Published 2022 by John Wiley & Sons Ltd.
Companion website: www.systematic-reviews3.org

A dose–response meta-analysis estimates the change of a response along the range of a quantitative exposure combining findings from multiple studies. In the most popular two-stage model, a dose–response analysis is taking place within each study [9–11]. A particular shape for the dose–response association is assumed (e.g. linear, quadratic), informed by content knowledge and epidemiological or clinical hypotheses in light of the available information. Then the within-study shape characteristics (e.g. the coefficients of a linear trend) are synthesized across studies. In a single-stage model or mixed-effects model, within- and across-studies dose–response shape is estimated in one step [12, 13]. Today, dose–response meta-analysis is conducted in a variety of disciplines (i.e. oncology, public health, nutrition, cardiology). Several methodological developments have taken place that enable flexible modeling of dose–response associations, assessment of publication bias, assignment of a typical dose to an exposure interval, assessment of the goodness of fit of the model, and a Bayesian approach based on hierarchical models [10, 12, 14–21].

In this chapter we provide an introduction to methods for summarizing aggregated dose–response data from multiple studies. We will illustrate how to investigate linear and nonlinear dose–response relationships using empirical data on coffee consumption and all-cause mortality as a motivating example.

14.1   EXAMPLE: COFFEE CONSUMPTION AND MORTALITY RISK

We illustrate the methods by re-analyzing the association between coffee consumption (cups/day) and all-cause mortality rates arising from 15 prospective cohort studies, including a total of 118 865 deaths [22]. Information was collected on sex, number of subjects (total number of deaths and total cohort size or total number of deaths and person-years of follow-up), coffee consumption, and estimated adjusted risk ratio (RR) with the studies' 95% confidence intervals. Since seven cohorts presented results by sex, the data include a total of 22 different tables of summarized dose–response data. Code (Stata, R) is available on this book's website (www.systematic-reviews3.org).

14.2   ESTIMATING DOSE–RESPONSE ASSOCIATION WITHIN A STUDY

Table 14.1 presents the data from the study by Klatsky et al. associating coffee consumption with mortality risk [23]. The reference dose category is zero cups/day, and the four estimated RRs, together with their standard errors, are presented. The shape implicit in this parametrization is a step function with jumps at the study-specific cut points used to categorize coffee consumption.

14.3   A LINEAR TREND FOR A SINGLE STUDY

The aim is now to associate the increase in the dose of coffee to the change in mortality risk using data in Table 14.1. The four empirical (log) RRs measure the estimated change in the mortality risk comparing 0.5, 2, 5, and 8 cups/day relative to 0 cups/

TABLE 14.1   Summarized data for the study by Klatsky et al. [23] including the number of deaths, total number of participants, adjusted RRs with 95% confidence intervals, the natural logarithm of the RRs with standard errors by levels of coffee intake measured in cups per day.

Level	Dose (cups/day)	Deaths	Total	RR (95% CI)	ln(RR)	SE(ln(RR))
0	0	832	34 755	1.00 (ref)		0 (ref)
1	0.5	564	18 106	0.96 (0.86, 1.08)	−0.041	0.059
2	2	2081	53 596	0.94 (0.86, 1.02)	−0.062	0.044
3	5	658	15 541	0.93 (0.83, 1.04)	−0.073	0.058
4	8	274	5522	0.88 (0.76, 1.02)	−0.128	0.075

day. We can specify a linear regression model, without an intercept, for the expected change in mortality RRs (on the natural log scale) according to changes in coffee consumption (cups/day) as follows:

$$E\left(\ln(RR_k) \mid dose_k \right) = \beta \left(dose_k - dose_{ref} \right).$$

The dose is centered about the reference dose because the dependent variable is an empirical change in responses. The exponentiated regression coefficient $\exp(\beta)$ represents the expected RR of mortality (or the relative increase/decrease in the outcome risk) associated with every one additional coffee cup per day in the kth study. As in meta-regression, each empirical estimate is weighted in the analysis by the inverse of the variance of $\ln(RR_k)$. Additionally, the four risk ratios are not independent, because they share the same reference category – 0 cups/day. Consequently, appropriate statistical methods, such as generalized least squares, need to be employed that account for the positive correlation of the $\ln(RR_k)$ [9, 16, 24]. These methods involve an estimate of the covariances between the log RRs. If the RRs were unadjusted, then the covariance between any two log RRs would be simply $\frac{1}{c_{ref}} - \frac{1}{t_{ref}}$, where c_{ref} and t_{ref} are the number of cases and total individuals in the reference group, respectively. If the $\ln(RR_k)$ are adjusted for potential confounding factors, then the covariances can be computed using the methods presented by Greenland and Longnecker [9], Hamling et al. [25], or Easton et al. [26, 27].

Using the Greenland and Longnecker method, the meta-regression coefficient estimated for the study by Klatsky et al. [23] is $\hat{\beta} = -0.014$ (95% CI 0.029–0.001). Figure 14.1 shows the estimated linear trend.

14.4   A QUADRATIC TREND FOR A SINGLE STUDY

The linear association above can be extended into a quadratic shape by adding a quadratic transformation of the dose. The model is then

$$E\left(\ln(RR_k) \mid dose_k \right) = \beta_1 \left(dose_k - dose_{ref} \right) + \beta_2 \left(dose_k^2 - dose_{ref}^2 \right)$$

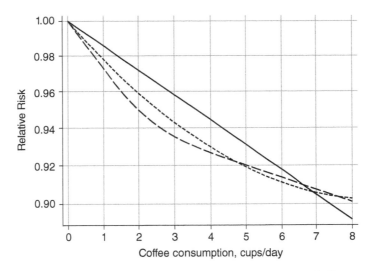

FIGURE 14.1 Dose–response association between coffee consumption and all-cause mortality risk estimated for the study by Klasky et al. [23]. Summarized data were fitted using a linear (solid), quadratic (short dash), and restricted cubic spline (long dash) function in an inverse variance/covariance weighted linear regression model. No coffee consumption (0 cups/day) served as referent.

where the two coefficients β_1 and β_2 jointly define the shape of the relationship. Of note is that any squared dose is centered about the squared reference dose. The centering of the dose transformations is done internally in the R dosresmeta and Stata drmeta programs. The same considerations regarding covariances apply as before, and then a multivariate meta-regression model with one quadratic transformation of the dose is fitted. Figure 14.1 shows the predicted quadratic relationship between coffee consumption and mortality risk for the Klatsky et al. study [23]. For this study we estimated $\hat{\beta}_1 = -0.024$ and $\hat{\beta}_2 = 0.001$. To illustrate this result, the predicted RR comparing 6 versus 0 cups/day can be computed as $\widehat{RR}_{6\,vs\,0} = \exp\left(-0.024\left(6-0\right) + 0.001\left(6^2 - 0^2\right)\right) = 0.90$. Statistical inference (confidence intervals, hypothesis tests) about the predicted RR can be conducted using the delta method.

14.5 A RESTRICTED CUBIC SPLINE MODEL FOR A SINGLE STUDY

The constant change, on the log scale, of the RR throughout the exposure range, i.e. the linearity assumption, is a strong assumption that may not be supported by the data or available knowledge. For instance, the dose–response association might be U shaped, hockey-stick shaped, or J shaped. In this situation, a model that allows for these nonlinearities would be in a better position to detect the mechanism underlying the empirical data. One option here is to use cubic splines.

To fit a restricted cubic spline model, first the number of knots is required. Here, knots are the dosages that separate the data into intervals. A restricted cubic spline requires at least three knots and splits the data into four dose intervals. Within each interval, a cubic polynomial is fitted, and the polynomials are forced to join smoothly at the knots. The additional constraint of being linear before and after the last knot greatly reduces the number of dose transformations to be included in the model. A restricted cubic spline model with three knots can be defined using two regression coefficients: β_1 for the linear part (the first spline is the dose) and β_2 for the nonlinear part (the second spline f is a nonlinear function that involves the dose and the knots):

$$E\left(\ln(RR_k)\mid dose_k\right) = \beta_1\left(dose_k - dose_{ref}\right) + \beta_2\left[f\left(dose_k\right) - f\left(dose_{ref}\right)\right],$$

where the two coefficients β_1 and β_2 jointly define the shape of the relationship, similar to the quadratic scenario [28]. In general, a comparison of predicted responses comparing any two dose levels will involve both regression coefficients. The first spline coefficient β_1 measures the relative increase in predicted response for an increase of 1 cup/day before the first knot. Interpretation of the second spline coefficient β_2 is not straightforward. To make predictions of the expected RR of the outcome comparing two particular doses, we need to involve both coefficients and the values of the splines. The estimated coefficients are $\hat{\beta}_1 = -0.028$ and $\hat{\beta}_2 = 0.018$. For example, the predicted RR comparing 6 versus 0 cups/day can be computed as $\widehat{RR}_{6vs0} = \exp\left(-0.028(6-0) + 0.018(4.135-0)\right) = 0.91$. The values 4.135 and 0 are the values of the second spline evaluated at 6 and 0 cups/day, respectively.

For the Klatsky et al. study [23], we fitted restricted cubic splines with three knots at 0.495, 2.000, 4.500 cups/day. The location of the knots is based on fixed percentiles of the exposure data points available from all the studies. The fitted curvilinear relationship between coffee intake and mortality risk is shown in Figure 14.1.

14.6 SYNTHESIZING DOSE–RESPONSE ASSOCIATION ACROSS STUDIES

A linear function, easy to fit and interpret, is often used to approximate the dose–response relationship that might be underlying multiple studies. In our example, the investigator may assume that every 1 cup/day increment of coffee consumption is conferring the same effect on (log) mortality risk in all studies. This single regression coefficient (slope) can be estimated as the weighted average of all study-specific coefficients (under the univariate fixed-effect model), or the mean of a distribution of different yet related study-specific coefficients (under the univariate random-effects model, see Chapter 9). Heterogeneity measures can then be estimated using quantities and tests as described in Chapter 9. The two-step approach can be extended to answer more complex dose–response questions involving more than one regression coefficient using multivariate meta-analytic models. For example, the dose–response relationship between alcohol intake and colorectal cancer rate can be modeled using splines of degree 0, 1, 3 or even some combination of them [24].

In Figure 14.2, we present the meta-analysis of the study-specific regression coefficients from all the studies using a random-effects linear dose–response model. The estimated mean linear trend is $\hat{\beta} = -0.033$ with a standard error $\widehat{SE}\left(\hat{\beta}\right) = 0.005$. Under the assumption of a linear dose–response function, every 1 cup/day increment in coffee consumption was associated with a 3% lower mortality risk (RR $= e^{-0.033 \pm 2(0.005)} = 0.97$; 95% CI 0.96–0.98; Figure 14.3 Panel a). The estimated heterogeneity variance of the linear

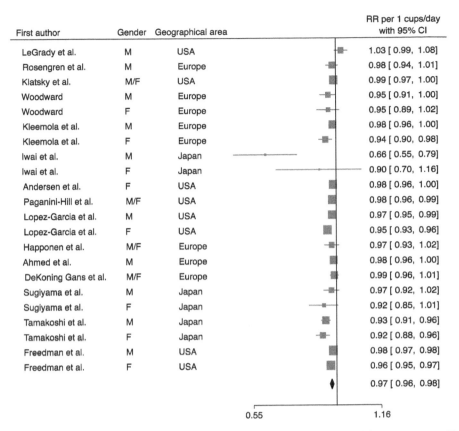

First author	Gender	Geographical area		RR per 1 cups/day with 95% CI
LeGrady et al.	M	USA		1.03 [0.99, 1.08]
Rosengren et al.	M	Europe		0.98 [0.94, 1.01]
Klatsky et al.	M/F	USA		0.99 [0.97, 1.00]
Woodward	M	Europe		0.95 [0.91, 1.00]
Woodward	F	Europe		0.95 [0.89, 1.02]
Kleemola et al.	M	Europe		0.98 [0.96, 1.00]
Kleemola et al.	F	Europe		0.94 [0.90, 0.98]
Iwai et al.	M	Japan		0.66 [0.55, 0.79]
Iwai et al.	F	Japan		0.90 [0.70, 1.16]
Andersen et al.	F	USA		0.98 [0.96, 1.00]
Paganini-Hill et al.	M/F	USA		0.98 [0.96, 0.99]
Lopez-Garcia et al.	M	USA		0.97 [0.95, 0.99]
Lopez-Garcia et al.	F	USA		0.95 [0.93, 0.96]
Happonen et al.	M/F	Europe		0.97 [0.93, 1.02]
Ahmed et al.	M	Europe		0.98 [0.96, 1.00]
DeKoning Gans et al.	M/F	Europe		0.99 [0.96, 1.01]
Sugiyama et al.	M	Japan		0.97 [0.92, 1.02]
Sugiyama et al.	F	Japan		0.92 [0.85, 1.01]
Tamakoshi et al.	M	Japan		0.93 [0.91, 0.96]
Tamakoshi et al.	F	Japan		0.92 [0.88, 0.96]
Freedman et al.	M	USA		0.98 [0.97, 0.98]
Freedman et al.	F	USA		0.96 [0.95, 0.97]
				0.97 [0.96, 0.98]

0.55   1.16

FIGURE 14.2 Summary of the study-specific (log) linear trends, expressed for every 1 cup/day increment, of the association between coffee consumption and all-cause mortality risk estimated using a two-stage random effects model. Study-specific trends were estimated using an inverse variance/covariance weighted linear regression model.

trends across studies is $\hat{\tau}^2 = 0.0003$. This quantity can be used to compute a plausible range of estimates (prediction interval) for future studies. About 95% of the studies are expected to have mortality RRs associated with every 1 cup/day between 0.93 and 1.00, that is $e^{-0.033 \pm 2\sqrt{0.005^2 + 0.0003}}$. The Cochran Q-test for residual heterogeneity was Q = 77 (df = 21), P value < 0.0001 and I^2 statistic = 75% (see Chapter 9). Possible explanations for heterogeneity are that coffee composition can vary substantially across populations, where differences may be related to different types of coffee powder, different methods of preparation, and different serving sizes [22]. Furthermore, in a dose–response meta-analysis another source of heterogeneity can be a poorly specified functional relationship. For example, the modeling assumption of a constant change in all-cause mortality risk associated with every additional cup of coffee contrasts with two previous meta-analyses where no further risk reduction was observed for high coffee consumption (≥4 cups/day) as compared with moderate coffee consumption (2–4 cups/day) [22].

Therefore, we next estimate a dose–response pattern with no particular constraints on its form. We specified a two-stage random-effects model with coffee consumption modeled using restricted cubic splines with three knots at fixed percentiles (0.5, 2, and 4.5 cups/day). The estimated mean mortality RR presented in Figure 14.3 Panel b does

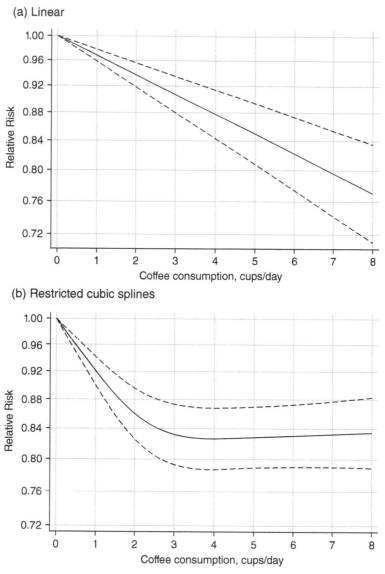

FIGURE 14.3   Mean dose–response association between coffee consumption and all-cause mortality in a dose–response meta-analysis of prospective cohort studies [22]. Coffee consumption was modeled with linear function (Panel a) and restricted cubic splines with three knots at 0.5, 2, and 4.5 cups/day (Panel b) in a two-stage random-effects dose–response model. Estimates obtained with the restricted maximum likelihood method. Dashed lines represent the 95% confidence intervals for the mean dose–response association (solid line). No coffee consumption (0 cups/day) served as the reference value.

not appear to be constant throughout the coffee consumption range. Compared with no coffee consumption, the mortality risk decreased up to 17% at 3 cups/day, with no material reduction above that level of coffee consumption. In comparing the two modeling strategies (splines versus linear function), the linear function underestimates the magnitude of the beneficial effect of moderate coffee consumption and overestimates the one for high coffee consumption. Selected mean RRs predicted by the random-effects model using either splines or linear functions are presented in Table 14.2.

TABLE 14.2 Mean risk ratio (*RR*) for all-cause mortality and 95% confidence intervals (*CI*) for various levels of coffee consumption (1–8 cups/day) versus no coffee consumption.

Coffee cups/day	Restricted cubic splines		Linear	
	RR	95% CI	RR	95% CI
0	1.000	Referent	1.000	Referent
1	0.920	0.900–0.941	0.968	0.958–0.978
2	0.860	0.825–0.895	0.937	0.918–0.956
3	0.832	0.793–0.873	0.907	0.880–0.935
4	0.826	0.787–0.868	0.878	0.843–0.914
5	0.828	0.789–0.869	0.849	0.808–0.893
6	0.830	0.790–0.873	0.822	0.774–0.873
7	0.832	0.790–0.877	0.796	0.741–0.854
8	0.834	0.789–0.883	0.770	0.710–0.835

Note: Estimates obtained with a two-stage random-effects dose–response model with restricted cubic splines with three knots at fixed percentiles of coffee consumption and a linear function. Estimates obtained with the restricted maximum likelihood method. The rounding to three digits after the decimal separator is for comparison of the two modeling strategies.

14.7 TESTING DEPARTURE FROM A LINEAR DOSE–RESPONSE RELATIONSHIP

Since the simpler linear dose–response relationship is nested within the restricted cubic spline model, a formal statistical test can be performed to detect a possible departure from linearity [24]. Consider the restricted cubic spline random-effects model with three knots involving two regression coefficients that we applied in our example in the previous section. The magnitude of the regression coefficient (β_2) reflects the degree of departure from a linear dose–response relationship. It should be noted that linearity is evaluated on the natural log scale when modeling multiplicative measures of association such as odds ratios, risk ratios, or hazard ratios. Under the scenario described by the null hypothesis $H_0 : \beta_2 = 0$ – a linear dose–response relationship – the sampling distribution of the Wald-type statistic $W = \left(\hat{\beta}_2 \,/\, \widehat{SE}\left(\hat{\beta}_2 \right) \right)^2$ follows approximately a χ^2 distribution with 1 degree of freedom. If the investigator is testing at a significance level of 5%, a value of the computed statistic W falling beyond the 0.95 quantile of a χ^2 distribution with 1 degree of freedom, that is 3.841, would be taken as indicative of disagreement (P value < 0.05) between the data and the null hypothesis. This is concisely and commonly reported as the "P value for nonlinearity."

The result of the statistical test should be interpreted with caution, keeping in mind common fallacies. Failing to reject the hypothesis of linearity with the data at hand because the P value is large (say, greater than 0.05) does not imply that the summary dose–response relationship is truly linear. Furthermore, rejecting the hypothesis of linearity because the P value is small (say, smaller than 0.05) does not provide insight into the possible shape of the relationship, the values of the dose for which this departure from linearity is occurring, or the subject-matter relevance of this departure.

In our example, the Wald-type statistic $\chi^2 = 37.6$ is well above the 0.95 quantile of the χ^2 distribution with 1 degree of freedom. So the test leads to a rejection of $H_0 : \beta_2 = 0$ (P value < 0.05), indicating that the data strongly disagree with a simpler monotonic linear trend between coffee consumption and mortality risk. A tabular (Table 14.2) or graphical presentation (Figure 14.3) is then important to interpret the estimated dose–response model and to determine what range of coffee consumption is associated with the lowest mortality risk.

14.8   EXTENSIONS, LIMITATIONS, AND DEVELOPMENTS

Although we have presented the model to combine results arising from prospective cohort studies, a similar approach can be employed with other study designs (randomized trials, case–control, cohort studies). Recent extensions for mean differences and standardized mean differences have been proposed in combining results of randomized trials on the effectiveness of different dosages of antipsychotic drugs in schizophrenia patients [19] and approaches to evaluate the goodness of fit for the various competing models have been developed [20].

An important limitation of the two-stage model is that the dose–response shape needs to be estimated within each study. When the assumed shape is non linear, then each study needs to examine at least three different doses so that two different effect sizes can be estimated and both coefficients are identifiable. This requirement might result in a reduction of the available number of studies: the studies that compare the outcome only between two doses must be excluded. Specification of a single mixed-effects dose–response model can overcome this limitation, through synthesis within and across studies in one step [12, 13].

Another limitation of assuming a common transformation for all the studies is that the chosen function may poorly fit the data in some studies, and combining dose–response coefficients may discard information about study-specific exposure range. For example, the typical coffee consumption in Japan may be lower than in Europe and the USA. Nevertheless, the regression coefficient estimated in Japan over a narrower exposure range would contribute to the overall combined dose–response relationship over the entire range of the exposure.

Although the typical dose (mean, median) within each interval is usually published, the assignment of the dose may represent an additional source of uncertainty in conducting dose–response meta-analysis. Sensitivity analysis varying the assignment of the dose values, particularly at the extremes of the distribution, may be required to examine the overall stability of the combined dose–response relationship.

The methods illustrated for dose–response meta-analysis have been implemented in major statistical packages, for example the `drmeta` command in Stata [29] or the `dosresmeta` package in R [30] (see also Chapters 25 and 26). Both the `dosresmeta` and `drmeta` procedures offer a one-stage approach [12], an extension to mean differences and standardized mean differences [19], and measures of goodness of fit [20]. Despite the various methodological and technical developments in the field, specialized training opportunities are still scarce, and reporting guidelines tailored to dose–response meta-analysis are lacking.

14.9   CONCLUSIONS

We have introduced dose–response meta-analysis through examples based on a previously published quantitative review of prospective cohort studies. Given summarized dose–response data arising from the categorization of a quantitative exposure, we have illustrated how to conduct inference on the dose–response pattern with single and multiple studies, how to summarize study-specific trends, how to detect a departure from linearity based on a spline model, and how to present the summary dose–response relationship in a tabular or graphical form.

Creating a table of summarized data is relatively quick, easy to share, and sustainable over a long period of time. Nevertheless, its careful analysis requires computational and statistical skills coupled with subject-matter knowledge. It is particularly important to know what defines the dependent and independent variables, how to relate them, and how to compare alternative models.

Modeling relative changes in estimated responses rather than absolute responses makes graphical comparison of alternative functional relationships particularly challenging. Sometimes a fitted trend will not even pass through the published estimates that are used as the dependent variable in the dose–response regression. An example is alcohol consumption and colorectal cancer rates when never drinkers are used as a comparison group [24]. The greater uncertainty in predicted responses due to sparse data at the extremes may incorrectly give the visual impression of a possible non-linear relationship. Dose–response models specified according to a plausible mechanism generating the data can overcome some of the misleading intuitions provided by naively graphing tables of summarized data points.

This is particularly important in case of flexible modeling using restricted cubic splines. Here the interpretation of the estimates may not be straightforward and typically a graphical presentation is required to appreciate the estimated functional relationship. On the other hand, a reasonable graph of the summary dose–response shape with related confidence bands requires the combination of the estimated parameters with the exposure data or some transformation of it that may not be available in the aggregated data.

Although the statistical methods are implemented in user-friendly packages, wise application of the methodology is likely to require more than one line of code and familiarity with the programming language. The computer practical associated with this chapter (see www.systematic-reviews3.org) provides a good starting point.

REFERENCES

1. Reynolds, A., Mann, J., Cummings, J., and et al (2019). Carbohydrate quality and human health: a series of systematic reviews and meta-analyses. *Lancet.* **393** (10170): 434–445.

2. Makgoeng, S.B., Bolanos, R.S., Jeon, C.Y. et al. (2018). Markers of immune activation and inflammation, and non-Hodgkin lymphoma: a meta-analysis of prospective studies. *JNCI Cancer Spectr.* 2 (4): pky082.

3. Du, Y., Lv, Y., Zha, W. et al. (2020). Association of body mass index (BMI) with critical COVID-19 and in-hospital mortality: a dose-response meta-analysis. *Metabolism* 16: 154373.

4. Hill, A.B. (2015). The environment and disease: association or causation? *J. R. Soc. Med.* 108 (1): 32–37.

5. White, I.R., Kaptoge, S., Royston, P., and Sauerbrei, W. (2019). Meta-analysis of non-linear exposure-outcome relationships using individual participant data: a comparison of two methods. *Stat. Med.* 38 (3): 326–338.

6. Turner, E.L., Dobson, J.E., and Pocock, S.J. (2010). Categorisation of continuous risk factors in epidemiological publications: a survey of current practice. *Epidemiol. Perspect. Innov.* **7**: 9.

7. Larsson, S.C. and Orsini, N. (2014). Red meat and processed meat consumption and all-cause mortality: a meta-analysis. *Am. J. Epidemiol.* 179 (3): 282–289.

8. Pelucchi, C., Bosetti, C., Galeone, C., and La Vecchia, C. (2015). Dietary acrylamide and cancer risk: an updated meta-analysis. *Int. J. Cancer* 136 (12): 2912–2922.

9. Greenland, S. and Longnecker, M.P. (1992). Methods for trend estimation from summarized dose-response data, with applications to meta-analysis. *Am. J. Epidemiol.* 135 (11): 1301–1309.

10. Shi, J.Q. and Copas, J.B. (2004). Meta-analysis for trend estimation. *Stat. Med.* 23 (1): 3–19. discussion 159–162.

11. Yu, W.W., Schmid, C.H., Lichtenstein, A.H. et al. (2013). Empirical evaluation of meta-analytic approaches for nutrient and health outcome dose-response data. *Res. Synth. Methods* 4 (3): 256–268.

12. Crippa, A., Discacciati, A., Bottai, M. et al. (2019). One-stage dose-response meta-analysis for aggregated data. *Stat. Methods Med. Res.* 28 (5): 1579–1596.

13. Sera, F., Armstrong, B., Blangiardo, M., and Gasparrini, A. (2019). An extended mixed-effects framework for meta-analysis. *Stat. Med.* 38 (29): 5429–5444.

14. Bagnardi, V., Zambon, A., Quatto, P., and Corrao, G. (2004). Flexible meta-regression functions for modeling aggregate dose-response data, with an application to alcohol and mortality. *Am. J. Epidemiol.* 159 (11): 1077–1086.

15. Rota, M., Bellocco, R., Scotti, L. et al. (2010). Random-effects meta-regression models for studying nonlinear dose-response relationship, with an application to alcohol and esophageal squamous cell carcinoma. *Stat. Med.* 29 (26): 2679–2687.

16. Berrington, A. and Cox, D.R. (2003). Generalized least squares for the synthesis of correlated information. *Biostatistics* 4 (3): 423–431.

17. Takahashi, K. and Tango, T. (2010). Assignment of grouped exposure levels for trend estimation in a regression analysis of summarized data. *Stat. Med.* 29 (25): 2605–2616.

18. Orsini, N., Li, R., Wolk, A. et al. (2012). Meta-analysis for linear and nonlinear dose-response relations: examples, an evaluation of approximations, and software. *Am. J. Epidemiol.* 175 (1): 66–73.

19. Crippa, A. and Orsini, N. (2016). Dose-response meta-analysis of differences in means. *BMC Med. Res. Methodol.* **16**: 91.

20. Discacciati, A., Crippa, A., and Orsini, N. (2017). Goodness of fit tools for dose-response meta-analysis of binary outcomes. *Res. Synth. Methods* 8 (2): 149–160.

21. Hamza, T., Cipriani, A., Furukawa, T.A. et al. (2021). A Bayesian dose-response meta-analysis model: a simulations study and application. *Stat. Methods Med. Res.* 27: 962280220982643.

22. Crippa, A., Discacciati, A., Larsson, S.C. et al. (2014). Coffee consumption and mortality from all causes, cardiovascular disease, and cancer: a dose-response meta-analysis. *Am. J. Epidemiol.* 180 (8): 763–775.

23. Klatsky, A.L., Armstrong, M.A., and Friedman, G.D. (1993). Coffee, tea, and mortality. *Ann. Epidemiol.* 3 (4): 375–381.

24. Orsini, N. and Spiegelman, D. (2020). Meta-analysis of dose-response relationships. In: *Handbook of Meta-Analysis*, Handbooks of Modern Statistical Methods, 1e (eds. C.H. Schmid, T. Stijnen and I. White), 395–428. London: Chapman & Hall/CRC.

25. Hamling, J., Lee, P., Weitkunat, R., and Ambühl, M. (2008). Facilitating meta-analyses by deriving relative effect and precision estimates for alternative comparisons from a set of estimates presented by exposure level or disease category. *Stat. Med.* 27 (7): 954–970.

26. Easton, D.F., Peto, J., Babiker, A.G. (1991). Floating absolute risk: an alternative to relative risk in survival and case-control analysis avoiding an arbitrary reference group. *Stat. Med.* 10: 1025–1035.

27. Orsini, N. (2010). From floated to conventional confidence intervals for the relative risks based on published dose-response data. *Comput. Methods Programs Biomed.* 98 (1): 90–93.

28. Harrell, F.E., Lee, K.L., and Pollock, B.G. (1988). Regression models in clinical studies: determining relationships between predictors and response. *J. Natl. Cancer Inst.* 80 (15): 1198–1202.

29. Orsini, N. (2021). Weighted mixed-effects dose-response models for tables of correlated contrasts. *Stata J.* **21** (2): 320–347.

30. Crippa, A. and Orsini, N. (2016). Multivariate dose-response meta-analysis: the dosresmeta R package. *J. Stat. Softw.* 72 (1): 1–15.

PART III

SPECIFIC STUDY DESIGNS

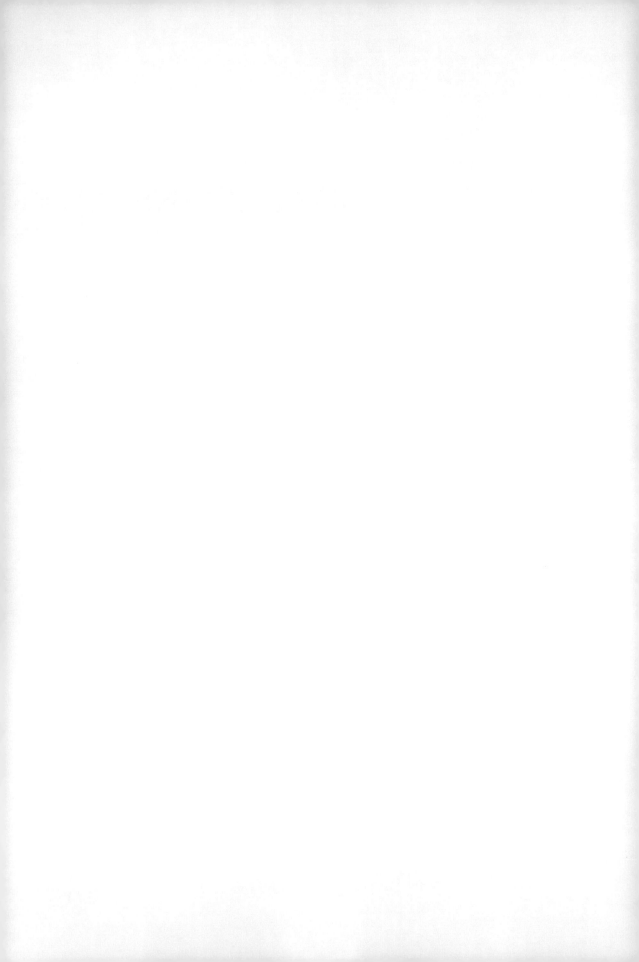

CHAPTER 15

Systematic Reviews of Nonrandomized Studies of Interventions

Jelena Savović, Penny F. Whiting, and Olaf M. Dekkers

This chapter concerns systematic reviews of nonrandomized studies of interventions (NRSIs) and systematic reviews that include both randomized and nonrandomized studies of interventions. An NRSI is a study that compares the effectiveness and/or safety of interventions in which interventions are not randomly allocated to participants (or to clusters of participants) [1]. This includes studies that are often described as **observational**. For example, a cohort study might compare remission of type 2 diabetes in participants with obesity who underwent gastric bypass surgery (intervention 1) compared with those following a supervised very low energy diet (intervention 2), where the allocation to surgery or diet did not involve randomization. The choice of the intervention received may have been made for one of several reasons. It may have been on the basis of participant suitability: for example, because surgery was considered to have a high risk of complications for the patient, or the patient was considered unlikely to adhere to a very strict diet. Alternatively, it may have been on the basis of the participant's preference for surgery versus diet; or perhaps as a consequence of the availability of the interventions (e.g. if different hospitals offer different approaches to management of diabetes in patients with obesity). In this example, two active interventions are compared; other NRSIs may compare outcomes in participants who received an intervention of interest (e.g. obesity surgery) with those who did not.

Observational studies are often used in the study of etiology (i.e. risk factors, or causes, of diseases and other health outcomes). Reviews of etiology are explored in Chapter 19; in the current chapter we restrict our attention to systematic reviews on the effects of health interventions. For example, a systematic review on the effects of obesity on type 2 diabetes investigates whether obesity is a risk factor for developing type 2 diabetes, so addresses a question of etiology. In contrast, a review evaluating the effects

Systematic Reviews in Health Research: Meta-Analysis in Context, Third Edition. Edited by Matthias Egger, Julian P.T. Higgins, and George Davey Smith.

of interventions to treat obesity (e.g. surgery vs. diet) on the remission of type 2 diabetes, as in our previous example, addresses a question about interventions [2]. In reality, interventions are a subset of the broad range of exposures that can be examined in observational studies, and the distinction between interventions and risk factors is not always clear. For instance, a review addressing the effect of taking nutritional supplements, or of eating more or less red meat, has features of both intervention and etiology reviews.

There are many situations in which NRSIs provide valuable evidence about effectiveness and safety of an intervention (see Section 15.1). Sometimes NRSIs are the only source of evidence, while in other situations they may supplement evidence from randomized controlled trials (RCTs). An early challenge when considering inclusion of NRSIs is to decide on the most appropriate study designs to include in the review to address the research question. There are many types of NRSIs. Cohort studies and case–control studies are the most widely used designs, but there are several variants of each of these, and numerous others, as we discuss in Section 15.2.2. When conducting an intervention review that includes both RCTs and NRSIs, the two categories may be used for different purposes. For example, a review might address questions of intervention effectiveness using only RCTs, but address potential harms of the intervention using both RCTs and NRSIs [3].

Many aspects of systematic reviews of NRSIs are similar to systematic reviews of RCTs that have already been covered in previous chapters. The absence of randomization poses a genuine threat to internal validity, making risk of bias assessment even more important than for RCTs. Other challenges include choosing the appropriate results to extract (e.g. from multiple statistical analyses arising from models adjusting for different variables), strategies for synthesis, and dealing with heterogeneity, all of which we address in this chapter.

15.1 THE IMPORTANCE OF NONRANDOMIZED STUDIES IN THE EVALUATION OF INTERVENTIONS

Systematic reviews of interventions aim to determine and quantify causal intervention effects on the outcomes of interest. If evidence comes from well-conducted RCTs, causality can generally be inferred. In situations where evidence from RCTs is incomplete, unavailable, or scarce, nonrandomized studies may provide valuable evidence. In particular, evaluation of the impact of interventions on rare events (including many important adverse effects) or long-term outcomes often requires larger sample sizes and longer follow-up time than is generally feasible in RCTs. In some cases, restricting a review to RCTs might lead to an inaccurate impression of long-term or rare effects of an intervention. In one such example, a systematic review of effectiveness of methylphenidate for attention deficit hyperactivity disorder (ADHD) in children included only RCTs and found no evidence of serious adverse effects linked to the drug [4]. However, observational studies have linked methylphenidate with rare, but serious, adverse events, including sudden death and psychosis. The reliance on RCT evidence had been insufficient, and a follow-up systematic review of NRSIs focusing on serious adverse events of methylphenidate found evidence of a potential increase in risk of some serious adverse events [5].

NRSIs may also be used to provide information on specific populations or settings that have not been evaluated in RCTs. Sometimes results of RCTs are difficult to generalize. This may be because their participants are atypical or unrepresentative due to strict inclusion criteria or low recruitment rates; or because health care settings or interventions involved in RCTs are atypical of routine care; or because some participant outcomes (e.g. quality of life or compliance) do not closely resemble what would be observed outside of the context of the RCT [6].

NRSIs are often the main source of evidence for public health interventions, because RCTs can be difficult to conduct in such settings. For example, the World Health Organization recommends introduction of taxes on sugary drinks as a measure to tackle obesity [7], based on nonrandomized intervention studies conducted in countries that have already introduced such taxes [8] and systematic reviews of nonrandomized studies [9].

Randomized evidence may not be available for some interventions, for a variety of other reasons. Ethical considerations may prevent the conduct of a randomized experiment, for example because of objections to random allocation of individuals to intensive care versus ward care [6]. Experimentation may be impossible (for example due to unwillingness of health professionals or patients to participate for lack of individual equipoise or for logistical reasons) or controversial (for example for political, legal, or commercial reasons) [6]. In other cases, randomized trials may be inappropriate because random allocation reduces the effectiveness of the intervention, for example when the effectiveness of the intervention depends on the participants' active participation (e.g. psychotherapy or physical exercise). However, it should be emphasized that the mere absence of RCTs does not add to the validity of NRSIs.

15.2 DEFINING THE RESEARCH QUESTION AND ELIGIBILITY CRITERIA FOR THE REVIEW

As described in Chapter 2, the key component to any systematic review of an intervention is a clearly defined research question, addressed in a PICO format – participants, intervention(s), comparator(s), outcome(s).

15.2.1 Specifying PICO in Reviews of Nonrandomized Studies of Interventions

Defining the participants or population of interest is usually similar to the same task for reviews of RCTs. The eligibility criteria for participants may be broader in individual NRSIs than in individual RCTs (which may exclude older or younger people, or people with comorbidities). This is often considered an advantage of NRSIs in terms of generalizability.

Defining the intervention of interest requires close attention in a review of NRSIs. In the absence of a predefined intervention protocol to follow, NRSI may group interventions into broader categories, and these may not be particularly well suited to guiding treatment policies. For example, NRSIs of the effects of exercise on back pain may have combined different forms of exercise (cycling, running, yoga, dog walking, strength training, etc.) into one broad category called "exercise," which addresses a somewhat broader question than an RCT of the effect of a "prescribed" exercise program (such as the implementation of a daily 30-minute yoga program). Even if a review of such NRSIs shows that those who exercise experience less back pain, the broad exposure categories cannot directly provide evidence for specific actions that could be taken to improve back pain in the population at large.

Comparator interventions are sometimes poorly defined in NRSIs, especially in studies focused on comparing outcomes in people who received an intervention of interest with those who did not. In many cases, those not receiving the intervention of interest may receive an array of different interventions that are often poorly described, and sometimes this information is not collected at all.

Outcomes collected in NRSIs may differ from those collected in RCTs. Most RCTs have clearly defined outcome measures, and one of the main challenges in a systematic review of RCTs is how to combine outcomes across studies. The situation is more complex with NRSIs. Some prospective NRSIs have predefined outcome measures, but others rely on routinely collected outcome data from administrative databases (e.g. electronic medical records, health insurance records, registries). It is important to consider what is the outcome of interest (e.g. presence or severity of depression) and what measures of this outcome are acceptable for the review (e.g. depression measured using a validated scale, or an ICD-10 code entered by the patient's doctor into the patient's electronic medical record).

15.2.2 Defining Types of Nonrandomized Study to Include

NRSIs comprise a broad range of study designs. Systematic reviews should consider at the protocol stage which study designs are the most appropriate for the review question and thus will be eligible for inclusion. Designs often used for studying intervention effects are cohort [10], case–control [10], and self-controlled studies [11], although some less common designs are increasingly used, including controlled before-and-after studies, interrupted time series (ITS), and regression discontinuity designs. Study design terminology is often confusing and inconsistently applied for NRSIs. Eligibility criteria should preferably be defined on the basis of desired study design features, e.g. consecutive recruitment of participants; identification of new users of a drug; comparisons made within the same participants over time, or between different groups receiving different interventions. Checklists are available to help identify study features to consider when determining eligibility criteria for NRSIs [12].

The most straightforward design is the **cohort study**, where participants receiving the intervention of interest and participants not receiving that intervention (either receiving a comparator intervention or no intervention) are followed up over time and their outcomes compared [10]. Such a design resembles the classic RCT, with one crucial distinction: intervention is not allocated by randomization but determined by some other factors, such as disease characteristics, or patient and clinician preferences. Cohort studies that are the most similar to RCTs will have a study protocol – including plans for collection of participant information and outcomes, and an analysis plan – developed before participants have received their interventions or been followed up.

Such studies can ensure that all known confounding characteristics are validly measured, and that researchers have control over which outcomes to measure and how.

It is possible to use existing sources of **routinely collected health data** for clinical research (e.g. electronic patient records, health insurance data, dispensing records). These large databases of patient data can be considered cohorts of participants. Using such data is efficient and low cost, but the type of data collected (interventions, outcomes, and confounders) may be limited by what has been routinely collected. Patient record data are often used to study adverse effects of drugs and other interventions. For example, Douglas et al. used a UK-based electronic database of patient records to explore whether the use of proton pump inhibitors (PPIs) decreases effectiveness of clopidogrel and aspirin (a drug combination taken to prevent myocardial infarction by people at high risk) [13]. The researchers identified a cohort of 24 471 patients receiving clopidogrel and aspirin prescriptions and linked them with data from other registries to identify cases of death and incident myocardial infarction. They compared outcomes occurring in people receiving a PPI with those not receiving a PPI, and found that PPI use was associated with a higher incidence of death or incident myocardial infarction (adjusted hazard ratio 1.37, 95% confidence interval [CI] 1.27–1.48). For this research question, a randomized study is not feasible as the sample size required is very large. To address it in an observational study, confounding should be carefully considered, as PPI use is related to lifestyle and body mass index (BMI), known risk factors for myocardial infarction.

In **self-controlled studies**, patients are compared with themselves under different interventions in different time periods. These studies may be reported under different names, such as "case-only" studies or "self-controlled series." Self-controlled designs are equipped to study intervention effects for acute outcomes when exact timings are available for intervention (e.g. drug use) and outcome occurrence [11]. The main advantage is that stable confounders (e.g. dietary patterns, socioeconomic status) are controlled by design. In addition to the cohort design described earlier for the effect of PPIs on the effectiveness of clopidogrel and aspirin, the researchers also used a self-controlled design, comparing periods of PPI use with periods of nonuse within the same participants. In contrast to the previous analysis, they found very weak evidence of a protective association between PPI use and myocardial infarction (rate ratio of 0.75, 95% CI 0.55–1.01). The authors concluded that the discrepancy between findings of the comparisons between and within people suggests that the observed associations in the standard cohort design are unlikely to be causal. This demonstrates the strengths of this self-controlled design in minimizing confounding [13].

Case–control studies are mainly used, in the context of intervention evaluations, to study rare adverse effects. An example is provided by the investigation of venous thrombosis risk due to oral contraceptive use, which was first studied in a case–control setting [14]. In this study, women who had developed deep venous thrombosis without any other underlying diseases were compared with healthy women sampled from the general population as controls. Analysis showed that the risk of thrombosis among users of oral contraceptives was increased fourfold. **Cross-sectional studies** are not well equipped to study intervention effects, because the temporal relation between intervention and outcome often cannot be established.

Some NRSIs rely on **instrumental variable** analysis, exploiting naturally occurring "randomness" in allocation of interventions [15]. An instrumental variable, or instrument, influences receipt of the intervention, but does not have an independent impact on the outcome. Any association between the instrument and the outcome is then assumed to have resulted from the impact of the intervention on the outcome. An instrumental variable sometimes used to study treatment effectiveness is physician preference, exploiting the variation that occurs when different doctors prescribe differently for exactly the same patient [16]. Such physician preferences have been used to study the effect of oral contraceptives on thrombosis risk [17]. Instrumental variable studies aim to circumvent (unmeasured) confounding. However, common causes of the instrument and the outcome can introduce confounding in these studies [18]. Instrumental variable studies harbor additional analytic complexities and assessing risk of bias requires in-depth understanding of the methodological complexities and assumptions of the design.

A **regression discontinuity** approach exploits opportunistic cut-offs, such as arbitrary eligibility criteria for intervention, which create a "discontinuity" that can be used to evaluate the effect of the intervention by comparing outcomes in groups of participants below and above the cut-off. In the region of the cut-off, intervention allocation is deemed to be made almost by chance. For example, a study investigated the effect of human papillomavirus (HPV) vaccination on participation in cervical cancer screening, by exploiting the recommended vaccination age cut-off (a "discontinuity") as an instrument for the effect of the HPV vaccine on taking up screening [19]. The hypothesis is that women aged just below and above the maximum age cut-off will be highly comparable in ways other than their eligibility to receive the vaccine. A narrower age range for participant selection into the study reduces the risk of confounding, but also reduces the available sample size and thus precision.

All of these examples are of studies in which interventions are applied, and outcomes measured, at the individual level. Further approaches are available where interventions are at an organizational level. Kontopantelis et al. [20] exploited a so-called **natural experiment** on the introduction of a pay-for-performance scheme in UK primary care in 2004–2005 by the UK government to reward general practices for achieving clinical and nonclinical targets to evaluate the scheme's effectiveness. This voluntary intervention was introduced nationally and was adopted almost universally by general practitioners due to its associated financial rewards. A simple before-and-after (or pre-post) analysis would not account for any trends in performance over time, so the researchers used ITS analysis to assess whether the performance on the incentivized targets improved. This approach involves measuring outcomes at multiple timepoints before and after the introduction of the intervention and comparing trends and patterns (e.g. regression slopes) before and after the intervention (the "interruption") (Figure 15.1).

There is increasing interest in using observational data (e.g. from electronic health records) to emulate a hypothetical "target trial." Eligibility criteria for the target trial are applied to the participants in the electronic records, along with the timepoint that would be appropriate for randomizing the individual into the target trial, which is used as the start of follow-up. Even in the presence of strong confounding by indication, some argue that this approach can lead to effect estimates that are consistent with those from randomized trials [21–23]. The target trial approach is not a panacea, however. There are examples in which this approach has yielded effect estimates different from those observed in RCTs. Danaei et al. attempted to emulate a target trial of

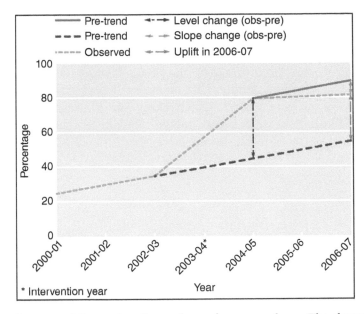

FIGURE 15.1   Interrupted time series of a pay-for-performance scheme. The observed performance increased more than was predicted based on pre-intervention trends ("pre-trend," dashed line), leading to a level change. Additionally, the subsequent observed slope was less than the slope predicted based on reapplying the pre-intervention trend after this level change ("pre-trend," solid line). *Source*: Kontopantelis et al. [20], reproduced under Creative Commons Attribution (CC BY 4.0) license.

antihypertensives versus no antihypertensives and found a 12% increase in death rate in the antihypertensives group, in contrast to data from RCTs that consistently show survival benefit of antihypertensives [21].

15.3   SEARCHING FOR NONRANDOMIZED STUDIES OF INTERVENTIONS

The general principles of searching for studies described in Chapter 3 also apply for systematic reviews of NRSIs. Searches of bibliographic databases will often focus on combining terms for intervention, population, and, where appropriate, outcomes and/ or comparisons (see Chapter 3, Section 3.5). These components of the search strategy will often be similar to those of RCTs of the same population and intervention(s). Chapter 3 (Section 3.4) provides some guidance for searching for studies other than RCTs. Restricting the search based on indexing terms for study designs (e.g. prospective cohorts) is problematic. Nonrandomized studies can be described in diverse ways in publications (e.g. "retrospective non-comparative interventional case series" [24]), which creates difficulties in identifying and indexing studies by their design. Moreover, study design labeling can be simply wrong: for example, a considerable proportion of studies labeled as case–control studies are in fact not case–control studies [25]. Applying study design filters is thus often discouraged, since it may compromise the sensitivity of the search. In practice, the omission of a study design filter will often result in a large number of retrieved records, of which only a small proportion may eventually meet eligibility criteria (i.e. the search has low specificity [26]), leading to a substantial workload at the record-screening stage of the review.

Studies indicate that the coverage of one single database will not be adequate for identification of observational studies [27], and searching a broader range of databases and nondatabase sources (e.g. reference checking and citation searches) can reduce the possibility of important studies being missed. Specific guidance is available to optimize search strategies for identification of adverse effects [28].

15.4   RISK OF BIAS

Potential for bias is a key consideration when including NRSIs in a review, because in the absence of randomization it is much more difficult to ascertain that the observed intervention effects are causal. In an RCT, randomization and concealment of allocation, if successfully implemented, ensure that the factors that predict the outcome (e.g. disease severity) do not influence the process of allocation to intervention groups. In the absence of randomization, NRSIs are prone to confounding. NRSIs are also vulnerable to selection biases that do not affect RCTs. Some types of bias are common to both RCTs and NRSIs. For example, while blinding is easier to apply in an RCT, especially when placebos are used, blinded assessment of outcomes may, in principle, be equally possible in NRSIs and RCTs. Loss to follow-up and selective outcome reporting are problems common to all types of prospective study. However, a detailed protocol is often not registered for an NRSI, which makes it difficult to assess whether results are reported selectively based on the findings.

15.4.1   Confounding

Confounding arises when there is a common cause of intervention and outcome. Its presence in an NRSI hampers the causal interpretation of effect estimates. For example, in a nonrandomized study evaluating the effect of statins on cardiovascular outcomes, higher cholesterol may increase the likelihood of statin treatment, while also being a risk factor for cardiovascular disease. The higher cholesterol levels of statin users at baseline could lead to different cardiovascular outcomes between the intervention groups being incorrectly attributed to the statin (Figure 15.2). This is an example of **confounding by indication**, where the indication for intervention (e.g. cholesterol level) is inherently a confounder in a study of the intended effects of an intervention (e.g. statin). Controlling for indication is often difficult in NRSIs, since it requires knowledge of all the indications involved in the decision to prescribe an intervention [29]. The extent of confounding is linked to the strength of the association between intervention allocation and prognosis [30]. When studying and comparing two (or more) treatments for the same indication, confounding may be less of an issue.

Randomization prevents confounding by breaking the link between intervention allocation and prognosis (outcome). However, some treatment decisions in clinical practice may not be related to prognostic factors. This can be the case for unintended outcomes of the intervention, including adverse events with physiological mechanisms that differ

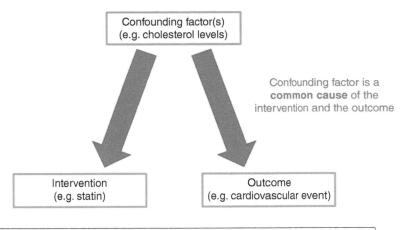

Confounding factor(s)
(e.g. cholesterol levels)

Confounding factor is a
common cause of the
intervention and the outcome

Intervention
(e.g. statin)

Outcome
(e.g. cardiovascular event)

Example:
In a non randomized study comparing cardiovascular events between statin and
non-statin users, results may be confounded by cholesterol levels, body mass
index, and socio economic status, as these factors predict the outcome and also
influence a doctor's decision whether to prescribe a statin.

FIGURE 15.2   Graphical representation of confounding in nonrandomized studies of
interventions shows that confounding factors influence both the intervention and the outcome.

from those leading to the clinical benefit for which the treatment was prescribed [29,
31]. For example, a urinary tract infection could be treated with a choice of two antibiotics. Although the severity of the condition or laboratory assessments of a pathogen's
sensitivity to various antibiotics may be considered in making a treatment decision, the
probability of an allergic reaction is unlikely to play a role in the treatment decision, as
allergic reactions from drugs cannot be predicted in a patient who has not received the
drug before. This means that there should be no link between prognosis and treatment in
an NRSI comparing the two antibiotics, so confounding is unlikely in relation to the risk
of an allergic reaction. There is empirical evidence that adverse events can sometimes be
studied validly in NRSIs [32–34], facilitating the investigation of some rare or long-term
adverse effects for which RCTs lack the required sample size or duration of follow-up.

This does not mean that NRSIs always provide unconfounded estimates for adverse
events. For example, a study assessing the risk of cardiovascular disease (adverse
event) associated with postmenopausal hormone replacement therapy (HRT) [35]
found that HRT halved the risk of cardiovascular disease. Although HRT is prescribed
to women to reduce their menopausal symptoms (indication), a decision whether to
prescribe it was likely influenced by a woman's general health, which was predictive
of subsequent cardiovascular disease risk. Indeed, a subsequent RCT has shown that
HRT in fact increased the risk of cardiovascular disease [36].

Confounding can also occur in prevention studies, when an intervention is taken
up preferentially by healthier individuals. One such example is a healthy vaccinee
bias, which occurs, for example, when healthy people are more likely to follow recommendations to take up seasonal influenza vaccination [37]. If the analysis is not adequately adjusted for markers of general health and health-seeking behavior, this may
lead to an overestimation of vaccine effectiveness. On the other hand, confounding by

indication is also likely to occur because people who are at higher risk of complications from disease are preferentially targeted by vaccination campaigns or encouraged by their doctors to get vaccinated, and this may lead to an underestimation of vaccine effectiveness. With these biases operating in opposite directions, the overall direction and magnitude of bias due to confounding may be difficult to predict [38].

A key task in a systematic review of NRSIs is to determine whether confounding has been adequately dealt with in the included studies. This requires subject matter knowledge (what are important confounding factors?) and methodological knowledge (are the statistical models used appropriate to deal with confounding?). Most statistical approaches (restriction, multivariable regression analysis, propensity score, inverse probability weighting, g-estimation) rely on the non-testable assumption that all important confounding factors have been (adequately) measured [39]. The full spectrum of characteristics that influence intervention decisions (prognostic factors, disease status and severity) is generally not completely recorded in a study dataset. For this reason, it is difficult to control completely for confounding by indication [39].

15.4.2   Selection Bias

Selection bias occurs if selection of either people or person-time into the study or into the analysis is related to both the intervention and the outcome under study. For example, selection bias will occur in a study of the harmful effect of corticosteroids on osteoporosis that is restricted to patients in whom bone mineral density is measured (thus selecting a subset of eligible patients). In routine care, patients taking corticosteroids will be monitored closely, often including measurements of bone mineral density or assessment for vertebral fractures. Patients not receiving corticosteroids will not generally have bone mineral density measured unless they have other risk factors for osteoporosis. Thus, selection into the study will be related to both corticosteroid use and risk of osteoporosis, introducing a selection bias leading to underestimation of osteoporosis risk in corticosteroid users. This type of bias is also sometimes referred to in epidemiological literature as "collider bias" [40]. To minimize this bias, a study was carried out comparing systemic corticosteroid users with nonsystemic corticosteroid users, assuming a similar follow-up with regard to osteoporosis and related fractures [41]. The magnitude of this bias can sometimes be so large that the observed effect is in the direction opposite to the causal effect (i.e. the study shows the intervention is protective when it is harmful).

In case–control studies, selection into the study is related to the outcome by design, i.e. cases and controls are selected because they have or have not experienced the outcome, respectively. Selection bias will occur if the selection of cases and controls is also related to whether they have received the intervention of interest. This is more common in case–control studies where controls are recruited from hospitals [42]. For example, in a case–control study of the efficacy of BCG revaccination for preventing tuberculosis, two different control groups were recruited: the first was selected from subjects presenting for routine prevention and care at the same health center where cases with tuberculosis had attended; the second was selected from the neighborhoods of the cases. Controls recruited from the health unit overrepresented exposure to BCG revaccination and would have resulted in overestimation of vaccine efficacy, so the investigators used the neighborhood controls for their analysis [43].

Selection biases due to exclusion of initial person-time of follow-up can arise in NRSIs when the start of the intervention and start of the follow-up time do not coincide. Such biases will not arise in RCTs (unless peculiar analysis strategies are followed). We will illustrate this type of selection bias using the Nurses' Health Study of HRT for menopausal symptoms (mentioned earlier). They assigned women to the HRT group if the women stated that they had been taking HRT. Thus, they were "prevalent users" of the intervention rather than new, "incident" users, as would be the case in an RCT [35]. Although residual confounding is likely to have occurred in this study, re-analyses of the data using the target trial approach indicate that the inclusion of prevalent HRT users was the main contributor to the incorrectly estimated effect of HRT on cardiovascular events [23]. Women who had started HRT but had already experienced an event before the start of their follow-up were excluded from the analysis, as were any who died before follow-up started. An early elevated risk of cardiovascular events after starting HRT was therefore missed due to selection bias. This type of selection bias is also referred to as prevalent user bias, survivor bias, or lead-time bias.

A different example of selection bias is provided by a study comparing patients taking beta-blockers after acute myocardial infarction with similar patients who were not prescribed beta-blockers. The investigators concluded that longer beta-blocker use was related to lower mortality risk [44]. Beta-blocker use was defined as at least two prescriptions after the myocardial infarction, so to be included in this group, patients could not have died in the period between myocardial infarction and the second prescription. Patients who only received one prescription, changed to a different beta-blocker, or had long intervals between prescriptions were excluded from the study. Thus, selection of participants into this study was related to both intervention (excluding those with only one prescription of beta-blockers) and outcome (not dying between myocardial infarction and second prescription), thereby introducing selection bias. The bias led to the underestimation of mortality risk in beta-blocker users. This type of selection bias is also referred to as immortal time bias [45]. Understanding of the mechanisms of selection bias, including its recognition in individual studies, requires in-depth understanding of epidemiological concepts.

15.4.3 Information Bias

Information bias occurs when there are errors in the measurement, collection, recording, or handling of information in a study. It can arise from assessment of intervention, outcome, and other characteristics, such as confounding factors. Intervention misclassification may occur, for example, in register-based studies where the registers rely on prescription information, which may not be an accurate indicator of actual drug use. Many outcomes are prone to misclassification. In RCTs, outcome assessment is often blinded, especially in placebo-controlled trials, which minimizes the risk of differential measurement error (errors that differ by intervention group). Even in trials where participants and care providers are not blinded, blinded outcome assessment is often implemented for specific outcomes, e.g. by a blinded endpoint committee. It is possible for outcome assessors to be unaware of the intervention in an NRSI – for example, researchers might score endpoints without knowledge of intervention status – but this is rarely implemented. A blinded outcome assessment will in general lower risk of measurement error for outcomes that require interpretation (e.g. reading an electrocardiogram or an X-ray). The extent and direction of bias due to misclassification and measurement errors should be judged separately for each estimate of effect.

15.4.4 Reporting Bias

Reporting biases occur when studies do not get published at all (e.g. because the result was undesirable to the investigators), or when study results are selectively reported in publications on the basis of the findings (see Chapter 5). The former is usually referred to as publication bias and the latter as selective reporting bias. The literature on publication bias is dominated by studies on RCTs, with less information on its effect on syntheses of NRSIs, but there is some evidence that the problem is more prevalent for studies other than RCTs [46]. The factors favoring or preventing publication might differ between RCTs and NRSIs. Since analyzing existing datasets is often quick and easy (and cheap), we might suspect that many such analyses never get reported, especially when they did not produce the results the investigators hoped for or journals were interested in. Publication bias and selective reporting may thus represent a substantial problem for reviews of NRSIs. However, Egger et al. argue that publication bias and reporting biases may be less important than confounding and other biases in terms of the heterogeneity of evidence available for syntheses of NRSIs [47].

Detailed assessment of the risk of selective reporting requires comparison of the original protocol and/or analysis plan with the final study report(s). Whereas a registered protocol is the norm for RCTs, it is still uncommon for NRSIs. Consequently, empirical evidence on the extent of deviations from study protocols and analysis plans in NRSIs is lacking, and systematic review authors will often be unclear whether the analyses presented in study reports had been pre-planned or are the results of a "fishing expedition" for statistically significant findings.

15.4.5 Assessing Risk of Bias in Nonrandomized Studies of Interventions Included in a Systematic Review: A Domain-Based Approach

Many tools have been developed to assess the quality or risk of bias of observational studies [48]. Most of these do not distinguish between etiological studies and NRSIs. Two widely used tools are the Downs and Black and Newcastle–Ottawa tools [49, 50]. As discussed in Chapter 4, methods for critiquing studies included in systematic reviews have shifted away from composite scales and summary scores measuring methodological quality, as in the Downs and Black and Newcastle–Ottawa tools, toward a component-based assessment of risk of bias, such as that adopted in the Cochrane Risk of Bias tools for RCTs [51, 52].

The ROBINS-I (Risk Of Bias In Non-randomized Studies of Interventions) tool was designed specifically to assess risk of bias in NRSIs [53]. It examines specific components of the study design, conduct, analysis, and aspects of reporting (referred to as "bias domains") and their potential to introduce bias in the estimate of the treatment effect. ROBINS-I approaches assessment of risk of bias in the results of an individual NRSI by comparing it with a "target" trial – a hypothetical, pragmatic, and unbiased randomized trial, whose results would validly answer the question addressed by the NRSI [53]. The benefits of this approach can be seen in relation to identifying selection bias in the Nurses' Health Study discussed in Section 15.4.2. In the target randomized trial for this study, the start of HRT and the start of follow-up would coincide for all participants. However, in this NRSI, some of the participants were already receiving HRT before they were included in the analysis, introducing bias. Comparison of the NRSI with the target trial allows the user to identify such differences, flagging up methods that could have led to bias in the comparison of the intervention groups.

ROBINS-I contains seven bias domains (Table 15.1). Each domain includes a set of "signaling questions," which are reasonably factual questions that aim to elicit information relevant to a judgment about the risk of bias in that domain. For example, questions include "Did the authors control for all the important confounding domains?" within the domain "Bias due to confounding," and "Were start of follow-up and start

TABLE 15.1   Risk of bias domains assessed in the ROBINS-I tool.

Domain	Explanation	Issues addressed	
Bias due to confounding	Confounding of intervention effects occurs when one or more prognostic factors (factors that predict the outcome of interest) also predict whether an individual receives one or the other intervention of interest	• Whether all known confounding domains are measured validly and reliably and controlled for using appropriate design or analytic approaches • Considers the use of negative controls	Peri-intervention domains for which risk of bias assessment is mainly distinct from assessments of randomized trials
Bias in classification of interventions	Bias introduced by either differential or nondifferential misclassification of intervention status	• Whether the intervention groups were clearly defined, based on the information recorded at the start of the intervention, and unaffected by knowledge of the outcome	
Bias in selection of participants into the study	Bias that arises when either all of the follow-up or an initial period of follow-up following initiation of intervention is excluded for some individuals	• Whether the selection of participants into the study/analysis was based on participant characteristics observed after the start of intervention • Whether prevalent user bias was likely • Whether immortal time bias was likely • Analytic approaches employed to avoid selection bias	

(Continued)

TABLE 15.1 *(Continued)*

Post-intervention domains for which there is substantial overlap with assessments of randomized trials

Domain	Explanation	Issues addressed
Bias due to deviations from intended interventions	Bias that arises when there are systematic differences between intervention and comparator groups in the care provided, which represent a departure from the intended intervention(s)	• Whether there were deviations from the intended intervention beyond those expected in usual practice, which differed between intervention groups (**effect of assignment**) • Whether any cointerventions were balanced across intervention groups, intervention implemented successfully, with adequate adherence, and appropriate analysis (**effect of adherence**)
Bias due to missing data	Bias that arises when later follow-up is missing for individuals initially included and followed (e.g. differential loss to follow-up that is affected by prognostic factors); bias due to exclusion of individuals with missing information about intervention status or other variables such as confounders	• Whether outcome data were available for all participants and avoided exclusion of participants due to missing intervention status or other variables • Whether, when there was missingness, the proportion and reasons were likely to be related to the true value of the outcome • Whether appropriate methods were used to impute any missing data
Bias in measurement of outcomes	Bias introduced by either differential or nondifferential measurement error in outcome data	• Whether the outcome measure was influenced by knowledge of the intervention received, or outcome assessors were aware of the intervention received • Whether methods of outcome assessment were comparable across intervention groups and systematic errors in measurement avoided
Bias in selection of the reported result	Selective reporting of results in a way that depends on the findings and prevents the estimate from being included in a meta-analysis (or other synthesis)	• Whether the reported effect estimate was likely to have been selected, on the basis of the results, from multiple outcome measurements, analyses, or subgroups

Source: Adapted from Sterne et al. [53].

of intervention the same for most participants?" within the domain "Bias in selection of participants into the study." The overall risk of bias judgment for each study result will usually be the highest risk of bias judgment for individual domains (e.g. if the study result was judged to have a serious risk of bias for confounding and low risk for all other domains, the overall risk of bias for that result would be a serious risk of bias). Like the risk of bias tool for RCTs (RoB 2), ROBINS-I differentiates between the effect of assignment and effect of adhering to the intervention (Chapter 4). Users of ROBINS-I are encouraged to seek out and interrogate all available information about an NRSI when assessing risk of bias, such as protocols, analysis plans, publications, and correspondence with investigators, to reduce the impact of poor or incomplete reporting on the accuracy of the risk of bias judgments.

15.5 SYNTHESIZING RESULTS

As with most systematic reviews, three considerations are key for the decision on whether and how to combine effect estimates from NRSIs: between-study heterogeneity; risk of bias in the results of individual studies; and potential for publication bias (and related reporting biases). Heterogeneity in effect estimates can be due to numerous features of the studies, including differences in the interventions examined, study populations, outcomes assessed, and risks of bias. Exploration of heterogeneity should be a central element of every review that includes NRSIs.

15.5.1   Exploring Heterogeneity

It is advisable to examine heterogeneity both in study characteristics and in study results. Differences in study characteristics can usefully be tabulated to enable readers to judge study diversity in detail. Statistical measures of heterogeneity (statistical tests, estimates of variability in effect size, and measures of consistency such as the I^2 statistic) are based on comparison of effect estimates across studies [54]. Methods to explore heterogeneity more formally include stratified analyses (comparing studies with and without a specific characteristic) and meta-regression (see Chapter 10). If there are sufficient studies, it may be informative to use such methods to explore whether differences in design, clinical characteristics, or risk of bias translate into different reported estimates. Unfortunately, differences in study characteristics do not necessarily translate into statistical heterogeneity, and explanations for statistical heterogeneity often cannot be found in the known differences in study characteristics. In any event, it is useful to examine whether all effect estimates point in the same direction and are of similar magnitude.

15.5.2   The Role of Meta-Analysis

After careful consideration of study diversity, statistical heterogeneity, risk of bias, and potential of publication bias, a decision will often be needed on whether it is sensible to combine all (or a subset of) studies quantitatively. As a general rule, results should only be combined in a meta-analysis if the studies are sufficiently similar in terms of populations, interventions, and outcomes for a combined result to be meaningful. The presentation of a combined estimate at the bottom of a forest plot will give the reader the impression that included studies are indeed combinable, even if the authors include notes of caution in their discussion. Unfortunately, there is no simple answer to the question "What amount of bias and heterogeneity is acceptable?" This must a be a careful and thoughtful decision made by the review team informed by their combined clinical, epidemiological, and statistical expertise.

Sources of diversity in study features such as interventions and study populations may be addressed by restricting the meta-analysis to studies that are very similar to each other, preventing large between-study heterogeneity, but possibly at the expense of the amount of evidence available to answer the research question.

With regard to risk of bias, authors should consider whether limitations of the included studies are acceptable to provide a combined estimate, or whether a subset of the studies were designed and conducted in a way that is likely to provide a more valid effect estimate for the intervention under study.

The potential of publication bias and the impact of missing studies on the overall evidence may be assessed following strategies described in Chapter 5. Funnel plots and similar methods may be helpful for larger meta-analyses [55, 56]. However, funnel plots may be less informative for NRSIs than for RCTs, since relationships between effect estimates and study sizes may not be the same. For example, a very large record linkage study may have limited information on confounding factors and thus may produce very precise but possibly biased estimates. In contrast, a small cohort study with meticulous attention to measurement of confounders and appropriate statistical modeling may provide a more accurate estimate, but with a wider confidence interval. If data from these two studies were to be combined in a meta-analysis, the data from the larger, biased study would dominate the meta-analysis, producing a biased summary estimate.

There may be further technical complications when including NRSIs in a meta-analysis. Different studies will most likely include a variety of different covariates in their analyses to adjust for confounding, and there will be several adjustment models presented in most studies. Selecting the best adjustment model to combine with other studies may be daunting. The ROBINS-I tool for assessing risk of bias recommends that the review team decide in advance the key confounding domains that will be relevant for all studies [53]. This is helpful for assessing risk of confounding, but it can also be useful to guide a decision on which adjusted result to select from each study for a formal meta-analysis. In addition, different studies may have reported different effect measures (e.g. hazard ratio, odds ratio, risk ratio, risk difference, or mean difference). When an event is rare, there is likely to be little difference between hazard ratios, odds ratios, risk ratios, and rate ratios. For some circumstances, statistical methods are available for converting various statistics to a common metric to use in the meta-analysis [57, 58].

If more than two intervention options for the same condition have been studied, network meta-analysis may be an option. This enables the mutual comparison and ranking of multiple interventions (see Chapter 13). An example is a network meta-analysis in which the authors combined results of observational studies – cohort or (nested) case–control studies – of healthy women to compare thrombosis risk for different oral contraceptives [59].

15.5.3   Combining Results from Randomized and Nonrandomized Studies

There are many instances where data from RCTs and NRSIs have produced conflicting results, and where combining these data would have been inappropriate. A striking example of this was a meta-analysis of beta-carotene and the risk of cardiovascular disease described by Egger et al. in 1998 (Figure 15.3) [47]. Data from NRSIs suggested a reduced risk of cardiovascular disease associated with beta-carotene. However, data from RCTs found a harmful effect of beta-carotene. Had only evidence from the NRSIs been available, the lack of heterogeneity in their results might have suggested that increasing beta-carotene would be beneficial. In this example, there are clear differences in the research questions asked by the cohort studies compared with the RCTs. The cohort studies compared groups with high and low beta-carotene dietary intake or serum beta-carotene concentration, whereas the trials examined beta-carotene supplementation. It is difficult to establish from the results in the forest plot whether it was high risk of bias in the cohort studies (or indeed the RCTs) or the differences in the research questions that led to the opposing conclusions from the different designs.

A second example is presented in Figure 15.4. It shows NRSIs and RCTs, collated in 2012, examining all-cause mortality after intensive surveillance including annual colonoscopy versus a less intensive surveillance (no or with less frequent colonoscopy), in patients who have had a curative resection for colorectal cancer. Here the

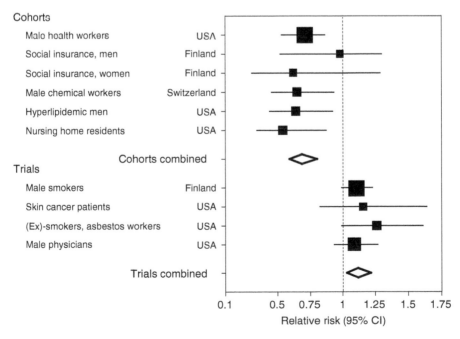

FIGURE 15.3   Forest plot showing relative risk of cardiovascular events for beta-carotene supplementation compared to nonuse. *Source*: From [47].

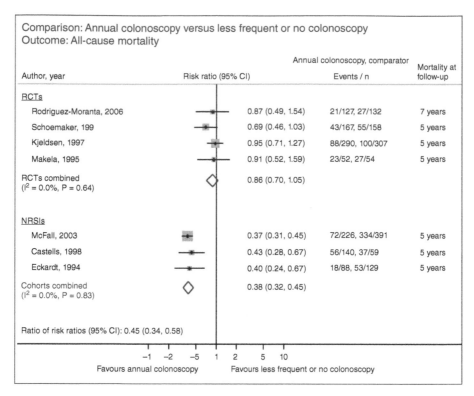

FIGURE 15.4   Forest plot showing risk ratios for all-cause mortality for a comparison of annual colonoscopy surveillance with less frequent or no colonoscopy in randomized and nonrandomized studies.

research questions were more similar, so it is likely that the differences were due to higher risk of bias in the NRSIs. In the RCTs, patients were randomized to intensive surveillance with annual colonoscopy versus a less intensive ("standard") surveillance program [60–63]. The NRSIs may be expected to be at risk of bias due to confounding. For example, in one NRSI, mortality was compared between patients who underwent surveillance compared with patients considered inappropriate for colonoscopic surveillance due to advanced malignancy, age, frailty, or severe comorbid conditions [64]. In the other two NRSIs, mortality was compared between those who adhered and did not adhere to intensive surveillance, who might have differed importantly in their prognostic factors [65, 66].

If both NRSIs and RCTs are included in a systematic review, we suggest that a stratified analysis by study design be performed before considering whether summary estimates for the different designs are sufficiently similar that an overall summary estimate would be appropriate. In Figure 15.4, the meta-analysis is stratified by study design, showing separate subgroup estimates for RCTs and NRSIs. A random-effects meta-regression is used to estimate the ratio of risk ratios comparing NRSIs with RCTs and its confidence interval. However, statistical comparisons across designs can be misleading, since there is often insufficient evidence to conclude that there is a difference, whereas lack of evidence of a difference cannot be taken as evidence of similarity of results across design.

15.6   CONCLUSIONS

Systematic reviews may need to include NRSIs to answer their research questions, especially when these questions concern long-term or rare outcomes, such as treatment harms (adverse events), or to evaluate interventions in fields where RCTs are difficult to conduct. However, the mere absence of RCTs does not add to the validity of NRSIs. Review methods for NRSIs are broadly similar to those for reviews of RCTs. Assessing risk of bias is a particularly important step for NRSIs, because NRSIs have an inherently greater risk of confounding, selection biases, and information biases than RCTs. The decision on whether to combine estimates from NRSIs statistically should be guided by the similarity of study designs, populations, interventions, and outcomes in included studies, and informed particularly by the risk of bias assessment. Statistical synthesis of results from studies of different designs should be approached with caution; careful consideration and exploration of difference in study characteristics and statistical heterogeneity are essential.

REFERENCES

1. Reeves, B.C., Deeks, J.J., Higgins, J.P.T., and Wells, G.A. (2017). Including non-randomized studies. In: *Cochrane Handbook for Systematic Reviews of Interventions*, 2e (eds. J.P.T. Higgins, J. Thomas, J. Chandler et al.) 595–621. Chichester: Wiley.

2. Hernán, M.A. and Taubman, S.L. (2008). Does obesity shorten life? The importance of well-defined interventions to answer causal questions. *Int. J. Obes. (Lond.)* 32 (Suppl. 3): S8–S14.

3. Peryer, G., Golder, S., Junqueira, D.R. et al. (2019). Adverse effects. In: *Cochrane Handbook for Systematic Reviews of Interventions*, 2e (eds. J.P.T. Higgins, J. Thomas, J. Chandler et al.), 493–506. Chichester: Wiley.

4. Storebo, O.J., Krogh, H.B., Ramstad, E. et al. (2015). Methylphenidate for attention-deficit/hyperactivity disorder in children and adolescents: Cochrane systematic review with meta-analyses and trial sequential analyses of randomised clinical trials. *BMJ* 351: h5203.

5. Storebo, O.J., Pedersen, N., Ramstad, E. et al. (2018). Methylphenidate for attention deficit hyperactivity disorder (ADHD) in children and adolescents – assessment of adverse events in non-randomised studies. *Cochrane Database Syst. Rev.* 5 (5): CD012069.

6. Black, N. (1996). Why we need observational studies to evaluate the effectiveness of health care. *BMJ* 312 (7040): 1215–1218.

7. World Health Organization (2017). *Taxes on Sugary Drinks: Why Do It?* Geneva: World Health Organization.

8. Colchero, M.A., Rivera-Dommarco, J., Popkin, B.M., and Ng, S.W. (2017). In Mexico, evidence of sustained consumer response two years after implementing a sugar-sweetened beverage tax. *Health Aff (Millwood).* 36 (3): 564–571.

9. Powell, L.M., Chriqui, J.F., Khan, T. et al. (2013). Assessing the potential effectiveness of food and beverage taxes and subsidies for improving public health: a systematic review of prices, demand and body weight outcomes. *Obes. Rev.* 14 (2): 110–128.

10. Vandenbroucke, J.P., von Elm, E., Altman, D.G. et al. (2007). Strengthening the reporting of observational studies in epidemiology (STROBE): explanation and elaboration. *Epidemiology* 18 (6): 805–835.

11. Petersen, I., Douglas, I., and Whitaker, H. (2016). Self controlled case series methods: an alternative to standard epidemiological study designs. *BMJ* 354: i4515.

12. Wells, G.A., Shea, B., Higgins, J.P.T. et al. (2013). Checklists of methodological issues for review authors to consider when including non-randomized studies in systematic reviews. *Res. Synth. Methods* 4: 63–77.

13. Douglas, I.J., Evans, S.J., Hingorani, A.D. et al. (2012). Clopidogrel and interaction with proton pump inhibitors: comparison between cohort and within person study designs. *BMJ* 345: e4388.

14. Vandenbroucke, J.P., Koster, T., Briet, E. et al. (1994). Increased risk of venous thrombosis in oral-contraceptive users who are carriers of factor V Leiden mutation. *Lancet* 344 (8935): 1453–1457.

15. Rassen, J.A., Brookhart, M.A., Glynn, R.J. et al. (2009). Instrumental variables I: instrumental variables exploit natural variation in nonexperimental data to estimate causal relationships. *J. Clin. Epidemiol.* 62 (12): 1226–1232.

16. Boef, A.G., le Cessie, S., Dekkers, O.M. et al. (2016). Physician's prescribing preference as an instrumental variable: exploring assumptions using survey data. *Epidemiology* 27 (2): 276–283.

17. Boef, A.G., Souverein, P.C., Vandenbroucke, J.P. et al. (2016). Instrumental variable analysis as a complementary analysis in studies of adverse effects: venous thromboembolism and second-generation versus third-generation oral contraceptives. *Pharmacoepidemiol. Drug Saf.* 25 (3): 317–324.

18. Hernán, M.A. and Robins, J.M. (2006). Instruments for causal inference: an epidemiologist's dream? *Epidemiology* 17 (4): 360–372.

19. Moghtaderi, A. and Dor, A. (2021). Immunization and moral hazard: the HPV vaccine and uptake of cancer screening. *Med. Care Res. Rev.* 78 (2): 125–137.

20. Kontopantelis, E., Doran, T., Springate, D.A. et al. (2015). Regression based quasi-experimental approach when randomisation is not an option: interrupted time series analysis. *BMJ* 350: h2750.

21. Danaei, G., Garcia Rodriguez, L.A., Cantero, O.F. et al. (2018). Electronic medical records can be used to emulate target trials of sustained treatment strategies. *J. Clin. Epidemiol.* 96: 12–22.

22. Danaei, G., Rodriguez, L.A., Cantero, O.F. et al. (2013). Observational data for comparative effectiveness research: an emulation of randomised trials of statins and primary prevention of coronary heart disease. *Stat. Methods Med. Res.* 22 (1): 70–96.

23. Hernán, M.A., Alonso, A., Logan, R. et al. (2008). Observational studies analyzed like randomized experiments: an application to postmenopausal hormone therapy and coronary heart disease. *Epidemiology* 19 (6): 766–779.

24. Habot-Wilner, Z., Sallam, A., Roufas, A. et al. (2010). Periocular corticosteroid injection in the management of uveitis in children. *Acta Ophthalmol.* 88 (8): e299–e304.

25. Grimes, D.A. (2009). "Case-control" confusion mislabeled reports in obstetrics and gynecology journals. *Obstet. Gynecol.* 114 (6): 1284–1286.

26. Fraser, C., Murray, A., and Burr, J. (2006). Identifying observational studies of surgical interventions in MEDLINE and EMBASE. *BMC Med. Res. Methodol.* 6: 41.

27. Lemeshow, A.R., Blum, R.E., Berlin, J.A. et al. (2005). Searching one or two databases was insufficient for meta-analysis of observational studies. *J. Clin. Epidemiol.* 58 (9): 867–873.

28. Golder, S. (2013). Optimising the retrieval of information on adverse drug effects. *Health Info. Libr. J.* 30 (4): 327–331.

29. Miettinen, O.S. (1983). The need for randomization in the study of intended effects. *Stat. Med.* 2 (2): 267–271.

30. Schneeweiss, S. (2007). Developments in post-marketing comparative effectiveness research. *Clin. Pharmacol. Ther.* 82 (2): 143–156.

31. Vandenbroucke, J.P. (2004). When are observational studies as credible as randomised trials? *Lancet* 363 (9422): 1728–1731.

32. Hemkens, L.G., Contopoulos-Ioannidis, D.G., and Ioannidis, J.P.A. (2016). Current use of routinely collected health data to complement randomized controlled trials: a meta-epidemiological survey. *CMAJ Open* 4 (2): E132–E140.

33. Hemkens, L.G., Contopoulos-Ioannidis, D.G., and Ioannidis, J.P.A. (2016). Routinely collected data and comparative effectiveness evidence: promises and limitations. *CMAJ* 188 (8): E158–E164.

34. Papanikolaou, P.N., Christidi, G.D., and Ioannidis, J.P.A. (2006). Comparison of evidence on harms of medical interventions in randomized and nonrandomized studies. *CMAJ* 174 (5): 635–641.

35. Stampfer, M.J., Colditz, G.A., Willett, W.C. et al. (1991). Postmenopausal estrogen therapy and cardiovascular disease. Ten-year follow-up from the nurses' health study. *N. Engl. J. Med.* 325 (11): 756–762.

36. Rossouw, J.E., Anderson, G.L., Prentice, R.L. et al. (2002). Risks and benefits of estrogen plus progestin in healthy postmenopausal women: principal results from the Women's Health Initiative randomized controlled trial. *JAMA* 288 (3): 321–333.

37. Benn, C.S., Fisker, A.B., Rieckmann, A. et al. (2018). How to evaluate potential non-specific effects of vaccines: the quest for randomized trials or time for triangulation? *Expert Rev. Vaccines* 17 (5): 411–420.

38. Remschmidt, C., Wichmann, O., and Harder, T. (2015). Frequency and impact of confounding by indication and healthy vaccinee bias in observational studies assessing influenza vaccine effectiveness: a systematic review. *BMC Infect. Dis.* 15: 429.

39. Bosco, J.L., Silliman, R.A., Thwin, S.S. et al. (2010). A most stubborn bias: no adjustment method fully resolves confounding by indication in observational studies. *J. Clin. Epidemiol.* 63 (1): 64–74.

40. Hernán, M.A., Hernandez-Diaz, S., and Robins, J.M. (2004). A structural approach to selection bias. *Epidemiology* 15 (5): 615–625.

41. Van Staa, T.P., Leufkens, H.G., Abenhaim, L. et al. (2000). Use of oral corticosteroids and risk of fractures. *J. Bone Miner. Res.* 15 (6): 993–1000.

42. Snoep, J.D., Morabia, A., Hernandez-Diaz, S. et al. (2014). Commentary: a structural approach to Berkson's fallacy and a guide to a history of opinions about it. *Int. J. Epidemiol.* 43 (2): 515–521.

43. Dantas, O.M., Ximenes, R.A., de Albuquerque, M.F. et al. (2007). Selection bias: neighbourhood controls and controls selected from those presenting to a health unit in a case control study of efficacy of BCG revaccination. *BMC Med. Res. Methodol.* 7: 11.

44. Rochon, P.A., Tu, J.V., Anderson, G.M. et al. (2000). Rate of heart failure and 1-year survival for older people receiving low-dose beta-blocker therapy after myocardial infarction. *Lancet* 356 (9230): 639–644.

45. Suissa, S. (2008). Immortal time bias in pharmaco-epidemiology. *Am. J. Epidemiol.* 167 (4): 492–499.

46. Scherer, R.W., Meerpohl, J.J., Pfeifer, N. et al. (2018). Full publication of results initially presented in abstracts. *Cochrane Database Syst. Rev.* 2018 (11): MR000005.

47. Egger, M., Schneider, M., and Davey, S.G. (1998). Spurious precision? Meta-analysis of observational studies. *BMJ* 316 (7125): 140–144.

48. Sanderson, S., Tatt, I.D., and Higgins, J.P.T. (2007). Tools for assessing quality and susceptibility to bias in observational studies in epidemiology: a systematic review and annotated bibliography. *Int. J. Epidemiol.* 36 (3): 666–676.

49. Downs, S.H. and Black, N. (1998). The feasibility of creating a checklist for the assessment of the methodological quality both of randomised and non-randomised studies of health care interventions. *J. Epidemiol. Community Health* 52 (6): 377–384.

50. Wells, G.A., Shea, B., O'Connell, D. et al. The Newcastle-Ottawa Scale (NOS) for assessing the quality of nonrandomised studies in meta-analyses. http://www.ohri.ca/programs/clinical_epidemiology/oxford.asp (accessed 21 February 2022).

51. Higgins, J.P.T., Altman, D.G., Gotzsche, P.C. et al. (2011). The Cochrane Collaboration's tool for assessing risk of bias in randomised trials. *BMJ* 343: d5928.

52. Sterne, J.A.C., Savović, J., Page, M.J. et al. (2019). RoB 2: a revised tool for assessing risk of bias in randomised trials. *BMJ* 366: l4898.

53. Sterne, J.A.C., Hernán, M.A., Reeves, B.C. et al. (2016). ROBINS-I: a tool for assessing risk of bias in non-randomised studies of interventions. *BMJ* 355: i4919.

54. Higgins, J.P.T., Thompson, S.G., Deeks, J.J., and Altman, D.G. (2003). Measuring inconsistency in meta-analyses. *BMJ* 327 (7414): 557–560.

55. Sterne, J.A., Sutton, A.J., Ioannidis, J.P.A. et al. (2011). Recommendations for examining and interpreting funnel plot asymmetry in meta-analyses of randomised controlled trials. *BMJ* 343: d4002.

56. Egger, M. and Davey Smith, G. (1998). Bias in location and selection of studies. *BMJ* 316 (7124): 61–66.

57. da Costa, B.R., Rutjes, A.W., Johnston, B.C. et al. (2012). Methods to convert continuous outcomes into odds ratios of treatment response and numbers needed to treat: meta-epidemiological study. *Int. J. Epidemiol.* 41 (5): 1445–1459.

58. Deeks, J.J., Higgins, J.P.T., and Altman, D.G. (2019). Analysisng data and undertaking meta-analyses. In: *Cochrane Handbook for Systematic Reviews of Interventions*, 2e (eds. J.P.T. Higgins, J. Thomas, J. Chandler et al.), 241–285. Chichester: Wiley.

59. Stegeman, B.H., de Bastos, M., Rosendaal, F.R. et al. (2013). Different combined oral contraceptives and the risk of venous thrombosis: systematic review and network meta-analysis. *BMJ* 347: f5298.

60. Kjeldsen, B.J., Kronborg, O., Fenger, C., and Jorgensen, O.D. (1997). A prospective randomized study of follow-up after radical surgery for colorectal cancer. *Br. J. Surg.* 84 (5): 666–669.

61. Makela, J.T., Laitinen, S.O., and Kairaluoma, M.I. (1995). Five-year follow-up after radical surgery for colorectal cancer. Results of a prospective randomized trial. *Arch. Surg.* 130 (10): 1062–1067.

62. Rodriguez-Moranta, F., Salo, J., Arcusa, A. et al. (2006). Postoperative surveillance in patients with colorectal cancer who have undergone curative resection: a prospective, multicenter, randomized, controlled trial. *J. Clin. Oncol.* 24 (3): 386–393.

63. Schoemaker, D., Black, R., Giles, L., and Toouli, J. (1998). Yearly colonoscopy, liver CT, and chest radiography do not influence 5-year survival of colorectal cancer patients. *Gastroenterology* 114 (1): 7–14.

64. McFall, M.R., Woods, W.G., and Miles, W.F. (2003). Colonoscopic surveillance after curative colorectal resection: results of an empirical surveillance programme. *Colorectal Dis.* 5 (3): 233–240.

65. Castells, A., Bessa, X., Daniels, M. et al. (1998). Value of postoperative surveillance after radical surgery for colorectal cancer: results of a cohort study. *Dis. Colon Rectum* 41 (6): 714–723; discussion 723–4.

66. Eckardt, V.F., Stamm, H., Kanzler, G., and Bernhard, G. (1994). Improved survival after colorectal cancer in patients complying with a postoperative endoscopic surveillance program. *Endoscopy* 26 (6): 523–527.

CHAPTER 16

Systematic Reviews of Diagnostic Accuracy

Yemisi Takwoingi and Jonathan J. Deeks

Tests are routinely used in medicine to screen for, diagnose, grade, and monitor the progression of disease. Diagnostic information is obtained from various sources, including imaging and biochemical technologies, pathological and psychological investigations, and signs and symptoms elicited during history-taking and clinical examinations [1]. Each item of information obtained from these sources can be regarded as a result of a separate diagnostic or screening **test**, whether it is obtained for the purpose of identifying diseases in sick people, or for detecting early disease in asymptomatic individuals. Systematic reviews of assessments of the reliability, accuracy, and impact of these tests are essential to guide optimal test selection and the appropriate interpretation of test results.

To make sense of a diagnostic investigation, a clinician needs to be able to make an inference regarding the probability that a patient has the disease in question according to the result obtained from the test. Tests rarely make a diagnosis 100% certain, but they may provide enough information to rule in or rule out a diagnosis in a pragmatic manner [2]. That is, they may make a diagnosis certain enough for the expected benefits of treating the patient to outweigh the expected consequences of not treating them. This chapter focuses on systematic reviews of studies of diagnostic accuracy that describe the probabilistic relationships between positive and negative test results and the presence or absence of disease, and therefore indicate how well a test can separate diseased from nondiseased patients.

Systematic Reviews in Health Research: Meta-Analysis in Context, Third Edition. Edited by Matthias Egger, Julian P.T. Higgins, and George Davey Smith.
© 2022 John Wiley & Sons Ltd. Published 2022 by John Wiley & Sons Ltd.
Companion website: www.systematic-reviews3.org

16.1   RATIONALE FOR UNDERTAKING SYSTEMATIC REVIEWS OF STUDIES OF TEST ACCURACY

Systematic reviews of tests are undertaken for the same reasons as systematic reviews of therapeutic interventions: to produce estimates of performance based on all available evidence, to evaluate the methodological quality of published studies, and to account for variation in findings between studies [3, 4]. It is the norm to observe variability in test accuracy between studies that is much more than would be expected due to chance alone. Measures of test accuracy are not fixed properties of a test and are not usually transferable across different populations and settings [5]. Other factors may affect test performance, including the threshold for defining a positive versus a negative test result, characteristics of the test and its conduct (including skill and experience of assessors or practitioners), and definition of the target condition. Reviews of diagnostic test accuracy (DTA) studies, in common with systematic reviews of randomized controlled trials (RCTs), involve key stages of question definition, literature searching, evaluation of studies for eligibility and quality, data extraction, and data synthesis (see Chapter 2). However, the details within many of the stages differ. In particular, the design of test accuracy evaluations differs from the design of studies that evaluate the effectiveness of treatments, which means that different criteria are needed when assessing study quality in terms of the potential for bias and applicability. Additionally, each study reports a pair of related summary statistics (for example, sensitivity and specificity) rather than a single statistic, requiring alternative statistical methods for combining study results.

In this chapter we provide an overview of the most established methods and current issues in undertaking systematic reviews of diagnostic accuracy. We also highlight recent methodological developments and areas where further research and evaluation are needed.

16.2   FEATURES OF STUDIES OF TEST ACCURACY

To ensure a representative sample, the people recruited into a test accuracy study should ideally be a consecutive (or randomly selected) series of patients/participants suspected of having the **target condition** (or disease) who are recruited from a clinical setting in which the test(s) will be used in practice. The terms "target condition" and "disease" are used interchangeably in this chapter for simplicity. Studies of test accuracy assess test results of patients with and without the target condition, each of whom undergoes one or more **index tests** (new or existing tests of interest) as well as the **reference standard**, sometimes known as the "gold" standard.

The relationship between the results of an index test and disease status is described using probabilistic measures, such as sensitivity, specificity, and likelihood ratios. It is important that the results of the reference standard are very close to the truth, or else the accuracy of an index test will be poorly estimated [6]. Therefore, the reference standard is the best available test for verifying true disease status. To achieve this, a reference standard may not be a single test, but rather a battery of clinical tests and other available clinical evidence (often termed a composite reference standard) [7], or may involve undertaking invasive procedures or lengthy periods of follow-up to ascertain disease status. If a composite reference standard is used, it should not include the index test, or else diagnostic accuracy will most likely be overestimated. Such an effect is known as **incorporation bias** [8].

16.3   SUMMARY MEASURES OF DIAGNOSTIC ACCURACY

16.3.1   Types of Data

A test may yield a nominal (binary), ordinal (ordered categories), discrete (count), or continuous result. Standard methods for assessing test accuracy rely on binary classification of the results of the index test and the reference standard. For nonbinary data, thresholds (cut-offs) are needed to dichotomize the data to define positive and negative test results. The threshold may be numeric (e.g. serum levels of prostate specific antigen, PSA) or may be non-numeric and based on subjective visual interpretation or judgment (e.g. qualitative interpretation of an ultrasound scan). The results of a test accuracy study are presented in a 2×2 table, with individuals classified as true positives (TP), true negatives (TN), false positives (FP), and false negatives (FN), based on cross-classification of the results of an index test against those of the reference standard (Table 16.1).

16.4   MEASURES OF DIAGNOSTIC ACCURACY

The most commonly used measures of test accuracy are defined in Box 16.1. Paired measures – sensitivity and specificity, positive and negative predictive values, and positive and negative likelihood ratios (LR+ and LR−) – are typically used to quantify test performance because of the need to distinguish between the presence and absence of the target condition. Probably the most commonly seen measures are **sensitivity**, which describes the proportion of those with the target condition who (correctly) have a positive test result, and **specificity**, which describes the proportion of those without the target condition who (correctly) have a negative test result. Note that calculations

TABLE 16.1   Cross-classification of index test and reference standard results in a diagnostic test accuracy study.

	Reference standard positive	Reference standard negative	Total
Index test positive	True positives (TP)	False positives (FP)	Test positives (TP + FP)
Index test negative	False negatives (FN)	True negatives (TN)	Test negatives (FN + TN)
Total	Disease positives (TP + FN)	Disease negatives (FP + TN)	Study total (TP + FP + FN + TN)

Box 16.1   Definition of Common Measures of Test Accuracy

Test accuracy measure	Formula[a]	Definition
Sensitivity	TP/(TP + FN)	Proportion of those with the target condition correctly identified as having the condition
Specificity	TN/(FP + TN)	Proportion of those without the target condition correctly identified as not having the condition
Positive predictive value	TP/(TP + FP)	Proportion of those with the target condition among the test positives
Negative predictive value	TN/(FN + TN)	Proportion of those without the target condition among the test negatives
Positive likelihood ratio (LR$^+$)	$\dfrac{TP/(TP+FN)}{FP/(FP+TN)}$	Ratio of the proportion of test positives among those with the target condition compared to the proportion of test positives among those without the target condition
Negative likelihood ratio (LR$^-$)	$\dfrac{FN/(TP+FN)}{TN/(FP+TN)}$	Ratio of the proportion of test negatives among those with the target condition compared to the proportion of test negatives among those without the target condition
Diagnostic odds ratio	$(TP \times TN)/(FP \times FN)$ or $\dfrac{\left(\dfrac{sensitivity}{1-sensitivity}\right)}{\left(\dfrac{specificity}{1-specificity}\right)}$ or LR$^+$/LR$^-$	Ratio of the odds of positivity in those who have the target condition compared to the odds of positivity in those without the condition

[a] Expressed using the notation in Table 16.1.

of sensitivity, specificity, and likelihood ratios are undertaken on the columns of Table 16.1, and give the same results if the numbers of participants with the disease and the numbers without the disease change. These values are therefore not *directly* affected by changes in the prevalence of the disease in a study sample.

In contrast to sensitivity and specificity, the calculations of predictive values are undertaken on the rows of the 2×2 table, and therefore *directly* depend on the prevalence of the disease in the study sample. The more common a disease is, the more likely it is that a positive result is right and a negative result is wrong. Clinicians often consider predictive values to be the most useful measures of diagnostic performance when interpreting the test results of a single patient. However, disease prevalence is rarely constant across studies included in a systematic review, so there is often an unacceptably high level of heterogeneity among positive and negative predictive values, making them an unsuitable choice of accuracy measures in systematic reviews and meta-analyses. There is an analogy here with the estimation of risk differences in systematic reviews of RCTs (Chapter 8), which are the easiest summary statistic to understand and apply, but are rarely the summary of choice for a meta-analysis as they are commonly heterogeneous across trials.

Different thresholds will produce different sensitivities and specificities. When several thresholds have been considered in a test accuracy study, the diagnostic accuracy of the test can be illustrated using a graph known as a **receiver operating characteristic** (ROC) plot of the TP rate (sensitivity) against the FP rate (1-specificity). For a test where presence of the target condition increases the value of a biomarker, e.g. PSA, as the threshold decreases, sensitivity increases while specificity decreases, and vice versa. The ROC plot (Figure 16.1) shows this trade-off between sensitivity and specificity across endometrial thickness thresholds used in endovaginal ultrasound for detecting endometrial cancer.

A likelihood ratio describes how many times more likely a person with disease is to receive a particular test result than a person without disease. Binary tests have two likelihood ratios: a **positive likelihood ratio** (LR+; usually a number greater than one) and a **negative likelihood ratio** (LR−; usually a number between zero and

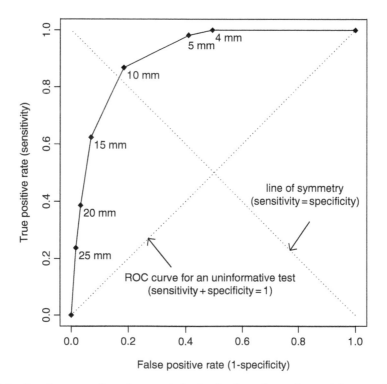

FIGURE 16.1   Receiver operating characteristic plot for detecting endometrial cancer by endovaginal ultrasound.

one). Likelihood ratios can be applied in clinical practice to update an individual's estimated chance of disease according to their test result using Bayes' theorem: the post-test odds that a patient has the disease are estimated by multiplying the pre-test odds by the likelihood ratio. The post-test odds are then converted to post-test probabilities (see Chapter 8 for an explanation of the differences between odds and probabilities). A nomogram (developed by Fagan) is a tool often used to calculate and graphically illustrate these post-test probabilities [9]. The predictive values of a test can be thought of as post-test probabilities, and hence estimated from likelihood ratios by application of Bayes' theorem [10]. In this situation the pre-test probability is estimated by the population prevalence: application of the positive likelihood ratio yields the positive predictive value. The negative predictive value can be calculated by application of the negative likelihood ratio, and subtracting the resulting post-test probability from one.

Sensitivities and specificities, and positive and negative likelihood ratios, can be combined into a single summary of diagnostic performance known as the **diagnostic odds ratio** (DOR) [11]. When a test provides no diagnostic evidence (sensitivity + specificity = 1), the DOR is 1. Note that while the DOR summarizes the results into a single number, crucial information contained in sensitivity and specificity or in likelihood ratios is discarded. Notably, the DOR cannot distinguish between tests with high sensitivity and low specificity and tests with low sensitivity and high specificity. For example, given two tests with an identical DOR of 14, one of the tests can have a sensitivity of 0.9 and specificity of 0.6 while the other test has a sensitivity of 0.6 and specificity of 0.9. This loss of information on the error rates in the diseased (FPs) and nondiseased groups (FPs) limits the clinical usefulness of the DOR. These error rates are important for judging the extent and likely impact of the downstream consequences of testing.

16.5 SYSTEMATIC REVIEWS OF STUDIES OF DIAGNOSTIC ACCURACY

A systematic review of DTA may summarize the accuracy of one or more tests individually, or compare their accuracy. There are three major ways in which systematically reviewing studies of diagnostic accuracy differs from reviewing therapeutic interventions: the choice of search terms for electronic literature searches, the criteria for the assessment of study quality, and the methods for the statistical combination of results.

16.5.1 Literature Searching

The identification of studies for a systematic review typically involves undertaking both electronic and manual searches. The manual searches may include hand-searching key or unindexed journals, reviewing reference lists and bibliographies, and contacting experts (see Chapter 3). This process is no different for systematic reviews of diagnostic accuracy than for reviews of RCTs.

However, electronic database searches for studies of diagnostic accuracy are more difficult than searches for RCTs because of inconsistent study design terminology and poor indexing due to lack of appropriate indexing terms. Occasionally a simple search using just the test name will prove to be sensitive, but many diagnostic technologies (such as ultrasound, X-rays, and serology tests) are used across a variety of fields in medicine, so that a mixture of appropriate and inappropriate studies will be retrieved, and the search will not be specific.

To reduce the risk of missing relevant studies, search strategies for identifying DTA studies usually include key elements of the review question such as the index test(s), target condition, and target population. Other terms such as the reference standard or measures of test accuracy may be included. However, care is needed to avoid retrieval of an overwhelming number of irrelevant records to screen. Methodological filters that can be added to target condition and index test(s) searches have been developed in an attempt to increase the precision of searches. These search filters consist of text words and database indexing terms. Beynon et al. have shown that search filters do not perform consistently, and should not be used as the only approach in formal searches to inform DTA systematic reviews [12]. This finding supports current recommendations in the *Cochrane Handbook for Systematic Reviews of Diagnostic Test Accuracy* [13].

Given the complexity of conducting searches for DTA studies, we recommend involving a librarian or information specialist who has previous experience of DTA reviews or expertise in designing complex systematic review search strategies. The combination of their technical expertise and clinical/content expertise from other members of the review team will aid in development of a comprehensive search strategy that captures the myriad ways in which the index test(s), target condition, and population are described in the literature. In future, text-mining techniques and other automation tools, coupled with better indexing in electronic databases, may improve the efficiency and accuracy of searches [14, 15].

16.5.2   Assessment of Methodological Quality

Flaws in the design and conduct of test accuracy studies can contribute to between-study variability and lead to biased results [16, 17]. Quality assessment is essential in systematic reviews of diagnostic accuracy studies to identify the potential for bias and the applicability of study results to the review question. The results of the quality appraisal may also guide investigations of heterogeneity and sensitivity analyses. The assessments should ideally be performed independently by at least two review authors, with a process for resolving disagreements.

The most commonly used tool is the Quality Assessment of Diagnostic Accuracy Studies (QUADAS), the more recent version being QUADAS-2 [18, 19]. This is the only tool recommended by Cochrane [20]. The QUADAS-2 tool explicitly addresses two aspects of study validity – risk of bias (internal validity) and applicability (external validity) – and consists of four domains: patient selection, index test, reference standard, and flow and timing. Each domain is assessed in terms of the risk of bias (low, high, or unclear risk), and the first three domains are also assessed in terms of concerns about applicability (low, high, or unclear concern) [19]. If a review evaluates more than one index test, the index test domain should be assessed separately for each index test, as there may be differences between tests. Signaling questions that

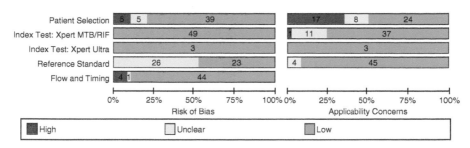

FIGURE 16.2   Summary of review authors' risk of bias and applicability concerns ratings presented as percentages across studies for each QUADAS-2 domain. *Source*: Reproduced with permission from Kay et al. [22].

address aspects of study design are used to facilitate risk of bias judgments within each QUADAS-2 domain. The QUADAS-2 tool must be tailored to each review by adding or omitting signaling questions and developing review-specific guidance on how to assess each signaling question. The QUADAS-2 tool is available from the QUADAS website (www.quadas.org). The tool was not designed for the assessment of test comparisons and an extension, QUADAS-C, for assessing risk of bias in comparative accuracy studies has been developed [21].

It is essential that the quality of the studies included in a review is assessed and reported so that appropriate inferences can be drawn. Results of methodological quality assessments may be tabulated or summarized graphically to show individual study results or across studies. Figure 16.2 summarizes the risk of bias and applicability concerns across 49 studies that evaluated Xpert MTB/RIF and Xpert Ultra for detection of active tuberculosis in children [22]. The numbers shown on the bars for each domain are the number of studies in each response category.

Assessments of methodological quality are often hindered by poor reporting, leading to ratings of "unclear" in one or more domains for several studies. For example, in Figure 16.2, the reference standard domain was rated "unclear" in 26 out of 49 (53%) studies. A study report should include clear descriptions of the reference and index tests, with definitions of positive and negative results for both, and descriptions of demographic characteristics, comorbidities, source, and referral history of patients. The Standards for Reporting Diagnostic Accuracy (STARD) statement aims to improve completeness and transparency in reporting of diagnostic accuracy studies [23].

16.6   META-ANALYSIS OF STUDIES OF DIAGNOSTIC ACCURACY

Based on the types of questions and objectives that can be addressed in a DTA review, the three main types of analyses are:

1. Analysis of the accuracy of a single test.
2. Analysis comparing the accuracy of multiple tests.
3. Investigations of heterogeneity to assess the effect of clinical and methodological characteristics on test accuracy [24].

Following an explanation of the general principles of DTA meta-analysis, we describe each type of analysis and illustrate them with examples. Further details and additional examples can be found in the *Cochrane Handbook for Systematic Reviews of Diagnostic Test Accuracy* [25].

16.7   GENERAL PRINCIPLES OF DIAGNOSTIC ACCURACY META-ANALYSIS

Diagnostic threshold is often a source of variation in meta-analyses of diagnostic accuracy because studies included in a systematic review may have used different thresholds to define positive and negative test results. Besides numeric thresholds, there may be naturally occurring variations in diagnostic thresholds between observers or between laboratories. Therefore, a general principle for synthesizing sensitivity and specificity across studies is to allow for potential correlation between these paired measures.

As with any statistical analysis, the first step is to understand the data. Estimates of sensitivity and specificity may be plotted on forest plots and in the ROC space for preliminary investigations of the data prior to meta-analysis. Figure 16.3 shows estimates of sensitivity and specificity at a particular threshold from each of the 30 studies included in a systematic review of the accuracy of the mood disorder questionnaire (MDQ) for detection of any type of bipolar disorder in mental health center settings [26]. The total score for the MDQ ranges from 0 to 15 points and the developers of the questionnaire recommend a threshold of 7 for defining test positivity [27].

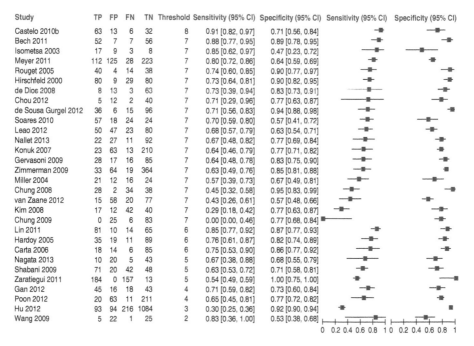

Study	TP	FP	FN	TN	Threshold	Sensitivity (95% CI)	Specificity (95% CI)
Castelo 2010b	63	13	6	32	8	0.91 [0.82, 0.97]	0.71 [0.56, 0.84]
Bech 2011	52	7	7	56	7	0.88 [0.77, 0.95]	0.89 [0.78, 0.95]
Isometsa 2003	17	9	3	8	7	0.85 [0.62, 0.97]	0.47 [0.23, 0.72]
Meyer 2011	112	125	28	223	7	0.80 [0.72, 0.86]	0.64 [0.59, 0.69]
Rouget 2005	40	4	14	38	7	0.74 [0.60, 0.85]	0.90 [0.77, 0.97]
Hirschfeld 2000	80	9	29	80	7	0.73 [0.64, 0.81]	0.90 [0.82, 0.95]
de Dios 2008	8	13	3	63	7	0.73 [0.39, 0.94]	0.83 [0.73, 0.91]
Chou 2012	5	12	2	40	7	0.71 [0.29, 0.96]	0.77 [0.63, 0.87]
de Sousa Gurgel 2012	36	6	15	96	7	0.71 [0.56, 0.83]	0.94 [0.88, 0.98]
Soares 2010	57	18	24	24	7	0.70 [0.59, 0.80]	0.57 [0.41, 0.72]
Leao 2012	50	47	23	80	7	0.68 [0.57, 0.79]	0.63 [0.54, 0.71]
Nallet 2013	22	27	11	92	7	0.67 [0.48, 0.82]	0.77 [0.69, 0.84]
Konuk 2007	23	63	13	210	7	0.64 [0.46, 0.79]	0.77 [0.71, 0.82]
Gervasoni 2009	28	17	16	85	7	0.64 [0.48, 0.78]	0.83 [0.75, 0.90]
Zimmerman 2009	33	64	19	364	7	0.63 [0.49, 0.76]	0.85 [0.81, 0.88]
Miller 2004	21	12	16	24	7	0.57 [0.39, 0.73]	0.67 [0.49, 0.81]
Chung 2008	28	2	34	38	7	0.45 [0.32, 0.58]	0.95 [0.83, 0.99]
van Zaane 2012	15	58	20	77	7	0.43 [0.26, 0.61]	0.57 [0.48, 0.66]
Kim 2008	17	12	42	40	7	0.29 [0.18, 0.42]	0.77 [0.63, 0.87]
Chung 2009	0	25	6	83	7	0.00 [0.00, 0.46]	0.77 [0.68, 0.84]
Lin 2011	81	10	14	65	6	0.85 [0.77, 0.92]	0.87 [0.77, 0.93]
Hardoy 2005	35	19	11	89	6	0.76 [0.61, 0.87]	0.82 [0.74, 0.89]
Carta 2006	18	14	6	85	6	0.75 [0.53, 0.90]	0.86 [0.77, 0.92]
Nagata 2013	10	20	5	43	5	0.67 [0.38, 0.88]	0.68 [0.55, 0.79]
Shabani 2009	71	20	42	48	5	0.63 [0.53, 0.72]	0.71 [0.58, 0.81]
Zaratiegui 2011	184	0	157	13	5	0.54 [0.49, 0.59]	1.00 [0.75, 1.00]
Gan 2012	45	16	18	43	4	0.71 [0.59, 0.82]	0.73 [0.60, 0.84]
Poon 2012	20	63	11	211	4	0.65 [0.45, 0.81]	0.77 [0.72, 0.82]
Hu 2012	93	94	216	1084	3	0.30 [0.25, 0.36]	0.92 [0.90, 0.94]
Wang 2009	5	22	1	25	2	0.83 [0.36, 1.00]	0.53 [0.38, 0.68]

FIGURE 16.3   Forest plot of the mood disorder questionnaire for detection of bipolar disorder in mental health center settings. FN, false negative; FP, false positive; TN, true negative; TP, true positive. The studies are sorted by threshold, sensitivity, and specificity in descending order. *Source*: Adapted from Takwoingi et al. [24].

Traditional univariate fixed-effect or random-effects meta-analytic methods (see Chapter 9) summarize sensitivity and specificity separately, thus ignoring potential correlation between the two measures. Such analyses can give misleading results [28]. The summary receiver operating characteristic (SROC) curve approach developed by Moses et al. [29] is a fixed-effect method that accounts for potential heterogeneity in threshold by combining sensitivity and specificity to produce an SROC curve. However, this SROC approach has methodological limitations that lead to inaccurate standard errors, making formal statistical inference invalid [30–32].

To overcome the limitations of simple univariate methods and the Moses SROC approach, hierarchical models (also known as mixed or multilevel models) are recommended [25, 33]. These hierarchical methods are more complex than methods routinely used for synthesizing the effects of interventions. The standard hierarchical models for meta-analysis of a pair of sensitivity and specificity from each included study are the bivariate model [34, 35] and the hierarchical summary receiver operating characteristic (HSROC) model [36]. The bivariate model focuses on estimation of a summary point (summary sensitivity and specificity), while the HSROC model focuses on estimation of a summary curve. Both models account for correlation between sensitivity and specificity across studies, as well as variability within and between studies. Between-study variation is modeled through the inclusion of random effects.

Although the parameters of the bivariate and HSROC models differ (Box 16.2), the models are mathematically equivalent when no covariates (e.g. test type) are included [37]. Therefore, SROC curves can be computed from bivariate models and summary points from HSROC models, and model choice for meta-analysis of a single test is unimportant [24, 25, 37]. However, when comparing test accuracy or investigating heterogeneity, model choice becomes important and is likely to be informed by variation in thresholds reported in the included studies, as well

Box 16.2 Basic Parameters of Hierarchical Models for Diagnostic Test Accuracy Meta-Analysis

Bivariate model	HSROC model
Mean logit sensitivity	Mean accuracy
Mean logit specificity	Mean threshold
Variance of random effects for logit sensitivity	Variance of random effects for accuracy
Variance of random effects for logit specificity	Variance of random effects for threshold
Correlation between the logits of sensitivity and logits of specificity	Shape of SROC curve

Each model has five parameters when no covariates are included.

as whether the focus of inference is a comparison of summary points or summary curves. Both classic and Bayesian hierarchical methods are available, but the latter are rarely used [38].

Extensions of these hierarchical models have been proposed to account for imperfect reference standard [39–43], disease prevalence [44–46], inclusion of multiple thresholds (i.e. multiple 2×2 tables from each study) [47–52], network meta-analysis of test accuracy [53–55], and other data complexities in a DTA meta-analysis [56–59]. However, the focus of this chapter is on recommended and well-established methods for meta-analysis based on a single 2×2 table from each study and assuming a perfect reference standard.

16.8   METHODS FOR META-ANALYSIS OF A SINGLE TEST

16.8.1   Estimation of a Summary Sensitivity and Specificity at a Common Threshold

The bivariate model enables joint inferences about sensitivity and specificity such that confidence and prediction regions can be plotted around the summary point. Confidence regions show the uncertainty around the point estimate (analogous to a confidence interval), while prediction regions illustrate the extent of between-study heterogeneity. This means that a 95% confidence region shows the region within which we are 95% certain the average sensitivity and specificity values will lie, while a 95% prediction region shows the region within which we are 95% certain the sensitivity and specificity of a new study will lie. Chu et al. have shown that a binomial likelihood should be used for modeling within-study variability [35, 60]. This bivariate generalized linear mixed model (GLMM) can be fitted in SAS, Stata, R, rjags, and WinBUGS.

For the interpretation of a summary sensitivity and specificity to be clinically meaningful, the meta-analysis should include only studies using thresholds that are the same or deemed to be similar. Using the MDQ data shown in Figure 16.3, bivariate meta-analysis of the 19 studies that used a common threshold of 7 gave a summary sensitivity (95% CI) of 0.65 (0.57 to 0.72) and summary specificity (95% CI) of 0.79 (0.72 to 0.84). Figure 16.4 shows an SROC plot with the summary point for the MDQ surrounded by 95% confidence and prediction regions. The scatter of study points on the SROC plot indicates substantial variation in the estimates of both sensitivity and specificity, even though only studies that used the same threshold were included in the analysis.

Bivariate meta-analysis of likelihood ratios and predictive values is possible. Zwinderman and Bossuyt [61] have shown that bivariate meta-analysis of likelihood ratios is not trivial and so they recommend meta-analysis of sensitivities and specificities. If likelihood ratios are required, they can be derived using functions of the parameters of the standard bivariate or HSROC models. Leeflang et al. [62] proposed bivariate meta-analysis of predictive values, but the main disadvantage is interpretation of the results and translation into practice, given the direct impact of prevalence on predictive values.

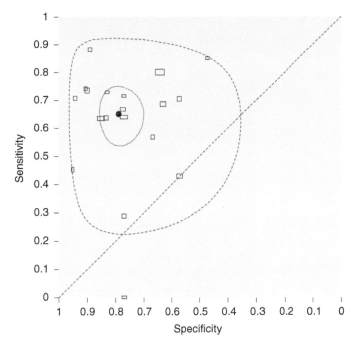

FIGURE 16.4 SROC plot of the mood disorder questionnaire (MDQ) at a common threshold of 7 for detection of bipolar disorder in mental health center settings. Each study point was scaled according to the precision of sensitivity and specificity in the study; the greater the height (or width) of a study point relative to other study points, the greater the precision of the estimate of sensitivity (or specificity). The solid circle (summary point) represents the summary estimate of sensitivity and specificity for the MDQ. The summary point is surrounded by a dotted line indicating the 95% confidence region and by a dashed line indicating the 95% prediction region. *Source*: Adapted from Takwoingi et al. [24].

16.8.2 Estimation of an SROC Curve

The Rutter and Gatsonis HSROC model is a nonlinear generalized mixed model that can be fitted in SAS, rjags, or WinBUGS. The model requires a 2×2 table from each eligible study for estimation of an SROC curve across different thresholds. Figure 16.5 shows the estimated SROC curve for the full set of 30 MDQ studies, drawn within the range of specificities (0.47 to 1.00) observed among the included studies to avoid extrapolating beyond the data. Given the relationship between the bivariate and HSROC models mentioned earlier [37], a clinically meaningful summary point can be estimated using the HSROC model by restricting the studies included in the meta-analysis to only those that reported a 2×2 table at the threshold of 7, thus reproducing the SROC plot shown in Figure 16.4.

An SROC curve can be numerically summarized using the DOR (exponent of the accuracy parameter) if the shape of the curve is symmetric, i.e. the shape parameter = 0, implying that accuracy does not depend on threshold. The DOR is not appropriate as a single summary if the curve is asymmetric, i.e. the shape parameter ≠ 0, because the DOR will be different at different points along the curve. One approach that can be used to aid in interpretation of the curve is to estimate sensitivity at fixed or clinically

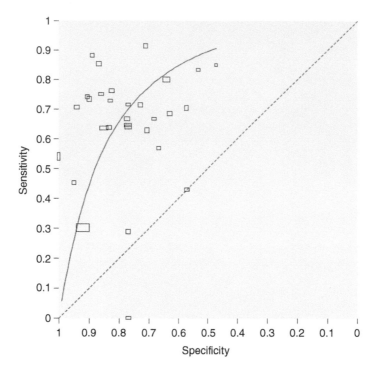

FIGURE 16.5   SROC plot of the mood disorder questionnaire (MDQ) across different thresholds for detection of bipolar disorder in mental health center settings. The size of each study point is relative to the precision of sensitivity and specificity in the study. *Source*: Adapted from Takwoingi et al. [24].

relevant values of specificity (or vice versa), e.g. at median and interquartile range (IQR) values of specificity from the included studies, as shown in Table 16.4.

16.9   QUANTIFYING AND INVESTIGATING HETEROGENEITY

The extent of heterogeneity in a meta-analysis can be quantified, but statistical approaches for assessing or describing heterogeneity in DTA meta-analysis are still developing. Unexplained heterogeneity is frequently described using the I^2 statistic proposed by Higgins et al. for traditional univariate meta-analysis (see Chapter 9) [63]. This I^2 statistic is not recommended for routine use in DTA meta-analysis because it does not account for potential threshold effects [25]. There are also issues with the I^2 statistic that could lead to misleading conclusions [64–66]. Multivariate and DTA-specific I^2 statistics have been proposed [64], but are yet to be used routinely. The estimates of between-study variance (Box 16.2) quantify heterogeneity and are akin to the quantity τ^2 in random-effects models for meta-analysis in Chapter 9. However, between-study variances are unlikely to be reliably estimated when there are sparse data and are also not easily interpreted because they represent variation in parameters expressed on log odds scales [25]. Therefore, these between-study variances are not usually reported in DTA reviews.

To investigate whether a study-level covariate is associated with test accuracy, exploratory analyses can be performed by visually inspecting forest plots and SROC plots to observe patterns in the data. Ideally, covariates should be pre-specified in the review protocol with a clear justification for their selection (see Chapter 10). Hierarchical models are regression models and so can be extended readily to meta-regression models by adding covariate terms to investigate association between test accuracy and a potential source of heterogeneity [34, 36].

16.9.1   Comparison of Summary Points

The bivariate meta-regression model enables assessment of the effect of covariates on sensitivity, specificity, or both. Kay et al. used bivariate meta-regression to investigate the effect of age group on the sensitivity and specificity of Xpert MTB/RIF (Figure 16.6) [22]. There was statistical evidence of a difference in sensitivity but not in specificity (Table 16.2). Comparing children aged 5–14 years with those

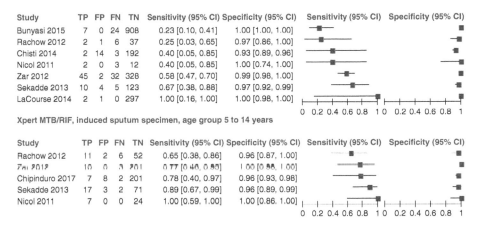

FIGURE 16.6   Accuracy of Xpert MTB/RIF for detecting pulmonary tuberculosis in children using induced sputum specimens, stratified by age group. FN, false negative; FP, false positive; TN, true negative; TP, true positive. Studies are sorted by sensitivity and specificity. *Source*: Data from Kay et al. [22].

TABLE 16.2   Effect of age group on sensitivity and specificity of Xpert MTB/RIF for detection of pulmonary tuberculosis using induced sputum specimens from children.

Age group	Studies	Number of children (cases)	Sensitivity (95% CI)	Specificity (95% CI)
5–14 years	5	627 (65)	0.80 (0.67 to 0.89)	0.98 (0.94 to 0.99)
0–4 years	7	2062 (143)	0.49 (0.32 to 0.65)	0.99 (0.97 to 1.00)
Absolute difference			0.32 (0.12 to 0.52), P = 0.002	−0.01 (−0.03 to 0.01), P = 0.34

Source: Adapted from Kay et al. [22]. P values reported for the absolute differences in sensitivity and specificity are from Wald tests.

aged 0–4 years, the absolute difference in sensitivity (95% CI) was 0.32 (0.12 to 0.52, P = 0.002), and the absolute difference in specificity (95% CI) was −0.01 (−0.03 to 0.01, P = 0.34).

16.9.2   Comparison of Summary Curves

The HSROC meta-regression model allows assessment of the effect of covariates on the accuracy, threshold, and/or shape parameters. If SROC curves are assumed to have the same shape (i.e. parallel curves) or are symmetric, differences in test accuracy can be expressed using the relative diagnostic odds ratio (RDOR), because the RDOR is constant across all values of the threshold parameter. However, when the shapes of the curves differ, the RDOR represents the relative accuracy of the points on the curves where they intersect the diagonal line in ROC space given by sensitivity = specificity, which may not be meaningful [25]. As stated in section 16.8.2, estimating sensitivity at fixed values of specificity (or vice versa) is a preferred approach.

Using HSROC meta-regression, Carvalho et al. investigated the effect of language (Asian versus non-Asian) on the accuracy of the MDQ by comparing SROC curves for the two subgroups of the covariate in one HSROC model [26]. By including covariate terms for only the accuracy and threshold parameters, the final model assumed the same shape for the two SROC curves. The RDOR (95% CI) of 0.55 (0.25 to 1.19) indicated that the DOR of Asian versions of the MDQ was 0.55 times that of the non-Asian versions, though there was little statistical evidence of a difference in accuracy (P = 0.13).

16.10   COMPARISONS OF THE ACCURACY OF TWO OR MORE TESTS

16.10.1   Test Comparison Strategy

For clinical and policy decision-making about test selection, it is important to know how the accuracy of a new test compares with that of an existing test or current practice. Ideally in primary studies, the diagnostic accuracy of competing tests should be compared in the same study population, but comparative studies are scarce [67]. There are two basic comparative accuracy study designs: a within-subject (paired) design in which all patients undergo all tests; and a randomized design in which patients are randomized to receive one of the index tests but all patients undergo the reference standard [67]. Such head-to-head evaluations from well-designed studies provide robust estimates of comparative accuracy.

Systematic reviews of comparative accuracy may undertake meta-analyses using indirect and/or direct comparisons [67, 68]. An indirect comparison includes all eligible studies that have evaluated at least one of the tests of interest, making the most of the available data, while a direct comparison includes only the comparative studies. Unlike adjusted indirect comparisons that are exploited in network meta-analyses of interventions (see Chapter 13), these naive indirect test comparisons do not use a common comparator test [69]. Since heterogeneity is the norm in test accuracy reviews, direct comparisons should provide the most reliable evidence on relative test accuracy by ensuring an unbiased comparison. However, such analyses may not always be feasible due to limited availability of comparative studies [67]. For example, in a systematic review comparing the diagnostic accuracy of computed tomography (CT) and magnetic resonance imaging (MRI) for clinically significant coronary artery disease, although 103 studies were included in the meta-analysis, only 5 of the studies evaluated both CT and MRI in the same study population [70]. Therefore, reviewers typically rely on indirect test comparisons. Takwoingi et al. provided empirical evidence of differences in the results from direct and indirect comparisons, although they found no evidence of a systematic direction in the differences [67].

16.10.2 Methods for Comparisons of Two or More Tests

Various methods have been used for comparing test accuracy in published systematic reviews [68, 71]. Network meta-analysis methods that extend either the bivariate or HSROC model have been proposed [72]. Cochrane currently recommends a hierarchical meta-regression approach to compare summary points or summary curves by adding test type as a covariate to the bivariate or HSROC model [20, 25]. This meta-regression approach, similar to the approach for investigating heterogeneity, is flexible, allowing the comparison of multiple tests. For example if there are N tests, N–1 indicator variables that take the value 0 or 1 are added to the model. Thus the effect of test type on model parameters can be estimated: the regression coefficients estimate the performance of one test relative to that of the test used as the reference category (note this test is not the reference standard, but another index test or comparator test) for the test type covariate. Additional variance terms for the random-effects parameters can also be added to either the bivariate or HSROC model to determine whether assumption of common variances is justified or separate variances for each test are needed [71]. It should be noted that as the models become increasingly complex, the number of additional parameters to estimate increases and can be difficult to fit, especially when there are few studies.

Figure 16.7 illustrates a comparison of summary points using bivariate meta-regression to compare the accuracy of CT and MRI. The indirect comparison shown in panel a included all 103 studies (84 CT studies,14 MRI studies, and 5 CT vs. MRI studies) in the analysis, while only the 5 paired studies of CT versus MRI were included in the direct comparison shown in panel b. Paired studies do not commonly report the joint classification of the results of two index tests within the diseased and nondiseased groups, but rather report a separate 2×2 table for each index test, ignoring the pairing of test results within individuals in each study. Therefore, the bivariate meta-regression described in this chapter is a conservative approach. A Bayesian bivariate model extension that accounts for paired data was proposed by Trikalinos et al. [74], but data availability and modeling complexities limit its use. Results from the indirect and direct comparisons of CT and MRI (Table 16.3) are consistent and show that CT is both more sensitive and more specific than MRI. However, the results of the direct comparison are less precise than the indirect comparison due to the limited number of studies.

When studies report different thresholds, a comparison of SROC curves is more appropriate than summary points. In addition, summary points can be estimated for

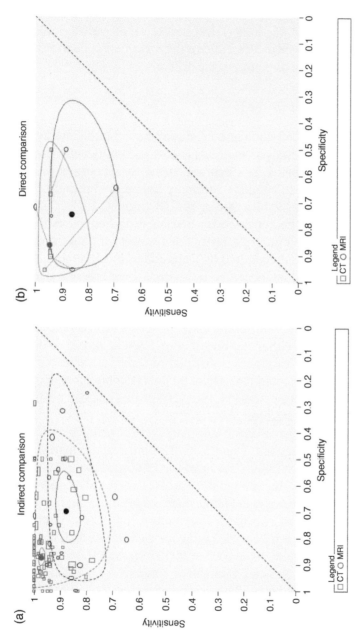

FIGURE 16.7 Comparison of summary points. (a) Indirect comparison. (b) Direct comparison. Panel a shows the indirect comparison of computed tomography (CT) and magnetic resonance imaging (MRI), while panel b shows the direct comparison. For each test on an SROC plot, each symbol represents the pair of sensitivity and specificity from a study. The size of each symbol was scaled according to the precision of sensitivity and specificity in the study. The solid circles (summary points) represent the summary estimates of sensitivity and specificity for each test. Each summary point is surrounded by a dotted line representing the 95% confidence region and a dashed line representing the 95% prediction region. Prediction regions are not shown in panel b due to the limited number of studies. In panel b, the pair of points from each comparative study is connected by a dotted line. *Source:* Adapted from Takwoingi et al. [73].

TABLE 16.3   Summary estimates from direct and indirect comparisons of computed tomography (*CT*) and magnetic resonance imaging (*MRI*) for coronary artery disease.

	Number of studies	Number of cases	Number of patients	Sensitivity (95% CI)	Specificity (95% CI)	P value[a]
Indirect comparison						
CT	89	4120	7526	0.97 (0.96, 0.98)	0.87 (0.84, 0.90)	<0.0001
MRI	19	523	978	0.88 (0.84, 0.91)	0.70 (0.59, 0.79)	
Direct comparison						
CT	5	159	334	0.94 (0.89, 0.97)	0.86 (0.72, 0.93)	0.02
MRI	5	142	307	0.86 (0.79, 0.91)	0.74 (0.56, 0.87)	

[a] Statistical significance of the difference in test performance was assessed using a likelihood ratio test comparing models with and without covariate terms for test type.

each test at clinically relevant thresholds for which data are available. Carvalho et al. compared the diagnostic accuracy of the bipolar spectrum diagnostic scale (BSDS), the hypomania checklist (HCL-32), and the MDQ for detecting bipolar disorder in mental health settings using indirect and direct test comparisons [26]. As the studies used various thresholds for each instrument, an HSROC meta-regression model was used to estimate and compare SROC curves.

The indirect comparison of BSDS, HCL-32, and MDQ included 44 studies. The effect of test type on the accuracy, threshold, and shape parameters of the model was assessed [26]. Using a likelihood ratio test to compare models with and without covariate terms for the shape parameter, there was statistical evidence that the shapes of the SROC curves differed (P = 0.002). Figure 16.8 (panel a) shows that the SROC curves for the three tests cross, implying that one test is not consistently more accurate than the other two. Therefore, the RDOR cannot be used to quantify relative accuracy. This is also evident in Table 16.4, which shows the sensitivities estimated from the curves at the median, lower, and upper quartiles of the observed specificities in the included studies. The direct comparison of the MDQ and HCL-32 included only eight studies (panel b). Three studies directly compared the BSDS and MDQ, but no study directly compared the HCL-32 and BSDS in a mental health setting.

16.11   SOFTWARE OPTIONS AND MODEL FITTING ISSUES

Several user-written macros and packages (e.g. MetaDAS, metandi, midas, bamdit) are available for fitting the models [73]. Further information and tutorials are available on the Cochrane Screening and Diagnostic Tests Methods Group website at https://methods.cochrane.org/sdt.

The GLMM implementation of the bivariate model reduces to two univariate random-effects logistic regression models for sensitivity and specificity when the

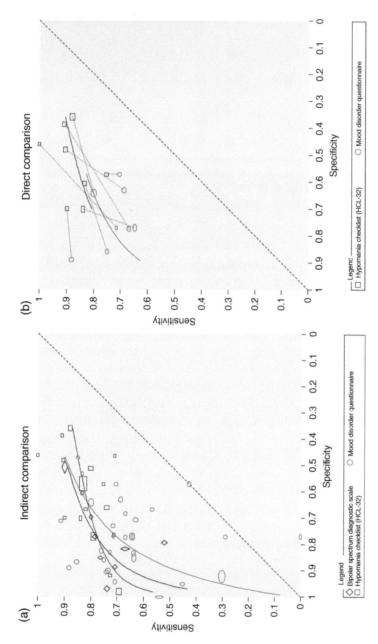

FIGURE 16.8 Comparison of summary curves. Panel a shows the indirect comparison of the three tests, while panel b shows the direct comparison of two of the tests. For each test on an SROC plot, each symbol represents the pair of sensitivity and specificity from a study. The size of each symbol was scaled according to the precision of sensitivity and specificity in the study. Each summary curve was drawn restricted to the range of specificities from the included studies for the test. In panel b, the pair of points from each comparative study is connected by a dotted line. BSDS, bipolar spectrum diagnostic scale; HCL-32, hypomania checklist; MDQ, mood disorder questionnaire. *Source:* Adapted from Carvalho et al. [26] and Takwoingi [71].

TABLE 16.4   Comparison of the accuracy of bipolar spectrum diagnostic scale (BSDS), hypomania checklist (HCL-32), and mood disorder questionnaire (MDQ) for detection of any type of bipolar disorder in mental health center settings.

Fixed value of specificity	Test	Estimated sensitivity (95% CI)
0.85	MDQ	0.58 (0.50 to 0.66)
	BSDS	0.71 (0.62 to 0.79)
	HCL-32	0.74 (0.68 to 0.80)
0.77	MDQ	0.70 (0.64 to 0.77)
	BSDS	0.78 (0.69 to 0.85)
	HCL-32	0.78 (0.73 to 0.82)
0.61	MDQ	0.83 (0.76 to 0.89)
	BSDS	0.86 (0.74 to 0.93)
	HCL-32	0.82 (0.78 to 0.85)

Source: Adapted from Carvalho et al. [26].

correlation parameter is dropped from the model (i.e. assumed to be zero). This simplification is sometimes necessary and appropriate when there are few studies or sparse data, which cause problems for the computationally intensive iterative process used to produce the estimates of the model parameters, leading to convergence issues or unreliable estimates [75]. Our experience suggests that the HSROC model can be successfully fitted with fewer studies and more extreme data more often than the bivariate model. An overview of approaches and pragmatic guidance for dealing with estimation problems and atypical data, such as when only 2×1 tables are available because false positives are impossible or only test positives are verified, are described in Takwoingi et al. [73].

16.12   INTERPRETATION AND REPORTING

Many researchers, health care professionals, and policymakers are unfamiliar with test accuracy statistics and systematic reviews of diagnostic accuracy [76, 77], let alone patients and the general public. Therefore, communicating review findings to a range of audiences is challenging. Reporting test accuracy using natural frequencies and visual aids may facilitate improved understanding and better estimation of the post-test probability of disease [76]. In their guidance on writing plain-language summaries, Whiting et al. [78] provided examples for presenting test accuracy results narratively and graphically, and gave equations for transforming results into natural frequencies using sensitivity, specificity, and prevalence. The calculations are illustrated in Box 16.3 using a prevalence or pre-test probability of 25% and summary estimates from the indirect comparison of CT and MRI presented in Table 16.3. Box 16.3 also gives a lay interpretation based on the natural frequencies. The calculations may be done manually, using a spreadsheet or online calculators that compute post-test probabilities. Confidence intervals can also be transformed into natural frequencies to communicate uncertainty. The numeric findings should

Box 16.3   Calculation of Natural Frequencies and Interpretation of the Results of a Diagnostic Test Accuracy Meta-Analysis

Calculation

Based on summary sensitivity of 0.97 for computed tomography (CT) and 0.88 for magnetic resonance imaging (MRI), and summary specificity of 0.87 for CT and 0.70 for MRI.

	CAD present	CAD absent	Total
CT positive	TP = sensitivity × (TP + FN) = 0.97 × 250 = 243	FP = 750–653 = 97	
CT negative	FN = 250–243 = 7	TN = specificity × (TN + FP) = 0.87 × 750 = 653	
Total	250	750	1000

	CAD present	CAD absent	Total
MRI positive	TP = sensitivity × (TP + FN) = 0.88 × 250 = 220	FP = 750–525 = 225	
MRI negative	FN = 250–220 = 30	TN = specificity × (TN + FP) = 0.70 × 750 = 525	
Total	250	750	1000

Interpretation

CT is more sensitive and more specific than MRI for detecting clinically significant coronary artery disease (CAD). Applying the summary estimates obtained from the 103 studies included in the comparison of CT and MRI to a hypothetical cohort of 1000 patients, if 250 (25%) of those presenting with suspected CAD have the disease, CT will miss 7 cases and MRI will miss 30 cases (false negatives). The number of people wrongly diagnosed with CAD (false positives) would be 97 with CT and 225 with MRI.

be discussed in the context of the quality of the evidence, and the consequences for FPs (e.g. overdiagnosis and overtreatment) and FNs (missed cases) should be considered. Further guidance is available in the *Cochrane Handbook for Systematic Reviews of Diagnostic Test Accuracy* [79].

A summary of findings (SoF) table that summarizes the main elements of a review's findings and provides information on the quantity, quality, and applicability of evidence as well as the accuracy of index test(s) also assists with accessibility [79]. An example of an SoF table can be found as a supplementary table in the PRISMA-DTA explanation and elaboration document [80]. PRISMA-DTA is an extension of PRISMA (Preferred Reporting Items for Systematic review and Meta-Analysis) statement (see Chapter 7) developed to improve the reporting quality of DTA systematic reviews [81]. The PRISMA-DTA checklist can facilitate complete and transparent reporting of reviews, and we encourage its use to make DTA reviews more useful.

16.13   DISCUSSION

While a health care practitioner desires valid summary estimates of the sensitivity and specificity of a diagnostic test, the presence of gross between-study heterogeneity can prohibit such estimates. Meta-analysis may not be appropriate because of clinical heterogeneity arising from differences in definition of the target condition, study populations, clinical settings, index test, reference standard, and other factors. We examined the Cochrane Library and found that of the 135 DTA reviews published up to July 31, 2020, 32 (24%) did not include a meta-analysis. Summarizing results of such reviews is challenging, especially if there are many studies and a variety of factors to consider. For example, Hanchard et al. included 33 studies in their Cochrane DTA review [82]. The studies assessed different index tests and used different reference standards and categories of the target conditions. In total, there were 170 target condition and index test combinations. No combination was assessed by more than two studies, and meta-analysis was considered inappropriate. The authors summarized the study-specific estimates of sensitivity and specificity on several forest plots, grouped according to target condition.

The review authors of the examples illustrated in this chapter considered meta-analysis appropriate despite the heterogeneity observed on forest and SROC plots. For example, to minimize clinical heterogeneity, Carvalho et al. did not lump all studies together but performed separate meta-analyses for different clinical settings to avoid a potential threshold effect that may occur due to a change in the spectrum of disease and alternative diagnoses on sensitivity and specificity [26]. They also investigated different subtypes of the target condition and the effect of potential sources of heterogeneity. Investigations of heterogeneity are often limited in practice due to the small number of included studies and/or poor or inconsistent reporting of the factors of interest. Although there have been improvements in the reporting quality of DTA studies since the introduction of the STARD statement [83], further improvements are needed to ensure information needed for assessing eligibility, quality assessment, and meta-analysis is available in published papers.

Publication bias and other reporting biases have been researched extensively for systematic reviews of RCTs of health interventions (see Chapter 5), but there is less understanding about mechanisms for such biases with respect to DTA studies. The limited evidence available suggests that failure to publish and selective reporting are prevalent in test accuracy studies [84]. Furthermore, time to publication was significantly shorter for studies reporting higher estimates of diagnostic accuracy compared to those reporting lower estimates (time-lag bias) [85]. Combined with failure to register many diagnostic accuracy studies in trial registries and the challenge of searching for DTA studies, estimates obtained from meta-analyses may thus be at risk of bias, i.e. included studies may systematically deviate from studies that are difficult to find, published later, or remain unpublished.

Standard funnel plots and statistical tests for detecting funnel plot asymmetry (see Chapter 5) should not be used in DTA reviews. Deeks et al. developed the effective sample size funnel plot and associated regression test of asymmetry for meta-analyses of diagnostic accuracy [86]. The statistical test assesses the association between the natural log of the DOR and the effective sample size (a function of the number of diseased and nondiseased individuals). However, when DORs are heterogeneous, this test also has low power, like all tests for funnel plot asymmetry [86].

The evaluation of the diagnostic accuracy of a test is one component of assessing whether it is of clinical value and does not capture the impact of tests on patients [87]. Therapeutic interventions can be recommended for use in health care only if they are shown on average to be of benefit to patients: the same criterion applies for the use of a diagnostic test, and even the most accurate of tests can be clinically useless and do more harm than good. Studies of diagnostic accuracy cannot prove that a diagnostic investigation is effective, but can discern whether the performance of a test is satisfactory for it to have the potential to be effective.

A reviewer should consider whether undertaking a systematic review of studies of diagnostic accuracy is likely to provide the most useful evidence of the value of a diagnostic test. Studies of patient outcomes, or the impact of using a test on therapeutic and diagnostic decisions, may provide more convincing evidence of the incremental benefit of using a new diagnostic test. However, such studies are not available for many tests, especially for new technologies and components of the clinical examination. Consequently, systematic reviews of diagnostic accuracy are often the main source of evidence for decision-making about the use of a test. Practical issues (such as the absence of good independent reference standards for some diseases) occasionally mean that reliable studies of diagnostic accuracy cannot be undertaken, and studies of test reliability, diagnostic yield, management decisions, and patient outcomes will provide the only evidence of the value of a diagnostic test.

While the basic methodology for undertaking rigorous systematic reviews of studies of diagnostic accuracy exists and more advanced methods continue to evolve, the greatest barrier to their practical application is the absence of appropriately designed, conducted, and reported primary studies [28]. In some fields, useful estimates of diagnostic accuracy can be obtained and many systematic reviews have informed national and international guidelines on diagnosis, yet in other fields the role of systematic reviews is limited to highlighting deficiencies in the primary studies.

REFERENCES

1. Sackett, D.L., Guyatt, G.H., and Tugwell, P. (1991). *Clinical Epidemiology: A Basic Science for Clinical Medicine*, 2e. Boston, MA: Little, Brown.

2. Pauker, S.G. and Kassirer, J.P. (1980). *The threshold approach to clinical decision making*. N. Engl. J. Med. 302 (20): 1109–1117.

3. Irwig, L., Tosteson, A.N., Garsonis, C. et al. (1994). *Guidelines for meta-analyses evaluating diagnostic tests*. Ann. Intern. Med. 120 (8): 667–676.

4. Leeflang, M.M., Deeks, J.J., Takwoingi, Y. et al. (2013). *Cochrane diagnostic test accuracy reviews*. Syst. Rev. 2: 82.

5. Irwig, L., Bossuvt, P., Glasziou, P. et al. (2002). *Designing studies to ensure that estimates of test accuracy are transferable. BMJ* 324 (7338): 669–671.

6. Valenstein, P.N. (1990). *Evaluating diagnostic tests with imperfect standards. Am. J. Clin. Pathol.* 93 (2): 252–258.

7. Naaktgeboren, C.A., Bertens, L.C., van Smeden, M. et al. (2013). *Value of composite reference standards in diagnostic research. BMJ* 347: f5605.

8. Ransohoff, D.F. and Feinstein, A.R. (1978). *Problems of spectrum and bias in evaluating the efficacy of diagnostic tests. N. Engl. J. Med.* 299 (17): 926–930.

9. Fagan, T.J. (1975). *Nomogram for Bayes theorem (letter). N. Engl. J. Med.* 293 (5): 257.

10. Glasziou, P. (2001). *Which methods for bedside Bayes? Evid. Based Med.* 6 (6): 164.

11. Glas, A.S., Lijmer, J.G., Prins, M.H. et al. (2003). *The diagnostic odds ratio: a single indicator of test performance. J. Clin. Epidemiol.* 56 (11): 1129–1135.

12. Beynon, R., Leeflang, M.M., McDonald, S. et al. (2013). *Search strategies to identify diagnostic accuracy studies in MEDLINE and EMBASE. Cochrane Database Syst. Rev.* 9: MR000022.

13. de Vet, H.C.W., Riphagen II, E.A., Aertgeerts, B., and Pewsner, D. (2008). Searching for studies. In: *Cochrane Handbook for Systematic Reviews of Diagnostic Test Accuracy*, Chapter 7. Version 0.4 (eds. J.J. Deeks, P.M. Bossuyt and C. Gatsonis). London: Cochrane Collaboration. https://methods.cochrane.org/sdt. (accessed February 21, 2022).

14. Thomas, J., McNaught, J., and Ananiadou, S. (2011). *Applications of text mining within systematic reviews. Res. Synth. Methods* 2 (1): 1–14.

15. Stansfield, C., O'Mara-Eves, A., and Thomas, J. (2017). *Text mining for search term development in systematic reviewing: a discussion of some methods and challenges. Res. Synth. Methods* 8 (3): 355–365.

16. Lijmer, J.G., Mol, B.W., Heisterkamp, S. et al. (1999). *Empirical evidence of design-related bias in studies of diagnostic tests. J. Am. Med. Assoc.* 282 (11): 1061–1066.

17. Rutjes, A.W., Reitsma, J.B., Di Nisio, M. et al. (2006). *Evidence of bias and variation in diagnostic accuracy studies. CMAJ* 174 (4): 469–476.

18. Whiting, P., Rutjes, A.W., Reitsma, J.B. et al. (2003). *The development of QUADAS: a tool for the quality assessment of studies of diagnostic accuracy included in systematic reviews. BMC Med. Res. Methodol.* 3: 25.

19. Whiting, P.F., Rutjes, A.W., Westwood, M.E. et al. (2011). *QUADAS-2: a revised tool for the quality assessment of diagnostic accuracy studies. Ann. Intern. Med.* 155 (8): 529–536.

20. Leeflang, M.M., Deeks, J.J., Gatsonis, C. et al. (2008). *Systematic reviews of diagnostic test accuracy. Ann. Intern. Med.* 149 (12): 889–897.

21. Yang, B., Mallett, S., Takwoingi, Y. et al. (2021). QUADAS-C: A tool for assessing risk of bias in comparative diagnostic accuracy studies. *Ann. Intern. Med.* 174 (11): 1592–1599.

22. Kay, A.W., Gonzalez Fernandez, L., Takwoingi, Y. et al. (2020). *Xpert MTB/RIF and Xpert MTB/RIF ultra assays for active tuberculosis and rifampicin resistance in children. Cochrane Database Syst. Rev.* 8: CD013359.

23. Liu, E., Nisenblat, V., Farquhar, C. et al. (2015). *Urinary biomarkers for the non-invasive diagnosis of endometriosis. Cochrane Database Syst. Rev.* (12): CD012019. https://doi.org/10.1002/14651858.CD012019.

24. Takwoingi, Y., Riley, R.D., and Deeks, J.J. (2015). *Meta-analysis of diagnostic accuracy studies in mental health. Evid. Based Ment. Health* 18 (4): 103–109.

25. Macaskill, P., Takwoingi, Y., Deeks, J.J. et al. (2021). Understanding meta-analysis, draft version 17 June 2021, For inclusion in: *Cochrane Handbook for Systematic Reviews of Diagnostic Test Accuracy Version 2* (eds. J.J. Deeks, P.M.M. Bossuyt, M.M.G. Leeflang and Y. Takwoingi). London: Cochrane Collaboration. https://methods.cochrane.org/sdt. (accessed 21 February 2022).

26. Carvalho, A.F., Takwoingi, Y., Sales, P.M. et al. (2014). *Screening for bipolar spectrum disorders: a comprehensive meta-analysis of accuracy studies. J. Affect. Disord.* 172C: 337–346.

27. Hirschfeld, R.M., Williams, J.B., Spitzer, R.L. et al. (2000). *Development and validation of a screening instrument for bipolar spectrum disorder: the mood disorder questionnaire. Am. J. Psychiatry* 157 (11): 1873–1875.

28. Irwig, L., Macaskill, P., Glasziou, P. et al. (1995). *Meta-analytic methods for diagnostic test accuracy. J. Clin. Epidemiol.* 48 (1): 119–130. discussion 131–2.

29. Moses, L.E., Shapiro, D., and Littenberg, B. (1993). *Combining independent studies of a diagnostic test into a summary ROC curve: data-analytic approaches and some additional considerations. Stat. Med.* 12 (14): 1293–1316.

30. Arends, L.R., Hamza, T.H., van Houwelingen, J.C. et al. (2008). *Bivariate random effects meta-analysis of ROC curves. Med. Decis. Making* 28 (5): 621–638.

31. Dinnes, J., Mallett, S., Hopewell, S. et al. (2016). *The Moses-Littenberg meta-analytical method generates systematic differences in test accuracy compared to hierarchical meta-analytical models. J. Clin. Epidemiol.* 80: 77–87.

32. Ma, X., Nie, L., Cole, S.R. et al. (2016). *Statistical methods for multivariate meta-analysis of diagnostic tests: an overview and tutorial. Stat. Methods Med. Res.* 25 (4): 1596–1619.

33. Harbord, R.M., Whiting, P., Sterne, J.A.C. et al. (2008). *An empirical comparison of methods for meta-analysis of diagnostic accuracy showed hierarchical models are necessary. J. Clin. Epidemiol.* 61 (11): 1095–1103.

34. Reitsma, J.B., Glas, A.S., Rutjes, A.W. et al. (2005). *Bivariate analysis of sensitivity and specificity produces informative summary measures in diagnostic reviews. J. Clin. Epidemiol.* 58 (10): 982–990.

35. Chu, H. and Cole, S.R. (2006). *Bivariate meta-analysis for sensitivity and specificity with sparse data: a generalized linear mixed model approach (letter to the editor). J. Clin. Epidemiol.* 59: 1331–1331.

36. Rutter, C.M. and Gatsonis, C.A. (2001). *A hierarchical regression approach to meta-analysis of diagnostic test accuracy evaluations. Stat. Med.* 20 (19): 2865–2884.

37. Harbord, R.M., Deeks, J.J., Egger, M. et al. (2007). *A unification of models for meta-analysis of diagnostic accuracy studies. Biostatistics* 8 (2): 239–251.

38. Dahabreh, I.J., Chung, M., Kitsious, G.D. et al., 2012 Comprehensive overview of methods and reporting of meta-analyses of test accuracy. Methods Research Reports. Rockville, MD: Agency for Healthcare Research and Quality.

39. Menten, J. and Lesaffre, E. (2015). *A general framework for comparative Bayesian meta-analysis of diagnostic studies. BMC Med. Res. Methodol.* 15: 70.

40. Chu, H., Chen, S., and Louis, T.A. (2009). *Random effects models in a meta-analysis of the accuracy of two diagnostic tests without a gold standard. J. Am. Stat. Assoc.* 104 (486): 512–523.

41. Dendukuri, N., Schiller, I., Joseph, L. et al. (2012). *Bayesian meta-analysis of the accuracy of a test for Tuberculous pleuritis in the absence of a gold standard reference.* Biometrics 68 (4): 1285–1293.

42. Liu, Y., Chen, Y., and Chu, H. (2015). *A unification of models for meta-analysis of diagnostic accuracy studies without a gold standard.* Biometrics 71 (2): 538–547.

43. Xie, X., Sinclair, A., and Dendukuri, N. (2017). *Evaluating the accuracy and economic value of a new test in the absence of a perfect reference test.* Res. Synth. Methods 8 (3): 321–332.

44. Hoyer, A. and Kuss, O. (2015). *Meta-analysis of diagnostic tests accounting for disease prevalence: a new model using trivariate copulas.* Stat. Med. 34 (11): 1912–1924.

45. Nikoloulopoulos, A.K. (2017). *A vine copula mixed effect model for trivariate meta-analysis of diagnostic test accuracy studies accounting for disease prevalence.* Stat. Methods Med. Res. 26 (5): 2270–2286.

46. Chu, H., Nie, L., Cole, S.R. et al. (2009). *Meta-analysis of diagnostic accuracy studies accounting for disease prevalence: alternative parameterizations and model selection.* Stat. Med. 28 (18): 2384–2399.

47. Riley, R.D., Ahmed, I., Ensor, J. et al. (2015). *Meta-analysis of test accuracy studies: an exploratory method for investigating the impact of missing thresholds.* Syst. Rev. 4 (1): 12.

48. Hamza, T., Arends, L., van Houwelingen, H. et al. (2009). *Multivariate random effects meta-analysis of diagnostic tests with multiple thresholds.* BMC Med. Res. Methodol. 9 (1): 73.

49. Dukic, V. and Gatsonis, C. (2003). *Meta-analysis of diagnostic test accuracy assessment studies with varying number of thresholds.* Biometrics 59 (4): 936–946.

50. Putter, H., Fiocco, M., and Stijnen, T. (2010). *Meta-analysis of diagnostic test accuracy studies with multiple thresholds using survival methods.* Biom. J. 52 (1): 95–110.

51. Steinhauser, S., Schumacher, M., and Rücker, G. (2016). *Modelling multiple thresholds in meta-analysis of diagnostic test accuracy studies.* BMC Med. Res. Methodol. 16 (1): 97.

52. Jones, H.E., Gatsonis, C.A., Trikalinos, T.A. et al. (2019). *Quantifying how diagnostic test accuracy depends on threshold in a meta-analysis.* Stat. Med. 38 (24): 4789–4803.

53. Nyaga, V.N., Aerts, M., and Arbyn, M. (2018). *ANOVA model for network meta-analysis of diagnostic test accuracy data.* Stat. Methods Med. Res. 27 (6): 1766–1784.

54. Nyaga, V.N., Arbyn, M., and Aerts, M. (2018). *Beta-binomial analysis of variance model for network meta-analysis of diagnostic test accuracy data.* Stat. Methods Med. Res. 27 (8): 2554–2566.

55. Owen, R.K., Cooper, N.J., Quinn, T.J. et al. (2018). *Network meta-analysis of diagnostic test accuracy studies identifies and ranks the optimal diagnostic tests and thresholds for health care policy and decision-making.* J. Clin. Epidemiol. 99: 64–74.

56. Bipat, S. and Zwinderman, A.H. (2010). *Multivariate fixed- and random-effects models for summarizing ordinal data in meta-analysis of diagnostic staging studies.* Res. Synth. Methods 1 (2): 136–148.

57. Bipat, S., Zwinderman, A.H., Bossuyt, P.M. et al. (2007). *Multivariate random-effects approach: for meta-analysis of cancer staging studies.* Acad. Radiol. 14 (8): 974–984.

58. Ma, X., Suri, M.F., and Chu, H. (2014). *A trivariate meta-analysis of diagnostic studies accounting for prevalence and non-evaluable subjects: re-evaluation of the meta-analysis of coronary CT angiography studies.* BMC Med. Res. Methodol. 14: 128.

59. Ma, X., Chen, Y., Cole, S.R. et al. (2016). *A hybrid Bayesian hierarchical model combining cohort and case-control studies for meta-analysis of diagnostic tests: accounting for partial verification bias. Stat. Methods Med. Res.* 25 (6): 3015–3037.

60. Chu, H., Guo, H., and Zhou, Y. (2010). *Bivariate random effects meta-analysis of diagnostic studies using generalized linear mixed models. Med. Decis. Making* 30 (4): 499–508.

61. Zwinderman, A.H. and Bossuyt, P.M. (2008). *We should not pool diagnostic likelihood ratios in systematic reviews. Stat. Med.* 27 (5): 687–697.

62. Leeflang, M.M., Deeks, J.J., Rutjes, A.W. et al. (2012). *Bivariate meta-analysis of predictive values of diagnostic tests can be an alternative to bivariate meta-analysis of sensitivity and specificity. J. Clin. Epidemiol.* 65 (10): 1088–1097.

63. Higgins, J.P.T., Thompson, S.G., Deeks, J.J. et al. (2003). *Measuring inconsistency in meta-analyses. BMJ* 327 (7414): 557–560.

64. Zhou, Y. and Dendukuri, N. (2014). *Statistics for quantifying heterogeneity in univariate and bivariate meta-analyses of binary data: the case of meta-analyses of diagnostic accuracy. Stat. Med.* 33 (16): 2701–2717.

65. Rücker, G., Schwarzer, G., Carpenter, J.R. et al. (2008). *Undue reliance on I(2) in assessing heterogeneity may mislead. BMC Med. Res. Methodol.* 8: 79.

66. Wetterslev, J., Thorlund, K., Brok, J. et al. (2009). *Estimating required information size by quantifying diversity in random-effects model meta-analyses. BMC Med. Res. Methodol.* 9: 86.

67. Takwoingi, Y., Leeflang, M.M., and Deeks, J.J. (2013). *Empirical evidence of the importance of comparative studies of diagnostic test accuracy. Ann. Intern. Med.* 158 (7): 544–554.

68. Takwoingi, Y., Partlett, C., Riley, R.D. et al. (2020). *Methods and reporting of systematic reviews of comparative accuracy were deficient: a methodological survey and proposed guidance. J. Clin. Epidemiol.* 121: 1–14.

69. Lumley, T. (2002). *Network meta-analysis for indirect treatment comparisons. Stat. Med.* 21 (16): 2313–2324.

70. Schuetz, G.M., Zacharopoulou, N.M., Schlattmann, P. et al. (2010). *Meta-analysis: noninvasive coronary angiography using computed tomography versus magnetic resonance imaging. Ann. Intern. Med.* 152 (3): 167–177.

71. Takwoingi, Y. (2016). Meta-analytic approaches for summarising and comparing the accuracy of medical tests. PhD thesis, University of Birmingham. https://etheses.bham.ac.uk/id/eprint/6759 (accessed February 21, 2022).

72. Rücker, G. (2018). *Network meta-analysis of diagnostic test accuracy studies.* In: *Diagnostic Meta-Analysis: A Useful Tool for Clinical Decision-Making* (ed. G. Biondi-Zoccai), 183–197. Cham: Springer.

73. Takwoingi, Y., Dendukuri, N., Schiller, I., Rücker, G., Jones, H.E., Partlett, C., Macaskill, P. (2021) Chapter 11: Undertaking meta-analysis. Draft version (27 September 2021) for inclusion in: Deeks JJ, Bossuyt PMM, Leeflang MMG, Takwoingi Y, editor(s). *Cochrane Handbook for Systematic Reviews of Diagnostic Test Accuracy Version 2.* London: Cochrane. https://methods.cochrane.org/sdt. (accessed 21 February 2022).

74. Trikalinos, T.A., Hoaglin, D.C., Small, K.M. et al. (2014). *Methods for the joint meta-analysis of multiple tests. Res. Synth. Methods* 5 (4): 294–312.

75. Takwoingi, Y., Guo, B., Riley, R.D. et al. (2017). *Performance of methods for meta-analysis of diagnostic test accuracy with few studies or sparse data. Stat. Methods Med. Res.* 26 (4): 1896–1911.

76. Whiting, P.F., Davenport, C., Jameson, C. et al. (2015). *How well do health professionals interpret diagnostic information? A systematic review. Br. Med. J. Open* 5 (7): e008155.

77. Zhelev, Z., Garside, R., and Hyde, C. (2013). *A qualitative study into the difficulties experienced by healthcare decision makers when reading a Cochrane diagnostic test accuracy review. Syst. Rev.* 2: 32.

78. Whiting, P., Leeflang, M., de Salis, I. et al. (2018). *Guidance was developed on how to write a plain language summary for diagnostic test accuracy reviews. J. Clin. Epidemiol.* 103: 112–119.

79. Bossuyt, P., Davenport, C., Deeks, J. et al. (2013). Interpreting results and drawing conclusions. In: *Cochrane Handbook for Systematic Reviews of Diagnostic Test Accuracy. Version 0.9*, Chapter 11 (eds. J.J. Deeks, P.M. Bossuyt and C. Gatsonis). London: Cochrane Collaboration.

80. Salameh, J.P., Bossuyt, P.M., McGrath, T.A. et al. (2020). *Preferred reporting items for systematic review and meta-analysis of diagnostic test accuracy studies (PRISMA-DTA): explanation, elaboration, and checklist. Br. Med. J.* 370: m2632.

81. McInnes, M.D.F., Moher, D., Thombs, B.D. et al. (2018). *Preferred reporting items for a systematic review and meta-analysis of diagnostic test accuracy studies: the PRISMA-DTA statement. J.Am. Med. Assoc.* 319 (4): 388–396.

82. Hanchard, N.C., Lenza, M., Handoll, H.H. et al. (2013). *Physical tests for shoulder impingements and local lesions of bursa, tendon or labrum that may accompany impingement. Cochrane Database Syst. Rev.* 4: CD007427.

83. Korevaar, D.A., van Enst, W.A., Spijker, R. et al. (2014). *Reporting quality of diagnostic accuracy studies: a systematic review and meta-analysis of investigations on adherence to STARD. Evid. Based Med.* 19 (2): 47–54.

84. Korevaar, D.A., Ochodo, E.A., Bossuyt, P.M. et al. (2014). *Publication and reporting of test accuracy studies registered in ClinicalTrials.gov. Clin. Chem.* 60 (4): 651–659.

85. Korevaar, D.A., van Es, N., Zwinderman, A.H. et al. (2016). *Time to publication among completed diagnostic accuracy studies: associated with reported accuracy estimates. BMC Med. Res. Methodol.* 16: 68.

86. Deeks, J.J., Macaskill, P., and Irwig, L. (2005). *The performance of tests of publication bias and other sample size effects in systematic reviews of diagnostic test accuracy was assessed. J. Clin. Epidemiol.* 58 (9): 882–893.

87. Ferrante di Ruffano, L., Hyde, C.J., McCaffery, K.J. et al. (2012). *Assessing the value of diagnostic tests: a framework for designing and evaluating trials. BMJ* 344: e686.

CHAPTER 17

Systematic Reviews of Prognostic Factor Studies

Richard D. Riley, Karel G.M. Moons, Douglas G. Altman, Gary S. Collins, and Thomas P.A. Debray

Prognosis research aims to examine and predict future outcomes (such as death, disease progression, or medical complications) in individuals with a particular health condition or startpoint (such as receiving a certain diagnosis or undergoing surgery). The PROGRESS framework defines four types of prognosis research objectives: (i) to summarize overall prognosis (e.g. overall risk or rate) of health outcomes for groups defined by a particular health condition [1]; (ii) to identify prognostic factors associated with changes in health outcomes [2]; (iii) to develop, validate, and examine the impact of prognostic models for individualized prediction of such outcomes [3]; and (iv) to identify predictors of an individual's response to treatment [4]. Each topic area requires specific methods and tools for conducting a systematic review and meta-analysis. Here, we focus on prognostic factors, i.e. variables that are associated with the risk of a subsequent health outcome in individuals with a particular health condition. Different values or categories of a prognostic factor are associated with a better or worse prognosis, i.e. of future health outcomes. For example, in many cancers, tumor grade at the time of histological diagnosis is a prognostic factor for recurrence and survival (Figure 17.1). Many routinely collected patient characteristics are prognostic, such as sex, age, body mass index (BMI), smoking status, blood pressure, comorbidities, and symptoms. However, in recent years the most examined prognostic factors have been biomarkers, which include a diverse range of blood, urine, imaging, electrophysiological, physiological, and genetic factors. In clinical practice, prognosis is rarely made on the basis of a single patient characteristic, marker, or imaging test result. Rather, the information from a particular prognostic factor is typically used and judged in combination with other prognostic factors, making prognostication in clinical practice generally a multivariable problem (see also Chapter 18).

Systematic Reviews in Health Research: Meta-Analysis in Context, Third Edition. Edited by Matthias Egger, Julian P.T. Higgins, and George Davey Smith.
© 2022 John Wiley & Sons Ltd. Published 2022 by John Wiley & Sons Ltd.
Companion website: www.systematic-reviews3.org

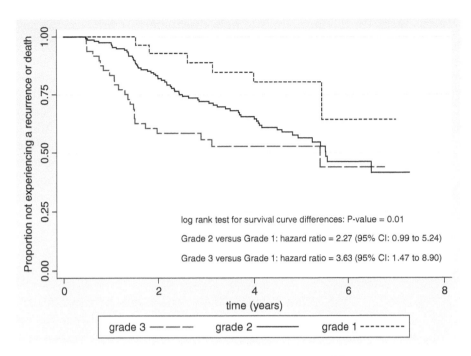

FIGURE 17.1   Tumor grade as a prognostic factor in breast cancer [2]. Kaplan–Meier curves for disease-free survival for three groups of breast cancer patients defined by tumor grade status (grade 1, 2 or 3). Curves are derived using 246 breast cancer patients treated with tamoxifen who had 94 recurrences or deaths over a possible seven years of follow-up [5]. The distinct curves, the statistically significant log-rank result, and the unadjusted hazard ratio estimates suggest that tumor grade is a prognostic factor, as it identifies three groups of patients with a different average prognosis.

Prognostic factors have many potential uses, including aiding in treatment decisions, improving outcome prediction, and enhancing the design and analysis of clinical trials [2]. This motivates research to identify prognostic factors (sometimes also called "predictor finding studies" [6]), with thousands of such studies published each year [7]. Prognostic factors are ideally studied using prospective cohort studies. These should involve a well-defined cohort of individuals with the health condition of interest, for which potential prognostic factors are measured at a relevant startpoint, with subsequent follow-up information recorded for relevant outcomes [2]. Prognostic factor studies may also use existing data from routine care databases, biobanks, or registries, which have been collected for a different purpose, but allow investigation of prognostic associations [8]. Furthermore, randomized trial data are often used to investigate prognostic factors, as these are essentially cohort studies with detailed baseline and follow-up information for individuals, albeit with potentially narrower inclusion criteria.

Unfortunately, prognostic factor studies often have variable quality and inconsistent findings [2]. This motivates the need for systematic reviews and meta-analyses that summarize the evidence about the prognostic value of particular factors [9–11]. In this chapter, we provide a guide to conducting such reviews, building on our previous work [9, 12]. Our aim is to help researchers understand the key principles, methods, and challenges of conducting reviews of prognostic factor studies, to produce robust evidence-based summaries about prognostic factors. Many of the issues discussed are also relevant to reviews of epidemiological studies of etiological or risk factor studies (as discussed in Chapter 19), and to reviews of prediction models (Chapter 18). There is a strong interest in factors that predict response to treatment (the fourth type of study in the PROGRESS framework) [4]. These factors are often referred to as predictive markers (or predictive factors) and are not the focus here, as they relate to an interaction between the factor and a particular treatment effect. Instead, we focus on the prognostic ability of a factor over and above that of treatment, although many of the issues discussed will also be relevant to reviews of studies of predictive markers.

17.1 DEFINING THE REVIEW QUESTION

The first step is to define the review question. Some reviews may be broad. For example, Riley et al. aimed to identify *any* prognostic factor for overall and disease-free survival in children with neuroblastoma or Ewing's sarcoma [13]. Other reviews may have a narrower focus. For example, Hemingway et al. summarized the evidence for whether C-reactive protein (CRP) is a prognostic factor for fatal and nonfatal events among patients with stable coronary disease [14]; this CRP review will be used as a running illustrative example throughout this chapter.

CHARMS (CHecklist for critical Appraisal and data extraction for systematic Reviews of prediction Modeling Studies) provides guidance for formulating a review question and a checklist for extracting data and critically appraising the eligible primary studies [15]. Though developed for reviews of prediction model studies [16], it has since been modified to define and frame the question for reviews of prognostic factor studies (CHARMS-PF) [12], and to inform data extraction (see Section 17.3). It proposes a modification (called PICOTS) of the traditional PICO system (Population, Intervention, Comparison, and Outcome) used in systematic reviews of therapeutic intervention studies (see Chapter 2), by additionally considering Timing and Setting (Box 17.1). In the context of prognostic factor reviews, the P of Population and O of Outcome remain largely the same as in the original PICO system, whereas the I refers to the Index prognostic factor(s).

The C in prognostic factor reviews needs careful thought. It is usually not defined by reference values of the factor itself, especially as most prognostic factors are continuous, such as age, BMI, blood pressure, and leucocyte count (and so do not have a reference group as such). Rather, C usually refers to other Comparator prognostic factors. For example, a typical prognostic factor review aims to investigate the prognostic value of a particular index factor adjusted for other (i.e. comparator) prognostic factors, and sometimes the review may aim to compare the prognostic value of a certain index factor with one or more other (i.e. comparator) prognostic factors. Only when the index factor is categorical, and its unadjusted prognostic effect is of interest, might C refer to the reference category of the index factor itself. For example, if the index factor is a comorbidity (present or absent) and is studied in isolation, then the I might

Box 17.1   Six Items to Help Define the Question for Systematic Reviews of Prognostic Factor Studies, Abbreviated as PICOTS, and Applied to a Review of the Added Prognostic Value of C-Reactive Protein

- **Population:** *define the target population in which the prognostic factor(s) under review are to be used.*

CRP review: patients with stable coronary disease, defined as clinically diagnosed angina pectoris or angiographic disease, or a history of previous acute coronary syndrome at least two weeks prior to prognostic factor (CRP) measurement.

- **Index factor:** *define the prognostic factor(s) under review.*

CRP review: CRP was the single biomarker reviewed for its prognostic value.

- **Comparators:** *if applicable,* define the other comparator prognostic factors. For example, a typical prognostic factor review aims to investigate the prognostic value of a particular index factor adjusted for other (i.e. comparator) prognostic factors, and sometimes the review may aim to compare the prognostic value of a certain index factor with one or more other (i.e. comparator) prognostic factors

CRP review: the focus was on the added prognostic value of CRP; i.e. its prognostic effect after adjusting for other prognostic factors. In particular, adjustment for the following conventional prognostic factors was of interest: age, sex, smoking status, obesity, diabetes, and one or more lipid variables (from total cholesterol, LDL cholesterol, HDL cholesterol, triglycerides), and inflammatory markers (fibrinogen, IL-6, white cell count).

- **Outcome:** *define the outcome(s) for which the prognostic ability of the factor(s) under review is of interest.*

CRP review: outcome events were defined as coronary (coronary death, sudden cardiac death, acute nonfatal myocardial infarction, primary percutaneous coronary intervention, unplanned emergency admissions with unstable angina), cardiovascular (where coronary events were reported in combination with heart failure, stroke, or peripheral arterial disease), and all-cause mortality.

- **Timing:** *define at what timepoints the prognostic factors are to be used and over what time period the outcome(s) are predicted.*

CRP review: there was no restriction on the timepoints and time period. The CRP measurement had to be done at least two weeks after diagnosis and all follow-up information on the outcomes (all time periods) was extracted from the studies.

- **Setting:** *define the intended role or setting of the prognostic factor(s) under review.*

CRP review: CRP measurement was studied in both primary and secondary care to provide prognostic information about patients diagnosed with coronary heart disease, and thus may be useful for health care professionals treating and managing such patients.

Source: Adapted from Hemingway H et al., 2010 [14].

be considered as one category (e.g. comorbidity present) and the C taken as the other reference category (e.g. comorbidity absent).

The T denotes Timing and refers to two concepts of time: (i) at what timepoint the prognostic factors under review are to be measured or assessed (i.e. the time-point at which prognosis information is required); and (ii) over what time period the outcome(s) are predicted by these factors. The S refers to Setting, which is the clinical setting or context for using the index prognostic factor(s); this is important, as the prognostic value of a factor may change across health care settings.

An important issue, and related to the I and C discussion, is whether unadjusted (crude) or adjusted prognostic factor effects (or both) will be summarized in a review. As mentioned, prognosis in health care is rarely based on a single factor, but on multiple prognostic factors. Hence, the prognostic ability of a single factor used in isolation is rarely of interest for prognostic factor reviews. Rather, the *adjusted* prognostic factor effect is needed to better reveal whether a factor contributes prognostic value after adjusting for the other prognostic factors that are routinely used in practice. In particular, usually for the clinical setting of interest there will be "established" or "conventional" prognostic factors that are routinely measured. Therefore, for index prognostic factors under review, it is important to understand whether they contribute additional prognostic information to these factors. The crude (unadjusted) prognostic relevance of a factor may completely disappear after adjustment and it may therefore be rather uninformative [3]. In addition, unadjusted prognostic effects may be highly dependent on population characteristics and therefore prone to substantial between-study heterogeneity.

Note that the driver to focus on adjusted effects is different from that within systematic reviews of etiological studies. In the latter, the focus is on estimating the causal effect of a certain risk factor, and adjustment for other risk factors is crucial as they may be confounders, so if left unadjusted would mask the true causal effect of the factor of interest. That is, adjustment is essential to help remove bias due to confounding factors. However, in situations where causality is not of interest, the notion of confounding is not relevant. In prognostic factor studies the typical aim is "simply" to identify whether certain factors are associated with (i.e. prognostic for) particular outcomes, and not whether they are causal for the occurrence of those outcomes. Nevertheless, adjusted results are still the clinically relevant results of interest, as the magnitude of a factor's prognostic effect usually depends on whether adjustment is made for other factors that are prognostic. Now the adjustment is not about removing bias, but rather about quantifying the added prognostic value of a factor. Therefore, whether a prognostic factor review should focus on estimating the adjusted (rather than the unadjusted) prognostic effect of a factor is more a matter of clinical relevance than removing risks of bias.

17.1.1   Application to the C-Reactive Protein Review

CRP is widely studied for its prognostic value in patients with coronary disease, but there is continued uncertainty as to whether it is useful. US and European clinical practice guidelines recommend measurement, but clinical practice varies widely. This motivated the systematic review by Hemingway et al. [14], for which the PICOTS system is shown in Box 17.1.

17.2   SEARCHING AND SELECTING ELIGIBLE STUDIES

The second step is to identify eligible primary studies, i.e. studies that address the defined review question as articulated using the PICOTS framework. It is more difficult to identify prognostic factor studies than randomized clinical trials (see Chapter 3). Prognosis studies do not tend to be indexed ("tagged") in bibliographic databases, and there is much variation in design (e.g. cohort studies, randomized trials, routine care registry data, and case–control study data can all be used), methods of statistical analysis, and the adjustment of other prognostic factors or covariates. Heterogeneity is thus the rule rather than the exception in prognostic factor research. It is therefore essential that the definition of inclusion criteria of studies for a systematic review is based on the PICOTS structure (Box 17.1), as it determines the search and study selection strategy.

Typically broad search and selection filters are required, combining terms related to prognosis research (such as "prognostic," "predict," "predictor," "factor," "independent") with clinical domain- or disease-specific terms and the names of prognostic factors [17]. Such a broad search comes at the expense of retrieving many irrelevant records. Geersing et al. [18] validated various search strategies for prognosis studies [17, 19, 20] and suggested a generic filter for identifying studies of prognostic factors, as shown in Box 17.2. When tested in a review of prognostic factors in acute stroke, this generic filter had a number needed to read (NNR) to identify one relevant study of 569, emphasizing the difficulty in targeting prognostic factor articles [18]. The NNR is reduced if specific factors or populations are added to the filter. Even then, care is needed to ensure inclusivity, as multiple terms may be used. For example, biomarker MYCN is also referred to as n-myc or nmyc [13].

Box 17.2   Generic Search String for Identifying Prognostic Model Studies, Which can Serve as a Good Starting Point for Identifying Prognostic Factor Studies

(Validat$ OR Predict$.ti. OR Rule$)

OR (Predict$ AND [Outcome$ OR Risk$ OR Model$])

OR ((History OR Variable$ OR Criteria OR Scor$ OR Characteristic$ OR Finding$ OR Factor$) AND (Predict$ OR Model$ OR Decision$ OR Identif$ OR Prognos$))

OR (Decision$ AND [Model$ OR Clinical$ OR Logistic Models/])

OR (Prognostic AND [History OR Variable$ OR Criteria OR Scor$ OR Characteristic$ OR Finding$ OR Factor$ OR Model$])

OR (Stratification OR "ROC Curve"[Mesh] OR Discrimination OR Discriminate

OR "c-statistic" OR "c statistic" OR "Area under the curve" OR AUC OR Calibration OR Indices OR Algorithm OR Multivariable)

Source: As proposed by Geersing et al. [18].

Once the search is complete, potentially relevant studies must be screened for eligibility. The study selection should first be based on screening of titles and abstracts, followed by full-text screening, both ideally done by two researchers independently. Any discrepancies should be resolved through discussion, and potentially with a third reviewer. To check if any relevant articles have been missed, it is helpful to share the list of identified studies with researchers in the field, to examine the reference lists of identified articles, and to perform a citation search.

17.2.1 Application to the C-Reactive Protein Review

Hemingway et al. included any prospective observational study that reported the risk of subsequent events among patients with stable coronary disease in relation to measured CRP values [14]. Eligible studies had to include patients with stable coronary disease, defined as clinically diagnosed angina pectoris or angiographic disease, or a history of previous acute coronary syndrome at least two weeks prior to CRP measurement. They searched MEDLINE between 1966 and November 25, 2009 and EMBASE between 1980 and December 17, 2009, using a search string containing terms for coronary disease, prognostic studies, and CRP. The search identified 1566 articles, of which 83 studies fulfilled the inclusion criteria, for a NNR of 19.

17.3 DATA EXTRACTION

Data extraction provides the necessary data from each study, which enables reviewers to examine their applicability and risk of bias. It also provides the information required for subsequent qualitative and quantitative (meta-analysis) synthesis of the evidence. The CHARMS checklist provides explicit guidance about which data should be extracted from primary studies of prediction models (see Chapter 18) [15]. Riley et al. modified this for prognostic factor studies, and refer to it as CHARMS-PF (Box 17.3) [12].

Box 17.3   The CHARMS-PF Checklist of Key Items to be Extracted from Primary Studies of Prognostic Factors, Modified from the Original CHARMS Checklist

Domain	Key items
Source of data	– Source of data (e.g. cohort, case–control, randomized trial participants, or registry data)
Participants	– Participant eligibility and recruitment method (e.g. consecutive participants, location, number of centers, setting, inclusion and exclusion criteria) – Participants description – Details of treatments received, if relevant – Study dates

Domain	Key items
Outcome(s) to be predicted	– Definition and method for measurement of outcome(s) – Was the same outcome definition (and method for measurement) used in all participants? – Type of outcome(s) (e.g. single or combined endpoints) – Was the outcome(s) assessed without knowledge of the candidate prognostic factors (i.e. blinded)? – Were candidate prognostic factors part of the outcome (e.g. when using a panel or consensus outcome measurement)? – Time of outcome(s) occurrence or summary of duration of follow-up
Prognostic factors (including candidate and established prognostic factors)	– Number and type of prognostic factors (e.g. obtained from demographics, patient history, physical examination, additional testing, disease characteristics) – Definition and method for measurement of prognostic factors – Timing of prognostic factor measurement (e.g. at patient presentation, at diagnosis, at treatment initiation, end of surgery) – Were prognostic factors assessed blinded for outcome, and for each other (if relevant)? – Handling of prognostic factors in the modeling (e.g. continuous, linear, nonlinear transformations or categorized)
Sample size	– Was a sample size calculation conducted and, if so, how? – Number of participants and number of outcomes/events – Number of outcomes/events in relation to the number of candidate prognostic factors (events per variable)
Missing data	– Number of participants with any missing value (in the prognostic factors and outcomes) – Number of participants with missing data for each prognostic factor of interest – Handling of missing data (e.g. complete-case analysis, imputation, or other methods)
Analysis	– Modeling method (e.g. linear, logistic, Cox, parametric survival, competing risks regression) – Modeling assumptions satisfied – Method for selection of prognostic factors **for inclusion** in multivariable modeling (e.g. all candidate prognostic factors considered, pre-selection of established prognostic factors, retain only those significant from univariable analysis) – Method for selection/exclusion of prognostic factors (including those of interest and those used as adjustment factors) *during multivariable modeling* (e.g. backward or forward selection, or full model approach including all factors regardless) and criteria used for any selection/exclusion (e.g. P value, Akaike information criterion) – Method of handling each continuous prognostic factor (e.g. dichotomization, categorization, linear, nonlinear), including values of any cut points used and their justification. For nonlinear trends, the method of identifying nonlinear relationships (e.g. splines, fractional polynomials)

(Continued)

Domain	Key items
Results	– Unadjusted and adjusted prognostic effect estimates (e.g. risk ratios, odds ratios, hazard ratios, mean differences) for each prognostic factor of interest, and the corresponding 95% confidence interval (or variance or standard error). Details of any nonlinear relationships – For each extracted adjusted prognostic effect estimate of interest, the set of adjustment factors used
Interpretation and discussion	– Interpretation of presented results – Comparison with other studies, discussion of generalizability, strengths, and limitations

Source: Adapted from Moons KG et al., 2014 [15].

Reviewers should extract key information from each selected study, such as the dates, setting, study design, definitions of startpoints, outcomes, follow-up length, and prognostic factors, where one should appreciate the likely large heterogeneity across studies in many aspects. The extracted information allows for summary tables of study characteristics. In addition, information that is more specific is needed for risk of bias and applicability assessment, such as methods of measurement of the prognostic factors and outcomes, the handling of missing data, and whether estimated associations of the prognostic factors under review were adjusted for other prognostic factors.

To enable meta-analysis of prognostic factor studies, the key elements to extract are estimates, and corresponding standard errors or confidence intervals, of the prognostic effect for each factor of interest; for example, the estimated risk ratio or odds ratio (for binary outcomes), the hazard ratio (for time-to-event outcomes), or mean difference (for continuous outcomes). As most prognostic factor studies consider time-to-event outcomes (including censored observations and different follow-up lengths for patients), hazard ratios are often the most suitable effect measure. Unfortunately, many prognostic factor studies do not adequately report estimated effect measures or their precision. Parmar et al. [21] and Tierney et al. [22] describe how to obtain unadjusted hazard ratio estimates (and their variances) when they are not reported directly. For example, one can use the number of outcomes (events) and an available P value (e.g. from a log-rank test or Cox regression) to indirectly estimate the unadjusted hazard ratio between two groups defined by a particular factor (e.g. "positive" versus "negative" levels). Perneger et al. [23] describe how to derive unadjusted hazard ratios from survival proportions. Even with such indirect estimation methods, not all results may be obtainable. For example, in a systematic review of 575 studies investigating prognostic factors in neuroblastoma [24], the methods of Parmar et al. were used to obtain 204 hazard ratio estimates and their confidence intervals, but this represented only 35.5% of the potential evidence.

Although indirect estimation methods help retrieve *unadjusted* prognostic effect estimates, they have limited value for obtaining *adjusted* effect estimates, which are the more clinically useful and thus preferred interest for meta-analysis.

Furthermore, even when multiple studies do provide the adjusted prognostic effect of a particular factor, then the set of adjustment factors will usually differ across studies. This complicates the interpretation of subsequent meta-analysis results. It may help the reviewer to pre-define a minimal set of established prognostic factors that is typically applied in the clinical context of interest (e.g. age and stage of disease in cancer patients), and include those studies that are least adjusted for this minimal set of other prognostic factors.

If the outcome is defined differently across studies, approaches to convert effect measures on different outcome scales might be useful [25]. Furthermore, the direction of effect will need standardizing if one study compares the risk or rate in a factor's "high" versus "normal" group, whereas another study compares the risk or rate in the factor's "normal" versus "high" group. A major issue is dealing with different cut point values for a particular continuous factor (i.e. the threshold value, above which defines "high" and below which defines "normal" [26]), and potentially converting prognostic effects of "high" versus "normal" to prognostic effects relating to a one-unit increase in the factor, based on an assumed distribution of the prognostic factor values. A concern is that the distribution of a prognostic factor may be unknown (or even vary across studies). Finally, it is also possible to derive standardized effect estimates by standardizing the corresponding regression coefficients [27].

17.3.1   Application to the C-Reactive Protein Review

Hemingway et al. [14] extracted background information such as year of study start, number of included patients, mean age, baseline coronary morbidity (e.g. proportion with stable angina), average levels of biomarker at baseline, method of CRP measurement, follow-up duration, and number and type of events. Basic information was often missing. For example, nearly a fifth of studies did not report the method of measurement, and only a quarter gave the number of patients included in the analyses and reasons for dropout. Prognostic effect estimates for CRP were extracted in terms of either the reported risk ratio, odds ratio, or hazard ratio, and their 95% confidence intervals. These effect estimates were then converted to a standardized scale comparing the highest third with the lowest third of the (log-transformed) CRP distribution. Where available, separate prognostic effect estimates were extracted for different degrees of adjustment for other prognostic factors.

17.4   EVALUATING APPLICABILITY AND QUALITY OF PRIMARY STUDIES

Once eligible studies have been identified and data extracted, an important next step is to assess the applicability and risk of bias (quality) of each study for the review. As for earlier steps, ideally this is done by two reviewers, independently, with any discrepancies resolved. **Applicability** refers to the extent to which a study matches the review question in terms of the population, startpoint, prognostic factors, and outcomes (endpoints) of interest. Just because a study is eligible for inclusion does not mean it is free from applicability concerns. A study may be applicable in some aspects (e.g. correct condition at startpoint, with prognostic factors of interest evaluated) but not others (e.g. incorrect population or setting, inappropriate outcome definition, different follow-up time, inappropriate choice of cut points, adjustment for an incomplete set of conventional prognostic factors used in the clinical context of interest for review, etc.).

Risk of bias refers to the extent to which flaws in the study design or analysis methods may lead to bias in estimates of the prognostic factor effects. Unfortunately, based on growing empirical evidence, many primary studies will be at high risk of bias [6, 24, 28–36]. For example, a common concern is the use of data-driven cut points to categorize continuous prognostic factors; this should lead to a high risk of bias, as the "optimal" cut point identified is unlikely to be replicated in new studies and leads to inflated prognostic effect estimates [37]. For prognostic factor studies, Hayden et al. developed the QUIPS checklist for examining risk of bias across six domains [38]: study participation, study attrition, prognostic factor measurement, outcome measurement, adjustment for other prognostic factors, and statistical analysis and reporting. Additional guidance may be found from general tools examining the quality of observational studies [39, 40], and the REMARK guideline for reporting of primary prognostic factor studies [41, 42].

17.4.1   Application to the C-Reactive Protein Review

Hemingway et al. [14] infer the quality of included studies by the quality of their reporting on 17 items derived from the REMARK guidelines [42]. The median number of study quality items reported was 7 out of a possible 17, and standards did not change between 1997 and 2009. Only two studies referred to a study protocol, with none referring to a statistical analysis plan. Hemingway et al. note that this "makes it difficult to know what the specific research objectives were at the start of cohort recruitment, at the time of CRP measurement, or at the onset of the statistical analysis" [14]. Only two studies reported the time elapsed between first lifetime presentation with coronary disease and assessment of CRP, raising applicability concerns. Studies reported 10 different ways of comparing CRP values, including continuous measures (per standard deviation [SD], tertile, quartile, unit [mg/L] on original or log 10 scale), equal-size groups (top versus bottom with group size 50%, 33%, or 25% for 2, 3, and 4 groups, respectively), unequal-size groups (top versus bottom; 2 or 3 groups defined by cut points), as well as measures on both log-transformed and untransformed CRP scales. The rationale for the choice of scale was stated in only a third of studies.

17.5   META-ANALYSIS

Meta-analysis of prognostic factor studies aims to summarize the (possibly adjusted) prognostic effect of each factor of interest. Aside from missing estimates, challenges for the meta-analyst include: (i) having different types of prognostic measures that are not comparable [23]; (ii) estimates without the standard errors that are required for meta-analysis (see Chapter 9); (iii) estimates relating to different timepoints; (iv) different methods of measurement for prognostic factors and outcomes; (v) different sets of adjustment factors; and (vi) different approaches to handling continuous prognostic factors, including the choice of cut point values.

Many of these issues lead to substantial heterogeneity, such that – if meta-analysis is performed – summary results are difficult to interpret. For this reason, it may be sensible not to undertake a meta-analysis, and indeed many authors reach this conclusion [2]. For example, Malats et al. conclude: "After 10 years of research, evidence is not sufficient to conclude whether changes in P53 act as markers of outcome in patients with bladder cancer. . .. That a decade of research on P53 and bladder cancer has not placed us in a better position to draw conclusions relevant to the clinical management of patients is frustrating" [43].

The quality of conduct and reporting of prognosis studies is gradually improving since the introduction of the REMARK and TRIPOD guidelines, and meta-analyses are thus becoming more often a sensible and achievable option [7, 41, 42, 44]. Meta-analyses will be most interpretable, and thus useful, when separate analyses are undertaken for groups of "similar" prognostic effect measures. In particular, we suggest separate meta-analyses for:

- Hazard ratios, odds ratios, and risk ratios.
- Unadjusted and adjusted associations.
- Prognostic factor effects at distinct cut points (or groups of similar cut points).
- Prognostic factor effects corresponding to a linear trend (association).
- Prognostic factor effects corresponding to nonlinear trends.
- Each method of measurement (for factors and outcomes).

Furthermore, ideally a meta-analysis of adjusted results should ensure that all included estimates are adjusted for the same set of other prognostic factors. This is unlikely, and a compromise could be to ensure that all estimates have been adjusted for a pre-defined minimum set of established prognostic factors.

Even when adhering to this guidance, unexplained heterogeneity is likely to remain. Therefore, if meta-analysis is performed, a random-effects approach is generally preferred to allow for unexplained heterogeneity across studies (see Box 17.4 and Chapter 9) [45]. This provides a summary estimate of the average prognostic effect of the factor, and the variability in effect across studies. Also potentially useful are dose–response meta-analysis methods to estimate the trend within studies, with each category compared to the reference category (see Chapter 14). These methods model the estimated prognostic effect in each category as a function of "exposure" level (e.g. midpoint or median prognostic factor value in the category), while accounting for within-study correlation and between-study heterogeneity [46–50]. To apply these methods, some additional knowledge of the factor's underlying distribution is usually needed to help define the "exposure" level, as the chosen value can influence the results (see Chapter 14) [48].

Advanced multivariate meta-analysis methods are available to jointly handle multiple cut points [51], multiple methods of measurement [51], or different adjustment factors in prognostic factor studies [52]. An introduction to multivariate meta-analysis is provided elsewhere [53]. Sometimes, rather than prognostic effect estimates, primary studies might report the change in the concordance index (also known as the

---

Box 17.4   Explanation of a Random-Effects Meta-Analysis of Prognostic Factor Effect Estimates

The true prognostic effect of a factor is likely to vary from study to study, and thus assuming a common (fixed) prognostic effect is not sensible. If Y_i and $\mathrm{var}(Y_i)$ denote the prognostic effect estimate – e.g. ln(hazard ratio), ln(odds ratio), ln(risk ratio), or mean difference – and its variance in study i, then a general random-effects meta-analysis model can be specified as:

$$Y_i \sim N(\mu, \mathrm{var}(Y_i) + \tau^2),$$

Most researchers use either restricted maximum likelihood or the approach of DerSimonian and Laird to estimate this model [57], but other options are available, including a Bayesian approach [58]. Of key interest is the summary (average) estimate, μ, which reveals the average prognostic effect of the factor. The standard deviation of the prognostic effect across studies is denoted by τ, and non-zero values suggest there is between-study heterogeneity. Confidence intervals for μ should ideally account for uncertainty in estimated variances (in particular τ) [59], and we have found the approach of Hartung–Knapp to be robust for this purpose in most settings [60, 61]. When synthesizing prognostic effects on the log scale, the summary results and confidence intervals require back-transformation (using the exponential function) to the original scale.

C statistic, area under the ROC curve) or change in Royston's D statistic when adding a particular factor [54, 55]. Pennells et al. discuss potential ways to synthesize such measures of change in discrimination performance [56].

17.5.1   Application to the C-Reactive Protein Review

Hemingway et al. [14] apply a random-effects meta-analysis to combine 53 adjusted prognostic effect estimates for CRP from studies that adjusted for at least one of six conventional risk factors (age, sex, smoking, diabetes, obesity, and lipids). The summary meta-analysis result was a risk ratio of 1.97 (95% CI: 1.78 to 2.17), which gives the average prognostic effect of CRP (for those in the top versus bottom third of CRP distribution), and suggests larger CRP values are associated with higher risk. Although there was substantial between-study heterogeneity, nearly all estimates were in the same direction (i.e. risk ratio >1). When restricting meta-analysis to just the 13 studies that adjusted for at least all six conventional prognostic factors, the summary risk ratio decreased to 1.65 (95% CI: 1.39 to 1.96) and the between-study heterogeneity was reduced. Using the 13 study-specific estimates provided by Hemingway et al., we repeated this meta-analysis using the Hartung–Knapp approach (Figure 17.2), obtaining the same summary result but a wider confidence interval (1.34 to 2.04) [60].

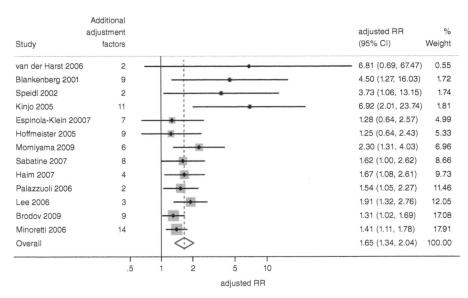

Study	Additional adjustment factors		adjusted RR (95% CI)	% Weight
van der Harst 2006	2		6.81 (0.69, 67.47)	0.55
Blankenberg 2001	9		4.50 (1.27, 16.03)	1.72
Speidl 2002	2		3.73 (1.06, 13.15)	1.74
Kinjo 2005	11		6.92 (2.01, 23.74)	1.81
Espinola-Klein 20007	7		1.28 (0.64, 2.57)	4.99
Hoffmeister 2005	9		1.25 (0.64, 2.43)	5.33
Momiyama 2009	6		2.30 (1.31, 4.03)	6.96
Sabatine 2007	8		1.62 (1.00, 2.62)	8.66
Haim 2007	4		1.67 (1.08, 2.61)	9.73
Palazzuoli 2006	2		1.54 (1.05, 2.27)	11.46
Lee 2006	3		1.91 (1.32, 2.76)	12.05
Brodov 2009	9		1.31 (1.02, 1.69)	17.08
Minoretti 2006	14		1.41 (1.11, 1.78)	17.91
Overall			1.65 (1.34, 2.04)	100.00

adjusted RR

FIGURE 17.2   Forest plot showing the study-specific estimates and meta-analysis summary result of the adjusted prognostic effect (risk ratio, *RR*) of C-reactive protein taken from the review of Hemingway et al. [14]; all 13 studies were adjusted for age, sex, smoking, diabetes, obesity, and lipids, plus up to 14 other variables. Meta-analysis results shown are based on a random-effects mcta-analysis model with DerSimonian and Laird estimation of the between-study variances. The summary result is identical to Hemingway et al. [14], but the confidence interval is wider as, here, we used the Hartung–Knapp approach to account for uncertainty in the estimate of between-study variance. Adapted from Hartung J et al. [60].

17.6   QUANTIFYING AND EXAMINING HETEROGENEITY

When meta-analysis is still performed in the face of heterogeneity, it is important to quantify and report the magnitude of heterogeneity itself, for example via the estimate of τ^2 (the between-study variance) [62], or an approximate prediction interval indicating the potential true prognostic effect of a factor in a new population (see Chapter 10) [45, 63]. Subgroup analyses and meta-regression can be used to examine or explore the causes of heterogeneity. A subgroup analysis performs a separate meta-analysis for categories defined by a particular characteristic, such as those with low risk of bias, those with a follow-up <1 year or ≥1 year, or those set in countries within Europe. A preferable approach is meta-regression (see Chapter 10), which extends the meta-analysis equation shown in Box 17.4 by including study-level covariates [64], and allows a formal comparison of how meta-analysis results differ across groups defined by covariates (e.g. low risk of bias studies versus studies at higher risk of bias). Unfortunately, subgroup analyses and meta-regression are often problematic. There will often be few studies per subgroup and low power to detect genuine causes of heterogeneity. Furthermore, study-level confounding will be rife, such that it is difficult to disentangle the associations for one covariate from another. For example, studies with a low risk of bias may also have a different length of follow-up, or a particular cut point level, compared with studies at higher risk of bias.

17.6.1   Application to the C-Reactive Protein Review

Hemingway et al. report that meta-regression identified four study-level covariates that explained some between-study heterogeneity in the prognostic effect of CRP: definition of comparison group, number of adjustment variables, (log) number of events, and proportion of patients with stable coronary disease [14]. Studies originally reporting unequal CRP groups had stronger effects than those reporting CRP on a continuous scale. For each additional adjustment factor the summary RR decreased by 3%. The summary RR was smaller among studies with more than the median number of outcome events, and smaller among studies confined to stable coronary disease. There was no evidence that the CRP effect differed according to study quality [14].

17.7   EXAMINING SMALL-STUDY EFFECTS

The term "small-study effects" refers to a systematic difference in prognostic effect estimates between small and large studies [65]. A particular concern is when small studies show larger prognostic effects than larger studies. This may be due to chance, but a major threat is publication bias and selective reporting (see Chapter 5), which are endemic in prognosis research [26, 62]. Smaller studies with statistically significant prognostic factor effects are more likely to be published (or reported in sufficient detail), and thus included in meta-analysis, than similar studies with nonsignificant results. As previously described, the implementation of variable selection procedures into the analysis (either for the prognostic factor of interest or the inclusion of adjustment factors) could be a cause of small-study effects. For example, it will typically lead to the smaller studies including fewer adjustment factors, and thus estimating larger effect estimates for the factors of interest. A related concern is that smaller prognostic factor studies are generally at higher risk of bias than larger studies, as they tend to be more exploratory in nature (e.g. investigating hundreds of potential factors and using arbitrary cut points for continuous factors) and based on a convenient sample, rather than a protocol-driven, prospective study [2].

The evidence for small-study effects is usually examined in a funnel plot, which shows the study estimates (x-axis) against their precision (y-axis). This is recommended if there are 10 or more studies [65]. The plot should show a symmetric shape, with results from larger studies at the top of the inverted funnel, and smaller studies spanning out in both directions equally. Asymmetry will arise if there are small-study effects, with a greater proportion of smaller studies in one particular direction. Statistical tests for asymmetry in risk, odds, and hazard ratios can be used, such as Peters' and Debray's tests (see Chapter 5) [66, 67]. Contour-enhanced funnel plots show the statistical significance of individual studies: "missing" studies will fall within regions of nonsignificance if publication bias was the cause of small-study effects.

Although publication bias is a threat for unadjusted results, it is arguably a larger concern for adjusted results; the adjusted prognostic effect of a factor is more likely to be reported if it is statistically significant. If some studies do report both adjusted and unadjusted (or partially adjusted) results of a particular factor, multivariate meta-analysis can be used to "borrow strength" from their correlation, to allow studies

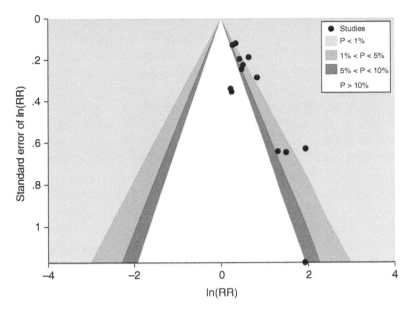

FIGURE 17.3   Evidence of funnel plot asymmetry (small-study effects) in the C-reactive protein meta-analysis shown in Figure 17.2. The smaller studies (those with higher standard errors) have adjusted RR estimates mainly to the right of the larger studies, and thus give the largest adjusted prognostic effect estimates. A concern is that this is due to publication bias, with "missing" studies potentially falling in the white area denoting nonsignificant RR estimates.

providing only unadjusted (or partially) adjusted results to contribute (via the correlation) toward the meta-analysis result for the fully adjusted effect [53]. This may reduce the impact of small-study effects. Note that the presence of small-study effects does not prove that publication bias exists. In particular, when there is between-study heterogeneity, the true prognostic effect of factor effects may genuinely differ between smaller and larger studies.

17.7.1   Application to the C-Reactive Protein Review

Figure 17.3 shows a funnel plot of the study estimates within the CRP meta-analysis shown in Figure 17.2. There is clear asymmetry, raising a concern of publication bias. When removing the four smallest studies (i.e. those with the largest standard errors), the summary meta-analysis result moves closer to 1 (summary RR = 1.51, 95% CI: 1.30 to 1.74), between-study heterogeneity becomes zero, and there is no longer any clear evidence of funnel plot asymmetry.

17.8   REPORTING AND INTERPRETATION OF RESULTS

As with all research studies, clear and complete reporting is essential for reviews of prognostic factor studies. Most of the reporting guidelines of PRISMA and MOOSE will be relevant [68, 69], but should be complemented by REMARK, which was aimed at primary prognostic factor studies.

Interpretation and translation of summary meta-analysis results form an important final step. The guidance in the previous steps is the essential input for this. Reviewers should discuss whether and how the prognostic factors identified may be useful in practice (i.e. translation of results to clinical practice), and what further research is necessary.

Further, for interpreting the *certainty* of the results of a review of randomized studies, Grades of Recommendation, Assessment, Development, and Evaluation (GRADE) was developed (see Chapter 22). This approach assesses the certainty of evidence for obtained summary results by addressing five domains using the information obtained by the tools and methods addressed in the above steps: risk of bias, inconsistency, imprecision, indirectness, and publication bias. Guidance is emerging for adapting GRADE to prognosis reviews [70, 71], including suggestions for rating the certainty of evidence for unadjusted prognostic factor effects in scenarios where clinicians use a single prognostic factor to inform their prognostication and subsequent shared decision-making [72]. As mentioned, such scenarios are uncommon, as most are informed by multiple prognostic factors.

17.8.1   Application to the C-Reactive Protein Review

In their discussion, Hemingway et al. downgrade the meta-analysis findings, due to a strong concern about the quality and reliability of the underlying evidence [14]. The absence of pre-specified protocols, poor and potentially biased reporting, and strong potential for publication bias prevented them from making firm conclusions about whether CRP adds prognostic value over and above existing prognostic factors. They state that the concerns "explicitly challenge the statement for healthcare professionals made by the Centers for Disease Control that measuring CRP is both 'useful' and 'independent' as a marker of prognosis" [73].

17.9   META-ANALYSIS USING INDIVIDUAL PARTICIPANT DATA

To address some of the methodological difficulties when using aggregate data from study publications, an alternative is to conduct a meta-analysis of individual participant data (IPD) (see Chapter 12) [11, 74–76]. In this approach, the raw individual-level data of each study are combined to estimate and summarize the (adjusted) factor–outcome associations of interest. Availability of IPD offers many advantages, such as having better-defined inclusion criteria, checking modeling assumptions, analyzing variables on their continuous scale with the possibility of assessing nonlinear relationships, and obtaining results adjusted (consistently) for other variables [74].

As described by Abo-Zaid et al. [77], IPD meta-analyses of prognosis studies are becoming increasingly common in the medical literature. The work of Trivella et al. [78] is notable in this context. They performed an IPD meta-analysis of 13 studies in non-small cell lung cancer, to examine the prognostic value of microvessel density. By obtaining IPD from published and unpublished studies, with consistent adjustment factors in each study, the authors show that microvessel density is not an additional prognostic factor for death, a conclusion different from that of previous single studies and meta-analyses based on published aggregate data with adjustment for fewer factors, which were also likely biased by the use of optimal cut points.

Researchers taking the IPD approach face many challenges [77], such as greater costs and time required to obtain and clean IPD, unavailable IPD for some studies, different sets of available prognostic (adjustment) factors in each study, and variability in study methods of measurement. For example, for the Trivella et al. review, "checking, validation and standardization of all datasets took nearly two years" and "for all but three centres some data corrections were necessary," making it altogether "a long, expensive, and rather laborious process" [79]. Furthermore, obtaining IPD does not necessarily make the quality of the original studies any better: there still needs to be improvement in primary studies and harmonization across new research in terms of design, methods, and data collection. Ideally, a prospective approach to IPD meta-analysis of prognostic factor studies is required [80]. More detailed discussion about IPD meta-analysis projects for prognosis and prediction research is provided by Riley et al. [8, 74]

17.10 CONCLUSIONS

We have described the key steps and methods for conducting a systematic review and meta-analysis of prognostic factor studies, building on our earlier work [12]. Current reviews are often limited by the quality and heterogeneity of primary studies, which in itself is an important finding [81]. We expect the number of prognostic factor reviews to grow rapidly in the coming years, especially with Cochrane (via the Cochrane Prognosis Methods Group: http://www.methods.cochrane.org/prognosis) currently embarking upon them (see Chapter 21). Lastly, we recommend that protocols for prognostic factor reviews are published, ideally at the same time as the review is registered, for example within PROSPERO (http://www.crd.york.ac.uk/PROSPERO) or the Cochrane database.

REFERENCES

1. Hemingway, H., Croft, P., Perel, P. et al. (2013). Prognosis research strategy (PROGRESS) 1: a framework for researching clinical outcomes. *BMJ* 346: e5595.
2. Riley, R.D., Hayden, J.A., Steyerberg, E.W. et al. (2013). Prognosis research strategy (PROGRESS) 2: prognostic factor research. *PLoS Med.* 10 (2): e1001380.
3. Steyerberg, E.W., Moons, K.G., van der Windt, D.A. et al. (2013). Prognosis research strategy (PROGRESS) 3: prognostic model research. *PLoS Med.* 10 (2): e1001381.
4. Hingorani, A.D., Windt, D.A., Riley, R.D. et al. (2013). Prognosis research strategy (PROGRESS) 4: stratified medicine research. *BMJ* 346: e5793.
5. Schumacher, M., Bastert, G., Bojar, H. et al. (1994). Randomized 2×2 trial evaluating hormonal treatment and the duration of chemotherapy in node-positive breast cancer patients. German breast cancer study group. *J. Clin. Oncol.* 12 (10): 2086–2093.

6. Bouwmeester, W., Zuithoff, N.P., Mallett, S. et al. (2012). Reporting and methods in clinical prediction research: a systematic review. *PLoS Med.* 9 (5): 1–12.

7. Moons, K.G., Altman, D.G., Reitsma, J.B. et al. (2015). Transparent reporting of a multivariable prediction model for individual prognosis or diagnosis (TRIPOD): explanation and elaboration. *Ann. Intern. Med.* 162 (1): W1–W73.

8. Riley, R.D., van der Windt, D., Croft, P. et al. (eds.) (2019). *Prognosis Research in Healthcare: Concepts, Methods and Impact.* Oxford: Oxford University Press.

9. Altman, D.G. (2001). Systematic reviews of evaluations of prognostic variables. *BMJ* 323 (7306): 224–228.

10. Altman, D.G. and Riley, R.D. (2005). An evidence-based approach to prognostic markers. *Nat. Clin. Pract. Oncol.* 2: 466–472.

11. Riley, R.D., Sauerbrei, W., and Altman, D.G. (2009). Prognostic markers in cancer: the evolution of evidence from single studies to meta-analysis, and beyond. *Br. J. Cancer* 100 (8): 1219–1229.

12. Riley, R.D., Moons, K.G.M., Snell, K.I.E. et al. (2019). A guide to systematic review and meta-analysis of prognostic factor studies. *BMJ* 364: k4597.

13. Riley, R.D., Burchill, S.A., Abrams, K.R. et al. (2003). A systematic review and evaluation of the use of tumour markers in paediatric oncology: Ewing's sarcoma and neuroblastoma. *Health Technol. Assess.* 7 (5): 1–162.

14. Hemingway, H., Philipson, P., Chen, R. et al. (2010). Evaluating the quality of research into a single prognostic biomarker: a systematic review and meta-analysis of 83 studies of C-reactive protein in stable coronary artery disease. *PLoS Med.* 7 (6): e1000286.

15. Moons, K.G., de Groot, J.A., Bouwmeester, W. et al. (2014). Critical appraisal and data extraction for systematic reviews of prediction modelling studies: the CHARMS checklist. *PLoS Med.* 11 (10): e1001744.

16. Debray, T.P., Damen, J.A., Snell, K.I. et al. (2017). A guide to systematic review and meta-analysis of prediction model performance. *BMJ* 356: i6460.

17. Ingui, B.J. and Rogers, M.A. (2001). Searching for clinical prediction rules in MEDLINE. *J. Am. Med. Inform. Assoc.* 8 (4): 391–397.

18. Geersing, G.J., Bouwmeester, W., Zuithoff, P. et al. (2012). Search filters for finding prognostic and diagnostic prediction studies in Medline to enhance systematic reviews. *PLoS One* 7 (2): e32844.

19. Haynes, R.B., McKibbon, K.A., Wilczynski, N.L. et al. (2005). Optimal search strategies for retrieving scientifically strong studies of treatment from Medline: analytical survey. *BMJ* 330 (7501): 1179.

20. Wong, S.S., Wilczynski, N.L., Haynes, R.B. et al. (2003). Developing optimal search strategies for detecting sound clinical prediction studies in MEDLINE. *AMIA Annu. Symp. Proc.*: 728–732.

21. Parmar, M.K., Torri, V., and Stewart, L. (1998). Extracting summary statistics to perform meta-analyses of the published literature for survival endpoints. *Stat. Med.* 17 (24): 2815–2834.

22. Tierney, J.F., Stewart, L.A., Ghersi, D. et al. (2007). Practical methods for incorporating summary time-to-event data into meta-analysis. *Trials* 8: 16.

23. Perneger, T.V. (2008). Estimating the relative hazard by the ratio of logarithms of event-free proportions. *Contemp. Clin. Trials* 29: 762–766.

24. Riley, R.D., Abrams, K.R., Sutton, A.J. et al. (2003). Reporting of prognostic markers: current problems and development of guidelines for evidence-based practice in the future. *Br. J. Cancer* 88 (8): 1191–1198.

25. Borenstein, M., Hedges, L.V., Higgins, J.P.T. et al. (2009). Converting among effect sizes. In: *Introduction to Meta-Analysis* (eds. M. Borenstein, L.V. Hedges, H. JPT, et al.). Chichester: Wiley.

26. Sadashima, E., Hattori, S., and Takahashi, K. (2016). Meta-analysis of prognostic studies for a biomarker with a study-specific cutoff value. *Res. Synth. Methods* 7 (4): 402–419.

27. Nieminen, P., Lehtiniemi, H., Vähäkangas, K. et al. (2013). Standardised regression coefficient as an effect size index in summarising the reported findings between quantitative exposure and response variables in epidemiological studies. *Epidemiol. Biostat. Public Health* 10: e8854.

28. Kyzas, P.A., Denaxa-Kyza, D., and Ioannidis, J.P. (2007). Almost all articles on cancer prognostic markers report statistically significant results. *Eur. J. Cancer* 43 (17): 2559–2579.

29. Kyzas, P.A., Denaxa-Kyza, D., and Ioannidis, J.P. (2007). Quality of reporting of cancer prognostic marker studies: association with reported prognostic effect. *J. Natl. Cancer Inst.* 99 (3): 236–243.

30. Kyzas, P.A., Loizou, K.T., and Ioannidis, J.P. (2005). Selective reporting biases in cancer prognostic factor studies. *J. Natl. Cancer Inst.* 97 (14): 1043–1055.

31. Mallett, S., Royston, P., Dutton, S. et al. (2010). Reporting methods in studies developing prognostic models in cancer: a review. *BMC Med.* 8: 20.

32. Collins, G.S., Mallett, S., Omar, O. et al. (2011). Developing risk prediction models for type 2 diabetes: a systematic review of methodology and reporting. *BMC Med.* 9: 103.

33. Collins, G.S., Omar, O., Shanyinde, M. et al. (2013). A systematic review finds prediction models for chronic kidney disease were poorly reported and often developed using inappropriate methods. *J. Clin. Epidemiol.* 66 (3): 268–277.

34. Burton, A. and Altman, D.G. (2004). Missing covariate data within cancer prognostic studies: a review of current reporting and proposed guidelines. *Br. J. Cancer* 91 (1): 4–8.

35. Collins, G.S., de Groot, J.A., Dutton, S. et al. (2014). External validation of multivariable prediction models: a systematic review of methodological conduct and reporting. *BMC Med. Res. Methodol.* 14: 40.

36. Mallett, S., Royston, P., Waters, R. et al. (2010). Reporting performance of prognostic models in cancer: a review. *BMC Med.* 8: 21.

37. Altman, D.G., Lausen, B., Sauerbrei, W. et al. (1994). Dangers of using "optimal" cut-points in the evaluation of prognostic factors. *J. Natl. Cancer Inst.* 86 (11): 829–835.

38. Hayden, J.A., van der Windt, D.A., Cartwright, J.L. et al. (2013). Assessing bias in studies of prognostic factors. *Ann. Intern. Med.* 158 (4): 280–286.

39. Sterne, J.A., Hernan, M.A., Reeves, B.C. et al. (2016). ROBINS-I: a tool for assessing risk of bias in non-randomised studies of interventions. *BMJ* 355: i4919.

40. Wells, G.A., Shea, B., O'Connell, D. et al. (2009). The Newcastle-Ottawa Scale (NOS) for assessing the quality of nonrandomized studies in meta-analyses. http://www.ohri.ca/programs/clinical_epidemiology/oxford.htm (accessed February 21, 2022).

41. Altman, D.G., McShane, L.M., Sauerbrei, W. et al. (2012). Reporting recommendations for tumor marker prognostic studies (REMARK): explanation and elaboration. *PLoS Med.* 9 (5): e1001216.

42. McShane, L.M., Altman, D.G., Sauerbrei, W. et al. (2005). REporting recommendations for tumour MARKer prognostic studies (REMARK). *Br. J. Cancer* 93 (4): 387–391.

43. Malats, N., Bustos, A., Nascimento, C.M. et al. (2005). P53 as a prognostic marker for bladder cancer: a meta-analysis and review. *Lancet Oncol.* 6 (9): 678–686.

44. Collins, G.S., Reitsma, J.B., Altman, D.G. et al. (2015). Transparent reporting of a multivariable prediction model for individual prognosis or diagnosis (TRIPOD): the TRIPOD statement. *Ann. Intern. Med.* 162: 55–63.

45. Riley, R.D., Higgins, J.P.T., and Deeks, J.J. (2011). Interpretation of random effects meta-analyses. *BMJ* 342: d549.

46. Berlin, J.A., Longnecker, M.P., and Greenland, S. (1993). Meta-analysis of epidemiologic dose-response data. *Epidemiology* 4 (3): 218–228.

47. Greenland, S. and Longnecker, M.P. (1992). Methods for trend estimation from summarized dose-response data, with applications to meta-analysis. *Am. J. Epidemiol.* 135 (11): 1301–1309.

48. Hartemink, N., Boshuizen, H.C., Nagelkerke, N.J. et al. (2006). Combining risk estimates from observational studies with different exposure cutpoints: a meta-analysis on body mass index and diabetes type 2. *Am. J. Epidemiol.* 163 (11): 1042–1052.

49. Shi, J.Q. and Copas, J.B. (2004). Meta-analysis for trend estimation. *Stat. Med.* 23 (1): 3–19. discussion 159–162.

50. Orsini, N., Li, R., Wolk, A. et al. (2012). Meta-analysis for linear and nonlinear dose-response relations: examples, an evaluation of approximations, and software. *Am. J. Epidemiol.* 175 (1): 66–73.

51. Riley, R.D., Elia, E.G., Malin, G. et al. (2015). Multivariate meta-analysis of prognostic factor studies with multiple cut-points and/or methods of measurement. *Stat. Med.* 34 (17): 2481–2496.

52. Fibrinogen Studies Collaboration (2009). Systematically missing confounders in individual participant data meta-analysis of observational cohort studies. *Stat. Med.* 28 (8): 1218–1237.

53. Riley, R.D., Jackson, D., Salanti, G. et al. (2017). Multivariate and network meta-analysis of multiple outcomes and multiple treatments: rationale, concepts, and examples. *BMJ* 358: j3932.

54. Royston, P. (2006). Explained variation for survival models. *Stata J.* 6: 83–96.

55. Royston, P. and Sauerbrei, W. (2004). A new measure of prognostic separation in survival data. *Stat. Med.* 23 (5): 723–748.

56. Pennells, L., Kaptoge, S., White, I.R. et al. (2014). Assessing risk prediction models using individual participant data from multiple studies. *Am. J. Epidemiol.* 179 (5): 621–632.

57. DerSimonian, R. and Laird, N. (1986). Meta-analysis in clinical trials. *Control. Clin. Trials* 7: 177–188.

58. Langan, D., Higgins, J.P.T., and Simmonds, M. (2015). An empirical comparison of heterogeneity variance estimators in 12 894 meta-analyses. *Res. Synth. Methods* 6 (2): 195–205.

59. Cornell, J.E., Mulrow, C.D., Localio, R. et al. (2014). Random-effects meta-analysis of inconsistent effects: a time for change. *Ann. Intern. Med.* 160 (4): 267–270.

60. Hartung, J. and Knapp, G. (2001). A refined method for the meta-analysis of controlled clinical trials with binary outcome. *Stat. Med.* 20 (24): 3875–3889.

61. Partlett, C. and Riley, R.D. (2017). Random effects meta-analysis: coverage performance of 95% confidence and prediction intervals following REML estimation. *Stat. Med.* 36 (2): 301–317.

62. Rucker, G., Schwarzer, G., Carpenter, J.R. et al. (2008). Undue reliance on I(2) in assessing heterogeneity may mislead. *BMC Med. Res. Methodol.* 8: 79.

63. Higgins, J.P.T., Thompson, S.G., and Spiegelhalter, D.J. (2009). A re-evaluation of random-effects meta-analysis. *J. R. Stat. Soc. Ser. A* 172: 137–159.

64. Berkey, C.S., Hoaglin, D.C., Mosteller, F. et al. (1995). A random-effects regression model for meta-analysis. *Stat. Med.* 14 (4): 395–411.

65. Sterne, J.A.C., Sutton, A.J., Ioannidis, J.P.A. et al. (2011). Recommendations for examining and interpreting funnel plot asymmetry in meta-analyses of randomised controlled trials. *BMJ* 342: d4002.

66. Debray, T.P.A., Moons, K.G.M., and Riley, R.D. (2018). Detecting small-study effects and funnel plot asymmetry in meta-analysis of survival data: a comparison of new and existing tests. *Res. Synth. Methods* 9 (1): 41–50.

67. Peters, J.L., Sutton, A.J., Jones, D.R. et al. (2006). Comparison of two methods to detect publication bias in meta-analysis. *J. Am. Med. Assoc.* 295 (6): 676–680.

68. Moher, D., Liberati, A., Tetzlaff, J. et al. (2009). Preferred reporting items for systematic reviews and meta-analyses: the PRISMA statement. *BMJ* 339: b2535.

69. Stroup, D.F., Berlin, J.A., Morton, S.C. et al. (2000). Meta-analysis of observational studies in epidemiology: a proposal for reporting. Meta-analysis of Observational Studies in Epidemiology (MOOSE) group. *J. Am. Med. Assoc.* 283 (15): 2008–2012.

70. Huguet, A., Hayden, J.A., Stinson, J. et al. (2013). Judging the quality of evidence in reviews of prognostic factor research: adapting the GRADE framework. *Syst. Rev.* 2: 71.

71. Iorio, A., Spencer, F.A., Falavigna, M. et al. (2015). Use of GRADE for assessment of evidence about prognosis: rating confidence in estimates of event rates in broad categories of patients. *BMJ.* 350: h870.

72. Foroutan, F., Guyatt, G., Zuk, V. et al. (2020). GRADE guidelines 28: use of GRADE for the assessment of evidence about prognostic factors: rating certainty in identification of groups of patients with different absolute risks. *J. Clin. Epidemiol.* 121: 62–70.

73. Pearson, T.A., Mensah, G.A., Alexander, R.W. et al. (2003). Markers of inflammation and cardiovascular disease: application to clinical and public health practice: a statement for healthcare professionals from the Centers for Disease Control and Prevention and the American Heart Association. *Circulation* 107 (3): 499–511.

74. Riley, R.D., Tierney, J.F., and Stewart, L.A. (eds.) (2021). *Individual Participant Data Meta-Analysis: A Handbook for Healthcare Research*. Chichester: Wiley.

75. Riley, R.D., Lambert, P.C., and Abo-Zaid, G. (2010). Meta-analysis of individual participant data: rationale, conduct, and reporting. *BMJ* 340: c221.

76. Debray, T.P.A., Riley, R.D., Rovers, M.M. et al. (2015). Individual participant data (IPD) meta-analyses of diagnostic and prognostic modeling studies: guidance on their use. *PLoS Med.* 12 (10): e1001886.

77. Abo-Zaid, G., Sauerbrei, W., and Riley, R.D. (2012). Individual participant data meta-analysis of prognostic factor studies: state of the art? *BMC Med. Res. Methodol.* 12: 56.

78. Trivella, M., Pezzella, F., Pastorino, U. et al. (2007). Microvessel density as a prognostic factor in non-small-cell lung carcinoma: a meta-analysis of individual patient data. *Lancet Oncol.* 8 (6): 488–499.

79. Altman, D.G., Trivella, M., Pezzella, F. et al. (2006). Systematic review of multiple studies of prognosis: the feasibility of obtaining individual patient data. In: *Advances in Statistical Methods for the Health Sciences* (eds. J.-L. Auget, N. Balakrishnan, M. Mesbah, et al.), 3–18. Boston, MA: Birkhäuser.

80. Blettner, M., Sauerbrei, W., Schlehofer, B. et al. (1999). Traditional reviews, meta-analyses and pooled analyses in epidemiology. *Int. J. Epidemiol.* 28 (1): 1–9.

81. Sauerbrei, W., Holländer, N., Riley, R.D. et al. (2006). Evidence-based assessment and application of prognostic markers: the long way from single studies to meta-analysis. *Commun. Stat.* 35: 1333–1342.

CHAPTER 18

Systematic Reviews of Prediction Models

Gary S. Collins, Karel G.M. Moons, Thomas P.A. Debray, Douglas G. Altman, and Richard D. Riley

Prediction model studies have proliferated across the medical literature, and policy-makers are increasingly recommending their use in clinical practice guidelines [1]. The clinical value of prediction models is closely linked to that discussed for prognostic factors in the previous chapter, but with the focus now more on absolute, rather than relative, risk estimates. Prediction models combine an individual's observed values of multiple predictors to estimate that individual's probability, which can be a diagnostic or a prognostic probability, depending on whether the model makes predictions for present or future outcomes.

Diagnostic prediction models combine values of multiple predictors (often called index tests or diagnostic determinants) to calculate the probability that an individual with particular symptoms or signs suspected of having a certain target disorder indeed has that condition or disease at this moment. For example, diagnostic models have been developed to determine the risk of a deep vein thrombosis in patients with a swollen, red, or painful leg [2], or to detect the presence of an ankle fracture in emergency patients with recent ankle trauma [3]. Diagnostic prediction models are often used to decide whether additional, usually more invasive or costly, tests are needed.

Prognostic prediction models combine values of multiple predictors (often called prognostic factors) to calculate the probability that an individual will develop a particular outcome in the future. Prognostic models are commonly used to predict the future course of an individual's diagnosed condition, such as predicting the risk of developing hearing deficits in children diagnosed with bacterial meningitis [4]. They can also predict the outcome for an individual undergoing an intervention (e.g. predicting mortality after cardiac surgery [5]), the development of a certain health outcome for apparently healthy

Systematic Reviews in Health Research: Meta-Analysis in Context, Third Edition. Edited by Matthias Egger, Julian P.T. Higgins, and George Davey Smith.
© 2022 John Wiley & Sons Ltd. Published 2022 by John Wiley & Sons Ltd.
Companion website: www.systematic-reviews3.org

individuals in the general population (e.g. predicting the 10-year risk of developing cardiovascular disease [6]), and the response of patients treated with a certain drug (e.g. predicting treatment response in breast cancer patients treated with tamoxifen [7]).

Primary studies of prediction models can be broadly categorized as model development, model validation, or a combination of the two [8–13], as explained in Box 18.1. Clearly, each prediction model can be developed only once, but validated more than once. Prediction models are being developed in increasing numbers, with many models developed to predict the same (or very similar) outcomes for the same target population. For example,

---

Box 18.1 Types of Prediction Model Studies

- **Prediction model development studies without external validation** aim to develop a prognostic or diagnostic prediction model using a dataset at hand, called the development set. Such studies commonly aim to identify important predictors for the outcome under study, assign mutually adjusted weights per predictor in a multivariable analysis, develop a final prediction model, and quantify the predictive performance (e.g. discrimination, calibration, and classification) of that model in the development set. As model overfitting can occur, particularly in small datasets, development studies ideally include **internal validation** using a data resampling technique such as bootstrapping, jack-knife, or cross-validation to quantify any optimism in the predictive performance of the developed model.

- **Prediction model development studies with external validation in independent data** have the same aim as the previous type. However, once the model has been developed, its predictive performance is quantified using participant data external to the development dataset. Validation can be done using participant data collected by the same investigators, commonly using the same predictor and outcome definitions and measurements, but from a later time period (**temporal** or **narrow validation**), or using data collected by other investigators in another hospital or country (**geographic** or **broad validation**).

- **External model validation studies with or without model updating** aim to assess and compare the predictive performance of an existing prediction model using participant data that were not used to develop the prediction model, and possibly to adjust or update the model using the results if the model performs poorly.

Prediction model studies that aim to quantify the impact of using a prediction model (on clinical decision-making, patient outcomes, or cost-effectiveness of care, for example) relative to not using the model can also be included in a systematic review of prognostic and diagnostic prediction models. However, these types of prediction model studies use very different data extraction and critical appraisal techniques, as they have different aims, designs, and reporting issues to studies that develop or validate prediction models. In this chapter we focus on reviews of studies that aim to develop, validate, or update a prediction model.

Source: Adapted from Moons et al. [21].

there are over 360 models for predicting the risk of cardiovascular events in the general population [14], over 100 models for diagnosing COVID-19 [15], predicting outcomes after brain trauma [16], predicting the course of patients with prostate cancer [17], and more than 40 models for predicting prevalent and incident type 2 diabetes [18]. For many models, validation studies are rare, while for a few models, multiple validations have examined their performance in different countries, populations, and settings [19, 20].

Alongside the accumulating profusion of development and validation studies of prediction models, clinical guidelines now increasingly recommend the use of these models. Clinical guidelines should be based on a thorough synthesis of all available evidence. We therefore need systematic reviews of prediction model studies, to identify, appraise, and synthesize the relevant evidence. Cochrane has recognized the need for good-quality evidence synthesis in the area of prognostic modeling. In 2008 it launched the Prognosis Methods Group to produce guidance on systematic reviews of prognosis studies [19, 20], and initiated exemplar reviews with a long-term view to including them within the Cochrane Library.

In this chapter, we examine the types of systematic reviews that can be conducted on prediction model studies and discuss the challenges faced in identifying, appraising, and qualitatively and quantitatively synthesizing these studies. We follow these steps, aligned with the processes described in Chapter 2 of this book:

1. Definition of a well-formulated review question.
2. Extensive search for studies.
3. Data extraction, critical appraisal, and risk of bias assessment.
4. Qualitative or quantitative synthesis of data (meta-analysis).
5. Interpretation and reporting.

18.1   FRAMING THE REVIEW QUESTION

Box 18.2 summarizes various systematic review questions and thus types of reviews of prediction models. The choice of review question type depends on the evidence available on the primary prediction model studies in the clinical context of interest. A well-defined review question delineates the types of prediction model studies (e.g. development or validation studies, see Box 18.1) to be retrieved and helps to focus the search (see also Chapter 3).

Many clinical areas have large numbers of prediction models, often for the same target population or outcome. A review can, for example, aim to summarize all existing models developed to predict a particular outcome in a particular target population (e.g. all models to predict five-year survival after diagnosis of breast cancer), or to simply review all existing models (regardless of the outcome or specific target population) in a clinical domain (e.g. in obstetrics). In both situations, we would proceed to retrieve all the model development studies and any corresponding validation studies.

Many prediction model studies evaluate (validate) the performance of a specific prediction model in another population or setting than that in which it was developed. Examples include the external validation of the EuroSCORE model [20], the ABCD2 model [31], the Framingham risk model [32], and the Wells model for diagnosing

Box 18.2   Examples of Types of Systematic Reviews of Prediction Model Studies

1. **Reviews of all models in a particular clinical field or target population**
   - Prediction models in the traumatic brain injury setting [16].
   - Prediction models in obstetrics [22].

2. **Reviews of all models for specific outcomes in a specific target population**
   - Models for predicting the risk of kidney failure, cardiovascular events, and death in patients with chronic kidney disease [23].
   - Models to predict the risk of developing asthma in preschool children with asthma-like symptoms [24].

3. **Reviews of the performance of one or more specific prediction models (external validation studies)**
   - Performance of the EuroSCORE II model for predicting the risk of all-cause mortality following cardiac surgery [25].
   - Performance of the ABCD2 model for predicting the 7- and 90-day risk of stroke in individuals after transient ischemic stroke [26].

4. **Reviews of methods and reporting of prediction models**
   - Quality of reporting and methods used to validate prediction models [27].
   - Quality of reporting of diagnostic and prognostic prediction models published in high-impact general medical journals [28].

5. **Reviews of the added value of a specific predictor to a specific model**
   - Value of adding C-reactive protein to the Framingham Risk Score [29].
   - Value of adding circulating and genetic markers to type 2 diabetes risk prediction models [30].

pulmonary embolism [33]. A review can therefore aim to quantitatively summarize (meta-analyze) the performance, or the heterogeneity in performance, of this single specific prediction model across all tested populations or settings. We would then need to review all validation studies of that specific model, and its original development study. Finally, a review may examine the methods and reporting of prediction models, or the added value of one or more predictors to an existing model (Box 18.2).

The CHARMS (CHecklist for critical Appraisal and data extraction for systematic Reviews of prediction Modelling Studies) guidance was developed to help reviewers define a clear review question or aim, and provides a checklist for extracting data and to assist critical appraisal of the included studies [21]. CHARMS includes a modification (called PICOTS) of the traditional PICO system (Population, Intervention, Comparison, and Outcome) used in systematic reviews of therapeutic intervention studies, by replacing "Intervention" with "Index models" and additionally considering Timing (the timepoint and time period of the prediction) and Setting. Table 18.1

TABLE 18.1 The PICOTS system, as presented in the CHARMS guidance and checklist [21], describes key items for framing the review aim, search strategy, and study inclusion and exclusion criteria.

Item	Comment and examples
Population	Define the target population in which the prediction models under review will be used. Examples: • Women with diagnosed breast cancer (prognostic model review) • Women with palpable node breast, suspected of breast cancer (diagnostic model review) • Healthy adult men in the general population (prognostic model review)
Index models	Define the prediction models under review. Examples: • All models in women with diagnosed breast cancer • A certain prognostic model (e.g. the Framingham risk model) to predict the 10-year risk of a cardiovascular event in adult men in the general population
Comparator	If applicable, one may aim to compare the predictive ability of two or more models for the target population under review. Example: • Comparison of the predictive ability of the Framingham risk model (index model) with that of the SCORE or QRISK model (comparator) to predict the 10-year risk of a cardiovascular event in adult men in the general population
Outcome	Define the outcome of interest to be predicted by the models under review. Examples: • Specific future event (prognostic models), such as fatal or nonfatal coronary heart disease • Specific target disease presence (diagnostic models), such as presence of breast cancer
Timing	Define at what moment or timepoint the prediction models under review are to be used in the targeted population, and over what time period the outcomes are predicted (the latter in case of prognostic models). Examples: • Preoperative prediction of postoperative nausea and vomiting occurring within 48 hours after surgery • Prediction in the first trimester of pregnancy of the risk of developing pre-eclampsia in the third trimester • Prediction of the presence of deep venous thrombosis after patient history, physical examination, and D-dimer testing
Setting	Define the intended role or setting of the prediction models under review. Examples: • Diagnostic models to diagnose deep venous thrombosis in primary setting in order to decide on hospital referral • Prognostic models to predict the 10-year risk of cardiovascular disease to be used in secondary care to determine whether to administer lifestyle advice only, or combined with medical therapy

describes these six key issues to help frame the prediction model review question. A focused review question enables researchers to define the inclusion and exclusion criteria – and thus the applicability – of the primary studies included in the review and to develop a tailored search strategy. Applicability refers to the extent to which the primary study matches the review question and thus is applicable for the intended use of the reviewed prediction models in the target population.

The reviewer needs to define the target population and thus scope of the review, which directly indicates whether the aim is to review prognostic or diagnostic models and which index and comparator model or models are reviewed (Table 18.1, items "P," "I," and "C"). The latter immediately indicates which types of prediction model studies given in Box 18.1, development, validation, or both, are needed. For example, if we aim to assess the predictive performance of a specific prediction model compared to another prediction model developed for the same target population, we need to review only the external validation studies of these two models, and also the two corresponding development studies (see type 3, Box 18.2). Defining the outcomes to be predicted and their timing (Table 18.1, items "O" and "T") indicates the potential usefulness and applicability of the models and thus the review results. Models most relevant for patients predict patient-relevant outcomes such as death, pain, disease recurrence, or enhanced quality of life, rather than process outcomes (e.g. drug dose reduction) or intermediate pathophysiological outcomes (e.g. tumor response). Long-term outcomes are often more relevant for patients. We also need to clarify when the model will be used (e.g. at diagnosis, during general practitioner consultation), to help define which models are relevant for the review (Table 18.1, item "S"). Models that incorporate predictors collected after this predefined timepoint should not be included. For example, if we aim to review prognostic models to preoperatively predict the risk of developing postoperative pain within 48 hours after hip surgery, studies including intraoperative characteristics are not useful [21]. Defining the setting of the prediction models under review is important, as the predictive ability of models often changes across settings (Table 18.1, item "S").

Systematic reviews of prediction model studies, like all systematic reviews, need a study protocol (Chapter 2). Protocols allow external parties to judge the review results according to how the review was planned [34]. Protocols of systematic reviews can be registered in registries such as the international Prospective Register of Systematic Reviews (PROSPERO; www.crd.york.ac.uk/prospero) [35].

18.2   IDENTIFYING RELEVANT PUBLICATIONS

It is challenging to identify prediction model studies via a literature search, as many different terms are used interchangeably to describe prediction models, such as prognostic models, prediction models, risk scores, prediction rules, and algorithms. Furthermore, many prediction model studies have uninformative titles, and abstracts often fail to indicate that the study involves the development or validation of a prediction model. Despite these difficulties, search strategies for identifying diagnostic and prognostic prediction model studies have been developed [36–38], validated, and refined [39]. Box 18.3 describes the recommended search filters for finding prediction model studies.

Box 18.3   Effective MEDLINE Search Strategies for Identifying Clinical Prediction Model Studies

Ingui filter [36]	(Validat$ OR Predict$.ti. OR Rule$) OR (Predict$ AND [Outcome$ OR Risk$ OR Model$]) OR ((History OR Variable$ OR Criteria OR Scor$ OR Characteristic$ OR Finding$ OR Factor$) AND (Predict$ OR Model$ OR Decision$ OR Identif$ OR Prognos$)) OR (Decision$ AND [Model$ OR Clinical$ OR Logistic Models/]) OR (Prognostic AND [History OR Variable$ OR Criteria OR Scor$ OR Characteristic$ OR Finding$ OR Factor$ OR Model$])
Haynes broad filter [37]	(Predict*[tiab] OR Predictive value of tests[mh] OR Scor*[tiab] OR Observ*[tiab] OR Observer variation[mh])
Geersing [39]	Combine the Ingui or Haynes filter using the Boolean "OR" operator with ("Stratification" OR "ROC Curve"[Mesh] OR "Discrimination" OR "Discriminate" OR "c-statistic" OR "c statistic" OR "Area under the curve" OR "AUC" OR "Calibration" OR "Indices" OR "Algorithm" OR "Multivariable")

See Chapter 3 for further resources.

A search strategy should always be defined using the review aim and scope (see Box 18.2 and Table 18.1, and Chapter 3). The generic search strategy in Box 18.3 is applicable for the more common types of reviews of prediction models, which includes reviews of types 1 and 4, and to some extent type 2, as described in Box 18.2. We can also use the search strategy in Box 18.3 for reviews of types 3 and 5, if we add keywords addressing the specific name or acronym of the targeted prediction model or marker, the clinical field or domain, or the targeted population or outcome (as defined in Table 18.1). We can find studies relating to a specific, well-known prediction model with good sensitivity by using a simple query that searches only for the name of the model (e.g. Framingham Risk Score, EuroSCORE, or ABCD2) in the title or abstract. If the model's performance in a particular population or subgroup is of interest, then specific terms relating to that population can be added to the search string. Additional studies can be found by identifying citations to the original article describing the development of the prediction model [39].

18.3   DATA EXTRACTION

The next step is to extract the key information from each included study. Data extraction provides the necessary data to enable reviewers to examine the risk of bias in each study. It also provides the information required for subsequent qualitative and quantitative (meta-analysis) synthesis of the data obtained. Reviewers should extract key information from each study, such as the dates, setting, study design, definitions of startpoints, outcomes, follow-up length, and prognostic factors. This allows a summary table of study characteristics to be produced. In addition, more specific information is needed for risk of bias assessment, such as methods of measurement of the outcomes, predictors, and handling of missing data.

A particular problem with all prediction model research is incomplete reporting and methodological shortcomings [18, 27, 28, 40, 41]. The Transparent Reporting of a multivariable prediction model for Individual Prognosis Or Diagnosis (TRIPOD) statement describes the details of model development and validation that authors of prediction model studies should report [42, 43]. Despite this important initiative, it is unlikely that future reports of published prediction models will always report the key details that researchers need to synthesize models in a systematic review, let alone to include them in a meta-analysis. A key finding from a systematic review of prediction models can therefore be that many of the primary studies available are methodologically weak and do not report key details about their prediction models [15, 18].

The CHARMS guidance includes a checklist to help reviewers define the key items that need to be extracted from each primary study, given their specific review question [21]. These key items are grouped in 11 domains, given in Box 18.4. Some key items or even whole domains may not be applicable, depending on the review aim or question. For example, if a review aims to synthesize the evidence on the predictive performance of a specific model or the value of adding a specific marker to an existing model, the items in the domain "model development" will not be relevant.

Box 18.4   Items to Consider Extracting from Primary Studies in a Systematic Review of Prediction Models (The CHARMS Checklist)

Domain	Key items
Source of data	– Source of data (e.g. cohort, case–control, randomized trial participants, or registry data)
Participants	– Participant eligibility and recruitment method (e.g. consecutive participants, location, number of centers, setting, inclusion and exclusion criteria) – Participant description – Details of treatments received, if relevant – Study dates
Outcome(s) to be predicted	– Definition and method for measurement of outcome – Was the same outcome definition (and method for measurement) used in all patients? – Type of outcome (e.g. single or combined endpoints) – Was the outcome assessed without knowledge of the candidate predictors (i.e. blinded)? – Were candidate predictors part of the outcome (e.g. in panel or consensus diagnosis)? – Time of outcome occurrence or summary of duration of follow-up

Domain	Key items
Candidate predictors (or index tests)	– Number and type of predictors (e.g. demographics, patient history, physical examination, additional testing, disease characteristics) – Definition and method for measurement of candidate predictors – Timing of predictor measurement (e.g. at patient presentation, at diagnosis, at treatment initiation) – Were predictors assessed blinded for outcome, and for each other (if relevant)? – Handling of predictors in the modeling (e.g. continuous, linear, non-linear transformations or categorized)
Sample size	– Number of participants and number of outcomes/events – Number of outcomes/events in relation to the number of candidate predictors (events per variable)
Missing data	– Number of participants with any missing value (include predictors and outcomes) – Number of participants with missing data for each predictor – Handling of missing data (e.g. complete-case analysis, imputation, or other methods)
Model development	– Modeling method (e.g. logistic, survival, neural network, or machine learning techniques) – Modeling assumptions satisfied – Method for selection of predictors for inclusion in multivariable modeling (e.g. all candidate predictors, pre-selection based on unadjusted association with the outcome) – Method for selection of predictors during multivariable modeling (e.g. full model approach, backward or forward selection) and criteria used (e.g. P value, Akaike information criterion) – Shrinkage of predictor weights or regression coefficients (e.g. no shrinkage, uniform shrinkage, penalized estimation)
Model performance	– Calibration (calibration plot, calibration slope, Hosmer–Lemeshow test) and discrimination (c statistic, D statistic, log-rank) measures with confidence intervals – Classification measures (e.g. sensitivity, specificity, predictive values, net reclassification improvement) and whether a priori cut points were used
Model evaluation	– Method used for testing model performance: development dataset only (random split of data, resampling methods, e.g. bootstrap or cross-validation, none) or separate external validation (e.g. temporal, geographic, different setting, different investigators) – In case of poor validation, whether model was adjusted or updated (e.g. intercept recalibrated, predictor effects adjusted, or new predictors added)

(Continued)

Domain	Key items
Results	– Final and other multivariable models (e.g. basic, extended, simplified) presented, including predictor weights or regression coefficients, intercept, baseline survival, model performance measures (with standard errors or confidence intervals) – Any alternative presentation of the final prediction models, e.g. sum score, nomogram, score chart, predictions for specific risk subgroups with performance – Comparison of the distribution of predictors (including missing data) for development and validation datasets
Interpretation and discussion	– Interpretation of presented models (confirmatory, i.e. model useful for practice versus exploratory, i.e. more research needed) – Comparison with other studies, discussion of generalizability, strengths, and limitations.

Source: Taken from Moons et al. [21].

The CHARMS guidance also suggests which numeric information should be extracted (e.g. the domain "Results") to facilitate a quantitative meta-analysis, including meta-regression. It is widely recommended that studies evaluating a prediction model should assess calibration and discrimination [42, 44]. Calibration and discrimination are fundamental characteristics of a model that capture its predictive ability on a particular dataset with a particular case mix. Calibration is the agreement between predictions from the model and observed outcomes. Discrimination is the prediction model's ability to differentiate between those who do and do not experience the outcome event. Box 18.5 summarizes the most common methods to evaluate calibration and discrimination, depending on whether binary, survival, or other outcomes are predicted.

Box 18.5   Performance Measures

The most important considerations regarding a model's performance are calibration and discrimination. **Calibration** reflects the agreement between the model's outcome predictions and the observed outcomes. Informally, a model is said to be well calibrated if, for every group of, say, 100 individuals, each with a mean predicted risk of x%, close to x people have (diagnostic model) or develop (prognostic model) the outcome. Calibration should be reported graphically with predicted outcome probabilities (on the x-axis) plotted against observed outcome frequencies (on the y-axis) – see Figure 18.1 for an example. The plot is commonly done by tenths of the predicted risk, with 95% confidence intervals (95% CI). It should be augmented with a smoothed (Loess) line over the entire predicted probability range, with shaded 95% confidence bands [45–47] (black line and shaded area in Figure 18.1). It displays

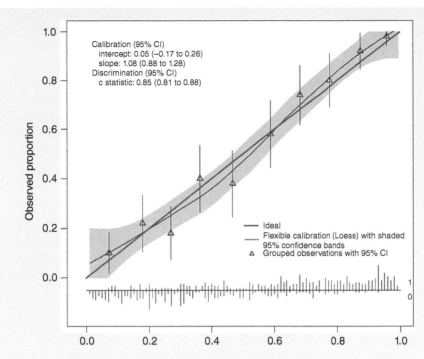

FIGURE 18.1   Example of calibration plot of a prediction model.

the direction and magnitude of model miscalibration across the probability range, which can be combined with estimates of the calibration slope and intercept [47]. A histogram may be added at the bottom of the plots, which shows the distribution of outcomes (1 = outcome occurred; 0 = outcome did not occur). A well-calibrated model shows predictions lying on or around the 45° line of the calibration plot (red line). Perfect calibration results in a slope of 1 and an intercept of 0. If calibration is poor, a prediction model will not be useful; however, good calibration does not guarantee that the model is unbiased or that prediction for an individual patient will be accurate [48].

Discrimination refers to the ability of a prediction model to differentiate between those who do or do not experience the outcome event. A model has perfect discrimination if the predicted risks for all individuals who have (diagnostic) or develop (prognosis) the outcome are higher than those for all individuals who do not experience the outcome. Discrimination is commonly estimated using the concordance statistic (c statistic) [49]. The c statistic is identical to the area under the receiver operating characteristic curve for models with binary endpoints. It can be generalized for time-to-event (survival) models accounting for censoring [50]. Extensions to the c statistic for models with more than two outcome categories [51], competing risks [52], and clustered data [53, 54] have been proposed for survival models.

Overall performance measures such as explained variation (R^2) [55–61] and the Brier score [62, 63] are sometimes reported alongside the traditional measures of discrimination and calibration, although they are less intuitive and informative.

Source: Adapted from Moons et al. [43].

Poor and inconsistent reporting of discrimination and calibration measures complicates meta-analysis of validation studies. However, it is still often possible to extract two common statistical measures: the concordance statistic (c statistic, also called c-index) and the overall observed–expected (O : E) ratio.

The c statistic measures a prediction model's discrimination. It ranges from 0.5, indicating no discriminative ability, to 1, indicating perfect discrimination. Concordance is most familiar from logistic regression models, where it is also known as the area under the receiver operating characteristics curve (AUC). C statistics are the most commonly reported estimates of prediction model performance and can if necessary be estimated from other reported quantities [64, 65]. Table 18.2 presents commonly used methods for estimating c statistics and their standard errors, and for implementing the logit transformations that are needed before a meta-analysis can be conducted. Care must be taken when extracting the performance of survival models from publications. For example, different adaptations of the c statistic have been proposed for use with time-to-event outcomes. Although Harrell's c statistic is the most commonly used, many other options are available [68]. For instance, the D statistic gives the log hazard ratio of a model's predicted risks dichotomized at the median value; it can be estimated from Harrell's c statistic when missing [69]. We recommend extracting all reported performance estimates and summarizing them through meta-analysis if possible (see below).

The overall O : E ratio provides a rough indication of overall model calibration across the entire range of predicted risks. It is directly related to the calibration-in-the-large statistic for logistic regression models [70]. Table 18.3 presents formulae using commonly reported quantities to calculate the overall O : E ratio and its standard

TABLE 18.2 Formulas for estimating the logit c statistic and its variance from other information in a primary study.[a]

What is reported?	Estimate for Var(logit(c))	Reference
C statistic and its confidence interval	$[logit(c_{ub}) - logit(c_{lb})] / (2 \times q)$	[66]
C statistic and its variance or standard error	$\dfrac{Var(c)}{(c(1-c))^2} = \left(\dfrac{SE(c)}{c(1-c)}\right)^2$	[67]
C statistic, the total sample size, and the total number of observed events	$\approx \dfrac{1 + \left(\frac{N}{2}-1\right)(1-c)/(2-c) + \left(\frac{N}{2}-1\right)c/(1+c)}{c(1-c)O(N-O)}$	[67]

[a] With logit(c) = ln(c) − ln(1-c), where ln is the natural log. The lower and upper bounds of the confidence interval of the c statistic are given by c_{lb} and c_{ub}, respectively. The value for q is given by the 100(1 − α) percentile of the Normal distribution, and corresponds to 1.96 for a 95% confidence interval. O represents the total number of observed events and N the total sample size. The linear predictor is the linear combination of the model predictors in the validation study weighted by the regression coefficients of the model in the development study.

TABLE 18.3   Formulas for estimating the ln(O : E) ratio from other information in a primary study.[a]

What is reported	Estimate for ln(O : E)	Estimate for Var(ln(O : E))	Reference
O : E with confidence interval	ln(O : E)	[logit(O:E$_{ub}$) − logit(O : E$_{lb}$)] / (2 × 1.96)	[66]
		$\left[\dfrac{\ln(O:E)}{-0.862 + \sqrt{0.743 - 2.404\ln(p)}} \right]^2$	[71]
O and E	ln(O) − ln(E)	$\dfrac{1}{O}$	
N, Po, and Pe	ln(P$_O$) − ln(P$_E$)	$\dfrac{NP_o(1-P_o)}{(NP_o)^2}$	
P$_O$, P$_E$, and Var(P$_O$)	ln(P$_O$) − ln(P$_E$)	$\dfrac{1}{P_0^2}\text{Var}(P_0)$	[67]
O and E across different risk strata	ln($\sum_i O_i$) − ln ($\sum_i E_i$)	$\sum_i\text{Var}(\ln(O:E)_i)$	[67]
N, Po, and Pe across different risk strata ([b])	$\ln\left(\sum_i P_{O_i}N_i\right) - \ln\left(\sum_i P_{E_i}N_i\right)$	$\sum_i\text{Var}(\ln(O:E)_i)$	[67]
Mean subject characteristics in the validation sample	Calculate P$_E$ by incorporating the mean values of the subject characteristics in the prediction model. Combine P$_E$ and P$_O$ to obtain O : E	See Var(ln(O : E)) when O and E are known	

[a] O : E$_{lb}$ and O : E$_{ub}$ are the lower and upper bounds of the 95% confidence interval of the overall O : E ratio, p is the P value of the overall O : E ratio, O is the total number of observed events, E is the total number of expected (predicted) events, P$_O$ is the observed event probability, P$_E$ is the expected event probability, N is the total sample size, and α is the calibration in the large.

[b] These numbers can sometimes also be extracted from a calibration plot. For instance, the horizontal axis of this plot usually depicts P$_E$ across the entire range of predicted risk. Conversely, the vertical axis of a calibration plot depicts P$_O$ across the entire range of predicted risk. Image editing tools can thus be used to extract values for P$_O$ and P$_E$ across different risk strata. Note that N is usually reported in published articles.

error [72]. The O : E ratio is sometimes also available for subgroups, for example those defined by tenths of predicted risk or for particular groups of interest (e.g. ethnic groups or regions); however, it is unlikely that every study will report the same subgroups. When summarizing the calibration performance of survival models, we recommend extracting O : E ratios (or their components) for all reported timepoints in each study, as O : E values are likely to differ across time. If some events are not observed due to censoring, the survival probability at a particular timepoint could be estimated from Kaplan–Meier analyses (and 1 minus this Kaplan–Meier estimate used to calculate the O : E ratio).

Meta-analysis requires a standard error for each extracted estimate of model performance. If standard errors cannot be retrieved from original articles, they should be calculated using the reported upper and lower limits of the confidence interval or the reported exact P value. The standard error of common performance measures can also sometimes be approximated from the sample size and numbers of observed and expected events, as described in Tables 18.2 and 18.3.

The discrimination and calibration of a prediction model are highly likely to vary between validation studies due to differences between the studied populations [73, 74]. In other words, heterogeneity in a model's predictive performance is to be expected. For instance, there may be differences in the overall predicted outcome frequency, otherwise known as differences in baseline risk or overall prognosis. Information about the case mix, or the distribution of individual characteristics, must therefore be extracted from each validation study. Examples include the mean and standard deviation of the key subject characteristics and of the linear predictor. Heterogeneity in reported performance can also appear when the predictor effects differ between studies (e.g. due to different methods of measuring the predictors) or when different definitions or derivations of the c statistic have been used.

18.4   ASSESSING METHODOLOGICAL QUALITY

Critical appraisal and assessing the risk of bias of primary studies are important aspects in any systematic review. **Risk of bias** in the context of prediction model studies refers to the extent to which flaws in design, conduct, and analysis may lead to biased, usually optimistic, estimates of predictive performance measures such as model calibration and discrimination. Many systematic reviews have shown that models are poorly developed in terms of their design, data quality, statistical methods, and reporting [18, 28, 40, 41, 75]. Unfortunately, these problems are even more marked for external validation studies that evaluate the performance of an existing model in other data (Box 18.1), which is unquestionably the most important aspect of a prediction model [27, 76].

Quality assessment of primary prediction model studies is a developing field. PROBAST is a tool designed specifically to assess and grade the risk of bias of primary studies on the development, validation, and extension or updating of prediction models, either diagnostic or prognostic, regardless of the type of outcomes, predictors, medical domain, and statistical methods used (see Box 18.6) [77, 78]. PROBAST includes four domains to cover key aspects of prediction model studies: participant selection, predictors, outcomes, and analysis (see Box 18.5). The risk of bias component of each domain comprises four sections: information used to support the judgment, 20 signaling questions (2–9 per domain), judgment of risk of bias, and rationale regarding the judgment. Signaling questions are rated as yes (Y), probably yes (PY), probably

Box 18.6   PROBAST Risk of Bias Tool

Domain 1: Participant Selection

    1.1 Were appropriate data sources used, e.g. cohort, randomized controlled trial, or nested case–control study data?

    1.2 Were all inclusions and exclusions of participants appropriate?

Domain 2: Predictors

    2.1 Were predictors defined and assessed in a similar way for all participants?

    2.2 Were predictor assessments made without knowledge of outcome data?

    2.3 Are all predictors available at the time the model is intended to be used?

Domain 3: Outcome

    3.1 Was the outcome determined appropriately?

    3.2 Was a pre-specified or standard outcome definition used?

    3.3 Were predictors excluded from the outcome definition?

    3.4 Was the outcome defined and determined in a similar way for all participants?

    3.5 Was the outcome determined without knowledge of predictor information?

    3.6 Was the time interval between predictor assessment and outcome determination appropriate?

Domain 4: Analysis

    4.1 Was there a reasonable number of participants with the outcome?

    4.2 Were continuous and categorical predictors handled appropriately?

    4.3 Were all enrolled participants included in the analysis?

    4.4 Were participants with missing data handled appropriately?

    4.5 Was selection of predictors based on univariable analysis avoided?

    4.6 Were important complexities in the data (e.g. competing risks, multiple events per individual) accounted for appropriately?

    4.7 Were relevant model performance measures evaluated, e.g. calibration and discrimination?

    4.8 Were model overfitting and optimism in model performance accounted for?

    4.9 Do predictors and their assigned weights in the final model correspond to the results from multivariable analysis?

Source: Taken from Wolff et al. [77].

no (PN), no (N), or no information (NI). Risk of bias is judged as "low," "high," or "unclear." All signaling questions are phrased so that "yes" indicates absence of bias. Any signaling question rated as "no" or "probably no" flags the potential for bias; and judgment will be required to determine whether the domain should be rated as "high", "low," or "unclear" risk of bias. A "no" rating does not automatically result in a "high" risk of bias rating.

18.5 META-ANALYSIS OF CLINICAL PREDICTION MODEL STUDIES

Once all relevant studies have been identified and the corresponding results have been extracted, the retrieved estimates of model discrimination and calibration can be summarized into a weighted average (see also Chapter 9). As validation studies are highly prone to heterogeneity, we recommend using random-effects meta-analysis to summarize estimates of model discrimination and calibration, to account for unexplained between-study heterogeneity. Furthermore, previous studies have demonstrated that performance measures such as the c statistic and O : E ratio should be transformed so that they are approximately normally distributed within and across the studies in a meta-analysis. We recommend using the logit transformation for the c statistic and the (natural) log transformation (ln) for O : E ratios. No transformations are needed for meta-analysis of "calibration in the large" or for calibration slopes.

For study i, let Y_i be the estimate of model performance of interest (e.g. logit c, log O : E), and let S_i^2 be its sample variance, which is assumed to be known. Then the meta-analysis can be written as

$$Y_i \sim N\left(\mu_i, S_i^2\right)$$

$$\mu_i \sim N\left(\mu, \tau^2\right)$$

assuming that that the Y_i are normally distributed about the ith study's true validation performance, μ_i, and the μ_i are also normally distributed with an average μ and a between-study standard deviation of τ. Estimation of this model (e.g. using restricted maximum likelihood, REML) produces an estimate of the average performance ($\hat{\mu}$) and the between-study variance in performance ($\hat{\tau}^2$) [79]. Confidence intervals for μ should also be produced, ideally accounting for the uncertainty in $\hat{\tau}^2$, for example using the Hartung–Knapp Sidik–Jonkman approach [80].

We need to be able to assess the performance (calibration and discrimination) of a particular prediction model in every tested setting to summarize its consistency across studies [81, 82]. However, carrying out a meta-analysis to produce a single measure of average performance ($\hat{\mu}$) is usually not helpful, as model performance is likely to vary according to differences in case mix and other study-level factors [73, 74]. A key focus of a meta-analysis should thus be to quantify the potential range of a prediction model's performance across different populations of interest, which vary due to a different case mix or setting (see also Chapter 10). For this goal, it is helpful to calculate an approximate $100(1-\alpha)\%$ prediction interval for the performance of the model in a new population [81–83], defined as

$$\hat{\mu} \pm t_{\alpha,N-2} \sqrt{\hat{\tau}^2 + \hat{\sigma}_\mu^2},$$

where $t_{\alpha,\,N-2}$ is the $100(1-\alpha/2)\%$ percentile of the t-distribution for $N-2$ degrees of freedom, N is the number of studies, $\hat{\sigma}_\mu$ is the standard error of $\hat{\mu}$, and $\hat{\tau}$ is the estimated between-study standard deviation. This equation is most accurate when I^2 is large (see Chapter 9) and the study sizes are similar [84]. When a meta-analysis involves a transformation, such as when summarizing the c statistic, the prediction interval should be derived on the transformed scale and then back-transformed. For instance, when meta-analyzing the logit c statistic, the $100(1-\alpha)\%$ prediction interval of the summary c statistic is given by $\mathrm{expit}\!\left(-\hat{\mu} \pm t_{\alpha,N-2} \sqrt{\hat{\tau}^2 + \hat{\sigma}_\mu^2}\right).$

If a meta-analysis reveals heterogeneity in model performance, the sources of this heterogeneity should ideally be investigated to suggest the circumstances under which model performance is adequate and those under which improvement is needed.

Sources of heterogeneity can be explored by performing a meta-regression analysis, using as the dependent variable the transformed estimate of the model performance measure. Study-level or summarized patient-level characteristics (e.g. mean age) are then used as explanatory or independent variables. Possible modifiers of model performance include differences in case mix or disease severity across the primary validation studies, differences in study characteristics (e.g. design, setting, follow-up time, and outcome definitions), differences in the statistical analysis, and characteristics related to selective reporting and publication (e.g. risk of bias and study size) [73].

Unfortunately, including aggregate patient information in a meta-regression (e.g. mean age) is problematic, as the process is susceptible to study-level confounding and aggregation bias (ecological fallacies) [85]. Systematic reviews often include only a few studies, so that robust conclusions cannot be drawn from a meta-regression. Limiting the number of covariates and pre-specifying these in the study protocol will help guard against false-positive conclusions [86]. Chapter 10 discusses in more detail when and how to investigate sources of heterogeneity.

18.6   CASE STUDY: META-ANALYSIS OF EUROSCORE II

Guida et al. described a meta-analysis of 22 studies that examined the predictive performance of the European system for cardiac operative risk evaluation (EuroS-CORE II) [25], which we have revised in this case study. Published in 2012, EuroS-CORE II was developed using logistic regression in a dataset comprising 16 828 adult patients undergoing major cardiac surgery from 154 hospitals in 43 countries over a 12-week period in 2010. EuroSCORE II was developed to predict in-hospital mortality for patients undergoing any type of cardiac surgery.

The authors reviewed validation studies that examined the predictive performance of EuroSCORE II in a narrower population, patients undergoing coronary artery bypass grafting (CABG). The review included 22 validation studies, including a further 145 592 patients from 21 external validation articles (one study included two validations [87]) and a split-sample validation contained within the original development article [5]; 23 validation studies in total. The included studies are summarized in Table 18.4. No risk of bias assessment was carried out, as no tool for this was available at the time of carrying out the review. The size of the validation studies ranged from 216 to 50 588 patients containing between 8 and 1071 deaths; 13 studies had fewer than the recommended 100 outcome events [108, 109].

The c statistic of EuroSCORE II was reported in all 23 validation studies (Table 18.4). Calibration was assessed using a variety of approaches, including the Hosmer–Lemeshow test, calibration plots, or comparing the observed mortality to the predicted EuroSCORE II (either overall or for groups of patients). As calibration was inconsistently assessed, for the purpose of this meta-analysis calibration was assessed by calculating the O : E ratio. While the O : E ratio itself was not explicitly reported in all studies, it could be calculated from other reported information in all validation studies; the log O : E was then used in the meta-analysis. Measures of uncertainty were often not reported for either discrimination or calibration. Standard errors or confidence intervals for the c statistic were reported in 19 validation studies; in the remaining 4 validation studies, the standard error of the logit c statistic was estimated using the equations described in Table 18.2. Similarly, the standard error of the overall log O : E ratio was approximated using the equations provided in Table 18.3. The resulting forest plots are shown in Figures 18.2 and 18.3.

We performed a random-effects meta-analysis using the models described above with REML estimation and Hartung–Knapp–Sidik–Jonkman confidence interval derivation [80]. For the discrimination of EuroSCORE II in the external validation studies, we found $\mu = 1.32$ (on the logit scale), which corresponds to a summary c statistic of $1/(1 + \exp.[-1.32]) = 0.79$. The average c statistic across the external validation studies was thus 0.79, with a 95% confidence interval 0.77 to 0.81 (Figure 18.2). There was substantial heterogeneity with $I^2 \approx 85\%$ ($\hat{\tau} = 0.26$). EuroSCORE II showed fairly consistent discrimination across the external validation studies (approximate 95% prediction interval: 0.72 to 0.87). To investigate whether case mix differences in the validation studies generated heterogeneity, we performed meta-regression analyses examining whether heterogeneity was explained by one or more of the following: the spread of the EuroSCORE II in each validation study, whether the study was a multicenter study, whether the study included patients before 2010 (i.e. before EuroSCORE II was developed), and the spread of the age of the patients as explanatory variables. The P values of the resulting coefficients were all larger than 0.05. We therefore did not find evidence that heterogeneity in the c statistic was explained importantly by these measures of case mix variation. However, the result may have been due to low power and adjusting for aggregate-level study characteristics.

TABLE 18.4 Summarized results of the 22 validation studies of the additive EuroSCORE II model included in our meta-analysis.

Study	Country	Enrolment (years)	Number of patients	Observed in-hospital deaths	Expected in-hospital deaths	C statistic	C statistic standard error
Nashef [5] (development)	43 countries	2010	5553	232	219.34	0.8095	0.014
Biancari [88]	Finland	2006–2011	1027	28	46.22	0.867	0.035
Di Dedda [89]	Italy	2010–2011	1090	41	33.79	0.81	0.036
Chalmers [90]	UK	2006–2010	5576	191	260.96	0.79	0.010
Grant [91]	UK	2010–2011	23 740	746	809.53	0.808	0.008
Carneo-Alcazar [92]	Spain	2005–2010	3798	215	169.39	0.85	0.010
Kunt [93]	Turkey	2004–2012	428	34	7.28	0.72	0.051
Kirmani [94]	UK	2001–2010	15 497	547	392.07	0.818	0.007
Howell [95]	UK/Netherlands	2006–2011	933	90	105.43	0.67	0.027
Wang (a) [96]	China	2008–2011	11 170	226	290.42	0.72	0.015
Borde [97]	India	2011–2012	498	8	10.01	0.72	0.076
Qadir [98]	Pakistan	2006–2010	2004	76	74.55	0.84	0.017
Spiliopoulos [99]	Germany	1999–2005	216	14	8.62	0.77	0.067
Wendt [100]	Germany	1999–2012	1066	45	34.11	0.72	0.034
Laurent [101]	France	2009–2011	314	18	7.22	0.77	0.061
Wang (b) [102]	New Zealand	2010–2012	818	13	13.09	0.642	0.071
Nishida [103]	Japan	1993–2013	461	33	34.11	0.7697	0.035
Barili (a) [87]	Italy	2006–2012	12 201	210	305.03	0.8	0.015
Barili (b) [87]	Italy	2006–2012	1670	125	103.54	0.82	0.020
Paparella [104]	Italy	2011–2012	6191	300	272.40	0.83	0.012
Carosella [105]	Argentina	2008–2012	250	9	4.10	0.76	0.056
Borracci [106]	Argentina	2012–2013	503	21	16.00	0.856	0.033
Osnabrugge [107]	US	2003–2012	50 588	1071	1568.23	0.77	0.010

study n events weight C index (95% CI)
Nashef 5553 232 5.68% 0.81 [0.78, 0.84]
Biancari 1027 28 3.86% 0.87 [0.80, 0.94]
Di Dedda 1090 41 3.78% 0.81 [0.74, 0.88]
Chalmers 5576 191 5.95% 0.79 [0.77, 0.81]
Grant 23740 746 6.05% 0.81 [0.79, 0.82]
Carneo 3798 215 5.95% 0.85 [0.83, 0.87]
Kunt 428 34 2.70% 0.72 [0.62, 0.82]
Kirmani 15497 547 6.09% 0.82 [0.80, 0.83]
Howell 933 90 4.57% 0.67 [0.62, 0.72]
Wang(a) 11170 226 5.61% 0.72 [0.69, 0.75]
Borde 498 8 1.60% 0.72 [0.57, 0.87]
Qadir 2004 76 5.45% 0.84 [0.81, 0.87]
Spiliopoulos 216 14 1.92% 0.77 [0.64, 0.90]
Wendt 1066 45 3.95% 0.72 [0.65, 0.79]
Laurent 314 18 2.17% 0.77 [0.65, 0.89]
Wang(b) 818 13 1.77% 0.64 [0.50, 0.78]
Nishida 461 33 3.86% 0.77 [0.70, 0.84]
Barilli(a) 12201 210 5.61% 0.80 [0.77, 0.83]
Barilli(b) 1670 125 5.20% 0.82 [0.78, 0.86]
Paparella 6191 300 5.82% 0.83 [0.81, 0.85]
Carosella 250 9 2.42% 0.76 [0.65, 0.87]
Borracci 503 21 4.03% 0.86 [0.79, 0.92]
Osnabrugge 50588 1071 5.95% 0.77 [0.75, 0.79]
Summary 100.00% 0.79 [0.77, 0.81]
95% prediction interval [0.72, 0.87]
0.5 0.7 0.9 1
C index

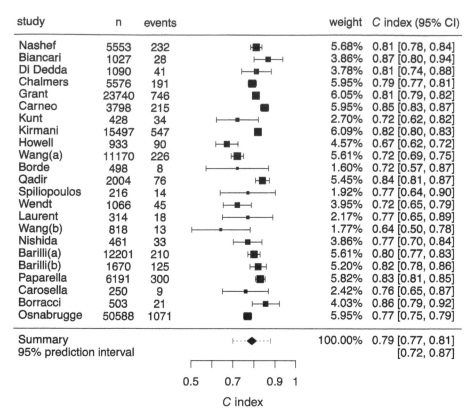

FIGURE 18.2 Forest plot of the extracted *c* indices from the 22 validation studies of EuroSCORE II included in our meta-analysis.

study n events weight O:E (95% CI)
Nashef 5553 232 4.79% 1.05 [0.92, 1.19]
Biancari 1027 28 4.16% 0.61 [0.42, 0.88]
Di Dedda 1090 41 4.37% 1.21 [0.89, 1.63]
Chalmers 5576 191 4.77% 0.73 [0.64, 0.84]
Grant 23740 746 4.86% 0.92 [0.86, 0.99]
Carneo 3798 215 4.78% 1.26 [1.10, 1.43]
Kunt 428 34 4.30% 4.86 [3.52, 6.71]
Kirmani 15497 547 4.85% 1.41 [1.30, 1.53]
Howell 933 90 4.65% 0.86 [0.70, 1.04]
Wang(a) 11170 226 4.79% 0.78 [0.69, 0.89]
Borde 498 8 3.01% 0.80 [0.40, 1.59]
Qadir 2004 76 4.60% 1.03 [0.82, 1.28]
Spiliopoulos 216 14 3.65% 1.56 [0.94, 2.58]
Wendt 1066 45 4.41% 1.32 [0.99, 1.76]
Laurent 314 18 3.87% 2.57 [1.64, 4.03]
Wang(b) 818 13 3.54% 0.62 [0.36, 1.06]
Nishida 461 33 4.28% 0.97 [0.70, 1.35]
Barilli(a) 12201 210 4.78% 0.69 [0.60, 0.79]
Barilli(b) 1670 125 4.71% 1.20 [1.02, 1.42]
Paparella 6191 300 4.81% 1.10 [0.99, 1.23]
Carosella 250 9 3.17% 2.25 [1.18, 4.27]
Borracci 503 21 3.97% 1.31 [0.86, 1.99]
Osnabrugge 50588 1071 4.87% 0.68 [0.64, 0.72]
Summary 100.00% 1.11 [0.91, 1.34]
95% prediction interval [0.55, 2.22]
0.2 0.5 1 2 7
O:E

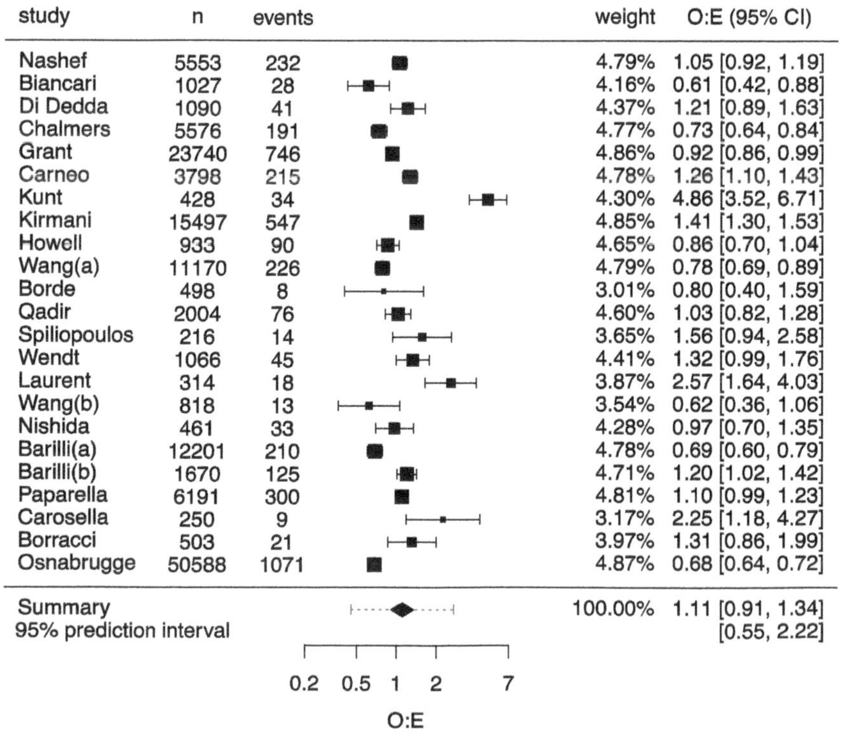

FIGURE 18.3 Overall calibration of EuroSCORE II, summarized from the 22 validation studies included in our meta-analysis.

We meta-analyzed the overall log O : E ratio in the validation studies and found $\mu = 0.11$, which corresponds to a summary total O : E ratio of exp.$(0.11) = 1.11$, with a 95% confidence interval of 0.91 to 1.34. EuroSCORE II therefore gives a slight underestimation of the risk of in-hospital 30-day mortality *on average*. There was a substantial amount of between-study heterogeneity, $I^2 \approx 97\%$ ($\hat{\tau} = 0.44$), leading to an approximate 95% prediction interval of 0.55 to 2.20. This wide prediction interval contains values well above and below the value of 1, indicating that in some populations the predicted probabilities are systematically too low (O : E >> 1) or too high (O : E << 1) [81]. The wide prediction interval illustrates the weakness of focusing solely on average performance, as calibration is good on average but is poor in some populations. A meta-regression using the same study-level characteristics for the meta-regression of the c statistic again found no evidence that this heterogeneity was explained by these measures of case mix variation. Figure 18.4 shows the association between the overall O : E mean and mean EuroSCORE II (P = 0.22).

We can conclude that although EuroSCORE II discriminates reasonably between mortality and survival in patients undergoing cardiac surgery, its overall calibration is unreliable. Predicted risks appear too low in low-risk patients, and vice versa. In this regard, the performance of EuroSCORE II appears to be similar to that of the original EuroSCORE [110] and to suffer from similar deficiencies. It would be helpful

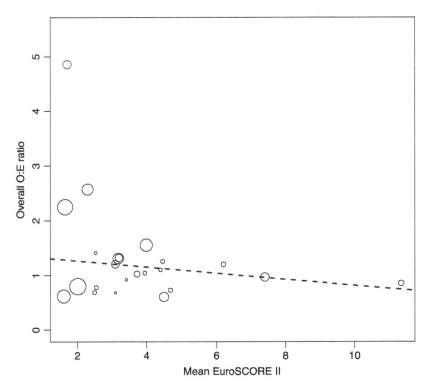

FIGURE 18.4   Association between mean EuroSCORE II and overall O : E. Circle size is proportional to the precision of the O : E estimate (that is, larger circles indicate O : E estimates with smaller standard errors, and thus more weight in the meta-regression, dashed line).

to evaluate possible causes of miscalibration and heterogeneity in model performance. Unfortunately, without individual participant data (IPD) of the development and validation studies, this is often infeasible [73, 81, 82, 111].

18.7 DISCUSSION

Systematic reviews are needed to identify and critically appraise prediction models, so that health care professionals and guideline developers can judge the evidence of the models' predictive abilities, applicability, and usefulness. A major limiting factor in conducting a meta-analysis of prediction model studies is the poor reporting of primary studies. Many reviews have shown that primary studies often fail to report key information on the performance of their prediction models [18, 27, 40]. Although discrimination, as measured by the c statistic, is frequently reported, model calibration measures, and certainly calibration slopes, are rarely and inconsistently evaluated and reported [27]. Furthermore, for a quantitative meta-analysis to be feasible, measures of uncertainty are needed that are often missing from primary reports of prediction models. When standard errors of the performance measures are not reported, an approximation will typically be required.

As illustrated in the EuroSCORE II case study, focusing on the average performance, in this instance calibration as measured by the overall observed–expected (O : E) ratio, can be misleading. The calibration meta-analysis of EuroSCORE II indicated reasonable overall calibration; however, there was substantial between-study heterogeneity, indicating that EuroSCORE II is over- and underpredicting the in-hospital mortality in many settings or populations. The source of this heterogeneity could not be identified using reported data at the aggregate level.

Meta-analysis based on IPD (see Chapter 12) opens up many new avenues of investigation in the context of prediction models [82, 111, 112]. When IPD are available, investigators can better explore sources of heterogeneity in model performance and identify subpopulations where a model works best (or worst) [111]. However, there are major challenges in obtaining and using IPD, for example convincing researchers to share their data, harmonizing predictor and outcome definitions, and dealing with missing data (e.g. completely missing predictors) [113, 114].

Individual prediction model studies are susceptible to many sources of bias that could influence and distort the results of a meta-analysis. Evaluation of study quality is thus essential, although it is not always done. Risk of bias assessment tools for prediction studies (e.g. PROBAST [77, 78]) allow authors to critically appraise the methodological conduct, and to assess the applicability of each individual study with respect to the review question. The results from a risk of bias assessment can then be used to decide which studies to include in the meta-analysis, or to perform sensitivity analyses (e.g. omitting studies rated at high risk of bias [115]). A more difficult problem arises when the prediction model study exhibits selective reporting, as noted above. Nonpublication is a concern too (see also Chapter 5). For most prediction models, validation studies are scarce. It is plausible that many studies go unpublished when there is poor model performance, particularly if conducted by the investigators who developed the original model.

REFERENCES

1. Rabar, S., Lau, R., O'Flynn, N. et al. (2012). Risk assessment of fragility fractures: summary of NICE guidance. *BMJ* 345: e3698.

2. Wells, P.S., Anderson, D.R., Bormanis, J. et al. (1997). Value of assessment of pretest probability of deep-vein thrombosis in clinical management. *Lancet* 350 (9094): 1795–1798.

3. Stiell, I.G., Greenberg, G.H., McKnight, R.D. et al. (1992). A study to develop clinical decision rules for the use of radiography in acute ankle injuries. *Ann. Emerg. Med.* 21: 384–390.

4. Koomen, I., Grobbee, D.E., Roord, J.J. et al. (2003). Hearing loss at school age in survivors of bacterial meningitis: assessment, incidence, and prediction. *Pediatrics* 112: 1049–1053.

5. Nashef, S.A., Roques, F., Sharples, L.D. et al. (2012). EuroSCORE II. *Eur. J. Cardiothorac. Surg.* 41 (4): 734–744. discussion 44-5. doi: https://doi.org/10.1093/ejcts/ezs043.

6. Hippisley-Cox, J., Coupland, C., Vinogradova, Y. et al. (2008). Predicting cardiovascular risk in England and Wales: prospective derivation and validation of QRISK2. *BMJ* 336: 1475–1482.

7. Linke, S.P., Bremer, T.M., Herold, C.D. et al. (2006). A multimarker model to predict outcome in tamoxifen-treated breast cancer patients. *Clin. Cancer Res.* 12: 1175–1183.

8. Steyerberg, E.W., Moons, K.G.M., van der Windt, D.A. et al. (2013). Prognosis research strategy (PROGRESS) 3: prognostic model research. *PLoS Med.* 10 (2): e1001381.

9. Royston, P., Moons, K.G.M., Altman, D.G. et al. (2009). Prognosis and prognostic research: developing a prognostic model. *BMJ* 338: b604. https://doi.org/10.1136/bmj.b604.

10. Steyerberg, E.W., Harrell, F.E. Jr., Borsboom, G.J.J.M. et al. (2001). Internal validation of predictive models: efficiency of some procedures for logistic regression analysis. *J. Clin. Epidemiol.* 54: 774–781.

11. Altman, D.G. and Royston, P. (2000). What do we mean by validating a prognostic model? *Stat. Med.* 19 (4): 453–473.

12. Altman, D.G., Vergouwe, Y., Royston, P. et al. (2009). Prognosis and prognostic research: validating a prognostic model. *BMJ* 338: b605.

13. Steyerberg, E.W., Pencina, M.J., Lingsma, H.F. et al. (2012). Assessing the incremental value of diagnostic and prognostic markers: a review and illustration. *Eur. J. Clin. Invest.* 42 (2): 216–228.

14. Damen, J.A.A.G., Hooft, L., Schuit, E. et al. (2016). Prediction models for cardiovascular disease risk in the general population: systematic review. *BMJ* 353: i2416. https://doi.org/10.1136/bmj.i2416.

15. Wynants, L., Van Calster, B., Collins, G.S. et al. (2020). Prediction models for diagnosis and prognosis of covid-19: systematic review and critical appraisal. *BMJ* 369: m1328. https://doi.org/10.1136/bmj.m1328.

16. Perel, P., Edwards, P., Wentz, R. et al. (2006). Systematic review of prognostic models in traumatic brain injury. *BMC Med. Inform. Decis. Mak.* 6: 38. https://doi.org/10.1186/1472-6947-6-38.

17. Shariat, S.F., Karakiewicz, P.I., Margulis, V. et al. (2008). Inventory of prostate cancer predictive tools. *Curr. Opin. Urol.* 18: 279–296.

18. Collins, G.S., Mallett, S., Omar, O. et al. (2011). Developing risk prediction models for type 2 diabetes: a systematic review of methodology and reporting. *BMC Med.* 9: 103.

19. Keogh, C., Wallace, E., Dillon, C. et al. (2011). Validation of the CHADS2 clinical prediction rule to predict ischaemic stroke. A systematic review and meta-analysis. *Thromb. Haemost.* 106 (3): 528–538. https://doi.org/10.1160/TH11-02-0061.

20. Parolari, A., Pesce, L.L., Trezzi, M. et al. (2010). EuroSCORE performance in valve surgery: a meta-analysis. *Ann. Thorac. Surg.* 89: 787–793.

21. Moons, K.G., de Groot, J.A., Bouwmeester, W. et al. (2014). Critical appraisal and data extraction for systematic reviews of prediction modelling studies: the CHARMS check-list. *PLoS Med.* 11 (10): e1001744. https://doi.org/10.1371/journal.pmed.1001744.

22. Kleinrouweler, C.E., Cheong-See, F.M., Collins, G.S. et al. (2016). Prognostic models in obstetrics: available, but far from applicable. *Am. J. Obstet. Gynecol.* 214 (1): 79–90. e36. doi: https://doi.org/10.1016/j.ajog.2015.06.013.

23. Tangri, N., Kitsios, G.D., Inker, L.A. et al. (2013). Risk prediction models for patients with chronic kidney disease: a systematic review. *Ann. Intern. Med.* 158: 596–603.

24. Smit, H.A., Pinart, M., Antó, J.M. et al. (2015). Childhood asthma prediction models: a systematic review. *Lancet Respir. Med.* 3: 973–984.

25. Guida, P., Mastro, F., Scrascia, G. et al. (2014). Performance of the European system for cardiac operative risk evaluation II: a meta-analysis of 22 studies involving 145,592 cardiac surgery procedures. *J. Thorac. Cardiovasc. Surg.* 148: 3049–3057.

26. Galvin, R., Geraghty, C., Motterlini, N. et al. (2011). Prognostic value of the ABCD² clinical prediction rule: a systematic review and meta-analysis. *Fam. Pract.* 28: 366–376.

27. Collins, G.S., de Groot, J.A., Dutton, S. et al. (2014). External validation of multivari-able prediction models: a systematic review of methodological conduct and reporting. *BMC Med. Res. Methodol.* 14: 40.

28. Bouwmeester, W., Zuithoff, N.P., Mallett, S. et al. (2012). Reporting and methods in clinical prediction research: a systematic review. *PLoS Med.* 9 (5): e1001221.

29. Tzoulaki, I., Liberopoulos, G., and Ioannidis, J.P. (2009). Assessment of claims of improved prediction beyond the Framingham risk score. *JAMA* 302: 2345–2352.

30. Echouffo-Tcheugui, J.B., Dieffenbach, S.D., and Kengne, A.P. (2013). Added value of novel circulating and genetic biomarkers in type 2 diabetes prediction: a systematic review. *Diabetes Res. Clin. Pract.* 101: 255–269.

31. Sanders, L.M., Srikanth, V.K., Blacker, D.J. et al. (2012). Performance of the ABCD2 score for stroke risk post TIA: meta-analysis and probability modeling. *Neurology* 79: 971–980.

32. D'Agostino, R.B. Sr., Vasan, R.S., Pencina, M.J. et al. (2008). General cardiovascular risk profile for use in primary care: the Framingham heart study. *Circulation* 117 (6): 743–753.

33. Geersing, G.J., Zuithoff, N.P., Kearon, C. et al. (2014). Exclusion of deep vein throm-bosis using the Wells rule in clinically important subgroups: individual patient data meta-analysis. *BMJ* 348: g1340.

34. Peat, G., Riley, R.D., Croft, P. et al. (2014). Improving the transparency of prognosis research: the role of reporting, data sharing, registration, and protocols. *PLoS Med.* 11: e1001671. https://doi.org/10.1371/journal.pmed.1001671.

35. Altman, D.G. (2014). The time has come to register diagnostic and prognostic research. *Clin. Chem.* 60: 580–582. https://doi.org/10.1373/clinchem.2013.220335.

36. Ingui, B.J. and Rogers, M.A.M. (2001). Searching for clinical prediction rules in MEDLINE. *J. Am. Med. Inform. Assoc.* 8 (4): 391–397.

37. Wong, S.S., Wilczynski, N.L., Haynes, R.B. et al. (2003). Developing optimal search strategies for detecting sound clinical prediction studies in MEDLINE. *AMIA Annu. Symp. Proc.* 2003: 728–732.

38. Keogh, C., Wallace, E., O'Brien, K.K. et al. (2011). Optimized retrieval of primary care clinical prediction rules from MEDLINE to establish a web-based register. *J. Clin. Epidemiol.* 64 (8): 848–860. https://doi.org/10.1016/j.jclinepi.2010.11.011.

39. Geersing, G.J., Bouwmeester, W., Zuithoff, P. et al. (2012). Search filters for finding prognostic and diagnostic prediction studies in Medline to enhance systematic reviews. *PLoS One* 7 (2): e32844.

40. Collins, G.S., Omar, O., Shanyinde, M. et al. (2013). A systematic review finds prediction models for chronic kidney were poorly reported and often developed using inappropriate methods. *J. Clin. Epidemiol.* 66: 268–277.

41. Mallett, S., Royston, P., Dutton, S. et al. (2010). Reporting methods in studies developing prognostic models in cancer: a review. *BMC Med.* 8: 20.

42. Collins, G.S., Reitsma, J.B., Altman, D.G. et al. (2015). Transparent Reporting of a multivariable prediction model for Individual Prognosis Or Diagnosis (TRIPOD): the TRIPOD statement. *Ann. Intern. Med.* 162 (1): 55–63.

43. Moons, K.G.M., Altman, D.G., Reitsma, J.B. et al. (2015). Transparent Reporting of a multivariable prediction model for Individual Prognosis Or Diagnosis (TRIPOD): explanation and elaboration. *Ann. Intern. Med.* 162 (1): W1–W73.

44. Steyerberg, E.W., Vickers, A.J., Cook, N.R. et al. (2010). Assessing the performance of prediction models: a framework for traditional and novel measures. *Epidemiology* 21 (1): 128–138.

45. Harrell, F.E. (2001). *Regression Modeling Strategies: With Applications to Linear Models, Logistic Regression and Survival Analysis*. New York: Springer.

46. Austin, P.C. and Steyerberg, E.W. (2014). Graphical assessment of internal and external calibration of logistic regression models by using loess smoothers. *Stat. Med.* 33 (3): 517–535. https://doi.org/10.1002/sim.5941.

47. Crowson, C.S., Atkinson, E.J., and Therneau, T.M. (2016). Assessing calibration of prognostic risk scores. *Stat. Methods Med. Res.* 25: 1692–1706. https://doi.org/10.1177/0962280213497434.

48. Vach, W. (2013). Calibration of clinical prediction rules does not just assess bias. *J. Clin. Epidemiol.* 66: 1296–1301.

49. Cook, N.R. (2008). Statistical evaluation of prognostic versus diagnostic models: beyond the ROC curve. *Clin. Chem.* 54: 17–23.

50. Pencina, M.J., D'Agostino, R.B., and Song, L. (2012). Quantifying discrimination of Framingham risk functions with different survival C statistics. *Stat. Med.* 31: 1543–1553.

51. Van Calster, B., Van Belle, V., Vergouwe, Y. et al. (2012). Extending the c-statistic to nominal polytomous outcomes: the polytomous discrimination index. *Stat. Med.* 31 (23): 2610–2626. https://doi.org/10.1002/sim.5321.

52. Wolbers, M., Blanche, P., Koller, M.T. et al. (2014). Concordance for prognostic models with competing risks. *Biostatistics* 15: 526–539. https://doi.org/10.1093/biostatistics/kxt059.

53. van Klaveren, D., Steyerberg, E.W., Perel, P. et al. (2014). Assessing discriminative ability of risk models in clustered data. *BMC Med. Res. Methodol.* 14: 5.

54. van Klaveren, D., Steyerberg, E.W., and Vergouwe, Y. (2014). Interpretation of concordance measures for clustered data. *Stat. Med.* 33: 714–716. https://doi.org/10.1002/sim.5928.

55. Akazawa, K. (1997). Measures of explained variation for a regression model used in survival analysis. *J. Med. Syst.* 21: 229–238.

56. Korn, E.L. and Simon, R. (1990). Measures of explained variation for survival data. *Stat. Med.* 9: 487–503.

57. Mittlböck, M. and Schemper, M. (1996). Explained variation for logistic regression. *Stat. Med.* 15: 1987–1997.

58. Royston, P. (2006). Explained variation for survival models. *Stata J.* 6 (1): 83–96.

59. Schemper, M. (2003). Predictive accuracy and explained variation. *Stat. Med.* 22: 2299–2308. https://doi.org/10.1002/sim.1486.

60. Schemper, M. and Henderson, R. (2000). Predictive accuracy and explained variation in Cox regression. *Biometrics* 56: 249–255.

61. Schemper, M. and Stare, J. (1996). Explained variation in survival analysis. *Stat. Med.* 15: 1999–2012.

62. Gerds, T. and Schumacher, M. (2006). Consistent estimation of the expected brier score in general survival models with right-censored event times. *Biom. J.* 6: 1029–1040.

63. Rufibach, K. (2010). Use of brier score to assess binary predictions. *J. Clin. Epidemiol.* 63 (8): 938–939; author reply 39. doi: https://doi.org/10.1016/j.jclinepi.2009.11.009.

64. Austin, P.C. and Steyerberg, E.W. (2012). Interpreting the concordance statistic of a logistic regression model: relation to the variance and odds ratio of a continuous explanatory variable. *BMC Med. Res. Methodol.* 12: 82.

65. Newson, R. (2002). Parameters behind 'nonparametric' statistics: Kendall's tau, Somers' D and median differences. *Stata J.* 2: 45–64.

66. Altman, D.G. and Bland, J.M. (2011). How to obtain the P value from a confidence interval. *BMJ* 343: d2304.

67. Debray, T.P., Damen, J.A., Snell, K.I. et al. (2017). A guide to systematic review and meta-analysis of prediction model performance. *BMJ* 356: i6460. https://doi.org/10.1136/bmj.i6460.

68. Austin, P.C., Pencinca, M.J., and Steyerberg, E.W. (2017). Predictive accuracy of novel risk factors and markers: a simulation study of the sensitivity of different performance measures for the Cox proportional hazards regression model. *Stat. Methods Med. Res.* 26: 1053–1077. https://doi.org/10.1177/0962280214567141.

69. Royston, P. and Sauerbrei, W. (2004). A new measure of prognostic separation in survival data. *Stat. Med.* 23: 723–748.

70. Steyerberg, E.W. and Vergouwe, Y. (2014). Towards better clinical prediction models: seven steps for development and an ABCD for validation. *Eur. Heart J.* 35: 1925–1931. https://doi.org/10.1093/eurheartj/ehu207.

71. Altman, D.G. and Bland, J.M. (2011). How to obtain the confidence interval from a P value. *BMJ* 343: d2090.

72. Dimitrov, B.D., Motterlini, N., and Fahey, T. (2015). A simplified approach to the pooled analysis of calibration of clinical prediction rules for systematic reviews of validation studies. *Clin. Epidemiol.* 7: 267–280. https://doi.org/10.2147/CLEP.S67632.

73. Debray, T.P., Vergouwe, Y., Koffijberg, H. et al. (2015). A new framework to enhance the interpretation of external validation studies of clinical prediction models. *J. Clin. Epidemiol.* 68 (3): 279–289. https://doi.org/10.1016/j.jclinepi.2014.06.018.

74. Vergouwe, Y., Moons, K.G., and Steyerberg, E.W. (2010). External validity of risk models: use of benchmark values to disentangle a case-mix effect from incorrect coefficients. *Am. J. Epidemiol.* 172 (8): 971–980.

75. Burton, A. and Altman, D.G. (2004). Missing covariate data within cancer prognostic studies: a review of current reporting and proposed guidelines. *Br. J. Cancer* 91 (1): 4–8.

76. Mallett, S., Royston, P., Waters, R. et al. (2010). Reporting performance of prognostic models in cancer: a review. *BMC Med.* 8: 21.

77. Wolff, R.F., Whiting, P.F., Mallett, S. et al. (2019). PROBAST: a tool to assess the risk of bias and applicability of prediction modelling studies. *Ann. Intern. Med.* 170 (1): 51–58.

78. Moons, K.G.M., Wolff, R.F., Riley, R.D. et al. (2019). PROBAST: a tool to assess the risk of bias of prediction model studies – explanation and elaboration. *Ann. Intern. Med.* 170 (1): W1–W33.

79. Hartung, J. and Knapp, G. (2001). A refined method for the meta-analysis of controlled clinical trials with binary outcome. *Stat. Med.* 20: 3875–2889.

80. Röver, C., Knapp, G., and Friede, T. (2015). Hartung-Knapp-Sidik-Jonkman approach and its modification for random-effects meta-analysis with few studies. *BMC Med. Res. Methodol.* 15: 99.

81. Snell, K.I.E., Hua, H., Debray, T.P.A. et al. (2016). Multivariate meta-analysis of individual participant data helped externally validate the performance and implementation of a prediction model. *J. Clin. Epidemiol.* 69: 40–50. https://doi.org/10.1016/j.jclinepi.2015.05.009.

82. Riley, R.D., Ensor, J., Snell, K.I.E. et al. (2016). External validation of clinical prediction models using big data from e-health records or IPD meta-analysis: opportunities and challenges. *BMJ* 353: i3140.

83. Riley, R.D., Higgins, J.P.T., and Deeks, J.J. (2011). Interpretation of random effects meta-analyses. *BMJ* 342: d549. https://doi.org/10.1136/bmj.d549.

84. Partlett, C. and Riley, R.D. (2017). Random effects meta-analysis: coverage performance of 95% confidence and prediction intervals following REML estimation. *Stat. Med.* 36: 301–317. https://doi.org/10.1002/sim.7140.

85. Lau, J., Ioannidis, J.P.A., and Schmid, C.H. (1998). Summing up evidence: one answer is not always enough. *Lancet* 351: 123–127.

86. Thompson, S.G. and Higgins, J.P.T. (2002). How should meta-regression analyses be undertaken and interpreted? *Stat. Med.* 21 (11): 1559–1573. https://doi.org/10.1002/sim.1187.

87. Barili, F., Pacini, D., Rosato, F. et al. (2014). In-hospital mortality risk assessment in elective and non-elective cardiac surgery: a comparison between EuroSCORE II and age, creatinine, ejection fraction score. *Eur. J. Cardiothorac. Surg.* 46 (1): 44–48. https://doi.org/10.1093/ejcts/ezt581.

88. Biancari, F., Vasques, F., Mikkola, R. et al. (2012). Validation of EuroSCORE II in patients undergoing coronary artery bypass surgery. *Ann. Thorac. Surg.* 93 (6): 1930–1935. https://doi.org/10.1016/j.athoracsur.2012.02.064.

89. Di Dedda, U., Pelissero, G., Agnelli, B. et al. (2013). Accuracy, calibration and clinical performance of the new EuroSCORE II risk stratification system. *Eur. J. Cardiothorac. Surg.* 43 (1): 27–32. https://doi.org/10.1093/ejcts/ezs196.

90. Chalmers, J., Pullan, M., Fabri, B. et al. (2013). Validation of EuroSCORE II in a modern cohort of patients undergoing cardiac surgery. *Eur. J. Cardiothorac. Surg.* 43 (4): 688–694. https://doi.org/10.1093/ejcts/ezs406.

91. Grant, S.W., Hickey, G.L., Dimarakis, I. et al. (2012). How does EuroSCORE II perform in UK cardiac surgery; an analysis of 23 740 patients from the Society for Cardiothoracic Surgery in Great Britain and Ireland National Database. *Heart* 98 (21): 1568–1572. https://doi.org/10.1136/heartjnl-2012-302483.

92. Carnero-Alcazar, M., Silva Guisasola, J.A., Reguillo Lacruz, F.J. et al. (2013). Validation of EuroSCORE II on a single-centre 3800 patient cohort. *Interact. Cardiovasc. Thorac. Surg.* 16 (3): 293–300. https://doi.org/10.1093/icvts/ivs480.

93. Kunt, A.G., Kurtcephe, M., Hidiroglu, M. et al. (2013). Comparison of original EuroSCORE, EuroSCORE II and STS risk models in a Turkish cardiac surgical cohort. *Interact. Cardiovasc. Thorac. Surg.* 16 (5): 625–629. https://doi.org/10.1093/icvts/ivt022.

94. Kirmani, B.H., Mazhar, K., Fabri, B.M. et al. (2013). Comparison of the EuroSCORE II and Society of Thoracic Surgeons 2008 risk tools. *Eur. J. Cardiothorac. Surg.* 44 (6): 999–1005. discussion 05. doi: https://doi.org/10.1093/ejcts/ezt122.

95. Howell, N.J., Head, S.J., Freemantle, N. et al. (2013). The new EuroSCORE II does not improve prediction of mortality in high-risk patients undergoing cardiac surgery: a collaborative analysis of two European centres. *Eur. J. Cardiothorac. Surg.* 44 (6): 1006–1011. discussion 11. doi: https://doi.org/10.1093/ejcts/ezt174.

96. Wang, L., Han, Q.Q., Qiao, F. et al. (2014). Performance of EuroSCORE II in patients who have undergone heart valve surgery: a multicentre study in a Chinese population. *Eur. J. Cardiothorac. Surg.* 45 (2): 359–364. https://doi.org/10.1093/ejcts/ezt264.

97. Borde, D., Gandhe, U., Hargave, N. et al. (2013). The application of European system for cardiac operative risk evaluation II (EuroSCORE II) and Society of Thoracic Surgeons (STS) risk-score for risk stratification in Indian patients undergoing cardiac surgery. *Ann. Card. Anaesth.* 16 (3): 163–166. https://doi.org/10.4103/0971-9784.114234.

98. Qadir, I., Alamzaib, S.M., Ahmad, M. et al. (2014). EuroSCORE vs. EuroSCORE II vs. Society of Thoracic Surgeons risk algorithm. *Asian Cardiovasc. Thorac. Ann.* 22 (2): 165–171. https://doi.org/10.1177/0218492313479355.

99. Spiliopoulos, K., Bagiatis, V., Deutsch, O. et al. (2014). Performance of EuroSCORE II compared to EuroSCORE I in predicting operative and mid-term mortality of patients from a single center after combined coronary artery bypass grafting and aortic valve replacement. *Gen. Thorac. Cardiovasc. Surg.* 62 (2): 103–111. https://doi.org/10.1007/s11748-013-0311-8.

100. Wendt, D., Thielmann, M., Kahlert, P. et al. (2014). Comparison between different risk scoring algorithms on isolated conventional or transcatheter aortic valve replacement. *Ann. Thorac. Surg.* 97 (3): 796–802. https://doi.org/10.1016/j.athoracsur.2013.09.012.

101. Laurent, M., Fournet, M., Feit, B. et al. (2013). Simple bedside clinical evaluation versus established scores in the estimation of operative risk in valve replacement for severe aortic stenosis. *Arch. Cardiovasc. Dis.* 106 (12): 651–660. https://doi.org/10.1016/j.acvd.2013.09.001.

102. Wang, T.K., Li, A.Y., Ramanathan, T. et al. (2014). Comparison of four risk scores for contemporary isolated coronary artery bypass grafting. *Heart Lung Circ.* 23 (5): 469–474. https://doi.org/10.1016/j.hlc.2013.12.001.

103. Nishida, T., Sonoda, H., Oishi, Y. et al. (2014). The novel EuroSCORE II algorithm predicts the hospital mortality of thoracic aortic surgery in 461 consecutive Japanese patients better than both the original additive and logistic EuroSCORE algorithms. *Interact. Cardiovasc. Thorac. Surg.* 18 (4): 446–450. https://doi.org/10.1093/icvts/ivt524.

104. Paparella, D., Guida, P., Di Eusanio, G. et al. (2014). Risk stratification for in-hospital mortality after cardiac surgery: external validation of EuroSCORE II in a prospective regional registry. *Eur. J. Cardiothorac. Surg.* 46 (5): 840–848. https://doi.org/10.1093/ejcts/ezt657.

105. Carosella, V., Mastantuono, C., Golovonevsky, V. et al. (2014). Prospective and multicentric validation of the ArgenSCORE in aortic valve replacement surgery. Comparison with the EuroSCORE I and the EuroSCORE II. *Rev. Argent. Cardiol.* 82 (1): 5–11.

106. Borracci, R.A., Rubio, M., Celano, L. et al. (2014). Prospective validation of EuroSCORE II in patients undergoing cardiac surgery in Argentinean centres. *Interact. Cardiovasc. Thorac. Surg.* 18 (5): 539–543. https://doi.org/10.1093/icvts/ivt550.

107. Osnabrugge, R.L., Speir, A.M., Head, S.J. et al. (2014). Performance of EuroSCORE II in a large US database: implications for transcatheter aortic valve implantation. *Eur. J. Cardiothorac. Surg.* 46 (3): 400–408. discussion 08. https://doi.org/10.1093/ejcts/ezu033.

108. Collins, G.S., Ogundimu, E.O., and Altman, D.G. (2016). Sample size considerations for the external validation of a multivariable prognostic model: a resampling study. *Stat. Med.* 35: 214–226. https://doi.org/10.1002/sim.6787.

109. Van Calster, B., Nieboer, D., Vergouwe, Y. et al. (2016). A calibration hierarchy for risk models was defined: from utopia to empirical data. *J. Clin. Epidemiol.* 74: 167–176. https://doi.org/10.1016/j.jclinepi.2015.12.005.

110. Siregar, S., Groenwold, R.H., de Heer, F. et al. (2012). Performance of the original EuroSCORE. *Eur. J. Cardiothorac. Surg.* 41 (4): 746–754.

111. Debray, T.P.A., Riley, R.D., Rovers, M.M. et al. (2015). Individual Participant Data (IPD) meta-analyses of diagnostic and prognostic modeling studies: guidance on their use. *PLoS Med.* 12 (10): e1001886. https://doi.org/10.1371/journal.pmed.1001886.

112. Debray, T.P., Moons, K.G., Ahmed, I. et al. (2013). A framework for developing, implementing, and evaluating clinical prediction models in an individual participant data meta-analysis. *Stat. Med.* 32: 3158–3180.

113. Jolani, S., Debray, T.P., Koffijberg, H. et al. (2015). Imputation of systematically missing predictors in an individual participant data meta-analysis: a generalized approach using MICE. *Stat. Med.* 34: 1841–1863. https://doi.org/10.1002/sim.6451.

114. Resche-Rigon, M., White, I.R., Bartlett, J.W. et al. (2013). Multiple imputation for handling systematically missing confounders in meta-analysis of individual participant data. *Stat. Med.* 32 (28): 4890–4905. https://doi.org/10.1002/sim.5894.

115. Christodoulou, E., Ma, J., Collins, G.S. et al. (2019). A systematic review shows no performance benefit of machine learning over logistic regression for clinical prediction models. *J. Clin. Epidemiol.* 110: 12–22. https://doi.org/10.1016/j.jclinepi.2019.02.004.

CHAPTER 19

Systematic Reviews of Epidemiological Studies of Etiology and Prevalence

Matthias Egger, Diana Buitrago-Garcia, and George Davey Smith

Systematic reviews of observational studies have become increasingly common in recent years. A search of PubMed for articles with "meta-analysis" in the title or abstract identified 915 publications for the year 2000 and 26 676 for 2020, reflecting the massive increase of publications reporting meta-analyses (see also Chapter 1). We randomly selected 100 articles published in 2000 or 2020 and examined them further (Table 19.1). Whereas in 2000 most meta-analyses were of controlled clinical trials, by 2020 observational studies had become the most common study type included in meta-analyses. In 2020, about a quarter of publications focused on epidemiological studies of etiology, and about 10% each on observational studies of interventions (see Chapter 15), diagnostic or prognostic studies (Chapters 16 and 17), or prevalence studies. This chapter focuses on systematic reviews of epidemiological studies of etiology and prevalence (see Box 19.1 for an overview of different study designs). We discuss the rationale for systematic reviews of epidemiological studies, highlight fundamental differences between observational studies and randomized controlled trials (RCTs), and address the steps from shaping the research question to defining the population, exposure, and outcome, exploring heterogeneity and interpreting results.

Systematic Reviews in Health Research: Meta-Analysis in Context, Third Edition. Edited by Matthias Egger, Julian P.T. Higgins, and George Davey Smith.
© 2022 John Wiley & Sons Ltd. Published 2022 by John Wiley & Sons Ltd.
Companion website: www.systematic-reviews3.org

TABLE 19.1 Characteristics of 100 articles sampled at random from articles published in 2000 or 2020 and included in PubMed.

	No. of publications	
Year	2000	2020
All publications	914	26 676
Random sample of publications	100	100
Meta-analysis of		
Controlled clinical trials	45[a]	43[b]
Observational studies, with focus on:	24[a]	55[b]
Etiology	9	23
Intervention effectiveness	8	12
Diagnostic accuracy or prognosis	6	10
Prevalence	1	10
Methodological article	7	0
Traditional review	12	0
Other	14[c]	9[c]

Based on a search of PubMed for articles with "meta-analysis" in the title or abstract, excluding publication types letter, comment, and editorial.

[a] Two meta-analyses included both clinical trials and observational studies.

[b] Seven meta-analyses included both clinical trials and observational studies.

[c] Other publications included study protocols, meta-analyses of animal experiments, agricultural or ecological studies or experimental studies in psychology, and systematic reviews without meta-analyses.

Box 19.1 Observational Designs and Approaches for Studying Etiology and Prevalence

Cohort study: Cohort studies follow a study population over time. An exposed and an unexposed group are compared regarding the risk of the outcome. Different levels of exposure and exposures that vary over time can be studied [1, 2]. Instrumental variable methods and self-controlled case series studies are types of cohort studies (see below and Chapter 15).

Instrumental variable methods: Instrumental variable (IV) analysis uses an external factor that determines the exposure of interest, but is not associated with the outcome other than through its effect on the exposure. In other words, the instrument is not associated with the factors that may confound the association between exposure and outcome. The instrument can be calendar time, geographic area, or treatment preferences [3, 4]. Mendelian randomization studies are examples of IV analyses using genetic factors as instruments [5] (see also Chapter 20).

Self-controlled designs: In self-controlled case series designs, the occurrence of the outcome is compared between time windows during which individuals are exposed to a risk factor, and time windows when they are not exposed. In contrast to standard cohort designs, the comparison is within individuals. The design is used to study transient exposures for which exact timings are available, such as infections, vaccinations, drug treatments, climatic exposures, or disease exacerbations [6] (see also Chapter 15).

Case–control study: In case–control studies, exposures are compared between people with the outcome of interest (cases) and people without (controls) [2]. The design is especially efficient for rare outcomes.

Cross-sectional studies: In cross-sectional studies, study participants are assessed at one point in time or during a short period to examine the prevalence of exposures, risk factors, or disease. The prevalence may be compared between exposure groups like in a cohort study, or the odds of exposure is compared between groups with and without disease like in a case–control study [2].

Ecological studies: In ecological studies, the association between an exposure and an outcome is studied and compared between populations that differ geographically or in calendar time. Limitations include the ecological fallacy, when associations observed at the aggregate level do not hold at the individual level, and confounding, which is often difficult to control.

Source: Adapted from Dekkers et al. [1] and Vandenbroucke et al. [2].

19.1   WHY DO WE NEED SYSTEMATIC REVIEWS OF EPIDEMIOLOGICAL STUDIES?

The RCT is the principal research design in the evaluation of medical interventions [7]. Etiological hypotheses, however, cannot generally be tested in randomized experiments. For example, does breathing other people's tobacco smoke promote the development of lung cancer, drinking coffee cause coronary heart disease, or eating a diet rich in unsaturated fat increase the risk of breast cancer? Studies of such "menaces of daily life" [8] often employ observational designs. In these situations, the risks involved are generally small. Still, once a large proportion of the population is exposed, the public health impact of these associations, if they are causal, can be striking [9].

The prevalence of disease or established determinants of disease at a given point in time (*point prevalence*) or during a specified period (*period prevalence*) are also of great importance for policymaking. Since the 1990s, the Global Burden of Diseases, Injuries, and Risk Factors study (GBD) has been integrating data on the prevalence of a given disease or risk factor with information on the harm it causes in order to estimate the burden of different diseases and risk factors [10, 11].

Systematic reviews of epidemiological studies play an important role in answering questions about etiology and prevalence. Epidemiological studies are also essential in medical effectiveness research, since the available evidence from clinical trials will rarely answer all the important questions [12]. Often the exposures in observational studies will be closely related or even identical to the interventions in RCTs (e.g. using vitamin E supplements for a few years), blurring the distinction between the two types of studies and raising the issue of combining data across them. These issues are discussed later in this chapter and in Chapter 15.

19.2   META-ANALYSIS OF EPIDEMIOLOGICAL STUDIES

It is always appropriate and desirable to review a body of data systematically, irrespective of the design and type of studies reviewed. Statistically combining results from separate studies in a meta-analysis may, however, be inappropriate (see also Chapter 1). Meta-analysis of RCTs is generally based on the assumption that each trial provides an unbiased estimate of the effect of an intervention: the variability in results between the studies is due mainly to random variation. The overall effect calculated from a group of sensibly combined RCTs should provide an unbiased estimate of the treatment effect, increasing its precision. Meta-analysis may seem attractive in etiological epidemiology, promising a precise and definite answer when the magnitude of the underlying risks is small, or in prevalence studies when the disease or condition of interest is rare. However, compared with RCT research, a fundamentally different situation arises in the case of epidemiological studies [13]. Epidemiological studies may yield estimates of causal effects that deviate systematically from the truth, beyond the play of chance. They may also produce precise but incorrect prevalence estimates. This may be due to the effects of bias in prevalence studies or confounding and bias in etiological epidemiology. Let us consider the example of smoking as a potential cause of suicide, and then examine biases in prevalence studies.

19.2.1   Bias and Confounding in Etiological Epidemiology: Does Smoking Cause Suicide?

Many cohort studies have shown a positive association between smoking and suicide, with a dose–response relationship being evident between the amount smoked and the probability of committing suicide [14]. Figure 19.1 illustrates this for four prospective studies of middle-aged men, including the large cohort of men screened for the Multiple Risk Factors Intervention Trial (MRFIT) [15]. Based on over 390 000 men and almost five million years of follow-up, a meta-analysis of these cohorts produces very precise and statistically robust estimates of the increase in suicide risk associated with smoking, after controlling for potential confounding factors: relative rate for 1–14 cigarettes 1.43 (95% confidence interval 1.06–1.93), for 15–24 cigarettes 1.88 (1.53–2.32), 25 or more cigarettes 2.18 (1.82–2.61).

Based on established criteria, such as Bradford Hill's classic considerations for assessing causality [16] or, more recently, the Grading of Recommendations, Assessment, Development and Evaluation (GRADE) methodology [17, 18] (see Chapter 22), many would consider that the dose–response relationship between smoking and suicide supports a causal association. However, it is improbable that smoking is causally related to suicide [14]. Instead, it may be the social and mental states predisposing to suicide that

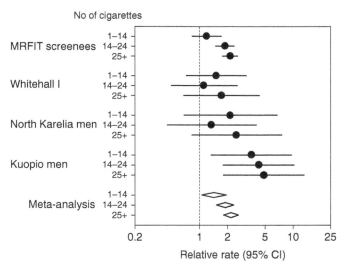

FIGURE 19.1   Adjusted relative rates of suicide among middle-aged male smokers compared to nonsmokers. Results from four cohort studies adjusted for age, and income, race, cardiovascular disease, diabetes (Multiple Risk Factor Intervention Trial: MRFIT), employment grade (Whitehall I), alcohol use, serum cholesterol, systolic blood pressure, and education (North Karelia and Kuopio). Meta-analysis by fixed-effects model. CI, confidence interval. Source: Adapted from [14].

are also associated with smoking. Factors that influence both the exposure and the disease under study (confounding factors) may thus have distorted the results. The usual approach is to adjust for confounding in the analysis. For example, any study assessing the influence of coffee consumption on the risk of myocardial infarction should make statistical adjustments for smoking. In many populations smoking is associated with drinking more coffee, and smoking is a cause of coronary heart disease [19, 20]. Even when confounding factors have been adjusted for in the analysis, as in the cohorts of smoking and suicide (Figure 19.1), *residual confounding* remains a potentially serious problem. Residual confounding arises whenever a confounding factor cannot be measured, or not be measured with sufficient precision, a situation that often occurs in epidemiological studies [21, 22]. Confounding is frequently the most important threat to the validity of results from cohort studies. Many additional difficulties, particularly selection biases, can influence cohort studies and, in addition, can be particular threats to the validity of case–control studies [23, 24]. When a disease process influences the apparent exposure, this can be especially problematic ("*reverse causality*"). Depression, for example, may make it harder to quit smoking, and since depression increases the risk of suicide, this will lead to an association between smoking and suicide.

19.2.2   Plausible but Spurious?

Implausible results, such as in the case of smoking and suicide, rarely prevent misleading conclusions: it is easy to produce plausible explanations for the results of observational research [13]. For example, researchers investigating cofactors in human immunodeficiency virus (HIV) transmission in a cohort of sex workers found a strong association between oral contraceptive use and HIV infection [25]. The authors hypothesized that the risk of transmission was higher due to "effects on the

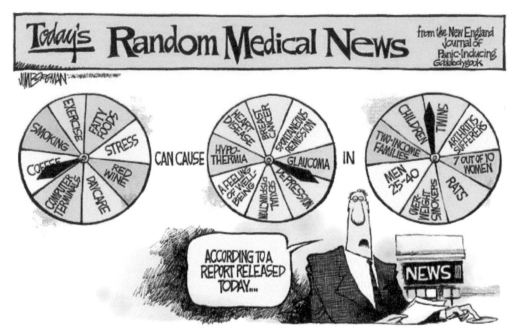

FIGURE 19.2 "Today's Random Medical News": Observational studies produce a large number of seemingly plausible associations. Some of these findings will be spurious due to bias and confounding, but they are nevertheless eagerly reported in the media. Source: Cartoon by Jim Borgman, © Hearst Corporation. Reproduced by permission.

genital mucosa, such as increasing the area of ectopy and the potential for mucosal disruption during intercourse." A cross-sectional study produced contradictory findings, indicating that contraceptives protect against the virus [26]. This finding was also considered plausible, "since progesterone-containing oral contraceptives thicken cervical mucus, which might be expected to hamper the entry of HIV." Confounding by sexual behavior or selection bias likely contributed to these discrepant findings. A cohort study among women in four African countries found no strong evidence for an association [27]. The women were asked about contraceptive use and sexual behaviors and underwent HIV testing at each quarterly visit, allowing better control of confounding. Epidemiological studies of etiology produce many seemingly plausible associations, and many are eagerly reported in the media. Figure 19.2 shows how cartoonist Jim Borgman envisages this situation.

19.2.3   Bias in Prevalence Studies: How Common Is Alcohol Consumption among Students?

Selection and information biases are central to the interpretation of prevalence studies. Selection bias will distort findings whenever the study population differs from the target population in characteristics related to the prevalence of the condition of interest [28]. Such bias is, for example, introduced when the individuals who refuse participation differ from those who participate in a study (*nonresponse bias*). For example, an alcohol consumption survey included a random sample of almost 2000 students at a university in New Zealand; 18% refused to participate [29]. More women than men participated, and the prevalence of alcohol consumption was probably underestimated because men drank more than women [29]. Among respondents, information bias may have distorted prevalence estimates due to *social desirability bias* [30]. Socially desirable responses may bias estimates due to over-reporting "good" or under-reporting "bad," undesirable behavior. Such bias is a problem in research based on self-reports of behaviors that are socially sanctioned, for example drug consumption or sexual behavior. *Recall bias* occurs when participants do not remember experiences or behaviors accurately [28]. A study of the lifetime prevalence of mental disorders in the United States found that older individuals may have had problems recalling past episodes: the prevalence of lifetime mental disorders was lower in older participants [31]. *Misclassification bias* for the measured condition is another issue in prevalence studies: the information on the presence or absence of a condition or symptom is rarely completely accurate. For example, in the case of COVID-19, the prevalence of asymptomatic SARS-CoV-2 infection depends on what symptoms are included in questionnaires [32]. In March 2020, symptoms such as loss of smell (anosmia) or taste (ageusia) were not recognized as typical for COVID-19 but were subsequently acknowledged as COVID-19 related. Patients with these symptoms may have been wrongly classified as asymptomatic in the early studies [32].

19.2.4   The Fallacy of Bigger Being Better

In a meta-analysis, the weight given to each study generally reflects the statistical power of the study: the larger the study, the greater the weight (see Chapter 9). In well-conducted RCTs, when the main problem is lack of precision in effect estimates, giving the greatest weight to studies that provide the most information is appropriate. However, in a meta-analysis of observational studies, the main problem is not lack of precision, but that some studies are more biased or confounded than others. Statistical power is not the best indicator of which study is likely to be most valid, and indeed the opposite may be the case [13]. Smaller studies can devote more attention to characterizing the exposure or condition of interest and confounding factors than can larger studies. Collecting more detailed data on fewer participants can be a better strategy for obtaining accurate results than collecting crude data on many [33]. The most informative studies are those that give the answer nearest to the correct one. This is unlikely for large but poorly conducted observational studies, including studies based on data collected for other purposes.

19.3   PREPARING THE SYSTEMATIC REVIEW

The principles and steps of systematic reviews outlined in Chapter 2 also apply to systematic reviews of observational studies of etiology or prevalence. A study protocol must be written in advance, which covers the steps and methodological approaches. A focused question needs to be formulated, inclusion and exclusion criteria defined, and studies located and assessed for eligibility. Then the risk of bias in included studies needs to be examined, and the relevant data extracted, analyzed, and reported. The confounder-adjusted estimates will be of greatest interest in etiological studies, but it is useful also to extract the unadjusted estimates [1]. In this section we discuss some aspects that are particularly relevant for systematic reviews of observational studies, drawing on COSMOS-E (Conducting Systematic Reviews and Meta-Analyses of Observational Studies of Etiology) and other guidance and literature [1, 13, 34–37].

19.3.1   Shaping the Research Question

A systematic review of observational studies requires a clear research question. It may initially be broad, but should later be narrowed down for clarity and feasibility. After formulating the question, the team should examine what evidence exists and what research has been done. This exploratory step clarifies whether the question has been addressed in a recent systematic review and whether that question should be refined and focused [1].

In line with the PICO framework (Participants, Interventions, Comparators, Outcomes) used in systematic reviews of RCTs (see Chapter 2), reviews of epidemiological studies of etiology should address a PECO (Population, Exposures, Comparators, Outcomes) framework [38]. The study population should reflect the target population to which the results should be applicable. Exposures, comparators (or comparisons), and outcomes should be clearly defined. Differences between studies in definition and measurement of exposures, such as socioeconomic position, diet, exercise, or environmental chemicals, and their comparability across studies need careful attention [1]. Similarly, many outcomes can be defined, classified, or measured differently, such as diseases (breast cancer, thrombosis, diabetes mellitus) or health-related states (quality of life, levels of risk factors).

A PC (Population, Condition) framework is appropriate for prevalence studies, carefully defining the (target) population and the condition of interest. The definition of the population should clearly distinguish between general population and health care settings. It should consider the setting in some detail, for example the level of health care (primary care, hospital etc.), the specific population (for example, an immigrant community), the geographic context (for example, urban or rural), or a season or calendar period (for example, a wave of SARS-Cov-2 infections) [34].

19.3.2   The Protocol

Plans for every systematic review should be described clearly and transparently in a protocol. For systematic reviews of observational studies, the protocol should always include a list of biases that could distort results, and for systematic reviews of etiological questions should include a *list of potential confounders* [1]. While reviewers should take care not to change the protocol based on study results, writing a protocol for a systematic review of observational studies will often be iterative, informed by scoping the literature and piloting procedures. Registering the protocol in the International Prospective Register of Systematic Reviews (PROSPERO) [39] or publishing it in advance in a journal or on a preprint server increases transparency.

19.3.3   Searching for Relevant Studies

Considerable progress has been made in identifying RCTs for systematic reviews (see Chapter 3). Procedures for identifying other types of studies are less well developed, but some general principles apply to any systematic review. Searches should be developed based on (i) the concepts in the review question (PECO or PC); (ii) the search terms that will capture the concepts; and (iii) the relevant bibliographic databases and other sources to be searched. Using all PECO concepts in a review of etiology risks missing relevant records: Population and Exposure should generally be covered, whereas Comparators and Outcomes may be left out to increase the sensitivity of the search. A concept to capture the study design may be added. The Information Specialists' Sub-Group (ISSG) Search Filter Resource collates search filters grouped by study design. Similarly, SuRe Info provides information on identifying different types of studies for systematic reviews [40]. Text mining tools are increasingly used to build search strategies [41]. Reviewers should seek advice from experienced librarians or information specialists to develop and implement the search strategy in different bibliographic databases. Chapter 3 provides details on and links to relevant resources.

19.3.4   Assessing Quality, Risk of Bias, and Study Sensitivity

The assessment of methodological aspects of studies is crucial in systematic reviews of observational studies. The term *study quality* is often used in this context, but it is important to distinguish between quality and *risk of bias* (see also Chapter 4). The quality will be high if the authors have performed the best possible study. However, a high-quality study may still be at high risk of bias. The above-mentioned study [27] of contraceptive use and HIV infection among African women had to rely on self-reported information on sexual behavior, potentially introducing (social desirability) bias [30].

How should the risk of bias in observational studies be assessed? The authors of a 2007 review of over 80 different tools concluded that there is no "single obvious candidate tool for assessing the quality of observational epidemiological studies" [42]. This is not surprising considering the many study designs, contexts, and research questions in observational research. As discussed in Chapter 15, the ROBINS-I (Risk Of Bias In Nonrandomized Studies of Interventions) tool was designed to assess the risk of bias in nonrandomized studies of interventions [43]. A similar instrument for longitudinal studies of exposures, ROBINS-E (Risk Of Bias In Nonrandomized Studies of Exposure), is under development [44]. The ROBINS tools illustrate that a one-size-fits-all approach is misguided. Instead, a set of criteria should be developed for each observational study design, guided by the general principles outlined in Box 19.2. Assessments of prevalence studies should focus on the degree of representativity of the sample, which may have been affected by nonresponse or other selection bias. Depending on the context, assessments should also consider information biases such as social desirability or misclassification bias.

Box 19.2   Seven Principles for Risk of Bias Assessment of Observational Studies

1. **The relevant types of bias should be identified**, separately for each review question and for different study designs, including potential confounding, selection bias, and information bias.

2. **The risk of bias should be assessed qualitatively**, for example as "low risk," "moderate risk," or "high risk." Quantitative assessments by assigning points should be avoided.

3. **Signaling questions may be helpful** to support judgments about the risk of bias. For example, addressing the question "Did the authors control for all the important confounders?" will help assess potential confounding. Signaling questions have been compiled for nonrandomized studies of interventions [43].

4. **Separate assessments may have to be made for different outcomes**. For example, bias in the ascertainment of death from all causes is less likely than for subjective outcomes, such as quality of life or pain, or an outcome that relies on clinical judgment, such as pneumonia.

5. **Assessments should be documented** by copying and archiving the text from the article on which an assessment is based. Such documentation increases transparency, facilitates discussion in case of disagreement, and allows replication of assessments.

6. **Summary scores should be avoided**. Typically, each scale item is weighted equally (0 or 1 point), but the importance of a bias will depend on the context [45]. The situation is made worse if the scale includes items that are not consistently related to bias, as in the case of the Newcastle–Ottawa Scale [46].

7. **Thinking about a hypothetical, unbiased trial may be helpful**. As a thought experiment, design a hypothetical RCT that would answer the review question posed in the systematic review [43]. Such a trial will often be unfeasible and unethical, but the thought experiment may help to sharpen the review question and clarify the potential biases in the observational studies.

Source: Adapted from Dekkers et al. [1].

The concept of *study sensitivity* [47] refers to the ability of studies to detect a true effect and is closer to study quality than the risk of bias. If the study is negative, does this really mean that there is no association between exposure and outcome? For example, were there sufficient numbers of exposed persons, and were the levels of exposure and length of follow-up adequate to detect an effect? Study sensitivity is particularly relevant in occupational and environmental epidemiology and of concern in pharmaco-epidemiology, for example in the context of adverse effects of drugs (Chapter 15). Reviewers should assess both the risk of bias and study sensitivity in reviews of observational studies.

19.3.5 Analysis and Interpretation

Some have argued that meta-analysis of observational studies should be abandoned altogether [48]. We disagree, but think that the statistical combination of studies in a meta-analysis should be a less prominent component of systematic reviews of observational studies, including reviews of etiology or prevalence. Instead, the thorough consideration of heterogeneity between study results will provide more insights than the mechanistic calculation of an overall measure of effect, which may often be biased.

19.3.5.1 Exploring Sources of Heterogeneity

Chapter 10 discusses the sources of clinical and methodological diversity that may lead to statistical heterogeneity and how to examine such heterogeneity in subgroup and meta-regression analyses. Here we illustrate the importance of methodological heterogeneity in meta-analyses of observational studies, using a few examples from the literature [13]. Consider etiological investigation of the effect of diet on breast cancer. The hypothesis arising from ecological analyses [49] that a higher intake of saturated fat could increase the risk of breast cancer generated much observational research, often with contradictory results. A meta-analysis [50] showed an association among case–control but not among cohort studies (Figure 19.3). This discrepancy was also shown in two separate meta-analyses of cohort and case–control studies [53, 54]. It seems likely that biases in the recall of dietary items and the selection of study participants produced a spurious association in case–control studies [54].

A meta-analysis of case–control studies of intermittent sunlight exposure and melanoma also showed evidence that differential recall of past exposures introduced bias [51] (Figure 19.3). Only a small effect was evident when combining studies in which some blinding to the study hypothesis was achieved. Conversely, in studies without blinding, the effect was considerably greater.

In occupational epidemiology, the quest to demonstrate a dose–response relationship can lead to very different groups of employees being compared. In a meta-analysis examining formaldehyde exposure and cancer, funeral directors and embalmers (higher exposure) were compared with anatomists and pathologists (intermediate exposure) and industrial workers (lower exposure) [52]. As shown in Figure 19.3, there is a striking deficit of lung cancer deaths among anatomists and pathologists, most likely due to a lower prevalence of smoking among this group. In this situation, few would argue that formaldehyde protects against lung cancer, but such selection bias may be less obvious in other instances.

The examples so far related to epidemiological studies of etiology and used subgroup analyses. The final example relates to studies of the prevalence of genital chlamydia infection in high-income countries, using meta-regression [55]. The authors examined whether estimated chlamydia prevalence differed according to the response rate in each population-based survey. There was evidence that chlamydia prevalence was lower in surveys with higher response rates in both women and men (Figure 19.4). The authors concluded that surveys of genital chlamydia prevalence are at risk of overestimating the prevalence of infection due to low response rates [55].

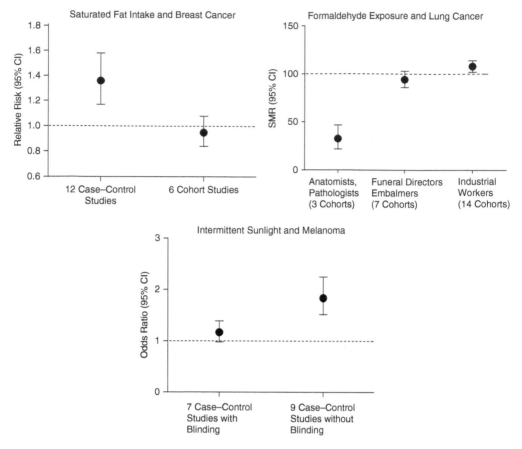

FIGURE 19.3   Examples of heterogeneity in published observational meta-analyses: saturated fat intake and breast cancer [50], intermittent sunlight and melanoma [51], and formaldehyde exposure and lung cancer [52]. CI, confidence interval; SMR, standardized mortality ratio. Source: Adapted from [13].

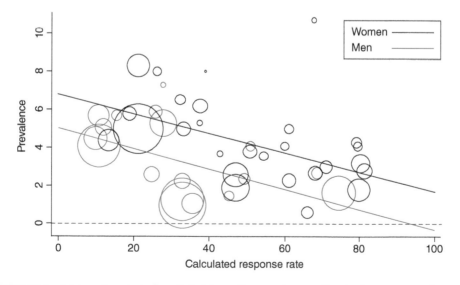

FIGURE 19.4   Meta-regression of genital chlamydia prevalence estimates in women and men against response rates in population-based studies from high-income countries (women, P = 0.003; men, P = 0.018 for slope). The size of the open circle corresponds to the precision of the prevalence estimate. Source: Adapted from [55].

In these examples, sources of methodological heterogeneity were explored at the level of study characteristics in sensitivity analyses (see Chapter 2) to test the stability of findings across different study designs, exposure assessments, and selection of study participants. Subgroup analysis and meta-regression based on averages of participant characteristics (such as the average age of all the participants) are also widely used. For example, the severity of COVID-19 was associated with the prevalence of right ventricular dysfunction in meta-regression [56]. Other meta-regression analyses found an exponential relationship between study-level average age and SARS-CoV-2 infection fatality [57], or an increase with average age of the length of median incubation [58]. As discussed in detail in Chapter 10, subgroup and meta-regression analyses based on study characteristics or participant characteristics aggregated at the level of the study may be affected by confounding or bias (for example, aggregation bias) and should be interpreted with caution. Analyzing individual participant data (IPD) from each study provides a stronger basis for exploring how effects vary according to participant characteristics such as age and disease severity (see Chapter 12).

19.3.5.2   Statistical Considerations

The general principles of meta-analysis and the commonly used statistical methods are discussed in Chapter 9 and are applicable to observational studies of etiology, with the provisos that between-study heterogeneity will often be pronounced and that the focus should be on exploring sources of heterogeneity. Similarly, the subgroup analyses and meta-regression approaches to explore sources of heterogeneity discussed in Chapter 10 are central in meta-analyses of etiological studies. A widespread issue in etiological studies is that results are presented as dose–response relationships or as associations for each of several ordered exposure categories in relation to a reference category. Methods for analyzing these data are discussed in Chapter 14.

Specific statistical issues arise in the context of prevalence studies [34, 59]. Due to the constrained range of proportions between 0 and 1, their mathematical properties are poor, and prevalence estimates from different studies need to be transformed, using, for example, the logit, arcsine, or double arcsine transformation. The proportions and confidence limits are then back-transformed to facilitate presentation and interpretation. There are advantages and disadvantages to different transformations, for example in the context of small sample sizes [59, 60]. Schwarzer and Rücker discuss these transformations in detail and provide relevant guidance [59]. Models that use the binomial distribution for the likelihood of the observed events have better properties than other models and are preferred to fit random-effects meta-analysis and meta-regression analysis of proportions extracted from prevalence studies [61]. One of these models is the binomial-normal model, which is available in many statistical software packages, including Stata and R (see Chapters 25 and 26).

19.4   TRIANGULATION OF EVIDENCE

Triangulation of different types of evidence is increasingly used in biomedical and other research [62, 63]. Triangulation embraces the variety of evidence thesis (VET) that inferential strength depends not only on the quantity of available evidence, but also on its variety: the greater the variety, the stronger the resulting support [64]. An essential condition is that the systematic errors and biases are unrelated across different study types [63, 65, 66]. For example, the effect of inhibiting HMGCoA reductase on the risk of coronary heart disease can be estimated from RCTs of statins or through Mendelian randomization using genetic variants related to HMGCoA activity. Both the results of RCTs (see Chapter 4) and Mendelian randomization studies could be biased [67, 68]. However, the potential biases in one study design would not influence estimates of the other approach: the biases are unrelated to each other.

When biases are unrelated, it may be possible to obtain two or more estimates using different estimation strategies from the same single study sample; these have been referred to as "evidence factors," which can be meta-analyzed to increase statistical power [69]. An example is a study based on the UK Biobank of the effect of years of education on health and health behavior [70]. Two different instrumental variables were used. The first was based on a natural experiment, the 1972 schooling reform in the UK, which raised the minimum school leaving age, and the second used Mendelian randomization. The two estimates could legitimately be meta-analyzed in these circumstances. The development of triangulation approaches is currently most advanced within epidemiology [62, 71, 72], but developing the methods for appropriately combining such data is still in its infancy.

19.5   CONCLUSION

The suggestion that formal meta-analysis of epidemiological studies of etiology or prevalence can be misleading and that insufficient attention is often given to heterogeneity does not mean that a return to the previous practice of highly subjective reviews is called for. Many of the principles of systematic reviews remain: a study protocol should be written in advance, complete literature searches should be carried out, and studies should be selected in a reproducible and objective fashion. The best practices and recommendations regarding the conduct of systematic reviews and meta-analyses of observational studies are less well defined than for RCTs, and there is substantial variability in practices [35–37]. Clearly, IPD will often be required to allow differences and similarities of the results found in different settings to be examined thoroughly, hypotheses to be formulated, and the need for future studies, including RCTs, to be defined.

ACKNOWLEDGMENTS

We thank Georgia Salanti, Nicola Low, and Julian Higgins for helpful comments on a previous version of this chapter. We are grateful to Jim Neaton (MRFIT Research Group), Juha Pekkanen, and Erkki Vartiainen (North Karelia and Kuopio Cohorts) and Martin Shipley (Whitehall Study) for providing additional data on suicides. This chapter draws on material published earlier in the *BMJ* [13] and on the guidance on Conducting Systematic Reviews and Meta-Analyses of Observational Studies of Etiology (COSMOS-E) [1].

REFERENCES

1. Dekkers, O.M., Vandenbroucke, J.P., Cevallos, M. et al. (2019). COSMOS-E: guidance on conducting systematic reviews and meta-analyses of observational studies of etiology. *PLoS Med.* 16: e1002742. https://doi.org/10.1371/journal.pmed.1002742.

2. Vandenbroucke, J.P., Von Elm, E., Altman, D.G. et al. (2007). Strengthening the reporting of observational studies in epidemiology (STROBE): explanation and elaboration. *PLoS Med.* 4: https://doi.org/10.1371/journal.pmed.0040297.

3. Hernan, M.A. and Robins, J.M. (2006). Instruments for causal inference: an epidemiologist's dream? *Epidemiology* 17: 360–372. https://doi.org/10.1097/01.ede.0000222409.00878.37.

4. Rassen, J.A., Brookhart, M.A., Glynn, R.J. et al. (2009). Instrumental variables I: instrumental variables exploit natural variation in nonexperimental data to estimate causal relationships. *J. Clin. Epidemiol.* 62: 1226–1232. https://doi.org/10.1016/j.jclinepi.2008.12.005.

5. Lawlor, D.A., Harbord, R.M., Sterne, J.A.C. et al. (2008). Mendelian randomization: using genes as instruments for making causal inferences in epidemiology. *Stat. Med.* 27: 1133–1163. https://doi.org/10.1002/sim.3034.

6. Petersen, I., Douglas, I., and Whitaker, H. (2016). Self controlled case series methods: an alternative to standard epidemiological study designs. *BMJ* 354: i4515. https://doi.org/10.1136/bmj.i4515.

7. Hariton, E. and Locascio, J.J. (2018). Randomised controlled trials—the gold standard for effectiveness research. *BJOG* 125: 1716. https://doi.org/10.1111/1471-0528.15199.

8. Feinstein, A.R. (1988). Scientific standards in epidemiological studies of the menace of daily life. *Science* 242: 1257–1263.

9. Rose, G. (1985). Sick individuals and sick populations. *Int. J. Epidemiol.* 14: 32–38.

10. Institute for Health Metrics and Evaluation (2014). GBD history. http://www.healthdata.org/gbd/about/history (accessed January 16, 2022).

11. IHME (2020). *Protocol for the Global Burden of Diseases, Injuries, and Risk Factors Study (GBD).* Seattle, WA: Institute for Health Metrics and Evaluation.

12. Black, N. (1996). Why we need observational studies to evaluate the effectiveness of health care. *Br. Med. J.* 312: 1215–1218.

13. Egger, M., Schneider, M., and Davey, S.G. (1998). Spurious precision? Meta-analysis of observational studies. *Br. Med. J.* 316: 140–145.

14. Davey Smith, G., Phillips, A.N., and Neaton, J.D. (1992). Smoking as "independent" risk factor for suicide: illustration of an artifact from observational epidemiology. *Lancet* 340: 709–711.

15. Multiple Risk Factor Intervention Trial Research Group. (1982). Multiple Risk Factor Intervention Trial. Risk Factor Changes and Mortality Results. *JAMA* 248: 1465–1477.

16. Hill, A.B. (1965). The environment and disease: association or causation? *Proc. R. Soc. Med.* 58: 295–300.

17. Guyatt, G.H., Oxman, A.D., Sultan, S. et al. (2011). GRADE guidelines: 9. Rating up the quality of evidence. *J. Clin. Epidemiol.* 64: 1311–1316. https://doi.org/10.1016/j.jclinepi.2011.06.004.

18. Shimonovich, M., Pearce, A., Thomson, H. et al. (2020). Assessing causality in epidemiology: revisiting Bradford Hill to incorporate developments in causal thinking. *Eur. J. Epidemiol.* https://doi.org/10.1007/s10654-020-00703-7.

19. Leviton, A., Pagano, M., Allred, E.N., and El Lozy, M. (1994). Why those who drink the most coffee appear to be at increased risk of disease: a modest proposal. *Ecol. Food Nutr.* 31: 285–293.

20. Bjorngaard, J.H., Nordestgaard, A.T., Taylor, A.E. et al. (2017). Heavier smoking increases coffee consumption: findings from a Mendelian randomization analysis. *Int. J. Epidemiol.* 46: 1958–1967. https://doi.org/10.1093/ije/dyx147.

21. Davey Smith, G., Phillips, A.N. (1992). Confounding in epidemiological studies: why "independent" effects may not be all they seem. *Br. Med. J.* 305: 757–759.

22. Fewell, Z., Davey Smith, G., and Sterne, J.A.C. (2007). The impact of residual and unmeasured confounding in epidemiologic studies: a simulation study. *Am. J. Epidemiol.* 166: 646–655. https://doi.org/10.1093/aje/kwm165.

23. Sackett, D.L. (1979). Bias in analytical research. *J. Chronic Dis.* 32: 51–63.

24. Kopec, J.A. and Esdaile, J.M. (1990). Bias in case-control studies. A review. *J. Epidemiol. Community Health* 44: 179–186. https://doi.org/10.1136/jech.44.3.179.

25. Plummer, F.A., Simonsen, J.N., Cameron, D. et al. (1991). Cofactors in male-female sexual transmission of human immunodeficiency virus type 1. *J. Infect. Dis.* 233: 233–239.

26. Lazzarin, A., Saracco, A., Musicco, M., and Nicolosi, A. (1991). Man-to-woman sexual transmission of the human immunodeficiency virus. *Arch. Intern. Med.* 151: 2411–2416.

27. Balkus, J.E., Brown, E.R., Hillier, S.L. et al. (2016). Oral and injectable contraceptive use and HIV acquisition risk among women in four African countries: a secondary analysis of data from a microbicide trial. *Contraception* 93: 25–31. https://doi.org/10.1016/j.contraception.2015.10.010.

28. Catalogue of Bias (2017). Welcome to the Catalogue of Bias. https://catalogofbias.org (accessed January 16, 2022).

29. Kypri, K., Stephenson, S., and Langley, J. (2004). Assessment of nonresponse bias in an internet survey of alcohol use. *Alcohol. Clin. Exp. Res.* 28: 630–634. https://doi.org/10.1097/01.ALC.0000121654.99277.26.

30. Tourangeau, R. and Yan, T. (2007). Sensitive questions in surveys. *Psychol. Bull.* 133: 859–883. https://doi.org/10.1037/0033-2909.133.5.859.

31. Kessler, R.C., Berglund, P., Demler, O. et al. (2005). Lifetime prevalence and age-of-onset distributions of DSM-IV disorders in the National Comorbidity Survey Replication. *Arch. Gen. Psychiatry* 62: 593–602. https://doi.org/10.1001/archpsyc.62.6.593.

32. Buitrago-Garcia, D., Egli-Gany, D., Counotte, M.J. et al. (2020). Occurrence and transmission potential of asymptomatic and presymptomatic SARS-CoV-2 infections: a living systematic review and meta-analysis. *PLoS Med.* 17: e1003346. https://doi.org/10.1371/journal.pmed.1003346.

33. Phillips, A.N. and Davey Smith, G. (1993). The design of prospective epidemiological studies: more subjects or better measurements? *J. Clin. Epidemiol.* 46: 1203–1211.

34. Munn, Z., Moola, S., Lisy, K. et al. (2015). Methodological guidance for systematic reviews of observational epidemiological studies reporting prevalence and cumulative incidence data. *Int. J. Evid. Based Healthc.* 13: 147–153. https://doi.org/10.1097/XEB.0000000000000054.

35. Hoffmann, F., Eggers, D., Pieper, D. et al. (2020). An observational study found large methodological heterogeneity in systematic reviews addressing prevalence and cumulative incidence. *J. Clin. Epidemiol.* 119: 92–99. https://doi.org/10.1016/j.jclinepi.2019.12.003.

36. Borges Migliavaca, C., Stein, C., Colpani, V. et al. (2020). How are systematic reviews of prevalence conducted? A methodological study. *BMC Med. Res. Methodol.* 20: 96. https://doi.org/10.1186/s12874-020-00975-3.

37. Mueller, M., D'Addario, M., Egger, M. et al. (2018). Methods to systematically review and meta-analyse observational studies: a systematic scoping review of recommendations. *BMC Med. Res. Methodol.* 18: 44. https://doi.org/10.1186/s12874-018-0495-9.

38. Morgan, R.L., Whaley, P., Thayer. K.A., and Schünemann, H.J. (2018) Identifying the PECO: a framework for formulating good questions to explore the association of environmental and other exposures with health outcomes. *Environ. Int.* https://doi.org/10.1016/j.envint.2018.07.015.

39. Booth, A., Clarke, M., Dooley, G. et al. (2012). The nuts and bolts of PROSPERO: an international prospective register of systematic reviews. *Syst. Rev.* 1: 2. https://doi.org/10.1186/2046-4053-1-2.

40. Ormstad, S. and Isojarvi, J. (2013). Keeping up to date with information retrieval research: summarized research in). *J. Eur. Assoc. Health Info. Libr.* 9: 17–19.

41. Paynter, R.A., Featherstone, R., Stoeger, E. et al. (2021). A prospective comparison of evidence synthesis search strategies developed with and without text-mining tools. *J. Clin. Epidemiol.* https://doi.org/10.1016/j.jclinepi.2021.03.013.

42. Sanderson, S., Tatt, I.D., and Higgins, J.P.T. (2007). Tools for assessing quality and susceptibility to bias in observational studies in epidemiology: a systematic review and annotated bibliography. *Int. J. Epidemiol.* 36: 666–676. https://doi.org/10.1093/ije/dym018.

43. Sterne, J.A., Hernán, M.A., Reeves, B.C. et al. (2016). ROBINS-I: a tool for assessing risk of bias in non-randomised studies of interventions. *BMJ (Online)* 355: i4919. https://doi.org/10.1136/bmj.i4919.

44. Risk of Bias (2021). Risk of bias tools. https://www.riskofbias.info/welcome (accessed January 16, 2022).

45. Juni, P., Witschi, A., Bloch, R., and Egger, M. (1999). The hazards of scoring the quality of clinical trials for meta-analysis. *JAMA* 282: 1054–1060. https://doi.org/10.1001/jama.282.11.1054.

46. Stang, A. (2010). Critical evaluation of the Newcastle-Ottawa scale for the assessment of the quality of nonrandomized studies in meta-analyses. *Eur. J. Epidemiol.* 25: 603–605. https://doi.org/10.1007/s10654-010-9491-z.

47. Cooper, G.S., Lunn, R.M., Agerstrand, M. et al. (2016). Study sensitivity: evaluating the ability to detect effects in systematic reviews of chemical exposures. *Environ. Int.* 92–93: 605–610. https://doi.org/10.1016/j.envint.2016.03.017.

48. Shapiro, S. (1994). Meta-analysis/Shmeta-analysis. *Am. J. Epidemiol.* 140: 771–778.

49. Armstrong, B. and Doll, R. (1975). Environmental factors and cancer incidence and mortality in different countries with special reference to dietary practices. *Int. J. Cancer* 15: 617–631.

50. Boyd, N.F., Martin, L.J., Noffel, M. et al. (1993). A meta-analysis of studies of dietary fat and breast cancer risk. *Br. J. Cancer* 68: 627–636. https://doi.org/10.1038/bjc.1993.398.

51. Nelemans, P.J., Rampen, F.H.J., Ruiter, D.J., and Verbeek, A.L.M. (1995). An addition to the controversy on sunlight exposure and melanoma risk: a meta-analytical approach. *J. Clin. Epidemiol.* 48: 1331–1342.

52. Blair, A., Saracci, R., Stewart, P.A. et al. (1990). Epidemiologic evidence on the relationship between formaldehyde exposure and cancer. *Scand. J. Work Environ. Health* 16: 381–393.

53. Howe, G.R., Hirohata, T., Hislop, T.G. et al. (1990). Dietary factors and risk of breast cancer: combined analysis of 12 case-control studies. *J. Natl. Cancer Inst.* 82: 561–569.

54. Hunter, D.J., Spiegelman, D., Adami, H.O. et al. (1996). Cohort studies of fat intake and the risk of breast cancer - a pooled analysis. *N. Engl. J. Med.* 334: 356–361.

55. Redmond, S.M., Alexander-Kisslig, K., Woodhall, S.C. et al. (2015). Genital chlamydia prevalence in Europe and non-European high income countries: systematic review and meta-analysis. *PLoS One* 10: e0115753. https://doi.org/10.1371/journal.pone.0115753.

56. Corica, B., Marra, A.M., Basili, S. et al. (2021). Prevalence of right ventricular dysfunction and impact on all-cause death in hospitalized patients with COVID-19: a systematic review and meta-analysis. *Sci. Rep.* 11: 17774. https://doi.org/10.1038/s41598-021-96955-8.

57. Levin, A.T., Hanage, W.P., Owusu-Boaitey, N. et al. (2020). Assessing the age specificity of infection fatality rates for COVID-19: systematic review, meta-analysis, and public policy implications. *Eur. J. Epidemiol.* 35: 1123–1138. https://doi.org/10.1007/s10654-020-00698-1.

58. Wei, Y., Wei, L., Liu, Y. et al. (2021). Comprehensive estimation for the length and dispersion of COVID-19 incubation period: a systematic review and meta-analysis. *Infection* https://doi.org/10.1007/s15010-021-01682-x.

59. Schwarzer, G. and Rücker, G. (2022). Meta-analysis of proportions. In: *Meta-Research: Methods and Protocols* (ed. E. Evangelou and A.A. Veroniki), 159–172. New York: Springer. https://doi.org/10.1007/978-1-0716-1566-9_10.

60. Barendregt, J.J., Doi, S.A., Lee, Y.Y. et al. (2013). Meta-analysis of prevalence. *J. Epidemiol. Community Health* 67: 974–978. https://doi.org/10.1136/jech-2013-203104.

61. Stijnen, T., Hamza, T.H., and Özdemir, P. (2010). Random effects meta-analysis of event outcome in the framework of the generalized linear mixed model with applications in sparse data. *Stat. Med.* 29: 3046–3067. https://doi.org/10.1002/sim.4040.

62. Lawlor, D.A., Tilling, K., and Davey Smith, G. (2016). Triangulation in aetiological epidemiology. *Int. J. Epidemiol.* 45: 1866–1886. https://doi.org/10.1093/ije/dyw314.

63. Kuorikoski, J. and Marchionni, C. (2016). Evidential diversity and the triangulation of phenomena. *Philos. Sci.* 83: 227–247. https://doi.org/10.1086/684960.

64. Hempel, C. (1966). *Philosophy of Natural Science*. Hoboken, NJ: Prentice Hall.

65. Hey, S.P. (2015). Robust and discordant evidence: methodological lessons from clinical research. *Philos. Sci.* https://doi.org/10.1086/678978.

66. Schupbach, J.N. (2016). Robustness analysis as explanatory reasoning. *Br. J. Philos. Sci.* axw008. https://doi.org/10.1093/bjps/axw008.

67. Davey Smith, G. and Ebrahim, S. (2003). "Mendelian randomization": can genetic epidemiology contribute to understanding environmental determinants of disease? *Int. J. Epidemiol.* 32: 1–22.

68. Skrivankova, V.W., Richmond, R.C., Woolf, B.A.R. et al. (2021). Strengthening the reporting of observational studies in epidemiology using mendelian randomisation (STROBE-MR): explanation and elaboration. *BMJ* n2233. https://doi.org/10.1136/bmj.n2233.

69. Karmakar, B., Small, D.S., and Rosenbaum, P.R. (2020). Using evidence factors to clarify exposure biomarkers. *Am. J. Epidemiol.* 189: 243–249. https://doi.org/10.1093/aje/kwz263.

70. Davies, N.M., Dickson, M., Davey Smith, G. et al. (2019). *The Causal Effects of Education on Adult Health, Mortality and Income: Evidence from Mendelian Randomization and the Raising of the School Leaving Age.* Rochester, NY: Social Science Research Network. https://doi.org/10.2139/ssrn.3390179.

71. Matthay, E.C., Hagan, E., Gottlieb, L.M. et al. (2020). Alternative causal inference methods in population health research: evaluating tradeoffs and triangulating evidence. *SSM - Popul. Health* 10: 100526. https://doi.org/10.1016/j.ssmph.2019.100526.

72. Hammerton, G. and Munafo, M.R. (2021). Causal inference with observational data: the need for triangulation of evidence. *Psychol. Med.* 51: 563–578. https://doi.org/10.1017/S0033291720005127.

Meta-Analysis in Genetic Association Studies

Gibran Hemani

There have been two major medical incentives for identifying genetic associations with complex traits and diseases. First, identification of genomic locations (loci) that influence a trait can provide information about the biological processes, or their disruptions, that lead to disease. Such knowledge can aid in the development of new drugs. Second, genetic variants can be used as predictors of disease. Complex traits are substantially heritable (typical range is 20–80%) [1–3], meaning that the total set of genetic variants that underlie the trait can explain that much of the trait variation or disease liability. As more genetic factors for a trait are identified, the accuracy of the genetic predictor improves. Genetic associations have value in other areas; for example, they can be used as instrumental variables in epidemiological studies to infer the causal relationships between different traits (see also Chapter 19).

Prior to genetic association studies, the predominant method for identifying genetic loci involved in phenotypes was linkage analysis [4]. Linkage studies are designed around genotyping markers in samples of related individuals. If a genetic locus is involved in the trait, then individuals within a family who share the same alleles at that marker will be more phenotypically similar. While linkage analysis is an elegant statistical formulation of the problem in comparison to population-based association studies, its statistical power is low [5].

The new millennium emerged from a decade of putative findings from linkage analysis that failed to be replicated [6]. In this chapter, we chart the transition from linkage to association-based study designs and then describe how meta-analysis has been central to the key successes that have emerged from the genome-wide association study (GWAS) era. Most importantly, meta-analysis has been crucial because of the combination of two factors: (i) complex traits and diseases are typically influenced

Systematic Reviews in Health Research: Meta-Analysis in Context, Third Edition. Edited by Matthias Egger, Julian P.T. Higgins, and George Davey Smith.
© 2022 John Wiley & Sons Ltd. Published 2022 by John Wiley & Sons Ltd.
Companion website: www.systematic-reviews3.org

by thousands of genetic variants, each of which has extremely small effects; and (ii) legal obstacles often prevent the sharing of individual-level genetic data from multiple studies. To enable the sample sizes of GWAS to grow to sufficient magnitudes that allow the detection of small genetic effects, results from many separate studies are meta-analyzed, generating overall results with sample sizes that now routinely exceed 100 000 individuals, and for some traits the sample sizes are numbered in the millions.

The practical implementation of meta-analysis for GWAS has been discussed elsewhere [7, 8]. GWAS meta-analyses are typically undertaken either within large consortia of primary researchers or based on online databases of aggregated data from multiple studies [9]. Of note is that such approaches are in contrast to the types of systematic reviews discussed in much of the rest of this book: GWAS meta-analyses are not usually based on systematic searches of the literature, and formal assessments of study quality or risk of bias are seldom undertaken.

20.1 STUDY DESIGNS FOR DETECTING GENETIC ASSOCIATIONS

20.1.1 Natural Genetic Variation

There are approximately 70 de novo mutations per newborn child, and these arise at random throughout the genome [10]. Over many generations, a new allele can replace the original allele within the population, or it can go extinct. The fate of an allele is determined by the effective population size, its response to natural selection, and chance. Statistical genetics is interested in those genomic positions that are polymorphic, where the new allele is present in the population alongside the original allele. By convention, we label the allele that is most frequent in the population as the major allele, and the other allele as the minor allele. Differences that involve a single base-pair change are known as a single-nucleotide polymorphism (SNP).

There are approximately 15 million known SNPs across the human genome, for which the least common allele is present in at least 1% of the chromosomes in the population [11]. An SNP with minor allele frequency (MAF) >1% is known as a common variant, whereas those with MAF <1% are known as rare variants. The major focus of GWAS has been on common variants, for three reasons. First, they can be assayed more reliably using SNP chip technology than rare variants [12]; second, they have greater statistical power for detecting associations [13]; and third, the common-disease common-variant hypothesis postulates that common SNPs contribute the majority of the genetic influence to common diseases [14].

20.1.2 Testing for Genetic Association Between a Trait and a Causal Variant

Genetic association studies are conducted using samples of "unrelated" individuals. The most widely used model to relate SNPs to traits is also the simplest, assuming that the alleles influence the phenotype in an additive manner. Supposing that a SNP has two alleles, A and G, with G being the minor allele. Because humans have two copies of each chromosome, there are three possible genotypes: AA, AG, and GG. An additive genetic model assumes that if the G allele influences the phenotype by some amount β, then individuals who are homozygous for the G allele (i.e. having two copies of the G allele) will have a mean value of 2β; and individuals who are heterozygous (i.e. only having one copy of the G allele) will have a mean value of β.

To conduct such a genetic association test, we re-code the genetic variant into "additive" (also known as "dosage") format. Here, instead of labeling individuals as AA, AG, or GG, we label them by counting how many G alleles the individual has. Those who are homozygous for the A allele will therefore have a numeric value of 0 G alleles, heterozygotes will have 1 G allele, and homozygotes for the G allele will have a value of 2. This numeric vector is regressed against the trait value, and the regression coefficient provides an estimate of β.

Age and sex are typically included as covariates to reduce residual variation and increase power. Covariates are also included to reduce the risk of confounding due to population structure. Here the concern is that subsets of individuals in a sample from distinct geographic regions can have different disease prevalence due to nongenetic factors. At the same time, they will have systematically different patterns of genetic polymorphisms due to ancestry. This confounding, known as population stratification, will lead to spurious genetic associations. To minimize the effects of confounding due to population stratification, we use the SNP data to estimate the geographic ancestry of each individual and include those estimates of ancestry as covariates [15].

20.1.3   Linkage Disequilibrium Aids Detection of Causal Variants

If genotyping technology fails to include the causal variant – the SNP that actually has the biological influence on the trait – then genetic association studies can still find an association [16]. The additive effect of an SNP can be estimated using a marker that is close to the causal variant. Genetic inheritance operates such that an individual receives one copy of a chromosome from their mother, and one from their father. However, due to the recombination during meiosis, neither of these copies is identical to a chromosome of a parent. Rather, the maternally inherited chromosome is a mixture of chromosome segments from the maternal grandparents. The same applies to the paternally inherited chromosome.

During meiosis, there are on average 100 recombination events across the genome. As a consequence, the chance that a particular causal variant on a chromosome is co-inherited with a genetic marker diminishes as the genetic marker gets further from the causal variant. This process of inheritance within families, when repeated over many generations in a randomly mating population, leads to a distinct correlation pattern between SNPs. A genetic marker on a different chromosome to the causal variant is completely uninformative about that causal variant; it is in linkage equilibrium, often denoted by $r_{LD}^2 = 0$. The closer together two SNPs are located on the same chromosome, the higher the chance that there is nonrandom association of the alleles at these loci. Complete nonrandomness, where each allele at one locus is only co-inherited with one allele at another locus, is known as complete linkage disequilibrium (LD), denoted $r_{LD}^2 = 1$.

If a marker is informative about a causal variant, then it depends on being in LD with the causal variant. In fact, the power to detect an association reduces linearly with decreasing LD [17].

20.1.4   The Failure of Candidate Gene Studies

Early genetic association analyses took the form of candidate gene studies [18]. Here, a few genotypes are assayed in a sample at a gene region with some a priori biological candidacy for involvement in the trait. This approach had two advantages over searching for loci across the whole genome in a hypothesis-free manner: (i) for a given financial cost, more samples could be genotyped at a few loci; and (ii) a high multiple-testing penalty could be avoided. And yet, though many associations were reported in the literature, like with linkage analysis independent replication was seldom achieved [19].

Many systematic reviews and meta-analyses were performed of these candidate gene studies [20], encouraged in part by the Human Genome Epidemiology Network [21]. However, the replication rate of candidate gene studies was poor. This was typically attributed to population stratification, as well as publication bias [22, 23]. These problems aside, with the benefit of hindsight, it is clear that the experimental design of candidate gene studies was not conducive to identifying genetic variants that influence complex traits. Genes earmarked for being biologically related to a trait are often based on gene knockout studies in model organisms. Even if this evidence translated to human traits, for genetic associations to identify such effects there must be (i) a genetic variant within the gene that has a sufficiently large effect size to be detectable; and (ii) a genetic marker used by the study that is in LD with the causal variant. Importantly, the vast majority of genetic variants are neutral with respect to their influences on gene function. It was soon realized that using a hypothesis-free search for genetic associations across the genome could mitigate these issues. Also of importance is that a GWAS is typically split into a discovery phase and a replication phase, the former performing a hypothesis-free scan of every available SNP, and the latter following up candidate loci for replication in an independent sample.

20.1.5   The Design of Genome-Wide Association Studies

Genotyping technology has become more cost-effective (the SNP density to price ratio), driven by competition between different companies offering similar products [24, 25]. The increasing number of SNPs assayed across the genome increases the chance of including a marker in high LD with the causal variant, or even the causal variant itself. Today, modern SNP chips use nano-arrays to assay genotypes at typically no lower than half a million positions in the genome.

Population sequencing studies identify up to 15 million common variants in human populations. Still, after accounting for LD between these variants, there are only around a million independent regions in the genome [26]. Therefore, $0.05/1\,000\,000 = 5 \times 10^{-8}$ is a conservative statistical threshold for correcting a *GWAS* for multiple testing. The gold standard for declaring a genetic association in a GWAS is to identify an SNP with $P < 5 \times 10^{-8}$ and then to replicate it in an independent sample [27].

Genotyping half a million markers in a European sample will capture up to 80% of the genetic variation due to common SNPs [28]. Studies can use more dense SNP chips or obtain sequence data to improve on this, but it can be prohibitively expensive. A widely used alternative approach is to impute missing common genetic variants.

This is achieved through a probabilistic process of matching partial chromosomal segments from the genotyped data (target data) with complete chromosomal segments in a sequenced dataset (reference data) (see Figure 20.1). While genetic imputation can boost the number of high-quality common SNPs in a dataset to around 10 million with MAF > 0.01 [29], it is important to note that there is uncertainty in the imputed SNPs.

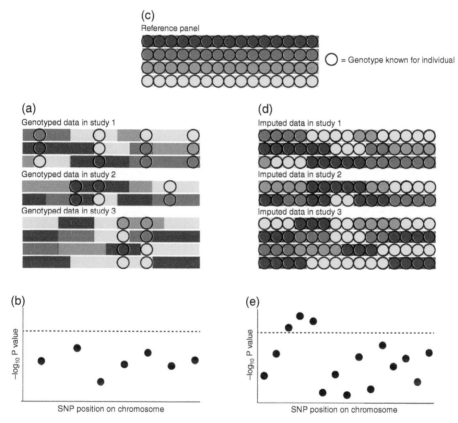

FIGURE 20.1   Schematic of how imputation aids in meta-analysis of genome-wide association studies. (a) Three studies are depicted where each row represents an individual in the study, and horizontal blocks represent a section of a chromosome. Circles represent positions on the chromosome that are genotyped in that study. (b) Performing meta-analysis across these studies is problematic because many of the single-nucleotide polymorphisms (SNPs) are not present in more than one study. The graph depicts the associations for each of the SNPs available. The y-axis is the –log10(P value) of the genetic association with the trait. The number of samples available for each SNP are labeled. The dotted horizontal line represents the significance threshold. (c, d) Imputation requires an external reference panel for which there is whole-sequence data, for example the 1000 Genomes Project. The haplotypes (colored blocks) in study data (a) are matched to haplotypes in the reference sample, and this provides information about the genetic background for each genotyped SNP. Inference of the nongenotyped variants can then be made. (e) If all studies have imputed their genotyped data to the same reference panel, then they will have the same set of imputed genotypes across the genome. Meta-analysis can now include each study for every variant, which improves power by increasing sample size and by potentially including the causal variant or SNPs closer to the causal variant. The sample sizes used here are illustrative; most studies will comprise at least several hundred individuals.

They are therefore typically reported as genotype probabilities rather than the discrete genotype calls that are obtained from SNP chips or sequencing. Association tests using imputed data are modified so that the contribution of an individual's data to the effect estimate is weighted by the level of certainty of the genotype imputation at that SNP [30].

The improved genome coverage achieved by genetic imputation increases power by increasing the likelihood that a causal variant is tagged by an SNP included in the study, or that the causal variant itself is included. However, the most crucial contribution that imputation has made to the success of GWAS is a practical one: through enabling meta-analysis. Different studies will invariably use different SNP chips to assay genotypes, and each SNP chip typically assays a unique set of SNPs. As a consequence, if one were to attempt to combine information from across studies, then only a fraction of the SNPs would benefit from a boost in sample size. If instead each cohort imputes to the same reference panel, then each will have (inferred) measures of millions of markers in common across the genome (Figure 20.1).

20.2   THE ROLE OF META-ANALYSIS IN GENOME-WIDE ASSOCIATION STUDIES

Sample sizes for GWAS have grown at a tremendous rate over the last decade, driven mainly by combining studies through meta-analysis [31]. Thousands of SNPs are now known to robustly associate with hundreds of complex traits (Figure 20.2). It is easy to understate the enormity of this success [32, 33]. In the following sections, we discuss the role of meta-analysis in the context of the missing heritability problem, the use of meta-analysis to overcome the winner's curse, and the most important sources of between-study heterogeneity.

20.2.1   The Missing Heritability

While GWAS identified robust genetic associations for complex traits, it quickly became apparent that the proportion of the phenotypic variance that could be explained by replicated genetic associations was much lower than the amount that was predicted to exist from heritability studies. This gap became known as the "missing heritability" [34] and several theories emerged to explain the phenomenon [35]. A study on psychiatric disorders made an important contribution by constructing genetic predictors using SNPs with P values that did not reach genome-wide significance [36]. As the significance threshold for including SNPs for prediction was relaxed, more SNPs were included in the model, and prediction accuracy in an independent dataset improved. This suggested that complex traits associate with a large number of independent causal variants across the genome, and therefore most genetic effects are small. Identifying more associations thus requires improved statistical power, which chiefly depends on increasing sample size.

There are three routes to increasing sample size. First, gather more samples in your cohort, record necessary phenotype information, and obtain genotype data. This comes at some expense, and certain cohorts will not be able to expand sample sizes due to their study designs. Second, combine data from across different cohorts. This is done occasionally, one prominent example being the Psychiatric Genetics Consortium [36].

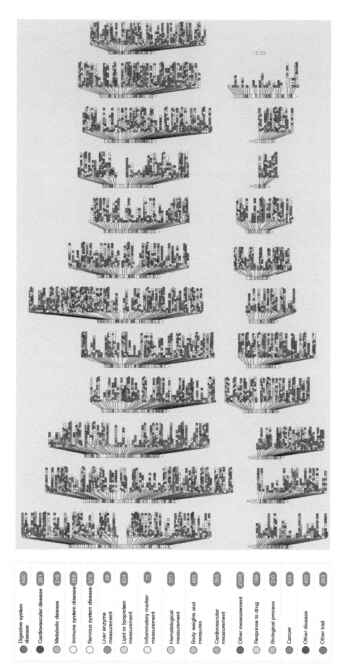

FIGURE 20.2 Schematic of known genetic associations. The NHGRI-EBI genome-wide association study (GWAS) catalog comprises known genetic associations for thousands of traits, from thousands of GWAS studies conducted over the last decade. The figure shows the 23 human chromosomes with known genetic associations mapped to each genome region. The take-home message is that regions right across the genome influence a range of different traits.

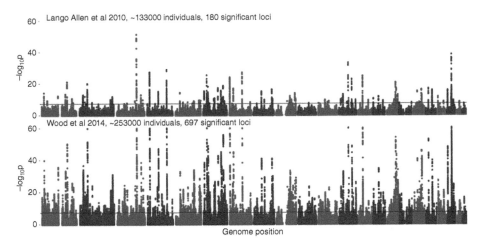

FIGURE 20.3   Improvements in genome-wide association study (GWAS) results as sample sizes increase. The figure shows two Manhattan plots. The *x*-axis represents the genome position, each point represents a single-nucleotide polymorphism (SNP) that has been analyzed in the GWAS, and the *y*-axis represents the strength of evidence of association. The horizontal line shows the significance threshold of $P < 5e{-}8$. The top graph is from a GWAS using approximately 133 000 individuals on height, and the bottom graph shows the analysis repeated but with over 250 000 samples.

However, the sharing of sensitive genetic and phenotypic data between researchers and across national borders comes with ethical and legal challenges that can take years to overcome [37]. The third route, which dominated GWAS in the past decade, is meta-analysis. GWAS is performed in each cohort separately, and the data shared among analysts are nondisclosive summary results, which typically include the effect size, standard error, and information about each SNP.

For example, in 2010, a GWAS meta-analysis on height was performed using over 130 000 samples from 46 independent study cohorts. This analysis yielded 180 independent loci, which together explained 3% of the phenotypic variation [38]. Yet heritability estimates signaled that 70% of the variation in height was due to genetic effects [6]. There was thus a huge gap between the known loci that influenced height as detected by GWAS and the number of loci remaining to be uncovered. By 2014, more than 250 000 samples from 79 studies had been analyzed through meta-analysis, increasing the yield to 697 independent loci, and explaining 10% of the heritability (Figure 20.3) [39]. These observations are in line with the so-called infinitesimal model of genetic architecture [40], which stipulates that there are many variants with small effects. A more detailed example of the GWAS meta-analysis process is presented in Box 20.1.

20.2.2   Replication, and the Use of Meta-Analysis to Overcome the Winner's Curse

If the objective of a GWAS is to identify areas of the genome that are relevant to a disease, then the size of the association is not important: we are only interested in the yes/no answer as to whether or not that locus is associated with the disease of interest.

Box 20.1   An Example of Genome-Wide Association Study Meta-Analysis used for Coronary Artery Disease

In 2011, the CARDIoGRAM (Coronary ARtery DIsease Genome-wide Replication And Meta-analysis) consortium performed a GWAS meta-analysis that identified 23 loci associated with coronary artery disease (CAD) [41]. Here we describe how meta-analysis was used in this study.

Discovery Analysis

The analysis comprised 14 studies in the discovery phase, including 22 233 cases (individuals with CAD) and 64 762 controls. Each study imputed their genotypes using a set of independent individuals in the HapMap2 study [42], resulting in 2.3 million genotypes in common across all studies. GWAS was performed within each study, and summary statistics were shared for meta-analysis. For each available SNP, the inverse variance-weighted (IVW) method was used to obtain a combined effect size, and Cochran's Q was also calculated to examine heterogeneity across studies.

For SNPs that had P values for $Q < 0.01$, an outlier test was performed for each study. If the outlier test gave $P < 0.01/14$ for any study, then it was excluded for that SNP, and the IVW estimate was recalculated. If heterogeneity remained even after outliers were removed, then the DerSimonian–Laird random-effects model was used to meta-analyze that SNP.

We note here that the outlier removal procedure based on contribution to heterogeneity is not generally recommended, as it could lead to artificially lower standard errors, raising the Type I error rate [43].

Replication Analysis

From the discovery stage, 30 SNPs were taken forward to the replication stage. These SNPs were selected because either they had $P < 5e–8$ for the association, or they had been previously implicated in CAD. The replication dataset comprised 56 682 samples, approximately half of which were cases, from 26 independent cohorts. Summary statistics for the 30 SNPs were shared for meta-analysis, following the same procedure as in the discovery sample.

Combined Analysis

Finally, the results from the discovery and replication samples for the 30 SNPs were combined in a concluding meta-analysis. Those with a combined $P < 5e–8$ *and* with a replication $P < 0.05/30$ were deemed significant.

In 2015, another GWAS meta-analysis for CAD was performed by the CARDIoGRAMplusC4D (CARDIoGRAM plus The Coronary Artery Disease (C4D) Genetics) consortium [44]. In this study, the entire analysis was performed using only a discovery sample of 185 000 cases and controls, with all cohorts imputed to the 1000 Genomes Project. This approach yielded 10 new loci.

The 2011 study has a set of replication effect sizes for each SNP, which are unbiased. Still, the authors did not capitalize on obtaining the least variance estimates by employing UMVUE (see the discussion of the winner's curse in the main text). The 2015 study demonstrates the pressure to detect novel causal variants – opting against using a replication sample to maximize discovery power. In the 2015 study, the effect size estimates will be biased upward due to the effect of the winner's curse.

However, if one aims to create a predictor of disease, or to use the SNP as an instrumental variable (see Chapter 19), it is crucial to obtain an unbiased effect size of the genetic association [45]. The GWAS design introduces a problem here. Due to the random variation around the estimates, some of the effects will be overestimated and others underestimated. By applying the significance threshold, we will tend to detect small effects that happened to be overestimated, thus introducing bias. Of note, such associations are not false positives: these SNPs have an impact on the trait. However, the use of a threshold to determine which SNPs we report will lead to overestimation of the effect sizes of some SNPs [46, 47], a problem akin to publication bias [48]. We can view this specific type of bias as an example of the "winner's curse" [49].

Approaches have been developed to correct biased estimates from discovery GWAS results [46, 50], but although the bias is reduced, none of the methods provides truly unbiased results [51]. Replication in a well-powered, independent sample is required to determine whether the association is robust. If no threshold is imposed in the replication study, it will provide an unbiased effect size estimate. A drawback of only using estimates of effect sizes from the replication sample is that the information from the discovery phase is discarded, thus reducing power. Some studies meta-analyze the discovery and replication datasets to obtain an overall effect size estimate (see Box 20.1). Although the meta-analysis includes the replication data, it does not protect the effect size estimate from bias due to the winner's curse. An alternative method is to weigh the contributions from the discovery and replication stages using information on the rankings of the effect sizes [52]. The advantage of this approach (known as the uniform minimum variance unbiased estimator, UMVUE) is that the statistical power is maximized while reducing bias.

20.2.3   Sources of Heterogeneity

The statistical methods used to perform meta-analysis in GWAS are not very different from standard meta-analysis methods described in Chapter 9. The only difference is that each SNP in the study is meta-analyzed separately, which means that several million meta-analyses are performed per study. Like in standard meta-analysis, steps must be taken to minimize heterogeneity. There are three main sources of heterogeneity in GWAS meta-analysis, outlined in the following.

20.2.3.1   Ancestral Differences

Studies with different population ancestries can introduce heterogeneity through both technical and biological processes. Technical effects can arise simply when a particular SNP is not polymorphic (has only one variant) in the population of one or several of the studies, in which case a full meta-analysis at that locus would be impossible. Another challenge is that LD patterns differ between studies [53]. If the causal variant is not present in all studies, then the level of LD between the markers and the causal variant should be consistent between studies. This is not guaranteed for different ancestral populations because haplotype structures have had independent historical trajectories.

Of more biological interest is that different effect sizes can exist between different studies simply because of ethnic differences, or because the SNP only manifests an effect in certain environments. The cross-population technical and biological differences can be addressed by modeling a study's expected contribution to heterogeneity based on its ancestral distance from the other studies in the analysis [54]. In an analysis of type 2 diabetes, it was shown that only 1 of 19 variants exhibited substantial heterogeneity after accounting for ancestry, suggesting that the effect size estimates were consistent between ethnicities at the remaining 18 loci [54].

20.2.3.2   Genotyping

From a biological perspective, genotypes are discrete measures. But genotype calls from array-based technologies are produced by probabilistic algorithms, and SNP calls from imputation can have considerable uncertainty around them. Genotyping error due either to failures in SNP chip assays or to imputation will lead to regression dilution bias, where effect size estimates are biased toward the null. The genotyping error rates from one study to the next are likely to differ, which can lead to issues in GWAS. If genotyping error rates between studies are not associated with the outcome (i.e. there is random measurement error in the exposure) then, at the meta-analysis stage, power may be reduced due to the increase in between-study heterogeneity [55].

A more problematic situation arises when batch effects differentially affect cases and controls, for example when cases and controls were genotyped on different platforms. In this situation, differential measurement error may introduce high Type I error rates. Combining studies in meta-analysis may exacerbate this problem by both increasing heterogeneity and producing high false discovery rates, similar to meta-analyses of observational studies, which may produce precise but spurious results due to confounding and bias [56].

There are some key variables to keep consistent between studies to minimize heterogeneity due to imputation: the sequenced reference panel that is being used, the software used for phasing the genotypes, software used for imputing, and filtering thresholds used for retaining SNPs [57]. Converting genotype probabilities to hard genotype calls is one way in which heterogeneity can be introduced, because it could introduce differential call accuracy by ignoring the uncertainty of the imputation.

A crucial technical consideration is ensuring that each study reports effects in reference to the same allele. DNA can be read in either a "forward" or a "reverse" direction, which can lead to two studies accidentally referring to the same allele differently, or to different alleles as being the same. Strand alignment procedures are necessary to avoid this problem [58].

20.2.3.3   Trait Definitions

The factors that lead to differential trait measures between epidemiological studies also influence GWAS. Many diseases and other complex traits require expert diagnosis, which may have different standards in different studies. Even if standardized scales or diagnostic tools are used, these often differ across studies to measure the same phenotype. Quality or calibration of measuring equipment could vary between studies or over time within a study. Batch effects are a pervasive problem with molecular traits such as gene expression or DNA methylation levels, and this is a particular problem with high-throughput phenotyping, which has been the focus of much recent attention. Some complex traits are well defined across studies, but if different studies adjust for different covariates, then their interpretation can be altered and heterogeneity introduced. For example, having a high body mass index is a cause of type 2 diabetes, and if analyzing type 2 diabetes, then adjusting for body mass index in some studies and not in others would introduce heterogeneity.

20.2.4   Random-Effects or Fixed-Effects Models?

Given the potential sources of heterogeneity, the use of a random-effects model seems like the natural default choice for meta-analysis (see Chapter 9). However, in practice it is far more common to use inverse variance-weighted fixed-effects meta-analysis, particularly in the discovery phase. The pressure to yield as many significant associations as possible, coupled with the perception that the fixed-effects model has greater statistical efficiency, is an argument against the random-effects approach, even though it is theoretically more justifiable. Often replication datasets will themselves combine studies, and it is more common to see the use of random-effects meta-analysis to obtain a replicated effect size estimate, using the DerSimonian and Laird [59] implementation.

20.2.5   Novel Approaches for Using Meta-Analysis with Genome-Wide Association Study Summary Data

20.2.5.1   Detecting Study Outliers

One advantage gained from GWAS meta-analysis is that many tests are performed, and therefore patterns can be unearthed to detect studies that are systematically introducing heterogeneity. A study examining the reliability of GWAS meta-analyses [60] explored how heterogeneity statistics could be used to identify such problematic studies. The authors proposed calculating the standardized predicted random effects (SPRE) for each study and for each of a set of independent variants, and then calculating the mean of the SPREs across the variants to obtain a statistic (the "M value") that is expected to be normally distributed with mean 0. Excluding studies that make a substantial contribution toward heterogeneity for a single test could be considered cherry-picking, with a danger of increasing Type I error rates. However, if a study systematically increases heterogeneity across many tests, then it is more likely that there is a problem with the study, and its exclusion would be justified to increase power.

20.2.5.2 Identifying Single-Nucleotide Polymorphisms that Influence Multiple Traits

Meta-analytical methods have been extended within the GWAS context to identify SNPs that influence two or more traits. Multitrait analysis of GWAS (MTAG) generalizes inverse variance-weighted meta-analysis to achieve this [61]. The idea is that if GWAS effects from two different traits are correlated, then effect estimates for each trait can be improved by incorporating information into one trait from the other traits. MTAG is performed by estimating the genetic correlation between a pair of traits and then evaluating the deviation from that genetic correlation due to each specific SNP.

20.3 FUTURE PROSPECTS

Meta-analysis in GWAS has brought tremendous success in identifying genetic factors for thousands of complex traits. Summary data from GWAS are now being stored in centralized repositories (e.g. MR-Base [9]), and making them easily accessible will fuel further developments that are likely to borrow methodology and ideas from meta-analysis.

One obvious area, discussed in detail elsewhere [62], is two-sample (or summary) Mendelian randomization [63], which is used to infer the causal relationships between traits. To this end, MR-Base, as a software and data repository, has integrated meta-analytic methods with GWAS summary data to automate causal inference for millions of pairwise trait combinations.

Though common genetic variation has been explored, there is also much interest in finding genetic associations between traits and rare variants – those that have allele frequencies below 1% [12]. These variants are much harder to impute [29]. Therefore, studies will depend on specific types of arrays that include rare variants, such as exome SNP chips that genotype them directly [64], or sequencing studies that capture both rare and common variations [65]. Another issue is that rare variants necessarily have a lower power to detect associations. Sufficiently large sample sizes of sequence data to routinely detect rare variants may become available soon, but until then, several methods exist that collapse rare variants in a region to improve power [66]. Aggregating the influences of multiple rare variants in a genomic region attempts to overcome the issue of low power, and meta-analysis of these aggregate scores is now also possible [67].

Finally, one potential future prospect for meta-analysis is that it will no longer be used! Several years of GWAS meta-analysis have demonstrated the requirement for very large sample sizes to obtain sufficient power in GWAS. Perhaps as a direct result, national and private efforts are now emerging that seek to genotype individuals on a much larger scale. The UK Biobank project and the China Kadoorie project, for example, have genotyped over half a million individuals each. The standard GWAS model still has a role for some traits, e.g. to ascertain cases for diseases that have low prevalence. But the major human resource required to conduct meta-analyses is largely sidestepped by these massive cohort studies. We may then see meta-analyses being performed on already published GWAS summary datasets from a few very large studies.

REFERENCES

1. Visscher, P.M., Hill, W.G., and Wray, N.R. (2008). Heritability in the genomics era – concepts and misconceptions. *Nat. Rev. Genet.* 9 (4): 255–266.

2. Zaitlen, N., Kraft, P., Patterson, N. et al. (2013). Using extended genealogy to estimate components of heritability for 23 quantitative and dichotomous traits. *PLoS Genet.* 9 (5): e1003520.

3. Polderman, T.J.C., Benyamin, B., De Leeuw, C.A. et al. (2015). Meta-analysis of the heritability of human traits based on fifty years of twin studies. *Nat. Genet.* 47 (7): 702–709.

4. Lander, E. and Kruglyak, L. (1995). Genetic dissection of complex traits: guidelines for interpreting and reporting linkage results. *Nat. Genet.* 11 (11): 241–247.

5. Risch, N. and Merikangas, K. (1996). The future of genetic studies of complex human diseases. *Science* 273 (5281): 1516–1517.

6. Hemani, G., Yang, J., Vinkhuyzen, A. et al. (2013). Inference of the genetic architecture underlying BMI and height with the use of 20 240 sibling pairs. *Am. J. Hum. Genet.* 93 (5): 865–875.

7. Thompson, J.R., Attia, J., and Minelli, C. (2011). The meta-analysis of genome-wide association studies. *Brief. Bioinform.* 12 (3): 259–269.

8. Evangelou, E. and Ioannidis, J.P. (2013). Meta-analysis methods for genome-wide association studies and beyond. *Nat. Rev. Genet.* 14 (6): 379–389.

9. Hemani, G., Zheng, J., Wade, K.H. et al. (2016). MR-base: a platform for systematic causal inference across the phenome using billions of genetic associations. *bioRxiv* 78: 972.

10. Scally, A. (2016). The mutation rate in human evolution and demographic inference. *Curr. Opin. Genet. Dev.* 41: 36–43.

11. The 1000 Genomes Project Consortium, GA, M.V., Altshuler, D.M. et al. (2012). An integrated map of genetic variation from 1092 human genomes. *Nature* 491: 56.

12. Lee, S., Abecasis, G.R., Boehnke, M., and Lin, X. (2014). Rare-variant association analysis: study designs and statistical tests. *Am. J. Hum. Genet.* 95 (1): 5–23.

13. The Wellcome Trust Case Control Consortium (2007). Genome-wide association study of 14 000 cases of seven common diseases and 3000 shared controls. *Nature* 447 (7145): 661–678.

14. Lander, E.S. (1996). The new genomics: global views of biology. *Science* 274 (5287): 536–539.

15. Price, A.L., Patterson, N.J., Plenge, R.M. et al. (2006). Principal components analysis corrects for stratification in genome-wide association studies. *Nat. Genet.* 38 (8): 904–909.

16. Schork, N.J., Nath, S.K., Fallin, D., and Chakravarti, A. (2000). Linkage disequilibrium analysis of biallelic DNA markers, human quantitative trait loci, and threshold-defined case and control subjects. *Am. J. Hum. Genet.* 67 (5): 1208–1218.

17. Weir, B.S. (2008). Linkage disequilibrium and association mapping. *Annu. Rev. Genomics Hum. Genet.* 9: 129–142.

18. Tabor, H.K., Risch, N.J., and Myers, R.M. (2002). Candidate-gene approaches for studying complex genetic traits: practical considerations. *Nat. Rev. Genet.* 3 (5): 391–397.

19. Pasche, B. and Yi, N. (2010). Candidate gene association studies: successes and failures. *Curr. Opin. Genet. Dev.* 20 (3): 257–261.

20. Sagoo, G.S., Little, J., and Higgins, J.P.T. (2009). Systematic reviews of genetic association studies. *PLoS Med.* 6 (3): e1000028.

21. Khoury, M.J. and Little, J. (2000). Human genome epidemiologic reviews: the beginning of something HuGE. *Am. J. Epidemiol.* 151 (1): 2–3.

22. Colhoun, H.M., McKeigue, P.M., and Smith, G.D. (2003). Problems of reporting genetic associations with complex outcomes. *Lancet* 361 (9360): 865–872.

23. Gaunt, T.R. and Davey, S.G. (2015). ENOS and coronary artery disease: publication bias and the eclipse of hypothesis-driven meta-analysis in genetic association studies. *Gene* 556 (2): 257–258.

24. Syvänen, A.-C. (2001). Accessing genetic variation: genotyping single nucleotide polymorphisms. *Nat. Rev. Genet.* 2 (12): 930–942.

25. Perkel, J. (2008). SNP genotyping: six technologies that keyed a revolution. *Nat. Methods* 5 (5): 447–453.

26. Dudbridge, F. and Gusnanto, A. (2008). Estimation of significance thresholds for genome-wide association scans. *Genet. Epidemiol.* 32 (3): 227–234.

27. Chanock, S.J., Manolio, T., Boehnke, M. et al. (2007). Replicating genotype–phenotype associations. *Nature* 447 (7145): 655–660.

28. Kruglyak, L. (1999). Prospects for whole-genome linkage disequilibrium mapping of common diseasegenes. *Nat. Genet.* 22 (2): 139–144.

29. Marchini, J. and Howie, B. (2010). Genotype imputation for genome-wide association studies. *Nat. Rev. Genet.* 11 (7): 499–511.

30. Marchini, J., Howie, B., Myers, S. et al. (2007). A new multipoint method for genome-wide association studies by imputation of genotypes. *Nat. Genet.* 39 (7): 906–913.

31. Hindorff, L.A., Junkins, H.A., Hall, P.N., Mehta, J.P., and Manolio, T.A. (2010). GWAS catalog. http://www.genome.gov/gwastudies (accessed February 25, 2022).

32. Visscher, P.M., Brown, M.A., MI, M.C., and Yang, J. (2012). Five years of GWAS discovery. *Am. J. Hum. Genet.* 90 (1): 7–24.

33. Visscher, P.M., Wray, N.R., Zhang, Q. et al. (2017). 10 years of GWAS discovery: biology, function, and translation. *Am. J. Hum. Genet.* 101 (1): 5–22.

34. Maher, B. (2008). The case of the missing heritability. *Nature* 456 (7218): 18–21.

35. Eichler, E.E., Flint, J., Gibson, G. et al. (2010). Missing heritability and strategies for finding the underlying causes of complex disease. *Nat. Rev. Genet.* 11 (6): 446–450.

36. Purcell, S.M., Moran, J.L., Fromer, M. et al. (2014). A polygenic burden of rare disruptive mutations in schizophrenia. *Nature* 506 (7487): 185–190.

37. Sorani, M.D., Yue, J.K., Sharma, S. et al. (2015). Genetic data sharing and privacy. *Neuroinformatics* 13 (1): 1–6.

38. Lango Allen, H., Estrada, K., Lettre, G. et al. (2010). Hundreds of variants clustered in genomic loci and biological pathways affect human height. *Nature* 467 (7317): 832–838.

39. Wood, A.R., Esko, T., Yang, J. et al. (2014). Defining the role of common variation in the genomic and biological architecture of adult human height. *Nat. Genet.* 46 (11): 1173–1186.

40. Fisher, R. (1918). The correlation between relatives on the supposition of Mendelian inheritance. *Trans. R. Soc. Edinb.* 52: 399–433.

41. Schunkert, H., König, I.R., Kathiresan, S. et al. (2011). Large-scale association analysis identifies 13 new susceptibility loci for coronary artery disease. *Nat. Genet.* 43 (4): 333–338.

42. The International Hapmap Consortium (2005). A haplotype map of the human genome. *Nature* 437 (7063): 1299–1320.

43. Cho, Y., Haycock, P.C., Sanderson, E. et al. (2020). Exploiting horizontal pleiotropy to search for causal pathways within a Mendelian randomization framework. *Nat. Commun.* 11: 1010.

44. Nikpay, M., Goel, A., Won, H.-H. et al. (2015). A comprehensive 1000 genomes–based genome-wide association meta-analysis of coronary artery disease. *Nat. Genet.* 47 (10): 1121–1130.

45. Wray, N.R., Goddard, M.E., and Visscher, P.M. (2007). Prediction of individual genetic risk to disease from genome-wide association studies. *Genome Res.* 17 (10): 1520–1528.

46. Göring, H.H., Terwilliger, J.D., and Blangero, J. (2001). Large upward bias in estimation of locus-specific effects from genome-wide scans. *Am. J. Hum. Genet.* 69 (Vc): 1357–1369.

47. Kraft, P. (2008). Curses – winner's and otherwise – in genetic epidemiology. *Epidemiology* 19 (5): 649–651.

48. Dickersin, K. (1990). The existence of publication bias and risk factors for its occurrence. *J. Am. Med. Assoc.* 263 (10): 1385–1389.

49. Capen, E.C., Clapp, R.V., and Campbell, W.M. (1971). Competitive bidding in high risk situations. *J. Petrol. Tech.* 23: 641–653.

50. Zollner, S. and Pritchard, J.K. (2007). Overcoming the winner's curse: estimating penetrance parameters from case–control data. *Am. J. Hum. Genet.* 80 (4): 605–615.

51. Stallard, N., Todd, S., and Whitehead, J. (2008). Estimation following selection of the largest of two normal means. *J. Stat. Plan. Inference* 138 (6): 1629–1638.

52. Bowden, J. and Dudbridge, F. (2009). Unbiased estimation of odds ratios: combining genome-wide association scans with replication studies. *Genet. Epidemiol.* 33 (5): 406–418.

53. The International Hapmap Consortium (2005). The international HapMap project. *Nature* 63 (Suppl 1): 29–34.

54. Morris, A.P. (2011). Transethnic meta-analysis of genome-wide association studies. *Genet. Epidemiol.* 35 (8): 809–822.

55. Lee, H., Yang, J., Chen, G.-B. et al. (2013). Estimation of SNP heritability from dense genotype data. *Am. J. Hum. Genet.* 93: 1151–1155.

56. Egger, M., Schneider, M., and Davey, S.G. (1998). Spurious precision? Meta-analysis of observational studies. *Br. Med. J.* 316: 140–145.

57. Zeggini, E., Scott, L.J., Saxena, R. et al. (2008). Meta-analysis of genome-wide association data and large-scale replication identifies additional susceptibility loci for type 2 diabetes. *Nat. Genet.* 40 (5): 638–645.

58. Deelen, P., Bonder, M.J., van der Velde, K.J. et al. (2014). Genotype harmoniser: automatic strand alignment and format conversion for genotype data integration. *BMC. Res. Notes* 7: 901.

59. DerSimonian, R. and Laird, N. (1986). Meta-analysis in clinical trials. *Control. Clin. Trials* 7 (3): 177–188.

60. Magosi, L.E., Goel, A., Hopewell, J.C. et al. (2017). Identifying systematic heterogeneity patterns in genetic association meta-analysis studies. *PLoS Genet.* 13 (5): e1006755.

61. Turley, P., Walters, R.K., Maghzian, O. et al. (2018). Multi-trait analysis of genome-wide association summary statistics using MTAG. *Nat. Genet* 50: 229–237.

62. Bowden, J., Holmes, M.V. (2019). Meta-analysis and Mendelian randomization: A review. *Res Synth Methods* 10: 486–496.

63. Pierce, B.L. and Burgess, S. (2013). Efficient design for Mendelian randomisation studies: subsample and 2-sample instrumental variable estimators. *Am. J. Epidemiol.* 178 (7): 1177–1184.

64. Khera, A.V., Won, H.-H., Peloso, G.M. et al. (2017). Association of rare and common variation in the lipoprotein lipase gene with coronary artery disease. *J. Am. Med. Assoc.* 317 (9): 1060–1068.

65. Hunt, K.A., Mistry, V., Bockett, N.A. et al. (2013). Negligible impact of rare autoimmune-locus coding-region variants on missing heritability. *Nature* 498: 232–235.

66. Wu, M.C., Lee, S., Cai, T. et al. (2011). Rare-variant association testing for sequencing data with the sequence kernel association test. *Am. J. Hum. Genet.* 89 (1): 82–93.

67. Lee, S., Teslovich, T.M., Boehnke, M., and Lin, X. (2013). General framework for meta-analysis of rare variants in sequencing association studies. *Am. J. Hum. Genet.* 93 (1): 42–53.

PART IV

COCHRANE AND GUIDELINE DEVELOPMENT

CHAPTER 21

Cochrane: Trusted Evidence. Informed Decisions. Better Health

Gerd Antes, David Tovey, and Nancy Owens

Health care professionals, researchers, policymakers, and people using health services are frequently overwhelmed with unmanageable amounts of information. As discussed in Chapter 1, systematic reviews are essential, although not sufficient, to make informed decisions about health and health care. They can prevent undue delays in the introduction of effective treatments and the continued use of ineffective or even harmful interventions. The Cochrane logo (see Figure 21.1) shows an example of a treatment in perinatal medicine whose effectiveness was not appreciated for many years because no systematic review had been performed. The logo has been used by The Cochrane Collaboration since its founding in 1993. Now referring to itself simply as "Cochrane," the organization has the ambitious aim to prepare, maintain, and promote the accessibility of systematic reviews across all areas of health care.

Cochrane is intrinsically linked to the development of the science of evidence synthesis, and much of the progress described in this book was to some extent influenced, if not driven, by the organization and its members. In this chapter we describe the historical developments that led to this unique enterprise, which has been compared to the Human Genome Project in its potential implications for modern health care [1]. We describe Cochrane's remit and structure, its current output, and its need to generate impact, and we discuss some of the existing challenges.

A description of Cochrane has always been a description of an organization in transition, because starting from scratch and developing into a formidable organization have required adaptation to accommodate ongoing growth, the continuous modernization of methods, and changing conditions and reader expectations.

Systematic Reviews in Health Research: Meta-Analysis in Context, Third Edition. Edited by Matthias Egger, Julian P.T. Higgins, and George Davey Smith.
© 2022 John Wiley & Sons Ltd. Published 2022 by John Wiley & Sons Ltd.
Companion website: www.systematic-reviews3.org

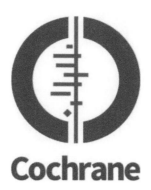

Cochrane

FIGURE 21.1   The Cochrane logo illustrates a systematic review of seven randomized controlled trials (RCTs) of a short, inexpensive course of a corticosteroid given to women about to give birth too early, comparing the intervention with placebo. A schematic representation of the forest plot (see Chapter 2) is shown. The first of these RCTs was reported in 1972, the last in 1980. The logo summarizes the evidence that would have been revealed had the available RCTs been reviewed systematically: it indicates strongly that corticosteroids reduce the risk of babies dying from the complications of immaturity. Because no systematic review of these trials was published until 1989, most obstetricians had not realized that the treatment was so effective, reducing the odds of the babies of these women dying from the complications of immaturity by 30–50%. As a result, tens of thousands of premature babies probably suffered and died unnecessarily, and needed more expensive treatment than was necessary. By 1991, seven more trials had been reported, and the picture had become still stronger.

21.1   BACKGROUND AND HISTORY

In 1972, the British epidemiologist Archie Cochrane drew attention to the great collective ignorance about the effects of health care in his influential book *Effectiveness and Efficiency: Random Reflections on Health Services* [2]. Cochrane recognized that people who want to make informed decisions about health care do not have ready access to reliable reviews of the available evidence [3]. His book, and the discussion stimulated by it, inspired what in retrospect can be seen as a pilot project for The Cochrane Collaboration [4]. Beginning in 1974, all controlled trials in perinatal medicine were systematically identified and assembled in a trials register. By 1985, the register contained more than 3500 reports of controlled trials, leading to the preparation of around 600 systematic reviews in the late 1980s. In 1987, the year before his death, Cochrane referred to a collection of systematic reviews of randomized controlled trials (RCTs) of care during pregnancy and childbirth, based on this work, as "a real milestone in the history of randomized trials and in the evaluation of care." He suggested that other specialties should follow this example [5]. In the same year, the scientific quality of the narrative reviews published in major medical journals was shown to leave much to be desired [6]. Subsequently, the need for systematically prepared reviews became increasingly recognized.

In response to Cochrane's call for systematic, up-to-date reviews of all relevant RCTs of health care, the Research and Development Programme, which was set up to support the British National Health Service (NHS), provided funding to establish a "Cochrane Centre" led by Iain Chalmers, to "facilitate the preparation of systematic reviews of randomized trials of health care." This center was opened in Oxford in October 1992 [7, 8]. Facilitated by a meeting organized by the New York Academy of Sciences six months later [9], the idea spread around the world and led to the formal launch of The Cochrane Collaboration at the first Cochrane Colloquium, which was held in Oxford in October 1993. By the end of 1994, six more Cochrane Centres had been founded in Europe, North America, and Australia. Ten groups were established to prepare reviews within different areas of health care, and groups were formed to address methodological issues. Cochrane was registered as a charity in May 1995. A steep increase in activities followed. New groups were established, attendance at the annual colloquia increased, and the number of Cochrane contributors grew rapidly. At the end of the twentieth century, more than 4000 health professionals, scientists, and consumers were participating in Cochrane, a remarkable number for an organization that had been founded formally only a few years earlier.

As described earlier, the Collaboration's mission was to help people make well-informed decisions about health care by preparing, maintaining, and promoting the accessibility of systematic reviews of the effects of health care interventions. Cochrane's work and organization in its efforts to achieve these aims were guided by 10 principles (see Box 21.1). These principles and a transparent structure were crucial in the

Box 21.1   Principles of the Cochrane Collaboration

1	Collaboration	by fostering global co-operation, teamwork and open and transparent communication and decision-making
2	Building on the enthusiasm of individuals	by involving, supporting and training people of different skills and backgrounds
3	Avoiding duplication of effort	by good management, co-ordination and effective internal communications to maximize economy of effort
4	Minimizing bias	through a variety of approaches such as scientific rigor, ensuring broad participation and avoiding conflicts of interest
5	Keeping up-to-date	by a commitment to ensure that Cochrane Reviews are maintained through identification and incorporation of new evidence
6	Striving for relevance	by promoting the assessment of health questions using outcomes that matter to people making choices in health and health care
7	Promoting access	by wide dissemination of our outputs, taking advantage of strategic alliances and by promoting appropriate access models and delivery solutions to meet the needs of users worldwide
8	Ensuring quality	by applying advances in methodology, developing systems for quality improvement and being open and responsive to criticism
9	Continuity	by ensuring that responsibility for reviews, editorial processes and key functions is maintained and renewed
10	Enabling wide participation	in our work by reducing barriers to contributing and by encouraging diversity

Source: https://www.cochrane.org/about-us

Box 21.2   Key Publications About Cochrane

The following articles provide useful descriptions of Cochrane and its development:

Chalmers, I. (1993). The Cochrane Collaboration: preparing, maintaining, and disseminating systematic reviews of the effects of health care. *Ann. N.Y. Acad. Sci.* 703: 156–165.

Bero, L., and Rennie, D. (1995). The Cochrane Collaboration: preparing, maintaining and disseminating systematic reviews of the effects of health care. *JAMA* 274: 1935–1938.

Chalmers, I., Sackett, D., and Silagy, C. (1997). The Cochrane Collaboration. In: *Non-random Reflections on Health Services Research* (eds. A. Maynard and I. Chalmers), 231–249. London: BMJ Publishing Group.

Bosch, F.X., and Molas, R. (eds.) (2003). *Archie Cochrane: Back to the Front*. Barcelona: published privately.

Cassels, A. (2015). *The Cochrane Collaboration: Medicine's Best Kept Secret*. Victoria, BC: Agio Publishing House.

light of the enormous diversity in disciplinary and cultural backgrounds of the people who were working together in Cochrane. The organization consisted of five types of "entities," described below (Review Groups, Geographic Groups/Centres, Methods Groups, Fields, and Consumer Network), in addition to the Steering Group. Entities had to register with Cochrane, and each entity acted as an independent unit and was responsible for its own management and for securing its own funding. Some sources of reading material about the history of Cochrane are listed in Box 21.2.

21.2   COCHRANE GROUPS

Cochrane's main work has for many years been overseen by around 50 Cochrane *Review Groups*. These manage the central task of preparing and maintaining Cochrane reviews. Each Review Group has an editorial base that includes a Co-ordinating Editor, a Managing Editor, and in most cases an Information Specialist and other support staff. The editorial base is responsible for maintaining a register of all relevant studies within the scope of the Review Group, coordinating and supporting the preparation and updating of reviews, and managing the Group's editorial processes. Cochrane Review Groups are further organized into eight networks, covering mental health and neuroscience; cancer; circulation and breathing; abdomen and endocrine; musculoskeletal, oral, skin, and sensory; acute and emergency care; children and families; and public health and health systems.

As of 2020 there were Cochrane *Geographic Groups or Centres* in more than 50 countries that act as regional representatives of Cochrane. They promote and support the use of Cochrane evidence in health policy and practice, and many of them are responsible for providing guidance, training, and support for the entities and individual contributors within the particular geographic area. The Centres are also responsible for providing information about the work of Cochrane and its products, and for promoting access to the Cochrane Library. Geographic Groups and Centres are heterogeneous, depending on their size, the funding situation, and especially their language and environment of the health research and health care system. As with all Cochrane entities, they have to identify their own funding sources. For the majority, funding is project based and therefore for a limited time. Groups in some countries are more fortunate than others. For example, Cochrane UK has received considerable support from the UK National Institute for Health Research (which has also funded more than 20 other groups). In 2017, Cochrane Germany secured funding for 10 years through a foundation financed by the Ministry of Health. The Centres can be involved in all activities where systematic reviews are providing synthesized knowledge as evidence input for evidence-based health care, decision-making, guideline development, health technology assessment (HTA) activities, and others.

Methods Groups advise Cochrane on the methods it uses to prepare, maintain, and promote the accessibility of systematic reviews. They promote and support relevant empirical methodological research and help to prepare and maintain systematic reviews of relevant methodological research. Methods Groups address almost 20 methodological areas, covering aspects of review methodology (e.g. information retrieval, bias assessment, statistical methods, use of the GRADE system, and using individual participant data) and different review types (e.g. screening and diagnostic tests, prognosis, and qualitative research). The outputs of methodological research are presented and discussed at the annual Cochrane Colloquia.

Fields are groups of people with a broad interest that cuts across a number of Review Groups. The focus can be on the setting of care (e.g. primary care), the type of consumer (e.g. children), the type of intervention (e.g. rehabilitation), or a broad category of condition (e.g. aging). They help to ensure that priorities and perspectives in their sphere of interest are reflected in the work of Review Groups, and liaise with relevant organizations within their area to promote knowledge translation and the use of evidence by decision-makers.

Engagement, input, and feedback from consumers are considered essential to fulfill Cochrane's aims. The *Consumer Network* was established to reflect consumer interests within Cochrane. It aims to provide information for consumers, and to encourage and support the involvement of consumers throughout Cochrane's activities. A significant result is the extension of Cochrane Reviews to include Plain Language Summaries, which complement the information provided in the abstract with a summary for patients and lay people.

Cochrane's membership historically consisted of all registered entities. Each entity, in turn, determined who among its own contributor base was eligible to vote for candidates to represent that type of entity on the Cochrane *Steering Group*. The Steering Group transitioned to the *Governing Board* in 2016 with 13 elected or appointed members, and this traditionally meets twice a year. The membership structure also transitioned to individual membership, and a majority of Governing Board members are elected as a result of individual voting. The Board has overall responsibility for overseeing the development and implementation of policy affecting Cochrane, and legal responsibility as the Board of Directors for The Cochrane Collaboration as a registered charity.

More information about the organization and its governance is available on the Cochrane website (http://cochrane.org) and the Cochrane Community website contained within it.

21.3   COCHRANE'S PRODUCT

Cochrane's efforts are focused on producing and maintaining up-to-date systematic reviews, which are available, together with other databases, in the Cochrane Library. The Cochrane Library (ISSN 1465–1858) is published online, currently by John Wiley & Sons.

For many years, the Cochrane Library included a collection of six databases containing different types of high-quality, independent evidence to inform health care decision-making, and a seventh database that provided information about Cochrane Groups. The databases could be searched simultaneously with the search engine provided. Since the databases previously produced by the Centre for Reviews and Dissemination – Database of Abstracts of Reviews of Effects (DARE) and the NHS Economic Evaluation Database (NHS EED) – and the Cochrane Methodology Register are not being updated, these are no longer available within the Cochrane Library. The Cochrane Library now includes the following:

- The *Cochrane Database of Systematic Reviews (CDSR)* is a rapidly growing collection of regularly updated, systematic reviews of the effects of health care, maintained by Cochrane. This is Cochrane's primary product.
- The *Cochrane Central Register of Controlled Trials (CENTRAL)* is a bibliography of controlled trials, downloaded from databases like Medline and Embase or identified as part of an international effort to handsearch the world's journals and create an unbiased source of data for systematic reviews.
- *Cochrane Clinical Answers* provide short, structured summaries of Cochrane Reviews that are aimed to be accessible to health professionals and to guide clinical decision-making.
- A federated search facility is available to enable readers to access high-quality non-Cochrane Reviews. Currently this function is available for the Epistemonikos platform, a large multilingual database of systematic reviews relevant for health decision-making [10].

21.4   COCHRANE IN THE TWENTY-FIRST CENTURY

Cochrane's growth is driven by the improved acceptance of systematic reviews in many countries around the globe, and their role as fundamental input in clinical guidelines, HTA reports, and patient information. However, the continuing international expansion has led to new challenges, by introducing greater diversity among the fast-growing number of contributors with respect to differences in cultural and social background, available resources, and language. The transformation of a group of enthusiastic individuals into an efficient international organization is at the heart of this process.

Between 2000 and 2021, the number of involved persons grew from around 4000 to more than 100 000. Inevitably, Cochrane Review Groups that have limited resources and are the recipients of public funding have to make decisions that prioritize the needs of readers and decision-makers, and that also represent the most effective use of resources. This means that the traditional approach of passive acceptance of review title requests from volunteer review teams has increasingly been replaced by active prioritization of research questions on the basis of end-user needs, and the development of funded and experienced teams.

Probably the biggest challenge has come from the ever-increasing number of RCTs being conducted, leading to a high demand for updating existing reviews to keep the reputation of the Cochrane Library as a database of up-to-date reviews. A substantial increase in the global funding of Cochrane would have been needed to meet the increase in growth, but could not be achieved. This again leads to an imperative for Cochrane Review Groups to make decisions on whether to update a review on the basis of the needs of users, and to investigate methods that will make systematic review processes more efficient.

In addition, demands from users have increased. The world of evidence synthesis has become increasingly large and competitive [11], and this has led to a situation where fewer than 20% of new systematic reviews are produced by Cochrane [12]. However, research has consistently shown that in terms of achieving high standards of quality and reporting, Cochrane Reviews are outperforming non-Cochrane reviews [12]. The criticism that Cochrane Reviews are inappropriately restricted to RCTs and that other study types should be considered has posed another challenge. In contrast to common perceptions, inclusion of nonrandomized studies of interventions has long been encouraged where appropriate. In 2008, Cochrane published its first systematic review of diagnostic test accuracy, and it is actively developing systems for reviewing other types of evidence, including studies of prognosis and qualitative research.

All of these factors initiated a comprehensive review of Cochrane and an intense discussion in all Cochrane entities with their members. This consultation has led to a gradual move from the "grass-roots" movement based on the work of volunteers toward professionalization.

21.5 COCHRANE IN TRANSITION: CHALLENGES AND OPPORTUNITIES

Cochrane retains an important place in the evidence synthesis eco-system. It comprises a large and disparate international community that includes many of the most prominent researchers and thinkers. Its Strategy to 2020 focused on four major areas of work, including the quality-efficient production of reviews, increasing their impact in the world, advocacy for evidence-informed health care, and the need to build a strong, diverse, and sustainable organization. Building on this, there are a number of important challenges that Cochrane will need to address:

- Whether and how the changes toward a more professional approach, and an expanded Central Executive Team (CET), will impact on the availability and motivation of researchers, authors, and other contributors to invest their personal resources in Cochrane. Academic researchers are increasingly expected to be able to demonstrate the benefits of their work in Cochrane to their host institutions, and are under increased pressure to generate income and research impact to ensure academic progression. Cochrane has to be better able to meet the needs of host institutions and their researchers to continue to attract and retain the most talented individuals.

- Cochrane processes are sometimes slow and bureaucratic, in some part due to increasing methodological complexity and the reliance on the work of volunteers. Changes are needed to accelerate the review process, including the exploitation of technology innovations, and Cochrane is investing heavily in this area.

- The ubiquitous expansion of interest in "Big Data" is another challenge. Promises from "Big Data" are sometimes unrealistic, epitomized by statements like "The end of theory" or "The era of causation is being replaced by correlation" [13]. Similarly, support for the use of observational "real-world evidence" in evaluations of health care interventions, embodied by the 21st Century Cures Act in the USA, is a clear challenge for Cochrane [14]. A "Big Data" or "real-world evidence" revolution may be a threat to controlled trials and consequently also to Cochrane.

- The global demand to increase accessibility to research output, as part of moves toward open science, has recently been reinforced by the European Parliament, following the US National Institutes of Health (NIH) and other organizations. Cochrane's CET and its technical infrastructure, including its content management systems and online learning programs, are currently dependent on the income from royalties from the publisher of the Cochrane Library. Cochrane has made important strides to develop its open access provision. Since the introduction of its green and gold open access models, the proportion of open access reviews has risen to 72%, and this figure will continue to rise. However, contemporary moves toward universal immediate open access will further challenge the financial sustainability of the organization in its current form.

This chapter has been completed during a period in which the world has been shaken by the novel coronavirus. This has been superimposed on a time of great transition in the wider scientific publishing world. Cochrane has many reasons for optimism, the greatest of which is the continuing enthusiasm, commitment, and skills of its community, but the challenges it faces from these developments are real and need to be taken seriously to allow the Cochrane success story to continue.

ACKNOWLEDGMENTS

We would like to acknowledge the generous efforts of the thousands of contributors to The Cochrane Collaboration, who together have helped turn a bright idea into a reality, and who collectively continue to define Cochrane and determine its development.

REFERENCES

1. Naylor, C.D. (1995). Grey zones of clinical practice: some limitations to evidence-based medicine. *Lancet* 345: 840–843.

2. Cochrane, A.L. (1972). *Effectiveness and Efficiency. Random Reflections on Health Services*, 35–36. London: Nuffield Provincial Hospital Trust.

3. Cochrane, A.L. (1979). 1931–1971: a critical review, with particular reference to the medical profession. In: *Medicines for the Year 2000* (eds. G.T. Smith and N. Wells), 1–11. London: Office of Health Economics.

4. Chalmers, I. (1991). The work of the national perinatal epidemiology unit. *Int. J. Technol. Assess Health Care* 7: 430–459.

5. Cochrane, A.L. (1989). Foreword. In: *Effective Care in Pregnancy and Childbirth* (eds. I. Chalmers, M. Enkin and M.J.N.C. Keirse). Oxford: Oxford University Press.

6. Mulrow, C.D. (1987). The medical review article: state of the science. *Ann. Intern. Med.* 106: 485–488.

7. Anon (1992). Cochrane's legacy. *Lancet* 340: 1131–1132.

8. Chalmers, I., Dickersin, K., and Chalmers, T.C. (1992). Getting to grips with Archie Cochrane's agenda. *Br. Med. J.* 305: 786–788.

9. Chalmers, I. (1993). The Cochrane collaboration: preparing, maintaining and disseminating systematic reviews of the effects of health care. *Ann. N. Y. Acad. Sci.* 703: 156–163.

10. Rada, G., Pérez, D., and Capurro, D. (2013). Epistemonikos: a free, relational, collaborative, multilingual database of health evidence. *Stud. Health Technol. Inform.* 192 (1–2): 486–490.

11. Ioannidis, J.P.A. (2016). The mass production of redundant, misleading, and conflicted systematic reviews and meta-analyses. *Milbank Q.* 94 (3): 485–514.

12. Page, M.J., Shamseer, L., Altman, D.G. et al. (2016 Mai). Epidemiology and reporting characteristics of systematic reviews of biomedical research: a cross-sectional study. *PLoS Med.* 13 (5): e1002028.

13. Anderson, C. (2008). The end of theory: the data deluge makes the scientific method obsolete. *Wired* June 23. https://www.wired.com/2008/06/pb-theory. Accessed 21 February 2022

14. Schwartz, J.L. (2017 Nov). Real-world evidence, public participation, and the FDA. *Hast. Cent. Rep.* 47 (6): 7–8.

CHAPTER 22

Using Systematic Reviews in Guideline Development

The GRADE Approach

Holger J. Schünemann

22.1 INTRODUCTION

Guidelines are systematically developed, evidence-based statements that help providers, patients, policymakers, and other stakeholders make informed decisions about health care and public health policy [1]. Systematic reviews are essential to producing trustworthy guidelines that make data and their interpretation fully transparent [1–8]. Expert opinion, defined as the combination of interpretation and assessment of relevant data, can be crucial too. The Grading of Recommendations Assessment, Development and Evaluation (GRADE) system also plays an important role in guideline development.

22.1.1 The Role of Systematic Reviews in Guidelines

Systematic reviews increase transparency by making sure that all members of a guideline panel discuss the same, comprehensive body of evidence. Systematic reviews are relevant to anything that influences the direction and strength of a recommendation. Questions such as those dealing with prognosis, test accuracy, or values and preferences related to different outcomes will need more than one systematic review. Figure 22.1 details the place of systematic reviews in the guideline development process [8].

The GRADE working group (www.gradeworkinggroup.org) is a collaboration of over 500 scientists, clinicians, and people with other backgrounds that has developed the GRADE approach to assessing the quality of or the certainty in the body of evidence summarized in systematic reviews [9, 10]. GRADE is used by over 100 organizations,

Systematic Reviews in Health Research: Meta-Analysis in Context, Third Edition. Edited by Matthias Egger, Julian P.T. Higgins, and George Davey Smith.
© 2022 John Wiley & Sons Ltd. Published 2022 by John Wiley & Sons Ltd.
Companion website: www.systematic-reviews3.org

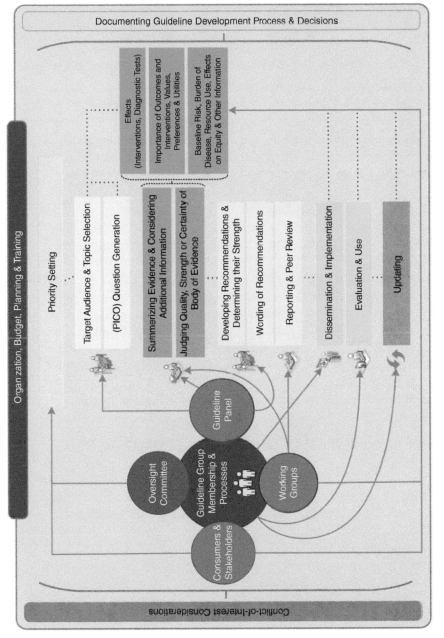

FIGURE 22.1 The guideline development process: summarizing the evidence and judging the quality, strength, or certainty of a body of evidence should be done through systematic reviews. The guideline panel and supporting groups (e.g. methodologist, health economist, systematic review team, a secretariat for administrative support) work collaboratively, informed through consumer and stakeholder involvement. They report to the oversight committee. PICO, Population, Intervention, Comparator, Outcome.

including the World Health Organization (WHO), the National Institute of Health and Care Excellence, the Canadian Task Force for the Preventive Services, numerous professional organizations, and Cochrane. GRADE is applicable to different types of evidence that include evidence on intervention effects (including multiple treatment comparisons), test accuracy, prognosis, resources and values, and preferences.

22.1.2   GRADE's Role in the Systematic Review Process and Guideline Development

GRADE defines certainty in the evidence as the "extent to which one can be confident that an estimate of the effect or association is correct." In the context of guideline development, certainty in the evidence reflects the confidence that the estimates of an effect are adequate to support a particular decision or recommendation [11–13]. GRADE uses the terms certainty in the evidence, quality of the evidence, strength of the evidence, and confidence in effect estimates interchangeably, but the preferred term is certainty in the evidence. Certainty in the evidence is one of several criteria used for grading the strength and direction of a recommendation or decision in GRADE Evidence to Decision (EtD) Frameworks [14–17] (see Section 22.3). These criteria consider risk of bias, imprecision, inconsistency, indirectness, and publication bias, which may downgrade certainty in the evidence, as well as the magnitude of effects, dose–response relations, and the impact of residual confounding and opposing bias, which may upgrade certainty in the evidence. Judgments consider specific items such as concealment of allocation, which is an important item to gauge the risk of bias in randomized trials, and the I^2 measure [18], which is important in the context of inconsistency (see also Chapters 4 and 9). A guideline development group will use GRADE assessments as the basis for its discussions to formulate recommendations. The group should have a basic understanding of GRADE. Figure 22.2 presents the detailed process of how GRADE is considered in the guideline development process.

22.1.3   Who Performs the Assessment of the Certainty in the Evidence?

Just as conducting a systematic review is a specialized task, assessing evidence and developing evidence summaries are best done by an experienced systematic review author or methodologist, with input from a multidisciplinary group and content experts. GRADE assessments have been found to be reproducible, in particular when done by assessors with training in health research methods [19, 20].

22.2   THE CERTAINTY IN THE EVIDENCE, QUALITY OF THE EVIDENCE, OR STRENGTH OF THE EVIDENCE

GRADE categorizes the certainty in the evidence as high, moderate, low, or very low (Table 22.1). These certainty levels apply to the body of evidence assessed for each key question, not to individual studies. However, an assessment of the risk of bias is

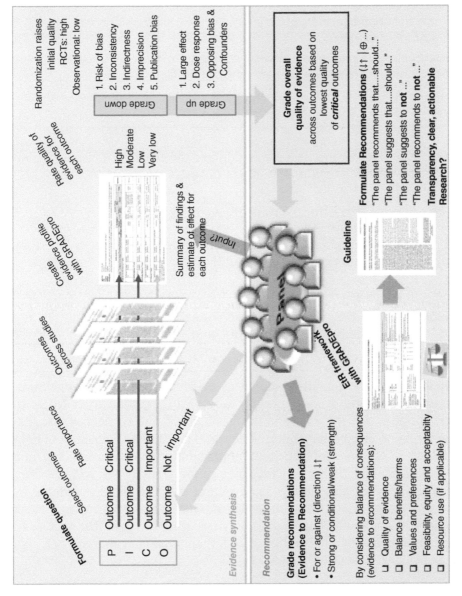

FIGURE 22.2 Integration of the GRADE approach into guideline development for interventions. There is a close relationship between systematic reviewers and guideline panels. The panels select critical and important outcomes. The evidence for these outcomes should be evaluated in systematic reviews. EtR, evidence to recommendation; PICO, Population, Intervention, Comparator, Outcome; RCT, randomized controlled trial.

TABLE 22.1   GRADE categories of certainty in the evidence.

Quality level	Definition
High	We are very confident that the true effect lies close to that of the estimate of the effect.
Moderate	We have moderate confidence in the effect estimate. The true effect is likely to be close to the estimate of the effect, but there is a possibility that it is substantially different.
Low	Our confidence in the effect estimate is limited. The true effect may be substantially different from the estimate of the effect.
Very low	We have very little confidence in the effect estimate. The true effect is likely to be substantially different from the estimate of effect.

needed for each study in order to assess the certainty in the evidence. This assessment can lead to lowering or increasing the certainty in the evidence.

22.2.1   Evidence on the Effects of Interventions

For interventions, the starting point for rating the certainty of the evidence is the study design, broadly separated into two types [13, 21, 22]:

- Randomized controlled trials (RCTs).
- Nonrandomized studies (NRSs) or observational studies (including but not limited to cohort studies, and case–control studies, cross-sectional studies, or case series and case reports).

Although RCTs are the preferred source of evidence to assess interventions, in many instances guideline developers must rely on information from NRSs, in particular to evaluate potential harms, and the feasibility of, and barriers and facilitators to, implementation of an intervention. Relevant data can be obtained from both RCTs and NRSs, with each type of evidence complementing the other. In GRADE, a body of evidence based on RCTs begins with a high certainty rating and evidence from NRSs begins with a low-certainty rating, as a result of the potential bias induced by the lack of randomization. However, if an assessment tool is used that covers the risk of bias due to lack of randomization (such as the new ROBINS-I tool: Risk Of Bias In Non-randomized Studies – of Interventions [23]), then all studies may start as high certainty in the evidence (see also Chapter 15).

22.2.2   Certainty in the Evidence from Randomized Controlled Trials and Nonrandomized Studies can be Lowered in Five Domains

The initial ratings are followed by detailed ratings across the five domains – risk of bias, inconsistency, indirectness, imprecision, and publication bias – which can lower certainty. The ratings in systematic reviews are conducted initially on a "per outcome" level. This requires detailed knowledge of the individual studies included in the body of evidence. Reasons for lowering the certainty in the evidence should be guided by GRADE [24]; for details readers are referred to the online GRADE Handbook [25] and the cited publications. The following provides a short description of the domains.

22.2.2.1   Risk of Bias

For RCTs, some of the main criteria for assessing the risk of bias are [26] (see also Chapter 4):

- Randomization methods, including concealment of allocation to intervention group.
- Blinding of participants and investigators and other relevant groups, particularly if the outcomes were measured subjectively and thus may be subject to bias.
- Appropriate use of intention-to-treat analysis.
- Examination of information about withdrawals of study participants.

For NRSs, the criteria depend on the design, but can be categorized as follows [26]:

- Application of appropriate eligibility criteria.
- Use of an unbiased approach to measurement and reporting of exposure and outcomes.
- Adequate control for confounding.
- Examination of information about withdrawals of study participants.

The assessment of the risk of bias is initially completed for each study and then summarized across studies for each outcome. Study limitations across the body of evidence for each outcome can be categorized as follows (Table 22.2):

- *No serious limitations* means that the majority of studies meet all the minimum quality criteria for the design.
- *Serious limitations* means that one of the minimum criteria for quality is not met by the majority of studies in the review. This results in lowering the overall quality rating (e.g. high becomes moderate for RCTs or low becomes very low for observational studies).
- *Very serious limitations* means that the risk of bias likely has a strong influence on the estimate of the effect, and potential study limitations are present in the majority of studies in the review. This typically results in lowering the quality by two levels.

22.2.2.2   Inconsistency

There is inconsistency if the results for an outcome are heterogeneous [27]. Inconsistency may arise from differences in the populations in the studies, in the interventions, comparators, or in outcomes. To explore inconsistency, sensitivity or subgroup

TABLE 22.2 Guidance for the risk of bias domain in a GRADE assessment: going from assessments of risk of bias to judgments about study limitations for main outcomes across all included studies.

Risk of bias	Across studies	Interpretation	Considerations	GRADE assessment of study limitations/risk of bias
Low risk of bias	Most information is from studies at low risk of bias	Plausible bias unlikely to seriously alter the results	No apparent limitations	No serious limitations, do not downgrade
Unclear risk of bias	Most information is from studies at low or unclear risk of bias	Plausible bias that raises some doubt about the results	Potential limitations are unlikely to lower confidence in the estimate of effect	No serious limitations, do not downgrade
			Potential limitations are likely to lower confidence in the estimate of effect	Serious limitations, downgrade one level
High risk of bias	The proportion of information from studies at high risk of bias is sufficient to affect the interpretation of results	Plausible bias that seriously weakens confidence in the results	Crucial limitation for one criterion, or some limitations for multiple criteria, sufficient to lower confidence in the estimate of effect	Serious limitations, downgrade one level
			Crucial limitation for one or more criteria sufficient to substantially lower confidence in the estimate of effect	Very serious limitations, downgrade two levels

analyses are useful. Three main criteria are used to assess the presence of important inconsistency [27]:

- Wide variation of the point estimates across studies.
- Minimal or no overlap of confidence intervals.
- If a meta-analysis was performed, a small P value from a test for heterogeneity, or a high I^2 value (see also Chapter 9).

If the confidence intervals of all the results overlap, the presence of important inconsistency is unlikely. If there is some inconsistency in the results, such as if the largest study shows results that contradict smaller studies, then the overall quality is lowered by one level. Evidence will be downgraded for an outcome by two levels if the results are very heterogeneous. If only one study is present, certainty in the evidence should not be lowered due to inconsistency. However, when there is only one study, certainty in the overall body of evidence likely will be lowered for risk of bias, publication bias, imprecision, or indirectness.

22.2.2.3   Indirectness

Directness, generalizability, external validity, transferability, and applicability of study results all refer to similar concepts that are addressed in GRADE in the domain of indirectness [28, 29].

Indirectness arises when the identified evidence differs with respect to the *PICO* questions (Population, Intervention, Comparator, Outcome) formulated by the guideline development group or the systematic reviewers. While all evidence is indirect to some degree [30], serious or very serious indirectness will lead to downrating the overall certainty in the evidence by one or two levels. However, certainty in the evidence should be lowered only if the effect is likely to differ between the target population and the identified evidence. This may be the case if there is evidence of relevant effect modification, if interventions are applied differently, or if there are differences in the comparator or the use of outcome measures that may not reflect the outcome of interest.

A special case of indirectness arises if direct comparisons between the intervention of interest and the comparator of interest are not available: for example, if the guideline panel is interested in a comparison of intervention A versus B, but studies only exist in which A was compared with C and B was compared with C. While these studies allow indirect comparisons of the magnitude of effect of A versus B, such indirect evidence may be of lower quality than direct comparisons and is therefore downrated. The results of network meta-analyses or multiple treatment comparisons are often subject to this indirectness [31] (see Chapter 13).

Systematic review authors should use GRADE's indirectness tables (Table 22.3), which provide a transparent record and starting point for evidence synthesis [24, 28]. The assessments of systematic reviewers may differ, though, from those of a guideline panel that uses systematic reviews. Guideline panels should discuss whether they agree with reviewers' judgments and may alter an overall certainty rating by reassessing indirectness in the context of their PICO questions.

22.2.2.4   Imprecision

Judgments about imprecision are made across studies and not at the level of an individual study [32]. In general, results are imprecise when the body of evidence includes few participants and few events, with wide confidence intervals around the estimate of the effect [22, 32]. GRADE suggests using the 95% confidence interval (95% CI) as the primary criterion to make judgments about imprecision, and the optimal information size (OIS) as a second criterion for determining adequate precision. If the confidence interval overlaps with a threshold for decision-making, then the body of evidence is imprecise for that outcome and certainty in the evidence is lowered [32].

TABLE 22.3   Judgments about indirectness by outcome.

Outcome: . . .					
Domain (original question asked)	Description (evidence found and included, including evidence from other studies) – consider the domains of study design and study execution, inconsistency, imprecision, and publication bias	Judgment – is the evidence sufficiently direct?			
		Yes	Probably yes	Probably no	No
Population:		□	□	□	□
Intervention:		Yes □	Probably yes □	Probably no □	No □
Comparator:		Yes □	Probably yes □	Probably no □	No □
Direct comparison:		Yes □	Probably yes □	Probably no □	No □
Outcome:		Yes □	Probably yes □	Probably no □	No □
Final judgment about indirectness across domains:		□ No indirectness	□ Serious indirectness	□ Very serious indirectness	

Source: Adapted from Schünemann et al. [28].

GRADE suggests that a guideline panel take the following steps to decide whether to downgrade the overall certainty in the evidence for imprecision:

- Consider the boundaries of the 95% CI: do they cross the health decision threshold between recommending and not recommending an intervention?
- If the answer is yes (i.e. the 95% CI crosses the threshold), downgrade for imprecision irrespective of where the point estimate and 95% CI lie.

The OIS is defined by a sample size calculation for a single, adequately powered trial to detect a worthwhile effect of interest [32, 33]. If the total number of patients included in a systematic review is less than the number of patients from a sample size calculation, one should consider downrating for imprecision. The OIS depends on a worthwhile effect that needs to be determined with input from decision-makers.

Indeed, guideline panels need to consider the context of a recommendation and other outcomes (for example, adverse effects), whereas judgments about specific outcomes in a systematic review are often free of that context. Another approach is to consider the review information size (RIS), which does not require defining a worthwhile effect but relies on plausible effects [17]. For continuous outcomes, a similar approach can be used that is based on a sample size calculation for plausible effects for continuous outcomes [32]. Generally speaking, if the sample size exceeds 400 for a continuous outcome, imprecision is unlikely to be present.

To formulate recommendations, all outcomes need to be considered together. Guideline panels will have to assess whether outcomes are critical, or important but not critical for decision-making. Downgrading for imprecision is dependent on both the decision threshold and consideration of the trade-off between desirable and undesirable effects and other consequences. Imprecision is therefore another domain where guideline panels may modify the judgments of systematic review authors [17].

22.2.2.5   Publication Bias

Publication bias is the systematic deviation of the effect estimated in a systematic review from the underlying true effect due to the selective publication of studies. The benefits of interventions typically are overestimated because negative studies remain unpublished (see Chapter 5). Statistical methods exist to detect the possibility of publication bias, but these should be applied and interpreted with caution (see Chapter 5). Systematic reviewers and guideline panels must often make assumptions about the extent of publication bias. Publication bias should be suspected in situations when published evidence is limited to a low number of small studies, or when all or almost all available studies were funded by a for-profit organization [34]. GRADE suggests downrating the certainty in the evidence in these situations. Of note is that selective outcome reporting bias is covered under the risk of bias domain (see above). Selective outcome reporting bias may arise when investigators fail to report outcomes that they have measured because of the direction of the results (see also Chapter 5).

22.2.3   Three Factors Can Increase the Certainty in the Evidence of Nonrandomized Studies

If and only if there are no further limitations, i.e. there is no reason for downgrading the quality of a body of evidence from NRSs, then upgrading the certainty in the evidence may be possible, within the following three domains [35].

22.2.3.1   Dose–Response Gradient

The presence of a dose–response gradient has long been recognized as supporting the causal nature of an association observed in NRSs [36]. Such a gradient will often increase confidence in the findings of NRSs, and thereby increase the certainty in the evidence. If there is evidence of a dose–response gradient, one may therefore upgrade the evidence for this outcome by one level.

22.2.3.2   Direction of Plausible Residual Confounding and Bias

It is possible that all plausible confounders or biases that could not be accounted for in a well-conducted NRS could result in an underestimate of an observed treatment effect. Consider the situation where sicker individuals tend to receive an experimental intervention, yet they still fare better. In this situation it is likely that the intervention effect is larger than the evidence suggests. If there is evidence that all of the plausible residual confounding or bias would influence the effect in this way, one can uprate the evidence for such an outcome by one level.

22.2.3.3   Magnitude of the Effect

Similar to the dose–response gradient, the strength of an association has long been proposed for consideration when assessing data from NRSs [35]. If a large or very large effect is observed, this will generally increase confidence in the results. GRADE suggests two thresholds when considering upgrading the evidence: a relative risk greater than 2.0 or smaller than 0.5 to upgrade by one level, and a relative risk of greater than 5.0 or smaller than 0.2 to upgrade by two levels [35]. Other aspects that should be considered in addition to the thresholds include the consistency of the effect across different studies and populations, and the precision of the effect estimate (as judged by the 95% CI). If the estimate is large but imprecise or inconsistent across populations, then the confidence in the evidence should not be upgraded.

22.2.4   Certainty in the Evidence by Outcome

A hypothetical assessment criterion for each of the eight GRADE domains in the certainty of evidence is shown in Table 22.4. This approach can be used to describe the findings of a systematic review and justify its judgments. A final rating of the evidence

TABLE 22.4   Domains for describing certainty in the evidence and justifying downgrading or upgrading.

Criteria for assessing certainty in the evidence by outcome	Results section	Examples of reasons for lowering or increasing the quality of evidence
Risk of bias	Describe the risk of bias based on the criteria used in the risk of bias table	Of eight randomized trials, five did not blind patients and caretakers and the other three trials had important loss to follow-up
Inconsistency	Describe the degree of inconsistency by outcome using one or more items (e.g. I^2 and P value), confidence interval overlap, and difference in point estimate	The proportion of the variability in effect estimates that is due to true heterogeneity rather than chance is not important ($I^2 = 0\%$, P values for heterogeneity >0.4), confidence intervals overlapping

TABLE 22.4   *(Continued)*

Criteria for assessing certainty in the evidence by outcome	Results section	Examples of reasons for lowering or increasing the quality of evidence
Indirectness	Describe if the majority of studies address the PICO – were they similar to the question posed? Use the GRADE directness table	The included studies were restricted to patients with advanced cancer and did not cover the full spectrum of cancer patients
Imprecision	Describe the number of events, and width of the confidence intervals	The confidence intervals for the effect on mortality are compatible with both an appreciable benefit and appreciable harm
Publication bias	Describe the possible degree of publication bias	1. The funnel plot of 19 randomized trials indicated that there were several small studies with a small positive effect, but small studies that showed no effect or harm may have been unpublished 2. There are only three small positive studies; it appears that studies showing no effect or harm have not been published. There also is for-profit interest in the intervention
Large effects (upgrading)	Describe the magnitude of the effect and the widths of the associated confidence intervals	The RR is 0.2 (95% CI 0.1 to 0.3) with a sufficient number of events
Dose–response (upgrading)	The studies show a clear relation of increases in the outcome frequency or severity with higher exposure or intervention levels	The dose–response relation shows a relative risk increase of 6% in never smokers, 10% in smokers of 10 pack-years, and 14% in smokers of 15 pack-years
Opposing plausible residual bias and confounding (upgrading)	Describe which opposing biases and confounders may not have been considered	An effect is observed between an intervention or exposure and an outcome. The estimate of effect is not controlled for the possible confounders smoking and degree of education, but the distribution of these factors in the studies is likely to lead to an underestimate of the true effect

CI, confidence interval; PICO, Population, Intervention, Comparator, Outcome; RR, risk ratio.

is obtained as shown in Figure 22.3. Judgments about one domain influence judgments about other domains; they need to be considered in context. For example, the domains of indirectness, inconsistency, and imprecision are closely related [12]. The final rating creates the transparency that allows others such as decision-makers to understand the judgments made in the systematic review.

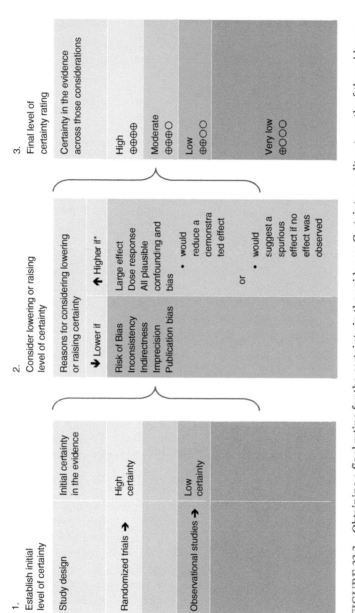

FIGURE 22.3 Obtaining a final rating for the certainty in the evidence. Certainty, quality, strength of the evidence, or the confidence in the estimate of effect are determined for each outcome based on a systematic review of the evidence for each outcome. For recommendations, the overall certainty is determined across outcomes based on the lowest-quality outcome among those critical for decision-making. *Criteria for upgrading the quality are usually only applicable to observational studies without any reason for downrating.

22.2.5   GRADE Evidence Profiles and Summary of Findings Tables

GRADE evidence profiles include detailed assessment of the quality or certainty in the evidence for each outcome [37]. Table 22.5 shows an example from a clinical practice guideline of the treatment of idiopathic pulmonary fibrosis (IPF) [38]. The effects of the intervention (pirfenidone, a drug that inhibits the production of growth factors and procollagens) are summarized both in relative terms and as absolute risk differences. The main reason for a quality assessment or other noteworthy points is documented in explanatory footnotes that constitute an essential part of GRADE tables [24, 39]. The summary of findings (SoF) table (Table 22.6) includes an assessment of the quality of evidence for each outcome, but not the detailed judgments on which that assessment is based. SoF tables are intended for a broader audience like users of guidelines; they provide a concise summary of the key information underlying a recommendation.

22.2.6   How is the Overall Certainty in the Evidence for a Decision or Recommendation Determined?

Guideline developers should assess all the information from the systematic review and make a final decision about which outcomes are critical and which are important given the recommendations they are dealing with. Panels then determine the overall certainty in the evidence across all the critical outcomes for a recommendation by providing a single grade of certainty in the evidence for every recommendation. Because certainty in the evidence is rated separately for each outcome, the certainty usually differs across outcomes. If the certainty in the evidence is the same for all critical outcomes, then this becomes the overall certainty in the evidence supporting the answer to the question. If the certainty in the evidence differs across critical outcomes, the overall certainty in the recommendation is not higher than the lowest certainty for any outcome that is critical for a decision. Therefore, the lowest certainty in the evidence for any of the critical outcomes determines the overall certainty in the evidence.

22.2.7   Assessing the Certainty in a Body of Evidence About Tests

The best evidence about the benefit of using a diagnostic or screening test comes from RCTs of test and intervention strategies that directly measure the relevant outcomes. Indeed, if a test fails to improve outcomes, there is no reason to use it whatever its accuracy [21]. The systematic review process should therefore begin with a search for intervention studies. If such studies are found, then the GRADE approach for interventions is used [16, 21].

In many situations, direct evidence from intervention studies is lacking and the evidence from studies of diagnostic test accuracy needs to be linked to other data to assess the likely effects on outcomes. This is a two-step process. In the first step, test accuracy studies are evaluated in systematic reviews and, where appropriate, combined in meta-analyses. The appropriate study design to measure test accuracy is observational, and the assessment of the certainty in the evidence therefore begins with a rating of high certainty. The evaluation follows the basic GRADE principles and the five domains for

TABLE 22.5 Example of a GRADE evidence profile.

Author(s): Schünemann HJ for the ATS/IPF Guideline Group
Date: January 30, 2016
Question: Pirfenidone compared to placebo for patients with Idiopathic pulmonary fibrosis (IPF)
Setting: inpatient and outpatient treatment
Bibliography: ATS/ERS guidelines on treatment of IPF [38]

		Quality assessment					Nº of patients		Effect		Quality	Importance
Nº of studies	Study design	Risk of bias	Inconsistency	Indirectness	Imprecision	Other considerations	Pirfenidone	Placebo	Relative (95% CI)	Absolute (95% CI)		
Mortality (follow-up: 72 weeks)												
5	Randomized trials	Not serious	Not serious	Not serious	Serious[a]	None	41/804 (5.1%)	59/763 (7.7%)	**RR 0.70** (0.47 to 1.02)	**23 fewer per 1000** (from 2 more to 41 fewer)	⊕⊕⊕○ MODERATE	CRITICAL
Acute exacerbation (follow-up: 72 weeks)												
4	Randomized trials	Serious[b]	Not serious	Not serious	Serious[c]	None	10/526 (1.9%)	14/486 (2.9%)	**RR 0.69** (0.20 to 2.42)	**9 fewer per 1000** (from 23 fewer to 41 more)	⊕⊕○○ LOW	CRITICAL

Disease progression (follow-up: 72 weeks; assessed with: Vital capacity [higher numbers are better])

№	Study design	Risk of bias	Inconsistency	Indirectness	Imprecision	Other	№ patients		Relative effect	Absolute	Certainty	Importance
4	Randomized trials	Not serious[d]	Not serious	Not serious	Not serious	None	521	–	–	SMD **0.23 more** (0.06 more to 0.41 more)	⊕⊕⊕⊕ HIGH	CRITICAL

Disease Progression (assessed with: DLCO [Higher numbers better])

№	Study design	Risk of bias	Inconsistency	Indirectness	Imprecision	Other	№ patients		Relative effect	Absolute	Certainty	Importance
4	Randomized trials[e]	Not serious	Not serious	Not serious	Serious[f]	None	526	486	–	See comment	⊕⊕⊕O MODERATE	CRITICAL

[a] Relatively wide confidence intervals. In the worst-case scenario one would not accept cost/side effects of drug.
[b] One trial stopped early (Azuma et al.) because of perceived benefit in regards to exacerbations.
[c] There are sparse data leading to imprecision. The confidence intervals are wide and compatible with important harm and benefit.
[d] Data were imputed in studies 004 and 006.
[e] It is not clear which patients had DLCO measured and the data provided in the primary publications do not allow for pooling of results.
[f] The importance of this outcome measure for patients and the relation to patient important outcomes is uncertain.
CI, confidence interval; DLCO, diffusing capacity of lung for carbon monoxide; MD, mean difference; RR, risk ratio; SMD, standardized mean difference.

TABLE 22.6 Example of a GRADE summary of findings table.

Pirfenidone compared to placebo for patients with idiopathic pulmonary fibrosis (IPF)

Bibliography: ATS/ERS guidelines on treatment of IPF [38]

Outcomes	Nº of participants (studies) Follow-up	Quality of the evidence (GRADE)	Relative effect (95% CI)	Anticipated absolute effects	
				Risk with placebo	Risk difference with Pirfenidone*
Mortality follow-up: 72 weeks	1567 (5 RCTs)	⊕⊕⊕⊖ MODERATE[a]	**RR 0.70** (0.47 to 1.02)	77 per 1000	**23 fewer per 1000** (41 fewer to 2 more)
Acute exacerbation follow-up: 72 weeks	1012 (4 RCTs)	⊕⊕⊖⊖ LOW[b,c]	**RR 0.69** (0.20 to 2.42)	29 per 1000	**9 fewer per 1000** (23 fewer to 41 more)
Disease progression assessed with: vital capacity (higher numbers are better) follow-up: 72 weeks	1006 (4 RCTs)	⊕⊕⊕⊕ HIGH[d]	–	–	SMD **0.23 more** (0.06 more to 0.41 more)
Disease progression assessed with: DLCO (higher numbers better)	1012 (4 RCTs)[e]	⊕⊕⊕⊖ MODERATE[f]	–	Not pooled	Not pooled

*The risk in the intervention group (and its 95% confidence interval) is based on the assumed risk in the comparison group and the **relative effect** of the intervention (and its 95% CI).

CI, confidence interval; **DLCO**, diffusing capacity of lung for carbon monoxide; **MD**, mean difference; **RCTs**, randomized controlled trials; **RR**, risk ratio; **SMD**, standardized mean difference.

GRADE Working Group grades of evidence

High quality: We are very confident that the true effect lies close to that of the estimate of the effect

Moderate quality: We have moderate confidence in the effect estimate. The true effect is likely to be close to the estimate of the effect, but there is a possibility that it is substantially different

Low quality: Our confidence in the effect estimate is limited. The true effect may be substantially different from the estimate of the effect.

Very low quality: We have very little confidence in the effect estimate. The true effect is likely to be substantially different from the estimate of effect.

[a] Relatively wide confidence intervals. In the worst-case scenario one would not accept cost/side effects of drug.
[b] One trial stopped early (Azuma et al.) because of perceived benefit with regard to exacerbations.
[c] There are sparse data leading to imprecision. The confidence intervals are wide and compatible with important harm and benefit.
[d] Data were imputed in studies 004 and 006.
[e] It is not clear which patients had DLCO measured and the data provided in the primary publications do not allow for pooling of results.
[f] The importance of this outcome measure for patients and the relation to patient important outcomes is uncertain.

downrating certainty. Domains for uprating may exist, but further work is required to better describe them.

In the second step, the best estimates of test accuracy are linked to other evidence such as data on the prevalence of the condition, its natural history, or the effectiveness of treatments. For recommendations based on linking different bodies of evidence, the overall certainty in the evidence involves an evaluation of which data are critical for decision-making. The overall rating is then based on the lowest certainty in any part of the evidence considered critical. For example, a WHO cervical cancer guideline panel had very low confidence in some of the critical evidence used to derive the estimates of benefit at the population level, despite the fact that the diagnostic test accuracy information was of moderate to high quality [40].

22.2.8   Prognosis, Resource Use, and Values and Preferences

Similar to evidence for intervention effects, the GRADE approach to rating certainty in the evidence can be used in systematic reviews of prognostic questions. Given that NRSs are the most appropriate design to assess prognosis, they start as high certainty in the evidence. While the operationalization of the domains differs for prognostic evidence, the domains for downrating the certainty in the evidence are the same. For details the reader is referred to the relevant guidance from the GRADE working group [41, 42]. Resource utilization can also be assessed using the GRADE approach [43, 44]. GRADE guidance on how to assess the certainty in the evidence about values and preferences is currently under review.

22.3   DEVELOPING RECOMMENDATIONS AND MAKING DECISIONS

The GRADE working group has developed EtD frameworks to help guideline panels use the available evidence and develop decisions and recommendations in a structured and transparent way [14, 45–48]. The EtD framework consists of three sections: the PICO questions, summaries of the evidence, and the conclusions.

Guideline panels typically use evidence from several systematic reviews to formulate their recommendations. These are usefully summarized in SoF tables (Table 22.5). The GRADE criteria that determine the direction and strength of the recommendation and a description of how they influence the recommendation are summarized in Table 22.7. An example of a detailed EtD framework can be found on the book's website at www.systematic-reviews3.org.

22.3.1   The Strength of the Recommendation

The strength of a recommendation reflects the confidence of a guideline development group in the balance of the desirable and undesirable consequences of implementing a recommendation:

TABLE 22.7 Criteria that influence the strength and direction in the GRADE Evidence to Decision frameworks.

Criteria	How the criterion influences the direction and strength of a recommendation
1. Problem	The judgment about the problem is determined by the importance and frequency of the health care issue that is addressed (burden of disease, prevalence, cost, or baseline risk). If the problem is of great importance, a strong recommendation may be more likely
2. Values and preferences or the importance of outcomes	This describes how important health outcomes are to those affected, how variable they are, and if there is uncertainty about this
3. Certainty in the evidence about the health benefits and harm	The higher the certainty in the evidence, the more likely is a strong recommendation
4. Health benefits and harms and burden and their balance	1. This requires an evaluation of the absolute effects of both the benefits and harms and their importance, including the judgment about the criterion 2. The greater the net benefit or net harm, the more likely is a strong recommendation for or against the option
5. Resource implications	This describes how resource intense an option is, if it is cost-effective, and if there is incremental benefit. The more advantageous or clearly disadvantageous these resource implications are, the more likely is a strong recommendation
6. Equity	The greater the likelihood of reducing inequities or increasing equity and the more accessible an option is, the more likely is a strong recommendation
7. Acceptability	The greater the acceptability of an option to all or most stakeholders, the more likely is a strong recommendation
8. Feasibility	The greater the acceptability of an option to all or most stakeholders, the more likely is a strong recommendation

- *Strong*: the guideline group is confident that the desirable effects outweigh any undesirable consequences.
- *Conditional or weak*: there is considerable uncertainty about the balance of desirable and undesirable effects.

Strong recommendations are not very common. Guideline panels often deal with low- or very low-quality evidence and therefore are reluctant to make strong recommendations [49].

The EtD framework (Table 22.7, Table S22.1 on www.systematic-reviews3.org) documents not only the evidence and the judgments leading to a recommendation, but also the justifications for the direction and strength of the recommendation and the process. Whether or not the panel voted on some or all of the recommendations and what the results of the vote were should be reported. Considerations regarding subgroups of patients, implementation of the recommendation, evaluation, and monitoring gaps may also be covered.

22.3.2   Research Gaps

The systematic assessment of certainty in the evidence in GRADE helps reviewers identify important gaps in the evidence base. Table 22.8 illustrates how review authors may interpret a body of evidence and draw conclusions about the need for future research. Guideline panels can then discuss these and formulate the concrete questions

TABLE 22.8   Interpretation of the certainty in a body of evidence according to individual GRADE domains.

By outcome	Implications for research	Examples	Implications for practice
Risk of bias	Need for methodologically better-designed and -executed studies	All studies suffered from lack of blinding of outcome assessors. Trials of this type are required	The estimates of effect may be biased because of a lack of blinding
Inconsistency	Unexplained inconsistency: need for individual participant data meta-analysis (IPDMA); need for studies in relevant subgroups	Studies in patients with small cell lung cancer are needed to understand if the effects differ from those in patients with pancreatic cancer	Unexplained inconsistency: consider and interpret overall effect estimates as for the certainty in a body of evidence Explained inconsistency (if results are presented in strata): consider and interpret effects estimates by subgroup
Indirectness	Need for studies that more directly address the PICO question of interest	Studies in patients with early cancer are needed because the evidence is from studies with advanced cancer	It is uncertain if the results directly apply to the patients or the way that the intervention is applied in your setting
Imprecision	Need for more studies with more participants to reach optimal information size	Studies with approximately 200 more events in the treatment and control group are required	Same as for certainty in a body of evidence

TABLE 22.8   (*Continued*)

By outcome	Implications for research	Examples	Implications for practice
Publication bias	Need to investigate and identify unpublished data; large studies might help resolve this issue		Same as for certainty in a body of evidence
Large effects	No implications	No implications	The effect is large in the populations that were included in the studies. The effect is going to be in the vicinity of the observed effect
Dose effects	No implications	No implications	The greater the reduction in the exposure, the larger is the expected benefit (harm)
Opposing bias and confounding	Studies controlling for the residual bias and confounding are needed	Studies controlling for following possible confounders are required: smoking, degree of education	The effect could be even larger than the one that is observed in the studies presented here

PICO, Population, Intervention, Comparator, Outcome.

for future research that will strengthen the evidence base underpinning their future recommendations. Guideline panels should be as specific as possible about what is needed and why the GRADE criteria are used in the EtDs.

22.3.3   GRADEpro Software

The GRADE process – from creating an SoF table to interactive EtD frameworks and full guidelines – is facilitated by the GRADEpro software (www.gradepro.org), which is used by Cochrane systematic review authors to produce SoF tables and by guideline developers to produce and publish recommendations online. GRADEpro can also be used to develop apps on handheld devices.

22.4   OUTLOOK

GRADE provides an approach to assess the certainty or quality of a body of evidence by outcome and across outcomes. GRADE also provides an approach to moving from evidence to a decision using EtD frameworks. The strength of the GRADE approach rests in its structured framework for the assessment of evidence independent of the actual intervention or question, and the requirement for explicit processes and transparent judgments. GRADE has been applied to a wide range of health care interventions, from clinical to public health and health policy questions [50]. The ease of applying the GRADE approach will vary according to the type of evidence being assessed, yet the circumstances in which GRADE cannot be usefully applied are rare. GRADE has been used for questions about prognosis, resource use, values and preferences, and tests. As in any such approach in science, GRADE is not perfect and will evolve with future research [51]. The GRADE working group currently hosts more than 20 project groups on issues such as how to assess certainty in the evidence for values and preferences, animal research, and how to formulate recommendations in fields such as environmental health.

ACKNOWLEDGMENTS

This chapter benefited from the many contributions of members of the GRADE working group to developing GRADE and its tools.

REFERENCES

1. World Health Organization (WHO) (2014). *WHO Handbook for Guideline Development*. Geneva: WHO. http://apps.who.int/iris/bitstream/10665/145714/1/9789241548960_eng.pdf (accessed 21 February 2022).

2. Canadian Task Force on Preventive Health Care (2020). *Procedure Manual*. Ottawa: Canadian Task Force https://canadiantaskforce.ca/methods (accessed 21 February 2022).

3. Oxman, A.D., Schünemann, H.J., and Fretheim, A. (2006). Improving the use of research evidence in guideline development: 8. Synthesis and presentation of evidence. *Heal. Res. Policy. Syst.* 4 (1): 20.

4. Institute of Medicine Committee on Standards for Developing Trustworthy Clinical Practice Guidelines (2011). *Clinical Practice Guidelines We Can Trust*. Washington, DC: National Academies Press.

5. Qaseem, A., Forland, F., Macbeth, F. et al. (2012). Guidelines International Network: Toward international standards for clinical practice guidelines. *Ann. Intern. Med.* 156 (7): 525. https://doi.org/10.7326/0003-4819-156-7-201204030-00009.

6. Karanicolas, P.J., Montori, V.M., Devereaux, P.J. et al. (2009). The practicalists' response. *J. Clin. Epidemiol.* 62 (5): 489–494. https://doi.org/10.1016/j.jclinepi.2008.08.013.

7. Woolf, S., Schünemann, H.J., Eccles, M.P. et al. (2012). Developing clinical practice guidelines: types of evidence and outcomes; values and economics, synthesis, grading, and presentation and deriving recommendations. *Implement. Sci.* 7 (1): 61. https://doi.org/10.1186/1748-5908-7-61.

8. Schünemann, H.J., Wiercioch, W., Etxeandia, I. et al. (2014). Guidelines 2.0: systematic development of a comprehensive checklist for a successful guideline enterprise. *CMAJ* 186 (3): E123–E142. https://doi.org/10.1503/cmaj.131237.

9. Atkins, D., Best, D., Briss, P.A. et al. Grading quality of evidence and strength of recommendations. *BMJ* 328: 1490. https://doi.org/10.1136/bmj.328.7454.1490.

10. Schünemann, H.J., Best, D., Vist, G. et al. (2003). Letters, numbers, symbols and words: how to communicate grades of evidence and recommendations. *CMAJ* 169 (7): 677–680. http://www.ncbi.nlm.nih.gov/pubmed/14517128.

11. Langer, G., Meerpohl, J.J., Perleth, M. et al. (2012). GRADE-Leitlinien: 1. Einführung – GRADE-Evidenzprofile und Summary-of-Findings-Tabellen. *Z Evid Fortbild Qual Gesundhwes* 106 (5): 357–368. http://www.ncbi.nlm.nih.gov/pubmed/22818160.

12. Guyatt, G., Oxman, A.D., Sultan, S. et al. (2013). GRADE guidelines: 11. Making an overall rating of confidence in effect estimates for a single outcome and for all outcomes. *J. Clin. Epidemiol.* 66 (2): 151–157. https://doi.org/10.1016/j.zefq.2012.05.017.

13. Balshem, H., Helfand, M., Schünemann, H.J. et al. (2011). GRADE guidelines: 3. Rating the quality of evidence. *J. Clin. Epidemiol.* 64 (4): 401–406. https://doi.org/10.1016/j.jclinepi.2010.07.015.

14. Alonso-Coello, P., Oxman, A.D., Moberg, J. et al. (2016). GRADE evidence to decision (EtD) frameworks: a systematic and transparent approach to making well informed healthcare choices. 2: clinical practice guidelines. *BMJ* 30: i2089. https://doi.org/10.1136/bmj.i2089.

15. Alonso-Coello, P., Schunemann, H., Moberg, J. et al. (2016). GRADE evidence to decision (EtD) frameworks: a systematic and transparent approach to making well-informed healthcare choices. 1. Introduction. *BMJ* 353 (11): i2016. https://doi.org/10.1136/bmj.i2089.

16. Schünemann, H.J., Mustafa, R., Brozek, J. et al. (2016). GRADE guidelines: 16. GRADE evidence to decision frameworks for tests in clinical practice and public health. *J. Clin. Epidemiol.* 76: 89–98. http://www.ncbi.nlm.nih.gov/pubmed/26931285.

17. Schünemann, H.J. (2016). Interpreting GRADE's levels of certainty or quality of the evidence: GRADE for statisticians, considering review information size or less emphasis on imprecision? *J. Clin. Epidemiol.* 75: 6–15. https://doi.org/10.1016/j.jclinepi.2016.01.032.

18. Higgins, J.P.T., Thompson, S.G., Deeks, J.J., and Altman, D.G. (2003). Measuring inconsistency in meta-analyses. *BMJ* 327 (7414): 557–560.

19. Mustafa, R.A., Santesso, N., Brozek, J. et al. (2013). The GRADE approach is reproducible in assessing the quality of evidence of quantitative evidence syntheses. *J. Clin. Epidemiol.* 66 (7): 736–742. -5. doi: https://doi.org/10.1016/j.jclinepi.2013.02.004.

20. Kumar, A., Miladinovic, B., Guyatt, G.H., and Schünemann, H.J. (2016). Djulbegovic B. GRADE guidelines system is reproducible when instructions are clearly operationalized even among the guidelines panel members with limited experience with GRADE. *J. Clin. Epidemiol.* 75: 115–118. https://doi.org/10.1016/j.jclinepi.2015.11.020.

21. Schünemann, H.J., Schünemann, A.H.J., Oxman, A.D. et al. (2008). Grading quality of evidence and strength of recommendations for diagnostic tests and strategies. *BMJ* 336 (7653): 1106–1110. https://doi.org/10.1136/bmj.39500.677199.AE.

22. Schünemann, H., Brozek, J., Guyatt, G., and Oxman, A. (eds.) (2013). *GRADE Handbook: Handbook for Grading the Quality of Evidence and the Strength of Recommendations Using the GRADE Approach.* Hamilton, ON: McMaster University http://gdt.guidelinedevelopment.org/app/handbook/handbook.html (accessed 21 February 2022).

23. Sterne, J.A.C., Hernán, M.A., Reeves, B.C. et al. (2016). ROBINS-I: a tool for assessing risk of bias in non-randomised studies of interventions. *BMJ* 355: i4919. https://doi.org/10.1136/bmj.i4919.

24. Santesso, N., Carrasco-Labra, A., Langendam, M. et al. (2016). Improving GRADE evidence tables part 3: detailed guidance for explanatory footnotes supports creating and understanding GRADE certainty in the evidence judgments. *J. Clin. Epidemiol.* 74: 28–39. https://doi.org/10.1016/j.jclinepi.2015.12.006.

25. GRADEpro GDT. (2020). GRADEpro Guideline Development Tool. https://gradepro.org (accessed 21 February 2022).

26. Guyatt, G.H., Oxman, A.D., Vist, G. et al. (2011). GRADE guidelines: 4. Rating the quality of evidence - study limitations (risk of bias). *J. Clin. Epidemiol.* 64 (4): 407–415.

27. Guyatt, G.H., Oxman, A.D., Kunz, R. et al. (2011). GRADE guidelines: 7. Rating the quality of evidence – inconsistency. *J. Clin. Epidemiol.* 64 (12): 1294–1302. https://doi.org/10.1016/j.jclinepi.2011.03.017.

28. Schünemann, H.J., Tugwell, P., Reeves, B.C. et al. (2013). Non-randomized studies as a source of complementary, sequential or replacement evidence for randomized controlled trials in systematic reviews on the effects of interventions. *Res. Synth. Methods* 4 (1): 49–62. https://doi.org/10.1002/jrsm.1078.

29. Guyatt, G.H., Oxman, A.D., Kunz, R. et al. (2011). GRADE guidelines: 8. Rating the quality of evidence – indirectness. *J. Clin. Epidemiol.* 64 (12): 1303–1310.

30. Schünemann, H.J. (2013). Methodological idiosyncrasies, frameworks and challenges of non-pharmaceutical and non-technical treatment interventions. *Z. Evid. Fortbild Qual. Gesundhwes* 107 (3): 214–220. https://doi.org/10.1016/j.zefq.2013.05.002.

31. Puhan, M.A., Schünemann, H.J., Murad, M.H. et al. (2014). A GRADE working group approach for rating the quality of treatment effect estimates from network meta-analysis. *BMJ* 349: g5630. https://doi.org/10.1136/bmj.g5630.

32. Guyatt, G.H., Oxman, A.D., Kunz, R. et al. (2011). GRADE guidelines 6. Rating the quality of evidence – imprecision. *J. Clin. Epidemiol.* 64 (12): 1283–1293.

33. Pogue, J.M. and Yusuf, S. (1997). Cumulating evidence from randomized trials: utilizing sequential monitoring boundaries for cumulative meta-analysis. *Control Clin. Trials* 18 (6): 580. 593–666.

34. Guyatt, G.H., Oxman, A.D., Montori, V. et al. (2011). GRADE guidelines: 5. Rating the quality of evidence – publication bias. *J. Clin. Epidemiol.* 64 (12): 1277–1282.

35. Guyatt, G.H., Oxman, A.D., Sultan, S. et al. (2011). GRADE guidelines: 9. Rating up the quality of evidence. *J. Clin. Epidemiol.* 64 (12): 1311–1316. https://doi.org/10.1016/j.jclinepi.2011.06.004.

36. Bradford, H.A. (1965). The environment and disease: association or causation? *Proc. R. Soc. Med.* 58: 295–300.

37. Guyatt, G., Oxman, A.D., Akl, E.A. et al. (2011). GRADE guidelines: 1. Introduction - GRADE evidence profiles and summary of findings tables. *J. Clin. Epidemiol.* 64 (4): 383–394.

38. Raghu, G., Rochwerg, B., Zhang, Y. et al. (2015). An official ATS/ERS/JRS/ALAT clinical practice guideline: treatment of idiopathic pulmonary fibrosis. An update of the

2011 clinical practice guideline. *Am. J. Respir. Crit. Care Med.* 192 (2): e3–e19. https://doi.org/10.1164/rccm.201506-1063ST.

39. Langendam, M., Carrasco-Labra, A., Santesso, N. et al. (2016). Improving GRADE evidence tables part 2: a systematic survey of explanatory notes shows more guidance is needed. *J. Clin. Epidemiol.* 74: 19–27. https://doi.org/10.1016/j.jclinepi.2015.12.008.

40. World Health Organization (2013). *Guidelines for Screening and treatment of Precancerous Lesions for Cervical Cancer Prevention.* Geneva: World Health Organization 60 p.

41. Spencer, F.A., Iorio, A., You, J. et al. (2012). Uncertainties in baseline risk estimates and confidence in treatment effects. *BMJ* 345: e7401. https://doi.org/10.1136/bmj.e7401.

42. Iorio, A., Spencer, F.A., Falavigna, M. et al. (2015). Use of GRADE for assessment of evidence about prognosis: rating confidence in estimates of event rates in broad categories of patients. *BMJ* 350: h870–h870. https://doi.org/10.1136/bmj.h870.

43. Guyatt, G.H., Oxman, A.D., Kunz, R. et al. (2008). Incorporating considerations of resources use into grading recommendations. *BMJ* 336 (7654): 1170–1173. https://doi.org/10.1136/bmj.39504.506319.80.

44. Brunetti, M., Shemilt, I., Pregno, S. et al. (2013). GRADE guidelines: 10. Considering resource use and rating the quality of economic evidence. *J. Clin. Epidemiol.* 66 (2): 140–150. https://doi.org/10.1016/j.jclinepi.2012.04.012.

45. Alonso-Coello, P., Schünemann, H.J., Moberg, J. et al. (2016). GRADE evidence to decision (EtD) frameworks: a systematic and transparent approach to making well informed healthcare choices. 1: introduction. *BMJ* 353: i2016. https://doi.org/10.1136/bmj.i2016.

46. Andrews, J., Guyatt, G., Oxman, A.D. et al. (2013). GRADE guidelines: 14. Going from evidence to recommendations: the significance and presentation of recommendations. *J. Clin. Epidemiol.* 66 (7): 719–725. https://doi.org/10.1016/j.jclinepi.2012.03.013.

47. Andrews, J.C., Schünemann, H.J., Oxman, A.D. et al. (2013). GRADE guidelines: 15. Going from evidence to recommendation – determinants of a recommendation's direction and strength. *J. Clin. Epidemiol.* 66 (7): 726–735.

48. Schünemann, H.J., Oxman, A.D., Akl, E.A. et al. (2012). ATS/ERS ad hoc committee on integrating and coordinating efforts in COPD guideline development. Moving from evidence to developing recommendations in guidelines: article 11 in integrating and coordinating efforts in COPD guideline development. An official ATS/ERS workshop report. *Proc. Am. Thorac Soc.* 9 (5): 282–292. https://doi.org/10.1513/pats.201208-064ST.

49. Neumann, I., Santesso, N., Akl, E.A. et al. (2016). A guide for health professionals to interpret and use recommendations in guidelines developed with the GRADE approach. *J. Clin. Epidemiol.* 72: 45–55. https://doi.org/10.1016/j.jclinepi.2015.11.017.

50. Akl, E.A., Kennedy, C., Konda, K. et al. (2012). Using GRADE methodology for the development of public health guidelines for the prevention and treatment of HIV and other STIs among men who have sex with men and transgender people. *BMC Public Health* 12 (1): 386. https://doi.org/10.1186/1471-2458-12-386.

51. Norris, S.L. and Bero, L. (2016). Methods for guideline development: time to evolve? *Ann. Intern. Med.* 165 (11): 810–811.

PART V

OUTLOOK

CHAPTER 23

Innovations in Systematic Review Production

Julian Elliott and Tari Turner

Systematic review methods seek to deliver an accurate summary of the available evidence for specific health questions. In practice, increasing methodological standards [1] and a deluge of primary studies challenge the ability of many review teams to produce high-quality systematic reviews that are timely, accurate, and useful, and are kept up to date [2].

Current systematic review production systems face several challenges. The time and resources required to complete many of the tasks of a systematic review are substantial (Table 23.1). In a study of systematic reviews in neurotrauma, reviews were published at medians of 2.5–6.5 years after the studies that were included in the respective systematic reviews, which is a substantial lag between publication of a primary study and its incorporation into a systematic review [3]. This lag typically reflects more than two years for the production of the systematic review [4] and more than one year from the date of the last search to review publication [5]. This slows the translation of research findings into guidelines and health practices. Furthermore, only a minority of reviews are updated within two years [6], and as new research is published in the intervening period these delays can lead to significant inaccuracies. One estimate is that 7% of systematic reviews are inaccurate the day they are published, and after two years 23% of reviews that are not updated will present incorrect conclusions [7].

Given these challenges, it is not surprising that innovations that seek to improve the production of systematic reviews often focus primarily on improving the efficiency of review production while maintaining existing methodological approaches and rigor.

Systematic Reviews in Health Research: Meta-Analysis in Context, Third Edition. Edited by Matthias Egger, Julian P.T. Higgins, and George Davey Smith.
© 2022 John Wiley & Sons Ltd. Published 2022 by John Wiley & Sons Ltd.
Companion website: www.systematic-reviews3.org

TABLE 23.1   Estimated time to perform specific tasks required to produce a systematic review.

Task	Unit	Number of units (mean)	Time per unit (minutes)	Total time (hours)
Search	Review	1	420	7.0
Citation screening	Citation	2475	2.6	107.3
Importing full-text articles	Article	100	9.2	15.3
Full-text article review	Article	100	12.5	20.8
Data extraction	Article	19	246	77.9
Risk of bias assessment	Article	19	40.8	12.9
TOTAL				241.2

Source: Unit time data generated during the Cochrane Fit For Purpose Project (Final report, July 2011). Volume data calculated from a one-year sample of Cochrane Reviews published between March 2013 and February 2014).

23.1   WORKFLOW PLATFORMS

Despite the fact that systematic reviews are important for the health of society, highly specialized, resource-intensive, and time-critical review production still relies largely on a fragmented mix of generic word-processing, spreadsheet, email, reference management, and statistical analysis tools [8]. A number of more specialized software tools are available that aim to improve the efficiency, quality, and experience of review production [9]. At the time of writing, the most widely used of these include Covidence, Distiller SR, EPPI-Reviewer, JBI-SUMARI, and Rayyan. In general, these tools are well adapted to the specific needs of systematic reviewers, but few independent evaluation data exist that concern their benefits to review production efficiency or quality.

23.2   SEMI-AUTOMATION

One of the most active areas of research in the field of systematic review production is the use of computerized systems to automate, or semi-automate, routine and time-consuming tasks [10]. The aim is usually to improve the efficiency of review production and redirect human effort to higher-level tasks [11]. Some have envisioned a future in which systematic reviews are fully automated, executed as computer programs defined by the review protocol [12]. This vision excludes human interpretation, currently a critical step in review production [13], and is not currently feasible. However, semi-automation systems are feasible and are beginning to be deployed in production systems.

Box 23.1   Natural Language Processing and Machine Learning

Natural Language Processing

Natural language processing is a process of deriving high-quality information from text. It takes the relatively unstructured data encapsulated in the natural language of text and creates structured data and new insights. The process typically involves collecting and organizing text, converting the text into structured forms (parsing), manipulating and transforming the text, analyzing (mining) the text, and evaluation and interpretation of the outputs of the analysis.

Machine Learning

Machine learning involves the creation of algorithms that learn from data to make predictions or decisions, rather than following static program instructions as is typical for conventional statistical models. The essential difference is that the performance of machine learning algorithms changes with exposure to data. Often the algorithm is given a set of inputs ("training data") and desired outputs, from which it derives a general rule ("learning"). This can be applied to a new set of inputs to predict outputs.

Given the substantial resources required to identify studies for inclusion in a systematic review, this task has received the most attention. Text presented in citations and full-text reports is commonly processed by computer systems using techniques known as natural language processing and machine learning. Natural language processing is the process of deriving high-quality, structured information from unstructured free text, and machine learning is the process by which analytic models learn from reference data and make predictions about new data (see Box 23.1).

23.2.1   Study Identification

The most recent systematic review of research on study identification was published in 2015 and identified 44 studies (Table 23.2) [14]. The reviewers were not able to perform a quantitative synthesis due to variability in the metrics and processes investigated in the studies. They concluded that although they were not able to establish which approaches were best, it was clear that substantial reductions in workload and efficiency gains were potentially achievable. Many studies suggested a 30–70% reduction in workload might be possible, although sometimes with a loss of approximately 5% of relevant studies (i.e. sensitivity or recall of 95%).

The issue of sensitivity or recall is an important challenge for semi-automation or automation of citation screening. Systematic reviewers value sensitivity/recall over specificity/precision, as is demonstrated by the use of highly sensitive search strategies that return large numbers of irrelevant citations. Various responses to this challenge have been proposed, including a "committee" approach in which multiple machine classifiers "vote" on each citation and the citation is selected if at least one,

TABLE 23.2   Approaches to semi-automation of study identification.

Purpose	Method	Description	Number of studies
Reduce the number of citations needing to be screened	Classifier	Explicit binary (include/exclude) decisions	23
	Ranking	Rank by likelihood of inclusion and exclude citations below a given threshold	7
	Active learning	Machine "learns" from ongoing interaction with reviewer screening decisions	9
Machine as a second screener	Classifier	Remove or significantly reduce need for second, independent screener using classifier as above	6
Increase the rate of screening	Visual data mining	Visual representation of document connections to speed up identification of studies more likely to be similar to one another	5
	Efficient citation assignment	Assignment of citations to expert and novice screeners based on estimated time to screen	1
Screening prioritization	Ranking	Order citations by likelihood of inclusion to improve the overall efficiency of the review team	4

Source: Adapted from [14].

or a majority, of the classifiers votes for inclusion; or weighting the classifiers to penalize false negatives more than false positives [14]. A related challenge is the imbalance between the number of includes and the number of excludes in a typical set of citations, which results in few relevant items to "train" the classifiers. Weighting and undersampling of nonrelevant citations are two approaches that have been used to address this issue.

Although the semi-automation of citation screening is an active research area, there are a number of limitations to the evidence base. As mentioned, a diversity of metrics and processes have been studied, limiting our ability to compare alternative approaches. Furthermore, there has been close to no replication of studies and very little use of common datasets. Many of the systems have been evaluated using relatively small, single-citation datasets and not tested across a diversity of citation set types (e.g. clinical and public health; interventions and diagnostic tests).

At the time of writing, few citation-screening semi-automation systems have been deployed. The review described earlier identified Abstrackr, EPPI-Reviewer, and Revis, and the generic text mining platform RapidMiner. The SRToolbox site [9] describes additional tools that use text mining to support study selection.

23.2.2   Data Extraction

"Extracting" (capturing) data reported in the abstract or full-text article is an important and time-consuming task in systematic review production (Table 23.1). A number of studies have investigated semi-automation of this process, including studies that focus on data contained in abstracts and those concerned with capturing data from full-text articles. Some studies have examined the ability of automation systems to identify text that refers to specific elements (e.g. PICO [Population, Intervention, Comparison, Outcome] descriptors), whereas other studies have pursued the capturing of these data (e.g. the specific details of the population included in the study).

A systematic review published in 2015 identified 26 studies in this field [15]. Overall, the review identified many studies with encouraging findings such as F-scores (mean of sensitivity and positive predictive value) above 70%. As with the review described above, the authors were unable to perform a quantitative synthesis due to the variety of datasets and metrics used in the included studies. They also highlighted the small number of data elements examined in the included studies and that many standard data elements have not been investigated in any study published to date. Very few deployed systems are available for use. One relevant example is the open-source tool Robot Reviewer [16, 17], which has demonstrated encouraging performance in a randomized trial [17].

23.3   CROWDSOURCING

The long history of citizen science, in which members of society contribute to a scientific endeavor, has recently been transformed by online platforms that engage large volunteer communities to help scientists and researchers efficiently and accurately deal with the flood of data that confronts them. Researchers working with Cochrane have evaluated this "crowdsourcing" approach for systematic review production.

For example, anonymous individuals (the "crowd") can indicate through an online interface (Cochrane Crowd [18]) whether a citation identified during a broad and sensitive search of bibliographic databases represent a report of a randomized trial. To date, a crowd of over 23 000 contributors has performed over six million classifications. The decisions of multiple crowd members are combined using "crowd algorithms" to derive final citation classifications. Evaluations of crowd performance have compared the performance of the crowd to that of an information specialist and a systematic reviewer acting as a reference standard [19]. In these studies, the sensitivity and specificity of crowd assessments were over 99 and 98%, respectively.

23.4   DATA STRUCTURES

At present, systematic reviews are usually disseminated as published full-text articles in academic journals. The data underlying the review findings are locked within the full-text pdf or html format, making them difficult for humans or machines to access or reuse. Furthermore, valuable data accrued during the production of the review (detailed study data or review process data) are usually not made available. These issues contribute to the wasteful aspects of systematic review duplication and often force groups with similar, but not identical, questions to repeat systematic reviews in very closely related topics.

In order to address these issues and make systematic review data more easily accessible and reusable, groups are pursuing the development of new data infrastructure. One step in this direction has been the development of a "linked data" project by Cochrane [20]. Linked data is a method of publishing structured data. It builds upon standard web technologies to share information in a way that computers can read automatically. This enables data from different sources to be connected and queried.

One aspect of Cochrane's linked data work has been the development of a "PICO Ontology." An ontology is a formal naming and definition of the types, properties, and interrelationships of entities that exist in a particular domain. Ontologies are used to limit complexity, organize information, and support problem-solving. The PICO Ontology [21] provides an overarching framework for the organization of data in systematic reviews, including studies included in the review, analyses conducted as part of the review, and the review itself. These data elements can then be annotated with metadata: terms from controlled vocabularies (e.g. Medical Subject Headings [MeSH] in MEDLINE/PubMed, SNOMED Clinical Terms) and other categories (e.g. COMET core outcome sets) to enable much richer data reuse options, for example finding and using data from across multiple systematic reviews, linking systematic review data to other relevant datasets, and using systematic review data within guideline development platforms (see below).

23.5   EVIDENCE USE

The systems described above enable more efficient production of structured, shareable systematic review data. This provides value for the production of other systematic reviews, but these data can also be used in "downstream" processes, including the development of guidelines, standards, decision aids, and clinical decision support systems. The key requirement is technical infrastructure that enables the easy transfer and reuse of data from systematic review tools and data repositories to systems supporting these downstream processes. At the time of writing, these links were only beginning to be established.

In turn, guideline development platforms are beginning to be linked to other downstream platforms, enabling the presentation of guideline recommendations within electronic medical records (EMRs) and online decision aids, and enabling more efficient production of decision support rules. Together, these interlinked systems may evolve into a much more efficient "ecosystem," extending from primary study data through systematic review and guideline development to decision support systems (Figure 23.1) [3]. Overall, it is likely the data generated during a systematic review will become at least as important as the systematic review report itself.

23.6   LIVING SYSTEMATIC REVIEWS

Interlinked platforms and systems that utilize the potential of automation and crowdsourcing are likely to make the production of systematic reviews more efficient (see Figure 23.2). This will reduce the resources required to produce reviews, but also

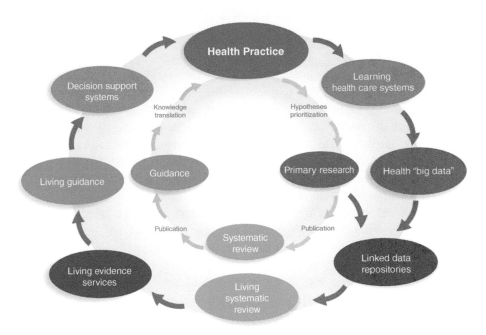

FIGURE 23.1   Current and emerging health knowledge ecosystems. The current health knowledge ecosystem (inner circle) is characterized by inefficiencies that hamper the flow of knowledge from health practice through primary research, systematic review, and guidelines, and finally back to impacts on health practice. The new health knowledge ecosystem that is emerging (outer circle) is characterized by a continuous flow of knowledge between efficient, living components, including the growing importance of learning health care systems, which together with traditional primary research will populate common data repositories. Living evidence services derived from these repositories, supporting living guidance and decision support systems, will close a "living" health knowledge loop. Source: Elliott et al. [3].

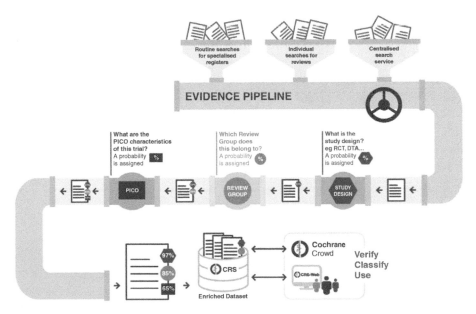

FIGURE 23.2   Cochrane's evidence pipeline. As an alternative to searching bibliographic databases for individual reviews and wholly manual screening, Cochrane's evidence pipeline uses the combination of broad searches of bibliographic databases for reports of controlled trials ("centralized search"), together with text mining and machine learning algorithms, combined with designations provided by the citizen science platform "Cochrane Crowd" to substantially reduce the resources required to identify reports of studies eligible for inclusion in Cochrane Reviews. Source: Cochrane.

improve the feasibility of review updating. Current challenges in review updating limit updating frequency and lead to considerable inaccuracy [7], to some extent undermining the value created through the use of rigorous methods.

Living systematic review (LSR) is an approach to the updating of systematic reviews that utilizes the emerging "evidence ecosystem" already described to keep review findings constantly up to date, even in fast-moving research areas [3]. LSRs are systematic reviews that are updated frequently, typically every month or so [22]. A number of LSR projects have demonstrated the feasibility of this approach for intervention and other review types [23–28] and its application in network meta-analysis has been proposed [29]. Box 23.2 describes some of its implementation during the COVID-19 pandemic.

The key areas in which LSRs differ from conventionally updated systematic reviews are team and workflow management and publication. Instead of the intense, sporadic effort of conventional systematic reviews and systematic review updates, LSRs require a continuous workflow, with a moderate amount of effort coordinated over long periods of time, and gradual evolution in the review team. Authors of LSRs should pre-specify the criteria that will be used to determine when new evidence will be incorporated into the review, and when the methods of the review will be revised (in light of, for example, changes to subject headings in databases searched, etc.)

Box 23.2   COVID-19 Living Systematic Reviews

The COVID-19 pandemic provided a clear example of the need for living, continually updated evidence syntheses to guide health decisions. In the early phase of the pandemic, there was little research to guide clinical practice and substantial uncertainty about which treatments were effective in treating people with COVID-19. However, research was rapidly produced, and static systematic reviews were almost immediately outdated. The value of living reviews in this context was very clear. Several groups applied living methods to develop evidence syntheses of evidence for treatments, which were frequently updated.

An international research group developed an LSR of drug treatments for COVID-19 that was first published on July 30, 2020, and by June 2021 had been updated and republished an additional three times [30]. This living review was used as the basis of a World Health Organization (WHO) living guideline, which was updated in line with updates to the systematic review [31].

Supported by WHO and Cochrane, the COVID-NMA initiative (https://covid-nma.com) undertook a living mapping and living systematic review of COVID-19 trials addressing preventive interventions, treatments, and vaccines for the virus [32]. By June 2021, the LSR included more than 300 randomized controlled trials, and the mapping of registered trials included more than 3000 studies.

The Australian National COVID-19 Clinical Evidence Taskforce (https://covid19evidence.net.au) used living evidence synthesis methods to develop living guidelines for treatment of people with COVID-19 [33]. These guidelines were first published in April 2020, and then updated weekly to reflect new research evidence. As of June 2021, the living guidelines had been updated more than 40 times and included over 140 recommendations.

Source: Adapted from Siemieniuk R et al. [30], Siemieniuk R et al. [31], Boutron I et al. [32], and Tendal B, et al. [33].

The publication of LSRs also requires some adaptation of existing norms. When a search does not identify any new studies for inclusion, only the published search date need be updated. If new studies are identified, a new publication may be generated with a new digital object identifier (DOI), bibliographic database listing, and citation.

23.7   DIVERSE DATA

The sources of data available for health decision-making are increasing in volume, velocity, and variety. From genomic sequences to clinical trial individual participant data, EMRs, mobile devices, wearables, and social networking applications [34], we face an increasing deluge of data and limited methods or technical infrastructure to manage and make sense of it, particularly within the evidence-based health care community. Conversely, many in data science fields, who are immersed in the combination and analysis of large and diverse datasets, are unaware of the approaches and methods of evidence synthesis, particularly the risks of bias associated with each data type and how to incorporate these risks into analyses [35].

As these fields evolve, evidence-based practice and other data science communities will benefit from better cross-talk and collaboration, developing a range of empirically verified and widely accepted methods for making sense of diverse data. Academic organizational structures, funding opportunities, and conferences may be reconfigured to encourage this interdisciplinary work. In the longer term, we may also see the emergence of a new type of data scientist, adept at appraising and combining diverse data.

23.8   DATA ANALYTICS

In parallel with the increasing availability of diverse datasets as already described, we are likely to see the emergence of increasingly sophisticated decision support systems that use artificial intelligence (AI) to make judgments and give recommendations to end users without the need for direct human input [36]. At present these systems learn from a wide range of data sources, including systematic reviews and guidelines, but it is conceivable that in the future these will not be necessary and a more direct connection from data to decisions will become prevalent. Also, over time it is likely that an increasing array of competing AI-based decision support systems will become available. The regulation and selection of systems will be complex, particularly given that at present it is virtually impossible to understand the reasoning used by the AI system to derive a specific statement or recommendation.

23.9   CONCLUSIONS

The science of evidence synthesis has provided incalculable benefit to human health and many other fields by helping to bridge the evidence–practice gap. However, less investment has been made in systems and processes than in methods; rigor has been emphasized more than currency. As such, the systems available to systematic reviewers have changed little over many years, hindering the production, updating, and availability of high-quality systematic reviews.

New systems are now emerging on several fronts. These range from improvements in workflow and collaboration platforms customized for the specific needs of systematic review teams, to the use of text mining, machine learning, and crowdsourcing to semi-automate or outsource specific tasks in the production of systematic reviews. Underlying these are new systems for structuring and organizing the data generated during a systematic review.

Altogether, these systems will have significant implications for other evidence processes, particularly guideline development and decision support systems. As the processing and synthesis of conventional data sources become more efficient, these downstream activities will benefit, creating an environment for more dynamic, interlinked synthesis and use of health data.

In parallel, there will be increasing complexity from the opportunities – and demand – for evidence syntheses incorporating a much wider range of data sources, including novel, large, and diverse data. This will occur in a context in which methodological approaches to the "analysis" and "synthesis" of these datasets will draw from a wide range of methods from statistics and machine learning.

REFERENCES

1. Higgins, J., Thomas, J., Chandler, J. et al. (eds.) (2019). *Cochrane Handbook for Systematic Reviews of Interventions*. Chichester: Wiley.
2. Bastian, H., Glasziou, P., and Chalmers, I. (2010). Seventy-five trials and eleven systematic reviews a day: how will we ever keep up? *PLoS Med.* 7 (9): e1000326.
3. Elliott, J.H., Turner, T., Clavisi, O. et al. (2014). Living systematic reviews: an emerging opportunity to narrow the evidence-practice gap. *PLoS Med.* 11 (2): e1001603.
4. Tricco, A.C., Brehaut, J., Chen, M.H., and Moher, D. (2008). Following 411 Cochrane protocols to completion: a retrospective cohort study. *PLoS One* 3 (11): e3684.
5. Sampson, M., Shojania, K.G., Garritty, C. et al. (2008). Systematic reviews can be produced and published faster. *J. Clin. Epidemiol.* 61 (6): 531–536.
6. Jadad, A.R., Cook, D.J., Jones, A. et al. (1998). Methodology and reports of systematic reviews and meta-analyses: a comparison of Cochrane reviews with articles published in paper-based journals. *JAMA* 280 (3): 278–280.
7. Shojania, K.G., Sampson, M., Ansari, M.T. et al. (2007). How quickly do systematic reviews go out of date? A survival analysis. *Ann. Intern. Med.* 147 (4): 224–233.
8. Ciapponi, A. and Glujovsky, D. (2012). Survey among Cochrane authors about early stages of systematic reviews. 20th Cochrane Colloquium. http://2012.colloquium.cochrane.org/abstracts/survey-among-cochrane-authors-about-early-stages-systematic-reviews.html (accessed February 21, 2022).
9. SRToolbox. http://systematicreviewtools.com (accessed February 21, 2022).
10. Tsafnat, G., Glasziou, P., Choong, M. et al. (2014). Systematic review automation technologies. *Syst. Rev.* 3: 74.
11. Adams, C., Polzmacher, S., and Wolff, A. (2013). Systematic reviews: work that needs to be done and not to be done. *J. Evid. Based Med.* 6: 232–235.

12. Tsafnat, G., Dunn, A., Glasziou, P., and Coiera, E. (2013). The automation of systematic reviews. *BMJ* 346: f139.

13. Elliott, J.H., Mavergames, C., Becker, L. et al. (2013). The efficient production of high quality evidence reviews is important for the public good. *BMJ* 346: f846.

14. O'Mara-Eves, A., Thomas, J., McNaught, J. et al. (2015). Using text mining for study identification in systematic reviews: a systematic review of current approaches. *Syst. Rev.* 4: 5.

15. Jonnalagadda, S., Goyal, P., and Huffman, M. (2015). Automating data extraction in systematic reviews: a systematic review. *Syst. Rev.* 4: 78.

16. RobotReviewer. https://www.robotreviewer.net/ (accessed February 21, 2022).

17. Marshall, I., Kuiper, J., and Wallace, B. (2016). RobotReviewer: evaluation of a system for automatically assessing bias in clinical trials. *J. Am. Med. Inform. Assoc.* 23 (1): 193–201.

18. Cochrane Crowd. http://crowd.cochrane.org/index.html (accessed February 21, 2022).

19. Noel-Storr, A., Dooley, G., Glanville, J., and Foxlee, R. (2015). The Embase project 2: crowdsourcing citation screening. 23rd Cochrane Colloquium. https://abstracts.cochrane.org/2015-vienna/embase-project-2-crowdsourcing-citation-screening (accessed February 21, 2022).

20. Cochrane Linked Data. http://linkeddata.cochrane.org/home (accessed February 21, 2022).

21. PICO Ontology. http://linkeddata.cochrane.org/pico-ontology (accessed February 21, 2022).

22. Elliott, J., Synnot, A., Turner, T. et al. (2017). Living systematic review: 1. Introduction – the why, what, when, and how. *J. Clin. Epidemiol.* 91: 23–30.

23. Badgett, R., Vindhyal, M., Stirnaman, J. et al. (2015). A living systematic review of nebulized hypertonic saline for acute bronchiolitis in infants. *JAMA Pediatr.* 169 (8): 788–789.

24. Cnossen, M., Scholten, A., Lingsma, H. et al. (2021). Adherence to guidelines in adult patients with traumatic brain injury: a living systematic review. *J. Neurotrauma* 38 (8): 1072–1085.

25. Synnot, A., Gruen, R.L., Menon, D. et al. (2015). A new approach to evidence synthesis in traumatic brain injury: living systematic reviews. *J. Neurotrauma* 38 (8): 1069–1071.

26. Hodder, R., Stacey, F., Wyse, R. et al. (2017). Interventions for increasing fruit and vegetable consumption in children aged five years and under. *Cochrane Database Syst. Rev.* 9: CD008552.

27. Akl, E., Kahale, L., Hakoum, M. et al. (2017). Parenteral anticoagulation in ambulatory patients with cancer. *Cochrane Database Syst. Rev.* 9: CD006652.

28. Counotte, M., Egli-Gany, D., Riesen, M. et al. (2018). Zika virus infection as a cause of congenital brain abnormalities and Guillain-Barré syndrome: From systematic review to living systematic review. *F1000Res* 7: 196.

29. Créquit, P., Trinquart, L., Yavchitz, A., and Ravaud, P. (2016). Wasted research when systematic reviews fail to provide a complete and up-to-date evidence synthesis: the example of lung cancer. *BMC Med.* 14: 8.

30. Siemieniuk, R., Bartoszko, J., Ge, L. et al. (2020). Drug treatments for covid-19: living systematic review and network meta-analysis. *BMJ* 370: m2980.

31. Siemieniuk, R., Bartoszko, J.J., Ge, L. et al. (2020). A living WHO guideline on drugs for covid-19 [update 3]. *BMJ* 370: m3379.

32. Boutron, I., Chaimani, A., Meerpohl, J.J. et al. (2020). The COVID-NMA project: building an evidence ecosystem for the COVID-19 pandemic. *Ann. Intern. Med.* 173: 1015–1017.

33. Tendal, B., Vogel, J.P., McDonald, S. et al. (2021). Weekly updates of national living evidence-based guidelines: methods for the Australian living guidelines for care of people with COVID-19. *J. Clin. Epidemiol.* 131: 11–21.

34. Weber, G., Mandl, K., and Kohane, I. (2014). Finding the missing link for big biomedical data. *JAMA* 311 (24): 2479–2480.

35. Elliott, J.H., Grimshaw, J., Altman, R. et al. (2015). Make sense of health data. *Nature* 527 (7576): 31–32.

36. IBM Watson. https://www.ibm.com/watson (accessed February 21, 2022).

CHAPTER 24

Future for Systematic Reviews and Meta-Analysis

Shah Ebrahim and Mark D. Huffman

The use of evidence in changing clinical and public health practice has increased greatly since the previous edition of this book [1] was published. Systematic reviews, too, have expanded from summarizing the randomized evidence of the effects of interventions to diagnostic and prognostic studies (see Chapters 16, 17, and 18), nonrandomized studies (Chapters 15, 19, and 20), and inclusion of public health interventions targeted at populations rather than individuals. This rapid growth in scope has resulted in the development of new methods and the involvement of many more people – biomedical and social scientists, research and health care funders, policymakers, patients, and the general public – and has created a complex environment within which systematic reviews are booming. This massive scope ensures there will be a future for systematic reviews, but it also engenders some challenges.

24.1   THE DEMAND FOR SYSTEMATIC REVIEWS

The major driver of demand for systematic reviews has been health care policymakers. The need to curb government spending on health care has resulted in several countries implementing processes to assess evidence of benefits of new (and old) health technologies and to conduct cost-effectiveness analyses to provide a rational approach to making decisions about which technologies deliver value. The UK's National Institute for Health and Care Excellence (NICE) has demonstrated how such approaches can transform health care delivery. The World Health Organization and the United States Preventive Services Task Force commission systematic reviews and support review groups to provide evidence required to inform policy. The US National Academy of Medicine has also set forth recommendations for providing reliable evidence to help the health sector make better decisions. Many other countries have similar agencies conducting this sort of work.

Systematic Reviews in Health Research: Meta-Analysis in Context, Third Edition. Edited by Matthias Egger, Julian P.T. Higgins, and George Davey Smith.
© 2022 John Wiley & Sons Ltd. Published 2022 by John Wiley & Sons Ltd.
Companion website: www.systematic-reviews3.org

Medical professional organizations and medical societies have also contributed demand for reviews as part of their role in continuing professional development. Guidelines produced by these organizations have moved from "expert opinion" to using systematic reviews where available to underpin recommendations for clinical practice. Clinical trials research funders have also played a role by requiring systematic reviews of previous evaluations of interventions before funding further trials. Patients and patient advocacy organizations are keen to get an understanding of their options for diagnosis and treatment, and the potential hazards of treatments. They, too, have increased demand for reviews.

Editors of medical journals are happy to publish high-quality systematic reviews. Systematic reviews can achieve higher citations, exceeding the citations of the primary studies. This results in a cycle in which authors find publishing reviews an excellent way of achieving high-profile publications that get cited and improve chances of career progression and research grants. Journals enjoy more citations, which results in a higher impact factor, and scientists in some countries are financially rewarded for publishing in higher impact factor journals. The massive growth in funding of medical science in China has spurred a huge output of systematic reviews focused not only on traditional Chinese medicine, but also conventional treatments. This growth raises problems of quality (see Box 24.1), though, it overloads journals, and may make it more difficult for readers to find reliable, high-quality systematic reviews. It seems likely that other low- and middle-income countries will follow suit and make investments in infrastructure for producing systematic reviews, which could potentially compound these problems.

24.2   INCREASING DEMAND IS GOOD

The demand for systematic reviews has broken down hierarchical structures of medical research, allowing small groups with limited resources to carry out systematic reviews that may challenge orthodox views. The historical failure of pharmaceutical companies to release all randomized controlled trial data and the selective reporting of findings

---

Box 24.1   Chinese Systematic Reviews and the Curious Case of the "Begger" Plot

A dramatic increase in systematic reviews archived in a complementary medicine database was noted in 2014, with 32 reviews written by 28 different groups in several Chinese universities. The papers had exactly the same structure and figures, including a "Begger's funnel plot. . . a surrealistic fusion of Begg and Egger (Colin Begg and Matthias Egger both gave their name to a test for publication bias)" [2]. On the basis of all these submissions having been made within only two months, this strange naming, and other grammatical errors, the best explanation for all these reviews was not plagiarism, but that the papers had been written by a ghostwriter or more likely ghostwriters working for a systematic review writing company in China.

focused on outcomes showing benefits and nonreporting of harms of treatment are now well known. Industry-funded research groups are beginning to respond to the demands for greater transparency and independent, verifiable summaries of the effects of drug treatments. The +AllTrials group, supported by over 700 institutions globally, previously reported that pension funds and asset managers worth more than €3.5 trillion have asked pharmaceutical companies to provide plans to register all clinical trials (past, present, and future) [3]. An "enlightenment" has spread across clinical medicine in many countries: systematic reviews are useful; they are more likely to give robust answers to clinical questions than single studies; they are essential tools for designing better trials; and sharing all the data is a *good thing*. Systematic reviews have democratized health sciences as entry into the field for researchers in low- and middle-income countries has become more feasible.

24.3   THE SUPPLY SIDE OF SYSTEMATIC REVIEWS

The demand side is clear about what it wants: timely, reliable evidence of the benefits and harms of interventions to aid in clinical and public health decision-making. And it is frequently if not always willing to pay for this evidence. The supply side, discussed in its various forms below, has been providing reviews of the evidence that exists. Systematic reviews (particularly Cochrane reviews, see also Chapter 21) have been placed at the top of the hierarchy of evidence tree. But this is to conflate "high methodological quality" of a systematic review with "high quality" of the source material. Most interventions of interest in modern medicine have small effect sizes, and the evidence available comprises small trials that are often not well designed and may be biased. Many Cochrane (and other) reviews – which aim to produce "trusted evidence, informed decisions, better health" – are comprised of trials that are of low quality (see Chapter 4), making the resulting pooled intervention effects of uncertain value. Future sustainability will depend on bridging the gap between what clinicians and patients want and what systematic reviewers are capable of providing. In spite of progress over the past few decades, improvements in the standards of both the conduct and publication of the primary studies making up the evidence base continue to be required. Many systematic reviews should be considered hypothesis generating, and tools for prioritizing research spending by exposing inadequate evidence in priority areas of health care.

24.4   NEW FRONTIERS FOR SYSTEMATIC REVIEWS

24.4.1   When will Basic Medical Sciences Embrace Systematic Reviews

Though the market for systematic reviews in basic medical sciences is still small, reviews from a somewhat different direction offer much potential. Animal experiments that evaluate the effects of treatments intended for future use in humans could benefit from systematic reviews of existing animal trial evidence before further experiments are embarked upon [4]. In part this is because much of the basic trial methodology used in animal experiments of interventions that might be useful for treating human diseases has not been well designed, conducted, or reported, and can introduce biases similar to those that occur in human trials. For example, the disappointing and expensive failures of animal studies to discover new treatments for acute ischemic stroke and Alzheimer's disease provide strong stimuli for changes in research practices.

Some animal experimenters have made the unwarranted assumptions that calls for systematic reviews of animal studies are misguided and are dominated by people who generally are hostile to animal experimentation. This simply is not true: many experiments have demonstrated the value of exploring pathophysiological mechanisms of disease in animals [5].

Even when systematic reviews of animal experiments are conducted, they may be oversimplistic, as shown by a recent meta-analysis of 53 rodent trials of maternal obesogenic diet on offspring appetite and body mass [6]. This meta-analysis concluded that "we found an effect on offspring body weight, consistent with permanent alterations of offspring metabolism in response to maternal diet." However, this interpretation is at odds with the heterogeneity between the effects observed in the studies, the strong evidence of small-study bias in body mass effects, and the lack of any grading of the quality of the trials included (see also Chapters 4 and 5).

Would guidelines similar to those widely adopted for randomized controlled trials in humans [7] help? A recent systematic review of the use of guidelines in animal experiments found 26 guidelines that made 55 recommendations for the design and conduct of in vivo animal experiments [8]. However, guidelines that may help reduce the discordance between preclinical animal findings and their effects in humans are not often implemented. It seems likely that there will be a major shift in basic medical sciences in the next decade, leading to a much greater acceptance of the value of (i) use of guidelines to aid in the design, conduct, and reporting of primary studies; and (ii) systematic reviews. Funding bodies such as national research councils have a responsibility to take a leadership role by providing training and grants to support such activities in both clinical and basic sciences.

24.4.2   Genetics and Novel Systematic Review Methods

Following early recognition of the study power required to generate robust estimates and the failure to replicate associations, the Human Genome Project has spawned a massive field of activity in which genome-wide association studies (GWAS) routinely use meta-analysis methodology (see also Chapter 20). Meta-analysis as used in many GWAS studies is simply a means of generating more power and reducing false-positive findings. Uniform standards of meta-analysis for GWAS will continue to be updated and more widely used, with greater attention given to sources of heterogeneity (phenotypic, ancestry-based, and population stratification), method of synthesis (fixed, random, and Bayesian), and correlated outcomes and genetic variants [9–11]. Extensions of these methods to epigenetics, metabolomics, and other fields that rely upon large data synthesis are underway. Novel uses of systematic review methodology have arisen with use of the Egger plot to assess pleiotropy in Mendelian randomization studies using multiple instruments (see Chapter 20) [12].

24.4.3   Wasted Resources, Duplication of Effort

The National Academy of Medicine's recommendations for the creation of trust-worthy clinical practice guidelines require high-quality systematic reviews that meet its Standards for Systematic Reviews of Comparative Effectiveness Research [13, 14]. Instead of using existing high-quality reviews, though, guideline panels often ask nuanced, different questions and create de novo systematic reviews for each new guideline. This is frequently inefficient and, worse, most guideline writers do not have the necessary skills to undertake high-quality systematic reviews within the typical guideline timeframe. To meet tight deadlines, systematic reviews conducted for clinical practice guidelines are outsourced to specialist teams. This dichotomization provides independence in the evidence synthesis process, but can also lead to disagreements between the review team and guideline writers based on the inevitable judgments required for evidence synthesis.

Overviews of existing, high-quality systematic reviews (see also Chapter 1) would save resources and be a better way to initiate a clinical guideline process than convening an expert committee, dividing up the topics, searching the literature (either independently or with the support of a systematic review group), and writing guidelines for which evidence is limited to opinion. For example, a 2009 analysis of American Heart Association/American College of Cardiology guidelines demonstrated that nearly half (48%) of clinical practice guidelines were based on expert opinion [15]. Not unexpectedly, recommendations based on expert opinion are less likely to be retained (74% retained) from one guideline to its next iteration when compared with observational studies (81% retained) or multiple randomized trials (91% retained) [16]. A 2019 update to this analysis demonstrated increases in the number of guidelines (from 17 to 28) and recommendations (from 3075 to 3509) over the previous decade, with only modest improvement in the proportion of recommendations supported by expert opinion (43%) [17].

In the current "mixed economy" of systematic reviews, one of the major Cochrane principles of reducing wasted effort is violated. In a review of systematic reviews conducted in 2010, two-thirds (49 of 73 reviews) had one or more overlapping reviews, with a maximum of 13 overlapping reviews [18]. The authors of this study commented, "While some independent replication of meta-analyses by different teams is possibly useful, the overall picture suggests that there is a waste of efforts with many topics covered by multiple overlapping meta-analyses" [18].

24.5   IS THE CURRENT WORLD OF SYSTEMATIC REVIEWS SUSTAINABLE?

There are four major ways of doing systematic reviews related to health care: under the auspices of Cochrane review groups, collaboration between randomized controlled trials investigators, independent groups, and commercial agencies. Each of these has strengths and weaknesses that affect its future sustainability. The Campbell Collaboration is an international research network that produces systematic reviews of the effects of social interventions, which also produces reviews of some health-related interventions (e.g. community rehabilitation, family therapy, improving reproductive health) [19].

24.5.1 Cochrane

Cochrane has been a spectacular success over the last two decades and has a reputation for methodologically high-quality, updated reviews (see Chapter 21). However, it is heavily dependent on funding from the UK National Institute for Health Research (NIHR), with over half the review groups based in the UK. Withdrawal of this funding for the Cochrane infrastructure would be highly damaging. The organization has established a new, expanded managerial structure, which has a daunting set of challenges ahead: improve quality, increase auditing, standardize reviews, innovate methodologically, engage with policymakers, update reviews more rapidly, involve more authors from developing countries, and retain the enthusiasm of a very large number of senior clinicians, academics, and patients – for all of whom participation is discretionary and not part of paid employment. Buy-in from governmental and nongovernmental agencies of other countries in supporting this collective international effort has grown in the last decade. Cochrane does not accept commercial or conflicted funding, as that could constrain its ability to produce authoritative and reliable reviews [20]. The commercial health services sector has played virtually no part in funding systematic reviews, yet it benefits from the evidence gained by public funding. Given the ongoing pressures on public-sector services and funding, it would be timely to explore ways in which the commercial sector could contribute to funding without jeopardizing the integrity and independence of Cochrane reviews. In the USA, Evidence Practice Centers funded by the Agency for Healthcare Research and Quality represent a parallel program to conduct evidence synthesis activities for governmental agencies [21]. The Cochrane US Network, established in 2019 and comprising existing Cochrane US review groups, fields, and affiliated institutions, will work collaboratively to promote evidence-based health care and public health [22].

24.5.2 Clinical Trial Collaborations

Collaborations between trialists have the great advantage of having access to all (at least in theory) the individual patient data from trials of the same intervention. In practice, collaboration will fall short of encompassing all trials of an intervention and not all the relevant data are shared or are available. Typically, collaborations present data on the intended benefit of interventions, but are much less likely to publish or have access to all the data on unintended consequences of interventions, which may be beyond the initial trial aim. The +AllTrials initiative and wider access to publicly and industry-funded trials may reduce this fundamental advantage of trialist collaborations as data from more and more trials are made freely available.

Another potential problem is that most collaborations between trialists are funded by the pharmaceutical industry; investigators who work on these trials and collaborations will, inevitably, be suspected of bias in favor of industry influence. Reducing possible bias in reviews conducted by trial collaborations is difficult to achieve, but may be assisted by partnerships with Cochrane review groups and other groups independent of pharmaceutical companies, as occurred with a systematic review of the unintended effects of statins in primary prevention of cardiovascular diseases [23]. Progress remains difficult, though, as evidenced by the uncovering of large amounts of unpublished data from trials evaluating the effect of neuraminidase inhibitors for patients with influenza [24].

24.5.3   Independent Systematic Review Groups

Groups of academic, independent systematic reviewers are increasing, particularly with the current investment in medical sciences in China. They often provide timely reviews of "hot" topics and give training opportunities to people who might not want the commitment required for Cochrane reviews and subsequent updates. But quality is variable, particularly with searching and assessment of risks of bias. Updating of reviews rarely happens, which is a major disadvantage. Moreover, huge duplication of effort is making it more difficult for patients, clinicians, and guideline developers to decide which of the many systematic reviews of the same intervention to use. Old reviews, particularly those published in major journals, remain in the public domain, but may be succeeded by more recent reviews conducted by other independent groups. Updates and reviews of old interventions lack novelty and may end up being published in minor journals. Doctors and patients doing quick searches on an intervention will almost certainly find the first relevant review in a major journal, but will not always find the review of unintended effects or an updated review including more recent trials. Partnerships between independent review groups and Cochrane groups may improve the situation and prove mutually beneficial. Novel strategies for such collaborations are explored later in this chapter.

24.5.4   Commercial Agencies

For-profit commercial agencies are not common, but have found a useful role in carrying out methodologically high-quality reviews quickly (though at a high price) for those who require evidence rapidly. Some Cochrane review groups have found it expedient to contract out updating of high-priority reviews to such agencies. It is quite possible that with open-access trial data and methodological developments discussed below for lowering costs, industrial-scale commercial systematic review agencies could become major players in the next decade.

24.6   METHODS FOR IMPROVING THE PROCESS OF CREATING AND UPDATING SYSTEMATIC REVIEWS

The number of randomized controlled trials published over the last decade has more than doubled and will double again in less than a decade [25]. The broad inclusion of diagnostics, prognosis, public health interventions, and nonrandomized studies in systematic reviews has only just begun in earnest. Open data mean that more information will be available for potential synthesis for some but not all trials, particularly older trials of interventions of common interventions that are the very trials for which open data would be most useful. Reviews that compare the effects of multiple interventions with multiple comparators can also be useful, but may be hampered by methodological complexity that can lead to misleading conclusions when not performed properly (see

Chapter 13). The growing mass of primary data also threatens to overwhelm our ability to synthesize and assimilate it in a timely fashion using our current methods of conducting systematic reviews.

The most important methodologies for the next decade will be those that reduce our reliance on individual searching, abstracting, cross-checking data, assessing bias, interpreting, writing up, and updating reviews. The human costs of reviewing are high and need to be minimized and shared. While people are not consistent and have their own biases, there can be wisdom in crowds given the right context. Such innovations will increase the sustainability of systematic review efforts and are discussed in detail in Chapter 23.

24.6.1   Informatics

Searching for trials related to a common patient group of interest is not straightforward when different reviewers are using different search terms. For example, a study of renal diseases demonstrated that using validated search terms improves retrieval of articles relevant to specific patient populations; used routinely this would improve the completeness of reviews [26]. Automated searching of biomedical databases by means of comprehensive search filters is also being researched at McMaster University, Canada in the HEDGES project. Such research could overcome the need to hand-search journals and reduce time taken to retrieve relevant articles [27].

Experts in information technology expect to see major gains from prospective registration of all trials, greater access to databases of regulatory bodies, the ability to search across databases automatically, and wider use of gateways (portals) and full-text databases (see also Chapter 3). Improvements in Google Scholar, Scopus, and Web of Science will occur and further assist with finding relevant articles. However, experts believe that searching will remain a major challenge despite technological advances in text analysis and data mining [28].

Empirical studies of automated or semi-automated systematic review processes are well underway. For example, risk of bias assessment (sequence generation, allocation concealment, and blinding) of trial reports has been done efficiently using machine learning. One-quarter of trial reports typically performed by two reviewers could thus be assessed by a single reviewer [29]. Natural language processing with machine learning represents an exciting possibility for automating systematic reviews (see Chapter 23). However, this field is in its infancy. A 2015 systematic review of automated methods for data extraction in systematic reviews found that there was no unified information extraction framework or standard, and most reports (out of only 26 total) focused on a small number of data elements (<7) compared with the total potential number of data elements in a typical systematic review of 52 [30]. Further investments in biomedical and health informatics are needed for these concepts to become mainstream tools.

24.6.2   Open Data

New data sources and data formats will also need to be incorporated into reviews. For example, while reviewers know how to extract and evaluate data from both published and unpublished sources, they have limited experience in handling new data elements such as clinical study reports. Doshi and colleagues have highlighted the opaque process of raw data filtering, distillation, and synthesis [31]. Clinical study reports represent a "new world of evidence" that will require methods of extraction, evaluation of risk of bias, and synthesis – as these investigators learned when they reviewed 22 000 pages of documents from published and unpublished neuraminidase inhibitor trials. They describe their methods of reviewing clinical study reports as "forensic," which sounds hard going for even the most experienced systematic reviewer.

The National Heart, Lung, and Blood Institute's Biologic Specimen and Data Repository Information Coordinating Center (BioLINCC) hosts observational, trial and other data that systematic reviewers are increasingly accessing. In 2016, there were more than 800 requests for data from 100 trials available in this dataset, though only 7% of requests were for meta-analysis and only two were for reproduction analyses [32]. As reviewers become more familiar with these platforms and as information specialists develop reproducible search methods for these data sources, these numbers should rise considerably. Despite the low overall numbers in 2016, organizations such as the European Medicines Agency started to provide clinical study reports and related data supporting drug applications – actions that are supported by European and US pharmaceutical trade organizations. Unfortunately, as a consequence of Brexit, the European Medicines Agency relocated from London to Amsterdam in March 2019, suspending the publication of clinical data in 2018, and this decision has extended into 2021 because of the COVID-19 pandemic [33]. Despite the European Medicines Agency's current position, reviewers will need to learn how to search, extract, evaluate, and synthesize in ways they have not previously imagined as a result of these sources providing data in new formats.

Doshi, Jefferson, and colleagues spent years pressuring companies to provide trial data; some companies have started to share their data more openly. Yale's Open Data Access (YODA) project [34] is one model by which an academic institution serves as the independent broker of the de-identified dataset and individual participant data for various companies. Important legal, ethical, and intellectual property issues need to be addressed, which include whether data sharing is permitted under informed consent procedures at the time of the trial. Nevertheless, clinical study reports are freely available on YODA [34], and data requests require only a data-use agreement and research protocol, though completing these relatively simple steps still takes considerable time [35]. Whether academic organizations will remain the primary data holder or whether companies might simply put their data on the web for open access remains to be seen. A 2014 report of the industry-supported website www.clinicalstudydatarequest.com demonstrated that only one quarter of requests (13 out of 53) led to data sharing in the first year. The experience of reviewers trying to access data from this site in 2015 also did not meet expectations [36], which may have contributed to a transfer of oversight to the Wellcome Trust. In 2019, the estimated time from submission to data access took, on average, 9 months and as of April 2021, only 84 (13%) reports from 633 requests had been published from a total of 3069 available trial datasets, demonstrating the continued challenges in operationalizing data sharing [37].

Some might describe these methods of outside reviewers re-evaluating trial data as "research voyeurism," particularly if outside investigators pursue analyses for personal rather than professional reasons. However, the openness of this process and replication of initial findings through independent analyses would seem more likely to strengthen the validity of results. While the challenges in re-analyzing trial data have been reported even by the trialists themselves, these challenges of re-analysis or reproducibility highlight the need for greater rather than less sharing of statistical analysis plans, statistical code, and case report forms with the original publication or on public sites such as GitHub (https://github.com).

The +AllTrials campaign is an effective activist organization, but a still more fundamental shift is required to change a fringe activity to a routine one. The National Academy of Medicine's 2015 report on open data calls for data sharing to be the "expected norm," including making complete datasets available 18 months after trial completion or 6 months after trial reporting [38]. The National Academy of Medicine further recommends that data holders should be responsible for risk mitigation and that sponsors should lead multistakeholder discussions to overcome infrastructure, technological, sustainability, and workforce challenges. This would represent a sea change for performing systematic reviews, but given recent history it seems improbable without binding regulatory action.

24.6.3   Leveraging the Power of the Crowd

Machine learning and open data represent top-down examples of the future of systematic reviews, whereas crowdsourcing represents a complementary, bottom-up approach that captures the grassroots spirit of groups such as Cochrane. Rather than creating overlapping reviews, systematic reviewers from all over the world can collaborate around topics of common interest. Cochrane's Project Transform, from 2015 to 2018, allowed reviewers to work in teams on projects and tasks that are matched to their interests [39]. Traditional methods will need to be adapted to fit this format (and new ones created), but crowdsourcing can speed up reviews as steps are performed almost in parallel rather than serially. Authorship will be tricky. The Cochrane and Campbell Collaborations might wish to set a trend by reviving the notion of "contributorship" rather than authorship, which in the future would make more sense [40, 41].

24.7   MULTIPLE INTERVENTIONS AND NETWORK META-ANALYSIS

Overviews (also called "umbrella" reviews) have been used to summarize the findings of multiple systematic reviews examining different treatments for the same condition using a narrative approach (see also Chapter 1). Overviews have developed in response to the clinical need to make choices among several treatments for the same condition in terms of potential benefits and harms. For example, in treating a child with nocturnal enuresis, the doctor, family, and child will want to know which of the following treatments is best: alarm systems, toileting during the night, a range of drugs, or psychological and complementary treatments [42]. Systematic reviews independently capture the effects of each of the treatments, reflecting the trial designs available to them and the ease of conducting a review of the effects of a single intervention. The overview pulled together findings from seven Cochrane reviews and presented the effect sizes from 13 treatment comparisons, with odds ratios ranging from 0.17 to 1.33 for failure to achieve 14 consecutive dry nights, and 11 of these estimates having an upper confidence interval below 1. The methodological quality of all the trials was rated as poor, but marked heterogeneity in most of the included meta-analyses was not explored. The authors considered that the "best buy" treatment was an alarm system, despite the effect of an alarm in conjunction with dry-bed training actually being greater than an alarm alone. Interestingly, this overview was re-analyzed using a network meta-analysis approach, which demonstrated that the conclusions of the original overview were not supported by the evidence. Furthermore, the network meta-analysis demonstrated marked inconsistency of direct and indirect treatment effects, making robust judgments on the best treatment impossible [43].

Attempting to trawl useful evidence from existing reviews is problematic not only because of reporting biases in the original trials, but also because of differences between reviews in their target populations, search methods, inclusion criteria, quality appraisal, and updating. A proposal that overviews should be conducted prospectively with a defined protocol has been made, on the grounds that this may be a more efficient approach than conducting reviews in an uncoordinated way [44].

There are still many areas in which small trials are conducted for pharmaceutical regulatory purposes to demonstrate the effectiveness of new drugs compared to "usual care" comparators or a placebo, or no treatment control if this is appropriate. These trials help neither the clinician nor the patient, who want to know which is the better of two treatments. Usually, head-to-head comparisons of new treatments do not get conducted for several years. For example, patients with atrial fibrillation might choose between aspirin, other more potent anti-platelet drugs, or anti-coagulants for the prevention of vascular events such as strokes and heart attacks. Trials of each treatment versus placebo exist, and there are head-to-head comparisons of some of the combinations. But how best to analyze these sources of data?

Methods of multiple treatment comparison through network meta-analysis have developed rapidly to tackle this problem over the last decade. Network meta-analysis (see Chapter 13) has grown in popularity, as it enables questions to be answered about best treatment options in the absence of direct head-to-head trials. Software applications have been developed that have made analysis more straightforward, which has also contributed to increased use. In many clinical areas network meta-analysis is not a panacea, as typically only small, underpowered trials exist comparing, for example, A versus placebo, B versus placebo, and A versus B. Pooling these data retains the inherent biases common to small trials and comparator biases. Moreover, heterogeneity of effects and incoherence between findings from direct and indirect comparisons may occur, making interpretation difficult. Investigators using these methods are advised to make cautious inferences [45].

24.8 IMPROVING TRIAL REGISTRATION, REPORTING AND DETECTING FRAUD

The failure of investigators to report trial findings or to delay publication has been an issue for decades, but continues despite efforts by funders and others to ensure prospective registration (see also Chapter 5). This problem includes nonpharmacological interventions just as much as pharmacological interventions. It is surprising that academic institutions and funders do not consider it part of their governance to monitor and enforce trial registration and publication. Better methods of assessing publication bias in systematic reviews are not a solution to this problem.

The poor reporting of randomized controlled trials remains a major issue for conducting systematic reviews and meta-analyses of the effects of interventions. It is difficult to distinguish between poor conduct of a trial and poor reporting of an adequately conducted trial. Guidelines for the reporting of trials produced by clinical trial methodologists, guideline developers, knowledge translation specialists, and journal editors aimed to solve this problem. The first CONSORT (CONsolidated Standards Of Reporting Trials) guidelines appeared in 1996 and comprehensive guidelines were published in 2010 (http://www.consort-statement.org/consort-2010). These guidelines have made it easier for investigators, journal editors, and peer reviewers to ensure that all relevant information is included in randomized trial reports. But they cannot deal with the "discrepancies" within and between reports of trials (e.g. in design: conflicting statements on randomization; in methods/baseline characteristics: percentages that could not be an integer number of patients; in results: conflicts between tables). In a study of 343 journal readers, of whom 260 agreed to read an article to identify discrepancies, remarkably 95% of discrepancies were missed by these readers, despite them having been asked specifically to look for them [46].

It might be thought that a few errors in numbers would not make any major difference – but that would be wrong. Bone marrow stem cells for heart disease are a cutting-edge treatment and trials have shown promising results. In a review of 49 trials with 133 reports, over 600 discrepancies were found [47]. What is worrying is that the more discrepancies detected in a trial, the greater was the effect size for the primary outcome of these trials – ejection fraction, a marker of how well the heart is pumping (see Figure 24.1). In the five trials with no discrepancies, the effect size was zero. Not a popular result for stem cell enthusiasts.

These problems of discrepancies are not isolated, and the analysis shown raises questions about the credibility of trial reports that incorporate errors. While many errors may be innocent, there are circumstances where fraudulent manipulation of

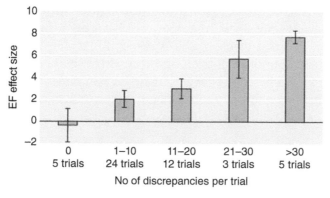

FIGURE 24.1   Relationship between discrepancies per trial and effect size (mean left ventricular ejection fraction). Source: Published with permission of the authors and BMJ Publications. Source: Nowbar et al. [47].

data has resulted in misleading findings that may have a huge influence on clinical practice if guidelines are adhered to. One outstanding example is the use of beta-blockade in patients undergoing non-cardiac surgery. The European Society of Cardiology guidelines [48] included a family of trials from the same scientific team that had discrepancies in reporting that were questioned, but action was not taken to remove these trials from the accumulated evidence. Indeed, these suspect trials contributed most of the evidence of benefit, with the remaining trials showing no benefit, but rather a 27% increase in mortality [49].

Surprisingly, in the 2014 update of these guidelines [50] the evidence that beta-blockers increased mortality was ignored, and their use was condoned [51]. A 2019 Cochrane review on this topic reported that beta-blockers may make little or no difference to the number of people who die within 30 days of surgery [52].

24.9   PRIORITIZATION OF REVIEWS AND UPDATES

The massive scope of health care that is now the remit for systematic reviews requires prioritization if it is to continue within finite resources, produce timely updates, and continue to engage the people who provide their time and energy to conduct systematic reviews, many for no financial gain. No clear strategy for prioritization of reviews and updates has emerged. Various ideas have been proposed within Cochrane. For example, they could implement rapid updates, which would be triggered on publication of a new major trial relevant to a specific systematic review. A Cochrane Agenda and Priority Setting methods group was established in 2011 [53] to develop policies and has produced empirical research [54–57], but no publications since 2017 have been logged on its website.

24.10   CONCLUSION

In the foreword to the last edition of this book, Sir Iain Chalmers, who established the Cochrane Collaboration, highlighted five developments he hoped to see before this next edition appeared (see also his foreword to the current edition) [58]. The first was the acknowledgment by researchers, funders, and journal editors of the central importance of research synthesis anticipated by Lord Rayleigh, in 1884, in the forward's epigraph: "discovery and explanation go hand in hand, in which not only are new facts presented, but their relation to old ones is pointed out." Second, more effort is needed to make bias less likely in studies contributing to reviews, and reporting biases should be reduced through registration of study protocols and full reporting of findings. Third, systematic reviews need to tackle etiology, diagnosis, risk prediction, and prognosis. Fourth, reviewers should be guided by systematic reviews of individual empirical studies addressing methodological questions. And fifth, social scientists, health researchers, and lay people will need to cooperate to improve both the science of research synthesis and the design of new studies. Gratifying progress has been made in all these areas, but much remains to be done.

Given the large and rapidly increasing number of studies worldwide, current methods of producing systematic reviews are not sustainable. Automation and crowdsourcing of generating systematic reviews of interventions will help. The role of systematic reviewers will move toward verification of the effects of high-priority interventions. A much stronger focus on the registration, publication, and quality of the primary studies will be needed. Metrics of success will focus on the hypothesis-generating role of most systematic reviews, rather than simply on their application in clinical practice guidelines or health technology assessments.

ACKNOWLEDGMENTS

We are very grateful to George Davey Smith, University of Bristol, and Juan Pablo Casas, Harvard Medical School, for their comments on this chapter.

REFERENCES

1. Egger, M., Davey Smith, G., and Altman, D. (2001). *Systematic Reviews in Health Care: Meta-Analysis in Context*, 2e. London: BMJ Publications.
2. Filion, G. (2014). A flurry of copycats on PubMed. *The Grand Locus*, October 4. http://blog.thegrandlocus.com/2014/10/a-flurry-of-copycats-on-pubmed (accessed January 7, 2022).
3. +AllTrials. (2015). Pharma company investors call for clinical trials transparency. http://www.alltrials.net/news/pharma-company-investors-call-for-clinical-trials-transparency (accessed January 7, 2022).
4. Pound, P., Ebrahim, S., Sandercock, P. et al. (2004). Where is the evidence that animal research benefits humans? *BMJ* 328: 514.
5. Royal Society. (2004). The use of non-human animals in research: a guide for scientists. London: Royal Society. https://royalsociety.org/~/media/Royal_Society_Content/policy/publications/2004/9726.pdf (accessed January 7, 2022).
6. Lagisz, M., Blair, H., Kenyon, P. et al. (2015). Little appetite for obesity: meta-analysis of the effects of maternal obesogenic diets on offspring food intake and body mass in rodents. *Int. J. Obes. (Lond)* 39 (12): 1669–1678. https://doi.org/10.1038/ijo.2015.160.
7. CONSORT Statement. http://www.consort-statement.org (accessed January 7, 2022).
8. Henderson, V.C., Kimmelman, J., Fergusson, D. et al. (2013). Threats to validity in the design and conduct of preclinical efficacy studies: a systematic review of guidelines for in vivo animal experiments. *PLoS Med.* 10 (7): e1001489. https://doi.org/10.1371/journal.pmed.1001489.
9. Barsh, G.S., Copenhaver, G.P., Gibson, G., and Williams, S.M. (2012). Guidelines for genome-wide association studies. *PLoS Genet.* 8 (7): e1002812. https://doi.org/10.1371/journal.pgen.1002812.
10. Evangelou, E. and Ioannidis, J.P.A. (2013). Meta-analysis methods for genome-wide association studies and beyond. *Nat. Rev. Genet.* 14: 379–389. https://doi.org/10.1038/nrg3472.
11. Little, J., Higgins, J.P.T., Ioannidis, J.P.A., et al. (2009). STrengthening the REporting of Genetic Association Studies (STREGA)— An Extension of the STROBE Statement. *PLOS Med.* 6: e1000022. https://doi.org/10.1371/journal.pmed.1000022.

12. Bowden, J., Davey Smith, G., and Burgess, S. (2015). Mendelian randomization with invalid instruments: effect estimation and bias detection through Egger regression. *Int. J. Epidemiol.* https://doi.org/10.1093/ije/dyv080.

13. IOM (Institute of Medicine) (2011). *Clinical Practice Guidelines We Can Trust.* Washington, DC: National Academies Press.

14. IOM (Institute of Medicine) (2011). *Finding What Works in Health Care: Standards for Systematic Reviews.* Washington, DC: National Academies Press.

15. Tricoci, P., Allen, J.M., Kramer, J.M. et al. (2009). Scientific evidence underlying the ACC/AHA clinical practice guidelines. *J. Am. Med. Assoc.* 301 (8): 831–841.

16. Neuman, M.D., Goldstein, J.N., Cirullo, M.A., and Schwartz, J. (2014). Durability of class I American College of Cardiology/American Heart Association clinical practice guideline recommendations. *J. Am. Med. Assoc.* 311 (20): 2092–2100.

17. Bevan, G.H., Kalra, A., Josephson, R.A., and Al-Kindi, S.G. (2019). Level of scientific evidence underlying the current American College of Cardiology/American Heart Association clinical practice guidelines. *Circ. Cardiovasc. Qual. Outcomes* 12 (2): e005293. https://doi.org/10.1161/CIRCOUTCOMES.118.005293. PMID: 30755028.

18. Siontis, K.C., Hernandez-Boussard, T., and Ioannidis, J.P.A. (2013). Overlapping meta-analyses on the same topic: survey of published studies. *BMJ.* 347: f4501.

19. Campbell Systematic Reviews. https://onlinelibrary.wiley.com/journal/18911803 (accessed January 7, 2022).

20. Cochrane Editorial Policies. https://training.cochrane.org/online-learning/editorial-policies/coi-policy/coi-policy-cochrane-library (accessed January 7, 2022).

21. Evidence-based Practice Center (EPC) Reports. https://www.ahrq.gov/research/findings/evidence-based-reports/index.html (accessed January 7, 2022).

22. Launch of Cochrane US Network. https://www.cochrane.org/news/launch-cochrane-us-network (accessed January 7, 2022).

23. Macedo, A.F., Taylor, F.C., Casas, J.P. et al. (2014). Unintended effects of statins from observational studies in the general population: systematic review and meta-analysis. *BMC Med.* 12: 51. https://doi.org/10.1186/1741-7015-12-51.

24. Jefferson, T., Jones, M., Doshi, P. et al. (2014). Heneghan CJ et al, Oseltamivir for influenza in adults and children: systematic review of clinical study reports and summary of regulatory comments. *BMJ* 348: g2545.

25. Viergever, R.F. and Li, K. (2015). Trends in global clinical trial registration: an analysis of numbers of registered clinical trials in different parts of the world from 2004 to 2013. *BMJ Open* 5: e008932. https://doi.org/10.1136/bmjopen-2015-008932.

26. Hildebrand AM, Iansavichus AV, Lee CW, Haynes RB, Wilczynski NL, McKibbon KA, et al. (2012). Glomerular disease search filters for Pubmed, Ovid Medline, and Embase: a development and validation study. *BMC Med Inform Decis Mak* 12: 49. https://doi.org/10.1186/1472-6947-12-49.

27. McMaster University. (2018). Hedges. http://hiru.mcmaster.ca/hiru/HIRU_Hedges_home.aspx (accessed January 7, 2022).

28. Lefebvre, C., Glanville, J., Wieland, L.S. et al. (2013). Methodological developments in searching for studies for systematic reviews: past, present and future? *Syst. Rev.* 2: 78.

29. Millard, L.A.C., Flach, P.A., and Higgins, J.P.T. (2016). Machine learning to assist risk of bias assessments of systematic reviews. *Int. J. Epidemiol.* 45 (1): 266–277. https://doi.org/10.1093/ije/dyv306.

30. Jonnalagadda, S.R., Goyal, P., and Huffman, M.D. (2015). Automating data extraction in systematic reviews: a systematic review. *Syst. Rev.* 4: 78.

31. Doshi, P., Jones, M., and Jefferson, T. (2012). Rethinking credible evidence synthesis. *BMJ* 344: d7898.

32. Giffen, C.A., Wagner, E.L., Adams, J.T. et al. (2017). Providing researchers with online access to NHLBI biospecimen collections: the results of the first six years of the NHLBI BioLINCC program. *PLoS One* 12 (6): e0178141. https://doi.org/10.1371/journal.pone.0178141.

33. European Medicines Agency. Brexit: the United Kingdom's withdrawal from the European Union. https://www.ema.europa.eu/en/about-us/brexit-united-kingdoms-withdrawal-european-union (accessed January 7, 2022).

34. Yale's Open Data Access. http://yoda.yale.edu (accessed January 7, 2022).

35. Gay, H.C., Baldridge, A.S., and Huffman, M.D. (2017). Feasibility, process, and outcomes of cardiovascular clinical trial data sharing: a reproduction analysis of the SMART-AF trial. *JAMA Cardiol.* 2 (12): 1375–1379. https://doi.org/10.1001/jamacardio.2017.3808.

36. Mayo-Wilson, E., Doshi, P., and Dickersin, K. (2015). Are manufacturers sharing data as promised? *Br. Med. J.* 351: h4169. https://doi.org/10.1136/bmj.h4169.

37. Clinical Study Data Request. https://www.clinicalstudydatarequest.com/Metrics.aspx (accessed January 7, 2022).

38. Institute of Medicine (IOM) (2015). *Sharing Clinical Trial Data: Maximizing Benefits, Minimizing Risk*. Washington, DC: National Academies Press.

39. Cochrane Project Transform. https://community.cochrane.org/help/tools-and-software/project-transform (accessed January 7, 2022).

40. Rennie, D., Yak, V., and Emanuel, L. (1997). When authorship fails: a proposal to make contributors accountable. *J. Am. Med. Assoc.* 278: 579–585.

41. Smith, R. (1997). Authorship: time for a paradigm shift? *BMJ* 314: 992.

42. Russell, K., Kiddoo, D., and The Cochrane Library and nocturnal enuresis (2006). An umbrella review. *Evid. Based Child Health* 1: 5–8.

43. Caldwell, D.M., Welton, N.J., and Ades, A.E. (2010). Mixed treatment comparison analysis provides internally coherent treatment effect estimates based on overviews of reviews and can reveal inconsistency. *J. Clin. Epidemiol.* 63: 875–882.

44. Ioannidis, J.P. (2009). Integration of evidence from multiple meta-analyses: a primer on umbrella reviews, treatment networks and multiple treatments meta-analyses. *CMAJ* 181: 488–493.

45. Mills, E.J. (2013). Demystifying trial networks and network meta-analysis. *BMJ* 346: f2914.

46. Cole, G., Shun-Shin, M.J., Nowbar, A.N. et al. (2015). Difficulty in detecting discrepancies in a clinical trial report: 260-reader evaluation. *Int. J. Epidemiol.* 44 (3): 862–869.

47. Nowbar, A.N., Mielewczik, M., Karavassilis, M. et al. (2014). Discrepancies in autologous bone marrow stem cell trials and enhancement of ejection fraction (DAMASCENE): weighted regression and meta analysis. *BMJ* 348: g2688.

48. Poldermans, D., Bax, J.J., Boersma, E. et al. (2009). Guidelines for pre-operative cardiac risk assessment and perioperative cardiac management in non-cardiac surgery. *Eur. Heart J.* 30 (22): 2769–2812.

49. Bouri, S., Shun-Shin, M.J., Cole, G.D. et al. (2014). Meta-analysis of secure randomised controlled trials of β-blockade to prevent perioperative death in non-cardiac surgery. *Heart* 100 (6): 456–464.

50. Kristensen, S.D., Knuuti, J., Saraste, A. et al. (2014). ESC/ESA guidelines on non-cardiac surgery: cardiovascular assessment and management. *Eur. Heart J.* 35: 2383–2431.

51. Cole, G.D. and Francis, D.P. (2014). Perioperative β blockade: guidelines do not reflect the problems with the evidence from the DECREASE trials. *BMJ* 349: g5210.

52. Blessberger, H., Lewis, S.R., Pritchard, M.W. et al. (2019). Perioperative beta-blockers for preventing surgery-related mortality and morbidity in adults undergoing non-cardiac surgery. *Cochrane Database Syst. Rev.* (9): CD013438. https://doi.org/10.1002/14651858.CD013438.

53. Cochrane Priority Setting Methods Group. http://capsmg.cochrane.org/welcome (accessed January 7, 2022).

54. Jamamillo, A., Welch, V.A., Ueffing, E. et al. (2013). Prevention and self-management interventions are top priorities for osteoarthritis systematic reviews. *J. Clin. Epidemiol.* 66 (5): 503–510.e4.

55. Bero, L.A. and Binder, L. (2013). The Cochrane collaboration review prioritization projects show that a variety of approaches successfully identify high-priority topics. *J. Clin. Epidemiol.* 66 (5): 472–473.

56. Clavisi, O., Bragge, P., Tavender, E. et al. (2013). Effective stakeholder participation in setting research priorities using a global evidence mapping approach. *J. Clin. Epidemiol.* 66 (5): 496–502.e2.

57. Nasser, M., Welch, V., Tugwell, P. et al. (2013). Ensuring relevance for Cochrane reviews: evaluating processes and methods for prioritizing topics for Cochrane reviews. *J. Clin. Epidemiol.* 66 (5): 474–482.

58. Chalmers, I. (2001). Foreword. Systematic reviews in health care. In: *Systematic Reviews in Health Care: Meta-Analysis in Context* (eds. M. Egger, G. Davey Smith and D.G. Altman), xii–xvii. London: BMJ Books.

PART VI

SOFTWARE

CHAPTER 25

Meta-Analysis in Stata

David J. Fisher, Marcel Zwahlen, Matthias Egger, and Julian P.T. Higgins

In this chapter we show how to perform meta-analysis using the statistical package Stata. There are more than 50 Stata commands to perform a meta-analysis, for different types of studies and data [1] (see https://www.stata.com/support/faqs/statistics/meta-analysis). In addition, Stata 16 (released in June 2019) includes built-in meta-analysis functionality for the first time.

We will describe how to perform a standard meta-analysis in Stata, and discuss how to examine the data in more detail, such as by looking at the accumulation of evidence in cumulative meta-analysis, using graphical and statistical techniques to look for evidence of bias, and using meta-regression to investigate possible sources of heterogeneity. We will also take a brief look at some more advanced topics, including network meta-analysis. To complement this chapter, Chapter 26 describes how to use the R software for meta-analysis and Chapter 27 introduces the Comprehensive Meta-Analysis software.

25.1 GETTING STARTED

Stata is a commercial, general-purpose, command-line-driven, programmable statistical package. Although Stata 16 introduced a built-in meta-analysis suite into the core package, at the time of writing it has limited functionality and it is unclear which directions its future development might take. Examples of its use will be given where appropriate, but otherwise we will concentrate on the numerous user-written routines for meta-analysis, which are freely available and are compatible with older versions of Stata. Hence, to follow the examples in this chapter, the reader should install these routines by downloading the relevant files from the internet. Throughout this chapter, Stata commands appear in **bold monospaced font**, and are followed by the Stata output that they produce in normal monospaced font. The easiest way to download user-writing commands is to type:

```
search commandname
```

then choose the latest version of the command, follow the appropriate links, and click on (click here to install). For example, at the time of writing, the most recent version of command **metareg** was published in *Stata Journal* volume 8, issue 4 (SJ-8-4). Clicking on the name of the package (sbe23_1) leads the user to the installation screen. All commands described here can be downloaded in this way. Often, the most recent version of a command is made available through the Statistical Software Components (SSC) archive (see **help ssc** in Stata). In that case, a more direct way is to type:

```
ssc describe commandname
ssc install  commandname
```

A more detailed description of the features and rationale of the commands (often with data examples) can be found in the help file of the command (type **help com-mandname** or go into the "Help" menu and click on the "Stata command. . ." option.). In addition, the book *Meta-Analysis in Stata: An Updated Collection from the Stata Journal* provides details of most of the key commands [1]. An overview of the commands we cover is given in Table 25.1. All the output shown in this chapter was produced using Stata version 16 although, as already stated, the featured user-written commands should produce similar output with earlier Stata versions. All the Stata data files are available from the book's website at www.systematic-reviews3.org.

TABLE 25.1   Summary of useful Stata commands for meta-analysis

Command	What the command does	Default data input	See also
metan	General-purpose meta-analysis command with a large number of features, including: • Fixed-effect inverse variance • Mantel–Haenszel and Peto fixed-effect analysis for 2 × 2 data • A variety of random-effects models including REML • Confidence intervals for heterogeneity parameters, including those suggested by Higgins and Thompson [2] • Cumulative and influence analysis	Any of the following: • Study effect estimates and standard errors • Numbers of events and nonevents in two groups • Means, standard deviations, and sample sizes in two groups • Numbers of events and sample sizes, for analysis of single-group proportions	Chapters 8, 9
metaan	Performs random-effects meta-analysis with several options for between-study variance, including REML	Study effect estimates and standard errors	Chapter 9
metareg	Performs random-effects meta-regression with several options for between-study variance, including REML	Study effect estimates and standard errors, and study-level covariates	Chapter 10
metabias	Test for funnel plot asymmetry using several regression-based methods	Depends on the choice of test (see documentation)	Chapter 5

TABLE 25.1   *(Continued)*

Command	What the command does	Default data input	See also
glst	Generalized least squares for trend estimation of summarized dose–response data for single or multiple summarized dose–response epidemiological studies	Effect estimates and standard errors per exposure level and per study; information for estimating within-study covariances	Chapter 14
metamiss	Meta-analysis of 2 × 2 (binary outcome) trials with missing data from some participants	Numbers of events, nonevents, and missing values in two groups	Chapter 11
metamiss2	Extension to metamiss, allowing binary, continuous, or generic outcome types and able to handle a broader range of missingness assumptions	Depends on the type of analysis (see documentation)	Chapter 11
metandi	Meta-analysis of diagnostic accuracy	Numbers of true positives, false positives, false negatives, and true negatives for each study	Chapter 16
mvmeta	Multivariate random-effects meta-analysis and meta-regression	Takes vectors and matrices as input	Chapters 9, 10
network	Suite of more than 10 commands for network meta-analysis	Depends on the command used within this suite	Chapter 13

Graphics commands (note that some of the above commands may also produce graphics)

Command	What the command does	Default data input	See also
forestplot	Produces generalized forest plots directly from source data, without analysis. Used by **metan** to produce its plots, but can also be used by itself	Effect estimates and confidence limits	Chapter 9
confunnel	Contour-enhanced funnel plots for meta-analysis	Effect estimates and standard errors	Chapter 5
metafunnel	Older command for producing funnel plots, with option to add fitted line from Egger's regression-based test	Effect estimates and standard errors or confidence limits	Chapter 5

All commands in this list are user written and maintained. For the built-in suite of meta-analysis commands introduced in Stata 16, see the official documentation.

25.2   COMMANDS TO PERFORM A STANDARD META-ANALYSIS

25.2.1   Example 1 – Intravenous Streptokinase in Myocardial Infarction

Table 25.2 gives data from 22 randomized controlled trials of streptokinase in the prevention of death following myocardial infarction [3–5].

TABLE 25.2   Data from 22 randomized controlled trials of streptokinase in the prevention of death following myocardial infarction.

Trial name	Publication year	Intervention group		Control group	
		Deaths	Total	Deaths	Total
Fletcher	1959	1	12	4	11
Dewar	1963	4	21	7	21
1st European	1969	20	83	15	84
Heikinheimo	1971	22	219	17	207
Italian	1971	19	164	18	157
2nd European	1971	69	373	94	357
2nd Frankfurt	1973	13	102	29	104
1st Australian	1973	26	264	32	253
NHLBI SMIT	1974	7	53	3	54
Valere	1975	11	49	9	42
Frank	1975	6	55	6	53
UK Collaborative	1976	48	302	52	293
Klein	1976	4	14	1	9
Austrian	1977	37	352	65	376
Lasierra	1977	1	13	3	11
N German	1977	63	249	51	234
Witchitz	1977	5	32	5	26
2nd Australian	1977	25	112	31	118
3rd European	1977	25	156	50	159
ISAM	1986	54	859	63	882
GISSI-1	1986	628	5860	758	5852
ISIS-2	1988	791	8592	1029	8595

Source: Adapted from Yusuf S et al. 1985 [2], GISSI 1986 [3] and ISIS-2 1988 [4].

We saved these data in the Stata dataset strepto.dta. We can list the variables contained in the dataset, with their descriptions (variable labels), by using the **describe** command:

```
describe

Contains data from strepto.dta
    obs:             22                      Streptokinase and mortality
   vars:              7
---------------------------------------------------------------------------
    1. trial     byte    %8.0g               Trial number
    2. trialnam  str14   %14s                Trial name
    3. year      int     %8.0g               Year of publication
    4. pop1      int     %12.0g              Treated population
    5. deaths1   int     %12.0g              Treated deaths
    6. pop0      int     %12.0g              Control population
    7. deaths0   int     %12.0g              Control deaths
---------------------------------------------------------------------------
Sorted by:   trial
```

25.2.2   The Metan Command

The **metan** command [6] (but more recently updated via the SSC archive) provides a variety of methods for combining results, all of which assume independence of the observations, as would be the case when each observation represents a different study. Results may be available in the form of an effect estimate together with its standard error or 95% confidence interval. Alternatively, where two groups have been compared in a randomized trial, more detailed information may be available such as means, standard deviations, and sample sizes for continuous outcomes; or the number of individuals in each group who did, and did not, experience a binary outcome. Single-group proportion data may also be analyzed. In all cases, either fixed-effect (sometimes called "common-effect") or random-effects models can be fitted.

In our streptokinase example, we have data from randomized trials with two groups with a binary outcome. The data in Table 25.2 comprise the number of individuals who experienced the event (death) and the totals, by group. To use **metan**, we need to create variables containing the number of individuals who *did not* experience the event, as follows:

```
generate alive1 = pop1 - deaths1
generate alive0 = pop0 - deaths0
```

With binary outcome data, the effect measure can be the difference between proportions (sometimes called the risk difference), the ratio of two proportions (risk ratio or relative risk), or the odds ratio. Here, we will use the **metan** command to perform a meta-analysis of risk ratios, derive a summary estimate using Mantel–Haenszel methods, and produce a forest plot. The options (following the comma) that we use are:

rr	Perform calculations using risk ratios (for which Mantel–Haenszel methods are the default)
label(namevar = trialnam)	Label the output and vertical axis of the graph with the trial name. The trial year may also be added by specifying **yearvar = year**

`forestplot(xlabel(.1 1 10))`   Label the *x*-axis in the forest plot (note that all options relating to the plot should be placed inside the **`forestplot()`** option)

The command and output of this analysis are as follows:

```
metan deaths1 alive1 deaths0 alive0, rr label(namevar=trialnam)
forestplot (xlabel(.1 1 10))
```

```
Studies included: 22
Participants included: 35834
```

```
Meta-analysis pooling of Risk Ratios
using the Mantel-Haenszel method
```

Trial name		Risk Ratio	[95% Conf. Interval]		% Weight
Fletcher	|	0.229	0.030	1.750	0.18
Dewar	|	0.571	0.196	1.665	0.30
1st European	|	1.349	0.743	2.451	0.64
Heikinheimo	|	1.223	0.669	2.237	0.75
Italian	|	1.011	0.551	1.853	0.78
2nd European	|	0.703	0.534	0.925	4.10
2nd Frankfurt	|	0.457	0.252	0.828	1.22
1st Australian	|	0.779	0.478	1.268	1.39
NHLBI SMIT	|	2.377	0.649	8.709	0.13
Valere	|	1.048	0.481	2.282	0.41
Frank	|	0.964	0.332	2.801	0.26
UK Collab	|	0.896	0.626	1.281	2.25
Klein	|	2.571	0.339	19.481	0.05
Austrian	|	0.608	0.417	0.886	2.68
Lasierra	|	0.282	0.034	2.340	0.14
N German	|	1.161	0.840	1.604	2.24
Witchitz	|	0.812	0.263	2.506	0.24
2nd Australian	|	0.850	0.537	1.345	1.29
3rd European	|	0.510	0.333	0.780	2.11
ISAM	|	0.880	0.619	1.250	2.65
GISSI-1	|	0.827	0.749	0.914	32.34
ISIS-2	|	0.769	0.704	0.839	43.86
Overall, MH	|	0.799	0.755	0.845	100.00

```
Test of overall effect = 1:  z =  -7.747  p = 0.000
```

```
Heterogeneity measures, calculated from the data
with Conf. Intervals based on non-central chi² (common-effect) distribution
for Q
```

Measure		Value	df	p-value
Mantel-Haenszel Q	|	30.41	21	0.084
	|		-[95% Conf. Interval]-	
H	|	1.203	1.000	1.545
I^2 (%)	|	30.9%	0.0%	58.1%

H = relative excess in Mantel–Haenszel Q over its degrees-of-freedom
I² = between-study variance (tau²) as a percentage of total variance (based on Q)

The output shows, for each study, the effect estimate (here the risk ratio) together with the corresponding 95% confidence interval (CI) and the percentage weight contributed to the overall meta-analysis. Underneath is the summary (pooled) treatment effect and 95% confidence interval, below which is a test for statistical significance of the summary effect, with a P value. The heterogeneity test and I² statistic (see Chapter 9) are also shown, along with related heterogeneity statistics. By default, Stata adds new variables to the dataset containing the effect estimate, its standard error, the 95% CI, study weights, and sample sizes.

The **metan** command also automatically produces a forest plot (see Chapter 9), shown in Figure 25.1. In a forest plot, the contribution of each study to the meta-analysis (its weight) is proportional to the area of a box whose center represents the effect estimate from that study (point estimate). The confidence interval for the effect estimate from each study is also shown, as a horizontal line. The summary effect estimate is shown by the middle of a diamond whose left and right extremities represent the corresponding confidence interval.

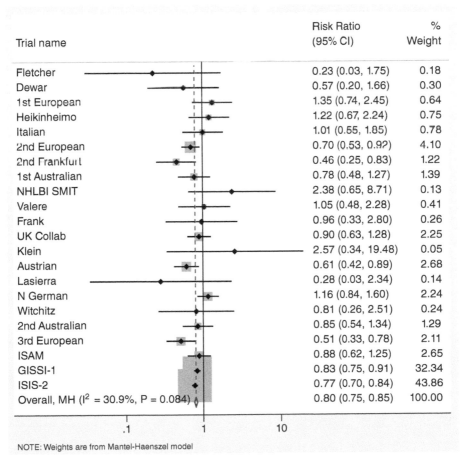

FIGURE 25.1   Forest plot of the data in Table 25.2 using **metan** with Mantel–Haenszel meta-analysis of risk ratios.

The following additional options are also likely to be useful:

`eform`	(Exponential form) display the output on the ratio scale
`effect(Relative risk)`	Label the effect size column differently
`or`	Perform calculations using odds ratios
`rd`	Perform calculations using risk differences
`counts`	Add columns of numbers of events and participants, by group
`lcols(trialnam year)`	Add columns containing a trial identifier and year; alternative to `label()`
`second(random)`	Add a second (random-effects) meta-analysis
`rfdist`	Add prediction interval for random-effects model

For a complete list of options, the help file can be consulted at any time within Stata by typing `help metan`.

Both the output text and the graph show that streptokinase protects against death following myocardial infarction. The meta-analysis is dominated by the large GISSI-1 and ISIS-2 trials, which contribute 76.2% of the weight in this analysis. We may choose to omit the weights or treatment effects from the graph, using the options `nowt` and `nostats`, respectively. The `metan` command will perform all the widely used fixed-effect and random-effects analyses (see Chapter 7).

As mentioned earlier, the `metan` command leaves behind new variables containing the calculated effect estimates and their standard errors. We can demonstrate how this works by calculating the summary log risk ratio and standard error for each study ourselves from our available data, using standard formulae. The log risk ratio is calculated as:

```
generate logrr = log((deaths1/pop1)/(deaths0/pop0))
```

and its standard error is approximately:

```
generate selogrr = sqrt((1/deaths1)-(1/pop1)+(1/deaths0)-(1/pop0))
```

It can easily be seen (for example using `list` or `browse`) that these variables contain the same values as the variables _ES and _seES left behind by `metan`.

25.2.3   Example 2 – Intravenous Magnesium in Acute Myocardial Infarction

Table 25.3 gives data from 16 randomized controlled trials of intravenous magnesium in the prevention of death following myocardial infarction. These trials are a well-known example where the results of a meta-analysis [7] were contradicted by a single large trial (ISIS-4) [8–10].

TABLE 25.3 Data from 16 randomized controlled trials of intravenous magnesium in the prevention of death following myocardial infarction.

Trial name	Publication year	Intervention group		Control group	
		Deaths	Total	Deaths	Total
Morton	1984	1	40	2	36
Rasmussen	1986	9	135	23	135
Smith	1986	2	200	7	200
Abraham	1987	1	48	1	46
Feldstedt	1988	10	150	8	148
Schechter	1989	1	59	9	56
Ceremuzynski	1989	1	25	3	23
Bertschat	1989	0	22	1	21
Singh	1990	6	76	11	75
Pereira	1990	1	27	7	27
Schechter 1	1991	2	89	12	80
Golf	1991	5	23	13	33
Thogersen	1991	4	130	8	122
LIMIT-2	1992	90	1159	118	1157
Schechter 2	1995	4	107	17	108
ISIS-4	1995	2216	29 011	2103	29 039

These data were saved in Stata dataset magnes.dta.

describe

```
Contains data from magnes.dta
  obs:            16                      Magnesium and CHD
  vars:            7
-------------------------------------------------------------------
storage   display    value
variable name   type    format    label    variable label
-------------------------------------------------------------------
trial           byte    %8.0g              Trial number
trialnam        str12   %12s               Trial name
year            int     %8.0g              Year of publication
pop1            int     %12.0g             Treated population
deaths1         double  %12.0g             Treated deaths
pop0            int     %12.0g             Control population
deaths0         double  %12.0g             Control deaths
-------------------------------------------------------------------
Sorted by: trial
```

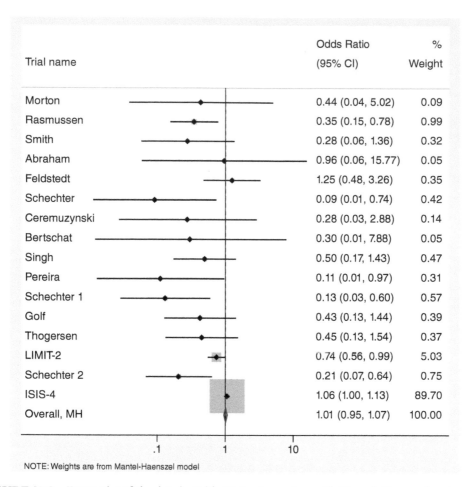

FIGURE 25.2 Forest plot of the data in Table 25.3 using **metan** with Mantel–Haenszel meta-analysis of odds ratios.

Let us run a meta-analysis of the 2×2 count data in Table 25.3. This time we request odds ratios as the effect measure, but otherwise the commands are very similar to those in our previous example. The forest plot appears in Figure 25.2.

```
generate alive1 = pop1-deaths1
generate alive0 = pop0-deaths0
metan deaths1 alive1 deaths0 alive0, or lcols(trialnam) nohet forestplot(xlabel(.1 1 10))

Studies included: 16
Participants included: 62607

Meta-analysis pooling of Odds Ratios
using the Mantel-Haenszel method

Continuity correction of 0.50 applied to studies with zero cells
for inclusion in summary table and forest plot (marked with *)
Mantel-Haenszel pooled effect is estimated from uncorrected counts
```

```
-----------------------------------------------------------------
                       |  Odds
Trial name             |  Ratio    [95% Conf. Interval]   % Weight
-----------------------+-----------------------------------------
Morton                 |  0.436    0.038    5.022         0.09
Rasmussen              |  0.348    0.154    0.783         0.99
Smith                  |  0.278    0.057    1.357         0.32
Abraham                |  0.957    0.058   15.773         0.05
Feldstedt              |  1.250    0.479    3.261         0.35
Schechter              |  0.090    0.011    0.736         0.42
Ceremuzynski           |  0.278    0.027    2.883         0.14
Bertschat *            |  0.304    0.012    7.880         0.05
Singh                  |  0.499    0.174    1.426         0.47
Pereira                |  0.110    0.012    0.967         0.31
Schechter 1            |  0.130    0.028    0.602         0.57
Golf                   |  0.427    0.127    1.436         0.39
Thogersen              |  0.452    0.133    1.543         0.37
LIMIT-2                |  0.741    0.556    0.988         5.03
Schechter 2            |  0.208    0.067    0.640         0.75
ISIS-4                 |  1.059    0.996    1.127        89.70
-----------------------+-----------------------------------------
Overall, MH            |  1.006    0.948    1.068       100.00
-----------------------------------------------------------------

Test of overall effect = 1:   z =    0.200   p = 0.841
```

The discrepancy between the results of the ISIS-4 trial and the earlier trials can be seen clearly in the forest plot. Note that because the ISIS-4 trial provides 89.7% of the total weight in the meta-analysis, the overall (summary) estimate of the odds ratio using the Mantel–Haenszel method is very similar to the estimate from the ISIS-4 trial alone. We will return to this point later, when we discuss influence analysis (Section 25.3.2).

25.2.4 Dealing with Zero Cells

If we look again at the output above, we see the message "Continuity correction of 0.50 applied to studies with zero cells (marked with *)" and that an asterisk was placed next to the Bertschat trial. For this trial, there were no deaths in the intervention group, so that if calculated using standard formulae the odds ratio would be zero and the standard error would be undefined.

When one arm of a study contains no events (or, alternatively, *all* events; that is, no *nonevents*), we have what is termed a "zero cell" in the 2×2 table. Zero cells can create problems in the computation of odds ratios or risk ratios, and of the standard error of any effect measure.

For an individual study, a common way to deal with this problem is to add what is termed a "continuity correction" of 0.5 to each cell of the 2×2 table for studies with zero cells, and then proceed with calculations in the usual way. We could then go on to perform an inverse-variance meta-analysis. However, there are alternative methods available such as Mantel–Haenszel (for odds ratios, risk ratios, or risk differences) or

Peto's method (for odds ratios only) for computing summary estimates and standard errors, even in the presence of zero cells, because they use the 2×2 cell counts in ways that avoid division by zero. With these methods, "continuity correction" is unnecessary and may even introduce bias [11]. (Note that if there are no events in either the intervention *or* control arms of the study – sometimes termed "double-zero" studies – then *any* measure of effect summarized as a ratio is undefined, and such studies would typically be discarded from the meta-analysis.)

The **metan** command deals with these issues automatically, by detecting studies with zero cells and, for inverse-variance meta-analysis, adding 0.5 where necessary before combining the results. For Mantel–Haenszel analysis, **metan** still adds 0.5 to "zero-cell" studies for the purpose of *presentation* (since otherwise those studies could not be listed in the table), but the summary estimate and standard error are computed from the original, uncorrected data, as the on-screen output makes clear. In either case, an asterisk is shown next to the name of studies with zero cells, such as the Bertschat trial in our magnesium example.

For commands that require summary statistics to be calculated (e.g. **metabias** and **metareg**), it may be necessary to correct manually for zero cells before calculating effect estimates and standard errors. Alternatively, as described in Section 25.2.2, summary statistics accounting for zero cells may be taken from the variables _ES and _seES left behind by **metan**, which will already have been corrected for zero cells.

25.2.5   Heterogeneity Variance and Random Effects

In this section, we will analyze the magnesium data from a different perspective. We will use summary statistics (`logor selogor`, accounting for zero cells as described in the previous section) instead of 2×2 counts (`deaths1 alive1 deaths0 alive0`). Furthermore, in this example we will compare results from two inverse-variance analyses: a fixed-effect and a random-effects analysis (see also Figure 25.3).

The next code follows on from the previous call to **metan**, first storing the meta-analytic log odds ratio and its standard error as variables `logor` and `selogor`, respectively.

```
rename _ES logor
rename _seES selogor
metan logor selogor, or random second(fixed) lcols(trialnam) nowt notable
  forestplot(xlabel(.1 1 10))

Studies included: 16
Participants included: Unknown

Meta-analysis pooling of Odds Ratios
using multiple analysis methods

Tests of overall effect = 1:
  DL              z =  -3.706  p = 0.000
  IV              z =   0.484  p = 0.629

Heterogeneity measures, calculated from the data
with Conf. Intervals based on Gamma (random-effects) distribution for Q
```

```
------------------------------------------------------------
Measure             |   Value     df       p-value
--------------------+---------------------------------------
Cochran's Q         |   47.06     15         0.000
                    |           -[95% Conf.  Interval]-
H                   |   1.771     1.000       3.026
I² (%)              |   68.1%     0.0%        89.1%
------------------------------------------------------------
H = relative excess in total variance over "typical" within-study variance
I² = between-study variance (tau²) as a percentage of total variance

Heterogeneity variance estimates
----------------------------------------
Method              |    tau²
--------------------+-------------------
DL                  |   0.2239
----------------------------------------
```

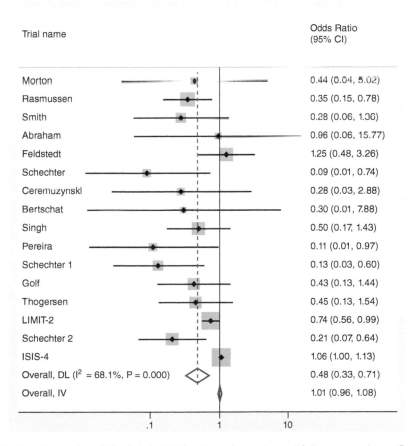

Trial name		Odds Ratio (95% CI)
Morton		0.44 (0.04, 5.02)
Rasmussen		0.35 (0.15, 0.78)
Smith		0.28 (0.06, 1.30)
Abraham		0.96 (0.06, 15.77)
Feldstedt		1.25 (0.48, 3.26)
Schechter		0.09 (0.01, 0.74)
Ceremuzynski		0.28 (0.03, 2.88)
Bertschat		0.30 (0.01, 7.88)
Singh		0.50 (0.17, 1.43)
Pereira		0.11 (0.01, 0.97)
Schechter 1		0.13 (0.03, 0.60)
Golf		0.43 (0.13, 1.44)
Thogersen		0.45 (0.13, 1.54)
LIMIT-2		0.74 (0.56, 0.99)
Schechter 2		0.21 (0.07, 0.64)
ISIS-4		1.06 (1.00, 1.13)
Overall, DL (I^2 = 68.1%, P = 0.000)		0.48 (0.33, 0.71)
Overall, IV		1.01 (0.96, 1.08)

FIGURE 25.3 Forest plot of the data in Table 25.3 using **metan** with inverse-variance fixed-effect meta-analysis and DerSimonian–Laird random-effects meta-analysis of odds ratios.

Note the dramatic difference between the fixed-effect and random-effects summary estimates, and the highly statistically significant test of heterogeneity using Cochran's Q statistic. Under a random-effects model, true effects across studies are assumed to follow a normal distribution, and the estimated mean of this distribution is taken as the summary estimate. The variance of the distribution – commonly referred to as "τ^2" – measures the *spread* of the study effects around this mean. The most popular random-effects estimation method, which **metan** will fit by default if a "random-effects model" is requested, is that of DerSimonian and Laird [12]. In our current example, using this method gives a value for τ^2 of 0.2239. One consequence of using a random-effects model is that study estimates are weighted much more equally: compare the weights in Figure 25.3 with the Mantel–Haenszel fixed-effect weights in Figure 25.2. Smaller studies are given more influence, and larger studies (such as ISIS-4) less, which largely explains the dramatic difference in summary effect size and statistical significance. Note that if τ^2 were to be estimated as zero, then the summary effect estimate would be the same as from the (inverse-variance) fixed-effect model. The **metan** command can fit a variety of other estimation methods suggested in the literature, some of which were developed for particular scenarios or rely upon particular assumptions. For example, and unlike at the time of its publication, the vast majority of methods included in a recent comprehensive review of meta-analysis models [13] are now able to be fitted by **metan**.

As discussed, τ^2 is an important component of the random-effects model, and may be used to compare meta-analysis results derived from similar types of data. However, as it is measured on the same scale as the effect estimates, it is unsuitable as a "universal" heterogeneity statistic (the value of τ^2 for meta-analysis based on mean differences cannot be compared to a value based on a meta-analysis of [log] odds ratios). In an attempt to resolve this issue, Higgins and Thompson suggested various other heterogeneity statistics, of which the most well-known is I^2, which expresses τ^2 as a percentage of total variance [2]. By default, the **metan** command reports these statistics, together with confidence intervals. In our current example, I^2 is estimated to be 68%, with 95% confidence limits of 0% to 89%, suggesting a moderate to large degree of heterogeneity (but note the wide confidence limits, reflecting the difficulties in accurately measuring such quantities).

25.2.6   The **meta** Command Suite in Stata 16

We will now briefly explain how to re-create the analyses we have so far performed using the built-in **meta** command suite available in Stata 16. The term "command suite" signifies that rather than carry out a full analysis with a single command (as with e.g. **metan**), we use several subcommands in a step-by-step fashion to set up, analyze, and plot our meta-analysis data. Recall that with **metan** we may analyze either counts from a 2×2 table, or generic effect estimates and standard errors (or, alternatively, the mean and standard deviation of a continuous outcome for each treatment group). With **meta**, we must specify the data structure *prior* to analysis, using either **meta esize** (for 2×2 counts or group means) or **meta set** (for generic effect estimates). At this time we also specify the outcome measure (e.g. odds ratio or risk ratio) and study name labels, and any other specifications such as adjustment for zero cells (see previous section). Then, having set up our data, we may use **meta summarize** to produce a summary analysis, and **meta forestplot** to produce a forest plot. Returning to our first example (streptokinase):

```
use "strepto.dta", clear
generate alive1 = pop1 - deaths1
generate alive0 = pop0 - deaths0
meta esize deaths1 alive1 deaths0 alive0, esize(lnrr) studylab(trialnam)
  common(mh)
```

Meta-analysis setting information

```
  Study information
      No. of studies:  22
         Study label:  trialnam
          Study size:  _meta_studysize
        Summary data:  deaths1 alive1 deaths0 alive0

         Effect size
                Type:  lnratio
               Label:  Log Risk-Ratio
            Variable:  _meta_es
   Zero-cells adj.:    None; no zero cells

           Precision
          Std. Err.:   _meta_se
                 CI:   [_meta_cil, _meta_ciu]
            CI level:  95%

    Model and method
               Model:  Common-effect
              Method:  Mantel-Haenszel
```

. meta summarize, eform

```
  Effect-size label:  Log Risk-Ratio
         Effect size:  _meta_es
           Std. Err.:  _meta_se
         Study label:  trialnam
```

Meta-analysis summary   Number of studies =   22
Common-effect model
Method: Mantel-Haenszel

Study	Risk Ratio	[95% Conf. Interval]		% Weight
Fletcher	0.229	0.030	1.750	0.18
Dewar	0.571	0.196	1.665	0.30
1st European	1.349	0.743	2.451	0.64
Heikinheimo	1.223	0.669	2.237	0.75
Italian	1.011	0.551	1.853	0.78
2nd European	0.703	0.534	0.925	4.10
2nd Frankfurt	0.457	0.252	0.828	1.22
1st Australian	0.779	0.478	1.268	1.39
NHLBI SMIT	2.377	0.649	8.709	0.13
Valere	1.048	0.481	2.282	0.41
Frank	0.964	0.332	2.801	0.26
UK Collab	0.896	0.626	1.281	2.25

```
           Klein |        2.571       0.339      19.481        0.05
        Austrian |        0.608       0.417       0.886        2.68
        Lasierra |        0.282       0.034       2.340        0.14
        N German |        1.161       0.840       1.604        2.24
        Witchitz |        0.813       0.263       2.506        0.24
  2nd Australian |        0.850       0.537       1.345        1.29
    3rd European |        0.510       0.333       0.780        2.11
            ISAM |        0.880       0.619       1.250        2.65
         GISSI-1 |        0.827       0.749       0.914       32.34
          ISIS-2 |        0.769       0.704       0.839       43.86
-----------------+-----------------------------------------------------
     exp(theta) |        0.799       0.755       0.845
-------------------------------------------------------------------------
Test of theta = 0: z = -7.75                      Prob > |z| = 0.0000
```

```
meta forestplot, eform nullrefline
```

(See Figure 25.4 for the forest plot.)

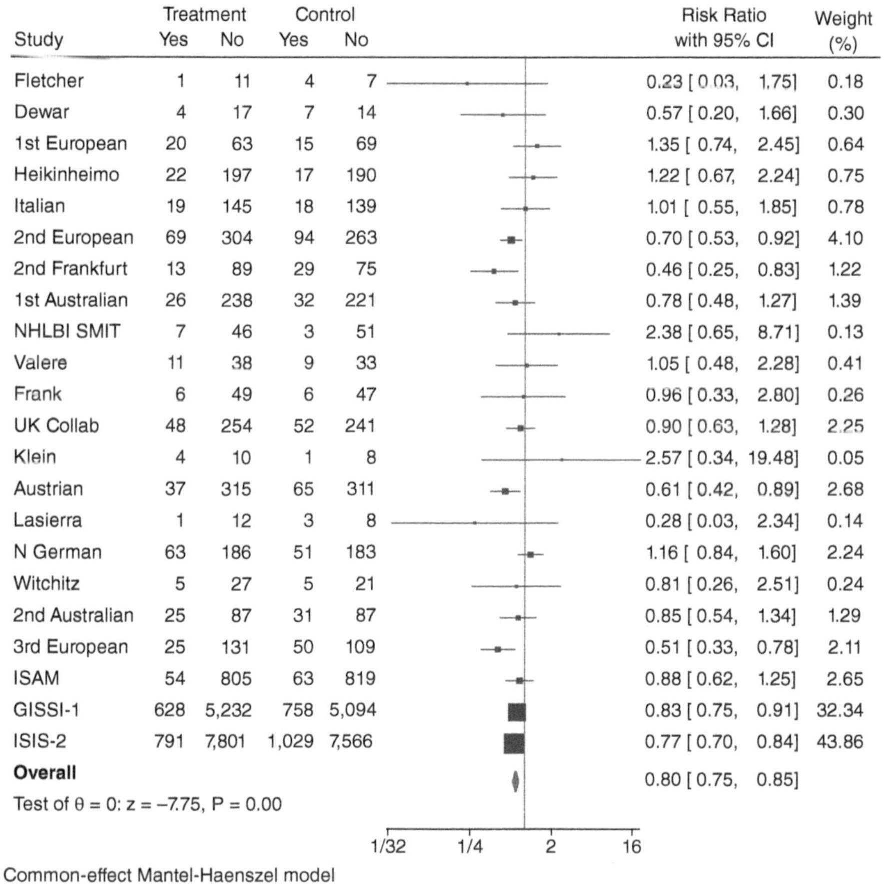

Study	Treatment Yes	No	Control Yes	No		Risk Ratio with 95% CI	Weight (%)
Fletcher	1	11	4	7		0.23 [0.03, 1.75]	0.18
Dewar	4	17	7	14		0.57 [0.20, 1.66]	0.30
1st European	20	63	15	69		1.35 [0.74, 2.45]	0.64
Heikinheimo	22	197	17	190		1.22 [0.67, 2.24]	0.75
Italian	19	145	18	139		1.01 [0.55, 1.85]	0.78
2nd European	69	304	94	263		0.70 [0.53, 0.92]	4.10
2nd Frankfurt	13	89	29	75		0.46 [0.25, 0.83]	1.22
1st Australian	26	238	32	221		0.78 [0.48, 1.27]	1.39
NHLBI SMIT	7	46	3	51		2.38 [0.65, 8.71]	0.13
Valere	11	38	9	33		1.05 [0.48, 2.28]	0.41
Frank	6	49	6	47		0.96 [0.33, 2.80]	0.26
UK Collab	48	254	52	241		0.90 [0.63, 1.28]	2.25
Klein	4	10	1	8		2.57 [0.34, 19.48]	0.05
Austrian	37	315	65	311		0.61 [0.42, 0.89]	2.68
Lasierra	1	12	3	8		0.28 [0.03, 2.34]	0.14
N German	63	186	51	183		1.16 [0.84, 1.60]	2.24
Witchitz	5	27	5	21		0.81 [0.26, 2.51]	0.24
2nd Australian	25	87	31	87		0.85 [0.54, 1.34]	1.29
3rd European	25	131	50	109		0.51 [0.33, 0.78]	2.11
ISAM	54	805	63	819		0.88 [0.62, 1.25]	2.65
GISSI-1	628	5,232	758	5,094		0.83 [0.75, 0.91]	32.34
ISIS-2	791	7,801	1,029	7,566		0.77 [0.70, 0.84]	43.86
Overall						0.80 [0.75, 0.85]	

Test of θ = 0: z = −7.75, P = 0.00

1/32   1/4   2   16

Common-effect Mantel-Haenszel model

FIGURE 25.4   Forest plot of the data in Table 25.2 using **meta** with Mantel–Haenszel meta-analysis of risk ratios.

Note that the two commands **meta** and **metan** have different default settings, and therefore different options need to be specified to achieve the same result. For example, the forest plot in Figure 25.4 includes columns of numbers of events and patients by treatment group by default, but requires the null-effect line to be requested explicitly, whereas **metan** is the opposite way around. More information is available in the help files.

25.3   CUMULATIVE AND INFLUENCE META-ANALYSIS

25.3.1   Cumulative Meta-Analysis

The **metan** command can also perform and illustrate meta-analyses in non-standard ways in order to draw out particular features of the data. One approach is cumulative meta-analysis [14, 15], where the summary effect is recalculated and displayed as each study in turn is added to the data set. The syntax is almost exactly the same as before: we just need to add the **cumulative** option, and to specify the order in which the studies should be accumulated using **sortby()**. We now return to the streptokinase trials (strepto.dta) and conduct a cumulative meta-analysis by year of publication (see also Figure 25.5). Note that test statistics and heterogeneity information are given for the final combined analysis using all the studies, which appears alongside the final study name, in this case ISIS-2 (compare with, for example, the output in Section 25.2.6).

```
generate alive1 = pop1 - deaths1
generate alive0 = pop0 - deaths0
metan deaths1 alive1 deaths0 alive0, or cumulative lcols(trialnam year)
  sortby(year) forestplot(xlabel(.1 1 10))

Studies included: 22
Participants included: 35834

Cumulative meta-analysis of Odds Ratios
using the Mantel-Haenszel method

Studies added cumulatively in order of year
```

Trial name		Odds Ratio	[95% Conf. Interval]		% Weight
Fletcher		0.159	0.015	1.732	0.18
Dewar		0.345	0.104	1.141	0.46
1st European		0.952	0.514	1.760	1.00
Heikinheimo		1.079	0.688	1.693	1.75
Italian		1.058	0.727	1.542	2.53
2nd European		0.806	0.624	1.040	6.29
2nd Frankfurt		0.737	0.580	0.936	7.49
1st Australian		0.740	0.594	0.921	8.91

```
NHLBI SMIT       |    0.765      0.616      0.950        9.03
Valere           |    0.776      0.629      0.959        9.39
Frank            |    0.781      0.635      0.962        9.65
UK Collab        |    0.798      0.662      0.963       11.78
Klein            |    0.807      0.670      0.972       11.82
Austrian         |    0.761      0.642      0.903       14.52
Lasierra         |    0.756      0.638      0.896       14.67
N German         |    0.808      0.691      0.946       16.55
Witchitz         |    0.808      0.691      0.945       16.77
2nd Australian   |    0.808      0.694      0.940       17.90
3rd European     |    0.769      0.664      0.889       19.89
ISAM             |    0.781      0.682      0.895       22.69
GISSI-1          |    0.796      0.730      0.868       55.18
ISIS-2           |    0.774      0.725      0.825      100.00
-----------------------------------------------------------------

Test of overall cumulative effect = 1:   z =  -7.757  p = 0.000

Heterogeneity measures, calculated from the data
with Conf. Intervals based on non-central chi² (common-effect) distribution
for Q
------------------------------------------------------------
Measure               |   Value      df     p-value
----------------------+-------------------------------------
Mantel-Haenszel Q     |   31.50      21      0.066
                      |          -[95% Conf. Interval]-
H                     |   1.225     1.000     1.569
I² (%)                |   33.3%      0.0%     59.4%
------------------------------------------------------------
H = relative excess in Mantel-Haenszel Q over its degrees-of-freedom
I² = between-study variance (tau²) as a percentage of total variance (based
on Mantel-Haenszel Q)
```

By the late 1970s, there was clear evidence that streptokinase prevented death following myocardial infarction. However, it was not used routinely until the late 1980s, when the results of the large GISSI-1 and ISIS-2 trials became known (see Chapter 1). The cumulative meta-analysis plot makes it clear that although these trials reduced the confidence interval width for the summary estimate, they did not change the estimated effect.

25.3.2   Examining the Influence of Individual Studies

The influence of individual studies on the summary effect estimate may also be examined using the **metan** command. With the **influence** option, **metan** will omit one study at a time from the sample and re-compute the meta-analysis estimates. The syntax is otherwise the same as in previous sections. We return to the magnesium data for this analysis.

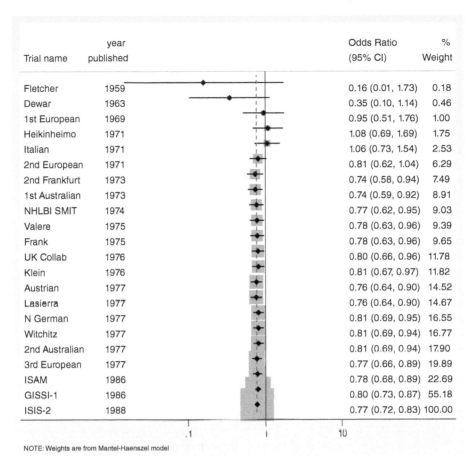

Trial name	year published	Odds Ratio (95% CI)	% Weight
Fletcher	1959	0.16 (0.01, 1.73)	0.18
Dewar	1963	0.35 (0.10, 1.14)	0.46
1st European	1969	0.95 (0.51, 1.76)	1.00
Heikinheimo	1971	1.08 (0.69, 1.69)	1.75
Italian	1971	1.06 (0.73, 1.54)	2.53
2nd European	1971	0.81 (0.62, 1.04)	6.29
2nd Frankfurt	1973	0.74 (0.58, 0.94)	7.49
1st Australian	1973	0.74 (0.59, 0.92)	8.91
NHLBI SMIT	1974	0.77 (0.62, 0.95)	9.03
Valere	1975	0.78 (0.63, 0.96)	9.39
Frank	1975	0.78 (0.63, 0.96)	9.65
UK Collab	1976	0.80 (0.66, 0.96)	11.78
Klein	1976	0.81 (0.67, 0.97)	11.82
Austrian	1977	0.76 (0.64, 0.90)	14.52
Lasierra	1977	0.76 (0.64, 0.90)	14.67
N German	1977	0.81 (0.69, 0.95)	16.55
Witchitz	1977	0.81 (0.69, 0.94)	16.77
2nd Australian	1977	0.81 (0.69, 0.94)	17.90
3rd European	1977	0.77 (0.66, 0.89)	19.89
ISAM	1986	0.78 (0.68, 0.89)	22.69
GISSI-1	1986	0.80 (0.73, 0.87)	55.18
ISIS-2	1988	0.77 (0.72, 0.83)	100.00

NOTE: Weights are from Mantel-Haenszel model

FIGURE 25.5 Forest plot of the data in Table 25.3 using **metan** with cumulative Mantel–Haenszel meta-analysis of odds ratios.

```
metan deaths1 alive1 deaths0 alive0, or influence lcols(trialnam year)
  nohet nograph

Studies included: 16
Participants included: 62607

Influence meta-analysis of Odds Ratios
using the Mantel-Haenszel method

Continuity correction of 0.50 applied to studies with zero cells
  for inclusion in summary table (marked with *)
```

Mantel-Haenszel pooled effect is estimated from uncorrected counts

```
-----------------------------------------------------------------
                    |  Odds
Trial name omitted  |  Ratio    [95% Conf. Interval]   % Weight
--------------------+--------------------------------------------
Morton              |  1.007    0.948     1.068         99.91
Rasmussen           |  1.013    0.954     1.075         99.01
Smith               |  1.008    0.950     1.070         99.68
Abraham             |  1.006    0.948     1.068         99.95
Feldstedt           |  1.005    0.947     1.067         99.65
Schechter           |  1.010    0.952     1.072         99.58
Ceremuzynski        |  1.007    0.949     1.069         99.86
Bertschat *         |  1.007    0.948     1.068         99.95
Singh               |  1.009    0.950     1.070         99.53
Pereira             |  1.009    0.951     1.071         99.69
Schechter 1         |  1.011    0.953     1.073         99.43
Golf                |  1.008    0.950     1.070         99.61
Thogersen           |  1.008    0.950     1.070         99.63
LIMIT-2             |  1.020    0.960     1.084         94.97
Schechter 2         |  1.012    0.954     1.074         99.25
ISIS-4              |  0.543    0.436     0.676         10.30
--------------------+--------------------------------------------
Overall, MH         |  1.006    0.948     1.068        100.00
-----------------------------------------------------------------
```

Test of overall effect = 1: z =   0.200 p = 0.841

The meta-analysis is dominated by the ISIS-4 study, so omission of other studies makes little or no difference. If ISIS-4 is omitted, then there appears to be a clear effect of magnesium in preventing death after myocardial infarction.

25.4   FUNNEL PLOTS AND TESTS FOR FUNNEL PLOT ASYMMETRY

A funnel plot is a plot of the standardized effect against standard error. It is commonly used to assess evidence of potential publication bias or other small-study biases, which may manifest as asymmetry in a funnel plot (see Chapter 5). The older **metafunnel** and the more recent **confunnel** commands both produce funnel plots, with slightly different option sets. For the magnesium data there is clear evidence of funnel plot asymmetry if the ISIS-4 trial is included. Therefore, it may be of greater interest to assess whether there was evidence of funnel plot asymmetry *before* the results of the ISIS-4 trial were known. Thus, in the following analysis we omit the ISIS-4 trial. The resulting funnel plot is shown in Figure 25.6.

```
use "magnes.dta", clear
generate alive1 = pop1 - deaths1
generate alive0 = pop0 - deaths0
generate logor   = log((deaths1/alive1) / (deaths0/alive0))
generate selogor = sqrt((1/deaths1)+(1/alive1)+(1/deaths0)+(1/alive0))
confunnel logor selogor if trialnam!="ISIS-4"
```

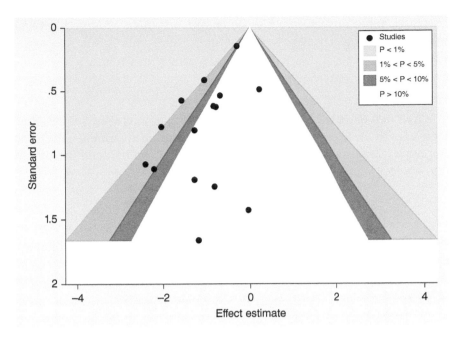

FIGURE 25.6   Funnel plot of the data in Table 25.3 using risk ratios.

The sloping lines indicate the expected 95% confidence intervals for a given standard error, assuming no heterogeneity between studies. Another command, **metabias**, provides a formal test for funnel plot asymmetry using one of several available methods, due to Begg et al. [16], Egger et al. [10], Harbord et al. [17], or Peters et al. [18]. For 2×2 count data, the Harbord test is recommended, with the Peters test a reasonable alternative. For other outcome types, the Egger test may be used. The Begg test is an older test that is no longer recommended. If we apply the Harbord test, we find significant funnel plot asymmetry even when excluding ISIS-4.

```
metabias deaths1 alive1 deaths0 alive0 if trialnam!="ISIS-4", harbord

Note: data input format tcases tnoncases ccases cnoncases assumed
Note: Odds ratios assumed as effect estimate of interest

Harbord's modified test for small-study effects:
Regress Z/sqrt(V) on sqrt(V), where Z is the efficient score and V is the
score variance
```

| Number of studies = 15 | | | | | Root MSE | = | 1.033 |

Z/sqrt(V)	Coef.	Std. Err.	t	P>|t|	[95% Conf. Interval]	
sqrt(V)	-.1975284	.1837316	-1.08	0.302	-.5944565	.1993997
bias	-1.207083	.4372929	-2.76	0.016	-2.151796	-.2623686

```
Test of H0: no small-study effects            P = 0.016
```

In Stata 16 there are also the built-in commands `meta funnelplot` and `meta bias` (note the spacing between the words).

25.5   META-REGRESSION

If there is heterogeneity in the treatment effect estimates between studies, then meta-regression can be used to analyze associations between treatment effect and study characteristics (see also Chapter 10). Meta-regression can be done in Stata by using the `metareg` command [19].

25.5.1   Example 3: Trials of BCG Vaccine Against Tuberculosis

Table 25.4 provides data from a meta-analysis by Colditz et al. [20], which examined the efficacy of the BCG vaccine against tuberculosis.

TABLE 25.4   Data from 11 studies of BCG vaccine to prevent tuberculosis (TB).

Trial name	Authors	Start year	Latitude[a]	Intervention group		Control group	
				TB cases	Total	TB cases	Total
Canada	Ferguson and Simes	1933	55	6	306	29	303
Northern USA	Aronson	1935	52	4	123	11	139
Chicago	Rosenthal et al.	1937	42	17	1716	65	1665
Georgia (School)	Comstock and Webster	1947	33	5	2498	3	2341
Puerto Rico	Comstock et al.	1949	18	186	50 634	141	27 338
UK	Hart and Sutherland	1950	53	62	13 598	248	12 867
Madanapalle	Frimont-Moller et al.	1950	13	33	5069	47	5808
Georgia (Community)	Comstock et al.	1950	33	27	16 913	29	17 854
Haiti	Vandeviere et al.	1965	18	8	2545	10	629
South Africa	Coetzee and Berjak	1965	27	29	7499	45	7277
Madras	TB Prevention Trial	1968	13	505	88 391	499	88 391

[a] = absolute value.
Source: Adapted from Colditz GA et al. 1994 [20].

The data were saved in Stata dataset bcgtrial.dta:

describe

```
Contains data from bcgtrial.dta
   obs:              11                          BCG and tuberculosis
  vars:              10
```

variable name	storage type	display format	value label	variable label
trial	int	%8.0g		Trial number
authors	str20	%20s		Authors
startyr	int	%8.0g		Year trial started
latitude	int	%8.0g		Latitude
trialnam	str14	%14s		Trial name
pop1	long	%12.0g		BCG vaccinated population
pop0	long	%12.0g		Unvaccinated population
cases1	int	%8.0g		BCG vaccinated cases
cases0	int	%8.0g		Unvaccinated cases
alloc	float	%33.0g	alloc	Allocation method

```
                                                        Sorted by: trial
```

Scientists had been aware of discordance between the results of these trials since the 1950s. The clear heterogeneity in the protective effect of BCG between trials can be seen in the forest plot in Figure 25.7 (we analyze this data set using risk ratios).

```
generate h1 = pop1   cases1
generate h0 = pop0 - cases0
```

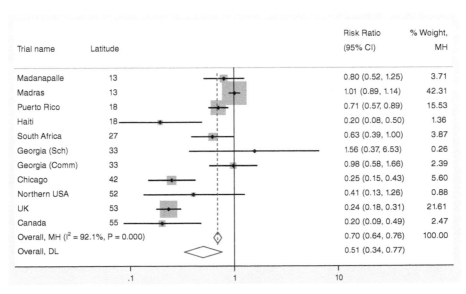

FIGURE 25.7 Forest plot of the data in Table 25.4 using **metan** with Mantel–Haenszel meta-analysis and random-effects meta-analysis of risk ratios.

```
metan cases1 h1 cases0 h0, rr label(namevar=trialnam) second(random)
  forestplot(xlabel(.1 1 10)) sortby(latitude startyr)
```

To use the **metareg** command, we need to derive the treatment effect estimate (in this case log risk ratio) and its standard error, for each study. As described previously, we can either calculate these using standard formulae, or make use of the variables left behind by **metan**:

```
generate logrr = log((cases1/pop1)/(cases0/pop0))
generate selogrr = sqrt(1/cases1 - 1/pop1 + 1/cases0 - 1/pop0)
```

or, following the previous call to **metan**:

```
rename _ES logrr
rename _seES selogrr
```

In their meta-analysis, Colditz et al. noted the pronounced heterogeneity between studies, and concluded that a random-effects meta-analysis was appropriate [20]. The authors then examined possible explanations for the clear differences in the effect of BCG between studies. The earlier studies may have produced different results than later ones. The latitude at which the studies were conducted may also be associated with the effect of BCG. As discussed by Fine [21], the possibility that BCG might provide greater protection at higher latitudes was first recognized by Palmer and Long [22], who suggested that this trend might result from exposure to certain environmental mycobacteria, more common in warmer regions, which impart protection against tuberculosis. In Figure 25.7, we have pre-emptively sorted the trials by latitude so that this trend can be clearly seen.

To use **metareg**, we provide a list of variables, the first of which is the treatment effect (here, the log risk ratio) and the rest of which are (one or more) study characteristics (additional variables in the dataset) hypothesized to be associated with the treatment effect. In addition, the standard error of the treatment effect must be provided, in the **wsse()** option. It is also possible to specify the method for estimating the between-study variance; here we use the default, which is using the restricted maximum likelihood (REML) method. To investigate the association with latitude we use the following code:

```
metareg logrr latitude, wsse(selogrr)
```

```
Meta-regression                                    Number of obs   =      11
REML estimate of between-study variance            tau2            =      .1
% residual variation due to heterogeneity          I-squared_res   =  61.80%
Proportion of between-study variance explained     Adj R-squared   =  72.99%
With Knapp-Hartung modification
------------------------------------------------------------------------------
     logrr |      Coef.   Std. Err.      t    P>|t|     [95% Conf. Interval]
-----------+------------------------------------------------------------------
  latitude | -.0288849   .0095887    -3.01   0.015    -.0505759   -.0071938
     _cons |  .2247162   .3215322     0.70   0.502    -.5026402    .9520726
------------------------------------------------------------------------------
```

The regression coefficients are the intercept and the estimated increase in the log risk ratio per unit increase in latitude. The log risk ratio is estimated to decrease by 0.0289 per unit increase in the latitude at which the study was conducted, with a log risk ratio of 0.2247 at zero latitude. The estimated between-study variance has been reduced from 0.37 (obtained from the **metareg** command without latitude) to 0.10. Similarly, the remaining I^2 is 61.8%, reduced from 92.0%. The estimated treatment effect given particular values of the covariates may be derived from the regression equation. For example, for a trial at latitude 50°, the estimated log risk ratio would be $0.2247 - 0.0289 \times 50 = -1.2203$, which corresponds to a risk ratio of exp.$(-1.2203) = 0.295$.

We might then proceed to investigate whether the log risk ratio differs according to any other recorded variables in the dataset, such as the year the trial started (`startyr`) or the type of random allocation (`alloc`).

25.6 MULTIVARIATE AND NETWORK META-ANALYSIS

25.6.1 Multivariate Meta-Analysis

Standard meta-analysis combines effect estimates on the assumption that they are independent, which will be the case when there is exactly one effect estimate from each study. Multivariate meta-analysis is an extension that can combine estimates of several related parameters from each study. For example, we may have estimates of treatment effects on two different outcomes in a series of randomized trials, or we may have estimates of the difference in outcome between "high," "medium," and "low" doses of treatment within each study. In both of these examples, estimates from the same study will be correlated, and therefore an analysis that encompasses the complete set of outcomes and their correlations will allow improved inference.

The user-written **mvmeta** command fits multivariate meta-analysis models. Recall that one of the input types for the **metan** command is an effect estimate and its standard error for each study. For **mvmeta**, the input can be seen as a generalization of this. First, we must rename all our desired effect sizes into the form `b1, b2, b3...` Next, we convert the associated standard errors into *variances*, and name them `V11, V22, V33, ...` Finally, if covariances are known, they should be held in variables named `V12, V13, V23, ...` Then a basic analysis may be run as follows:

```
mvmeta b V
```

Further information is given in White [23] and White [24].

25.6.2 Network Meta-Analysis

Network meta-analysis, also called "multiple treatments meta-analysis" or "mixed-treatment comparisons," is a method of combining evidence from studies that do not all compare the same two (treatment) groups (see Chapter 13). For example, some studies might compare treatment B with A, while others might compare C with A, or C with B. Any number of treatments may be included, as can studies comparing more than two treatments (e.g. "multi-arm trials"). Most often, a network meta-analysis model makes an assumption of *consistency*; that is, that the summary effect of treatment C versus A is equal to the effect of C versus B plus that of B versus A. Such models may be fitted in Stata as extensions to multivariate meta-regression [25] (Section 25.6.1). However, getting the data into the correct format can be tricky. There are two user-written commands, `network setup` and `network import`, for achieving this; following which a model may be fitted using the command `network meta consistency`. Further information is given in White [25].

REFERENCES

1. Palmer, T.T. and Sterne, J.A.C. (2016). *Meta-Analysis in Stata: An Updated Collection from the Stata Journal.* College Station, TX: Stata Press.
2. Higgins, J.P.T. and Thompson, S.G. (2002). Quantifying heterogeneity in a meta-analysis. *Stat. Med.* 21: 1539–1558.
3. Yusuf, S., Collins, R., Peto, R. et al. (1985). Intravenous and intracoronary fibrinolytic therapy in acute myocardial infarction: overview of results on mortality, reinfarction and side-effects from 33 randomized controlled trials. *Eur. Heart J.* 6: 556–585.
4. Gruppo Italiano per lo Studio della Streptochinasi nell'Infarto Miocardico (GISSI) (1986). Effectiveness of intravenous thrombolytic treatment in acute myocardial infarction. *Lancet* 1: 397–402.
5. ISIS-2 (Second International Study of Infarct Survival) Collaborative Group (1988). Randomised trial of intravenous streptokinase, oral aspirin, both, or neither among 17 187 cases of suspected acute myocardial infarction: ISIS-2. *Lancet* 2: 349–360.
6. Harris, R.J., Bradburn, M.J., Deeks, J.J. et al. (2008). Metan: fixed- and random-effects meta-analysis. *Stata J.* 8.
7. Teo, K.K., Yusuf, S., Collins, R. et al. (1991). Effects of intravenous magnesium in suspected acute myocardial infarction: overview of randomised trials. *BMJ.* 303: 1499–1503.
8. ISIS-4 (Fourth International Study of Infarct Survival) Collaborative Group (1995). ISIS-4: a randomised factorial trial assessing early oral captopril, oral mononitrate, and intravenous magnesium sulphate in 58 050 patients with suspected acute myocardial infarction. *Lancet* 345: 669–685.
9. Egger, M. and Davey, S.G. (1995). Misleading meta-analysis [editorial]. *BMJ.* 310: 752–754.
10. Egger, M., Davey Smith, G., Schneider, M., and Minder, C. (1997). Bias in meta-analysis detected by a simple, graphical test. *BMJ.* 315: 629–634.
11. Bradburn, M.J., Deeks, J.J., Berlin, J.A., and Localio, A.R. (2006). Much ado about nothing: a comparison of the performance of meta-analytical methods with rare events. *Stat. Med.* 26: 53–77.
12. DerSimonian, R. and Laird, N. (1986). Meta-analysis in clinical trials. *Control. Clin. Trials* 7: 177–188.
13. Veroniki, A.A., Jackson, D., Bender, R. et al. (2019). Methods to calculate uncertainty in the estimated overall effect size from a random-effects meta-analysis. *Res. Synth. Methods* 10: 23–43.

14. Lau, J., Antman, E.M., Jimenez-Silva, J. et al. (1992). Cumulative meta-analysis of therapeutic trials for myocardial infarction. *N. Engl. J. Med.* 327: 248–254.

15. Antman, E.M., Lau, J., Kupelnick, B. et al. (1992). A comparison of results of meta-analyses of randomized control trials and recommendations of clinical experts: treatments for myocardial infarction. *J. Am. Med. Assoc.* 268: 240–248.

16. Begg, C.B. and Mazumdar, M. (1994). Operating characteristics of a rank correlation test for publication bias. *Biometrics* 50: 1088–1101.

17. Harbord, R.M., Egger, M., and Sterne, J.A. (2006). A modified test for small-study effects in meta-analyses of controlled trials with binary endpoints. *Stat. Med.* 25: 3443–3457.

18. Peters, J.L., Sutton, A.J., Jones, D.R. et al. (2006). Comparison of two methods to detect publication bias in meta-analysis. *J. Am. Med. Assoc.* 295: 676–680.

19. Harbord, R.M. and Higgins, J.P.T. (2008). Meta-regression in Stata. *Stata J.* 8: 493–519.

20. Colditz, G.A., Brewer, T.F., Berkey, C.S. et al. (1994). Efficacy of BCG vaccine in the prevention of tuberculosis: meta- analysis of the published literature. *J. Am. Med. Assoc.* 271: 698–702.

21. Fine, P.E. (1995). Variation in protection by BCG: implications of and for heterologous immunity. *Lancet* 346: 1339–1345.

22. Palmer, C.E. and Long, M.W. (1966). Effects of infection with atypical mycobacteria on BCG vaccination and tuberculosis. *Am. Rev. Respir. Dis.* 94: 553–568.

23. White, I.R. (2009). Multivariate random-effects meta-analysis. *Stata J.* 9: 40–56.

24. White, I.R. (2011). Multivariate random-effects meta-regression. *Stata J.* 11: 255–270.

25. White, I.R. (2015). Network meta-analysis. *Stata J.* 15: 951–985.

CHAPTER 26

Meta-Analysis in R

Guido Schwarzer

This chapter describes how to use the general statistical package R to conduct basic meta-analysis tasks. We start with a short introduction to R and show how to install R packages. R functions for meta-analysis with binary outcomes are introduced and applied to two classic meta-analysis examples. We describe meta-regression with R using another classic meta-analysis example, and illustrate methods to evaluate small-study effects. We conclude with an overview of R packages and functions for more advanced statistical methods like network meta-analysis. The interested reader can find a more comprehensive introduction in a Use-R! book on meta-analysis with R [1].

We use the following syntax conventions: R packages are printed in **bold**, R functions are printed in `monospaced`, R commands are printed in **`bold monospaced`**, and the output from R commands is also printed in `monospaced`.

26.1 GETTING STARTED

R [2] is a general-purpose statistical package that is based on the statistical programming language S developed in the 1970s. R has been available since 1993, and is actively developed, maintained, and supported by the R Foundation for Statistical Computing (https://www.r-project.org). Distinguishing features of R compared with other general statistical packages are (i) release under the GNU General Public License, (ii) free of charge, and (iii) more than 15 000 add-on packages provided and maintained by community members/scientists that are available on the Comprehensive R Archive Network (CRAN) (https://cloud.r-project.org/web/packages). Additional R packages are available on other repositories like Bioconductor (http://bioconductor.org), which

Systematic Reviews in Health Research: Meta-Analysis in Context, Third Edition. Edited by Matthias Egger, Julian P.T. Higgins, and George Davey Smith.
© 2022 John Wiley & Sons Ltd. Published 2022 by John Wiley & Sons Ltd.
Companion website: www.systematic-reviews3.org

provides software for bioinformatics, and GitHub (https://github.com), a website offering access to the distributed revision control system git.

Further resources are *The R Journal*, an open access journal of the R project with peer review, and several mailing lists, including R-help for discussions about general problems and solutions, and R-package-devel to support the package development process. R is inherently command-line driven, which is an initial hurdle for many users. RStudio (www.rstudio.com) is an advanced integrated development environment (IDE) for R that is popular with beginners. RStudio provides menu-driven tools for plotting, a history of previously run R commands, data management, and the installation and update of R packages.

An overview of R packages for meta-analysis available on CRAN is provided by a Task View (https://cloud.r-project.org/web/views/MetaAnalysis.html). In this chapter we will focus on two general R packages for meta-analysis: **meta** [3] and **metafor** [4].

26.2   INSTALLING R PACKAGES FOR META-ANALYSIS

During initial setup of R only a limited set of R packages is installed. This is no drawback, as the installation of R packages available on CRAN is easily done by using the `install.packages` function. The following R command installs the **meta** and **metafor** packages that will be used in this chapter. In RStudio it is possible to use the following menu items for this task: *Tools – Install Packages...*

```
install.packages(c("meta", "metafor"),
                 repos = "https://cloud.r-project.org/")

Installing packages into '/Users/sc/R/library/R-4.0.4'
(as 'lib' is unspecified)
trying URL 'https://cran.rstudio.com/bin/macosx/contrib/4.0/meta_4.18-0.tgz'
Content type 'application/x-gzip' length 1570096 bytes (1.5 MB)
==================================================
downloaded 1.5 MB

trying URL 'https://cloud.r-project.org/bin/macosx/contrib/4.0/metafor_2.4-0.tgz'
Content type 'application/x-gzip' length 2988307 bytes (2.8 MB)
==================================================
downloaded 2.8 MB
... (output truncated)
```

This first R command already describes several aspects of R. First, we have to use brackets "( )" in order to execute an R command. Without these brackets, the command `install.packages` would print the definition, i.e. the R code, of this R function. Second, commands can receive a list of options, known as "arguments", which appear inside the brackets, separated by commas. Third, the first argument in the command is provided without specifying its name. Using R command `args(install.packages)` one can see that the first argument of this function is called pkgs, which refers to the names of R packages to install. In the line above we omit the name of this argument.

The other argument `repos` is given its name because this is not the second argument of R function `install.packages`. Fourth, when specifying the arguments we can use additional functions. In the above command we use R function `c` to combine values into a vector, i.e. we provide names of the two R packages **meta** and **metafor** in a single vector. Fifth, after command execution, the output is printed directly below the R command; note, we use ". . ." to truncate the printout of R commands in the following.

The above R command installs the R packages **meta** and **metafor** as well as additional R packages that are required for their use, i.e. that provide R functions that are essential for **meta** and **metafor** to work properly. In addition to mandatory R packages, an additional list of *suggested* R packages can be defined by the maintainer of an R package in order to extend the functionality. R package **meta** defines **metafor** as mandatory because R functions from **metafor** are used to calculate some estimators of between-study variance, as well as to conduct meta-regression and to fit generalized linear mixed models (GLMM). Accordingly, specifying "metafor" in the command **install.packages** is not strictly necessary.

26.3   LOADING META-ANALYSIS PACKAGES

In order to make installed R packages available in the R session, either R function `library` can be used directly or one has to click on *Tab: Packages – Select Package* in RStudio.

```
library(meta)
Loading 'meta' package (version 4.18-0).
Type 'help(meta)' for a brief overview.
library(metafor)
Loading required package: Matrix
Loading 'metafor' package (version 2.4-0). For an overview
and introduction to the package please type: help(metafor).
```

The version numbers of the installed packages are provided and informative messages to provide a brief overview of the R packages are given.

Most of the following R commands will only work if the respective R package is available. Thus, before conducting a meta-analysis with **meta** or **metafor**, the **library** command has to be executed once to make the package available for the current R session.

26.4   GETTING HELP

R has an extended help system. Manuals and FAQs can be found on the R website, https://www.r-project.org; for beginners, the manual *An Introduction to R* is a good starting point. Furthermore, each R package provides its own documentation with help pages for individual R functions and datasets as a minimum requirement; the existence of these help pages is checked during submission of a package update to CRAN. In addition, more detailed information can be provided by the maintainer of an R package.

The command `help.start()` opens a local website in the standard web browser. This website contains HTML versions of R manuals and FAQs, as well as help pages for all installed R packages. RStudio users can access the same information by opening the help window (menu: *Help – R Help*).

The R command `help(meta)` prints summary information for R package **meta**. This help page can also be accessed by typing *meta* in the search of the RStudio help window. A screenshot of the first part of this help page as provided by RStudio is shown in Figure 26.1. A brief description is followed by details of the meta-analysis methods available in **meta**, including names of corresponding R functions. We see that several R functions are available to conduct a fixed-effect or random-effects meta-analysis for specific outcomes. For example, a meta-analysis with binary outcomes can be conducted using the `metabin` function. Clicking on any of the links directs us to the corresponding help page with further information.

A similar introduction for R package **metafor** can be accessed using the R command `help(metafor)`. Furthermore, a portable document format (pdf) file of [4] can be opened using R command `vignette("metafor")`. Note that quotes can optionally be used in the `help` command, but are mandatory in the `vignette` command. The

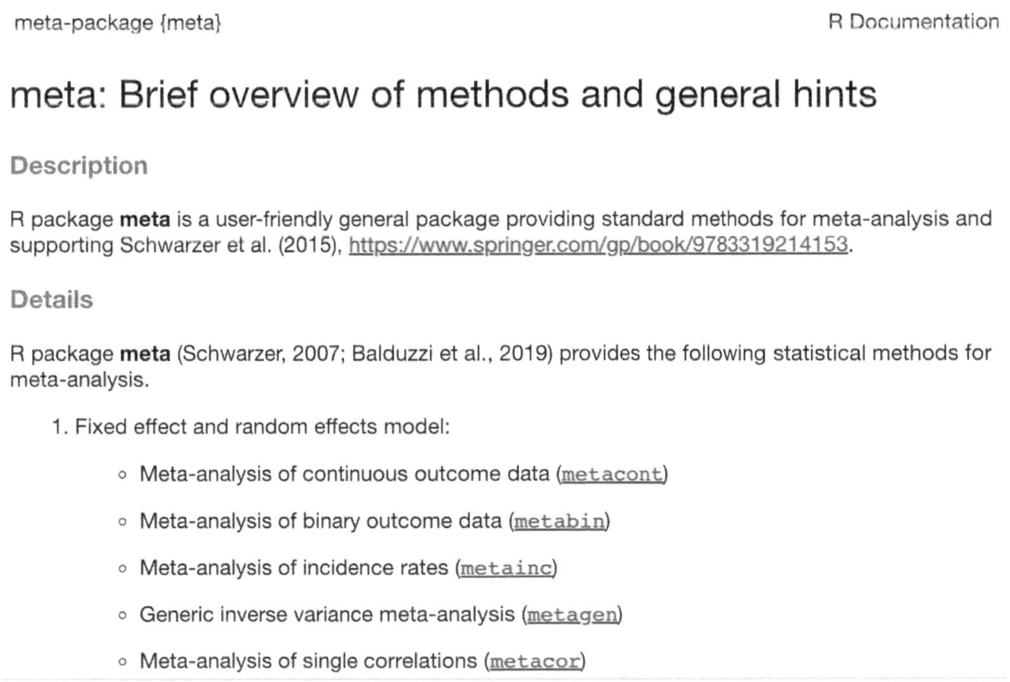

meta-package {meta}   R Documentation

meta: Brief overview of methods and general hints

Description

R package **meta** is a user-friendly general package providing standard methods for meta-analysis and supporting Schwarzer et al. (2015), https://www.springer.com/gp/book/9783319214153.

Details

R package **meta** (Schwarzer, 2007; Balduzzi et al., 2019) provides the following statistical methods for meta-analysis.

1. Fixed effect and random effects model:

   - Meta-analysis of continuous outcome data (metacont)

   - Meta-analysis of binary outcome data (metabin)

   - Meta-analysis of incidence rates (metainc)

   - Generic inverse variance meta-analysis (metagen)

   - Meta-analysis of single correlations (metacor)

FIGURE 26.1   Help page with brief overview of R package **meta**.

`help` function can also be used to get information on a single R function, e.g. for the `metabin` function. Here, we show the text version of this help page to describe important parts.

```
help(metabin)
metabin                  package:meta                  R Documentation
```

Meta-analysis of binary outcome data

Description:

```
    Calculation of fixed effect and random effects estimates
    (risk ratio, odds ratio, risk difference or arcsine
    difference) for meta-analyses with binary outcome data.
    Mantel-Haenszel, inverse variance, Peto method, generalised
    linear mixed model (GLMM), and sample size method are
    available for pooling. For GLMMs, the 'rma.glmm' function
    from R package metafor (Viechtbauer 2010) is called
    internally.
```

Usage:

```
    metabin(event.e, n.e, event.c, n.c, studlab,
            data = NULL, subset = NULL,
Arguments:
  event.e: Number of events in experimental group or true
           positives in diagnostic study.
     n.e: Number of observations in experimental group or number
          of ill participants in diagnostic study.
  ...
Details:
    Calculation of fixed and random effects estimates for
    meta-analyses with binary outcome data.


    The following measures of treatment effect are available
    (Rücker et al., 2009):


  ...
```

A short description of the R function is provided first, followed by the function call and its arguments. As we can see, the first four arguments of R function **metabin** are the number of events and observations in the two treatment groups or from a diagnostic test accuracy study. More details on statistical methods are typically provided under Details, followed by a list of references, related R functions, and examples. These examples can be run using the following command:

```
example(metabin)
metabn> metabin(10, 20, 15, 20, sm = "OR")
     OR           95%-CI       z p-value
 0.3333 [0.0874; 1.2716] -1.61  0.1078

Details:
- Mantel-Haenszel method ...
```

Here, we only show the result of the first example, which calculates the odds ratio for a single study. In addition to the odds ratio, a 95% confidence interval as well as Z statistic and P value for a test for an overall treatment effect are printed.

26.5   ASPIRIN IN PREVENTING DEATH AFTER MYOCARDIAL INFARCTION (EXAMPLE 1)

Our first example is a meta-analysis on the use of aspirin in comparison with placebo to prevent death after myocardial infarction. Data from this meta-analysis have been extracted from Table 3 in [5] and are part of R package **meta**. The following commands can be used to make dataset Fleiss93 available in the current R session and to print summary information on the structure of Fleiss93.

```
data(Fleiss93)
str(Fleiss93)
```

```
'data.frame': 7 obs. of  6 variables:
 $ study   : chr  "MRC-1" "CDP" "MRC-2" "GASP" ...
 $ year    : int  1974 1976 1979 1979 1980 1980 1988
 $ event.e : int  49 44 102 32 85 246 1570
 $ n.e     : int  615 758 832 317 810 2267 8587
 $ event.c : int  67 64 126 38 52 219 1720
 $ n.c     : int  624 771 850 309 406 2257 8600
```

The str command shows that Fleiss93 is a data frame – essentially a dataset – with seven observations (studies) and six variables. For each variable the actual values are printed. All but the first variable with study labels are of type integer.
We can also print the whole dataset by simply typing its name.

```
Fleiss93
```

	study	year	event.e	n.e.	event.c	n.c.
1	MRC-1	1974	49	615	67	624
2	CDP	1976	44	758	64	771
3	MRC-2	1979	102	832	126	850
4	GASP	1979	32	317	38	309
5	PARIS	1980	85	810	52	406
6	AMIS	1980	246	2267	219	2257
7	ISIS-2	1988	1570	8587	1720	8600

Here, we can see that all seven studies are rather large, with total sample sizes between about 600 and 17 000 patients (variable n.e + n.c). Furthermore, numbers of events (variables event.e, event.c) are much larger than zero; we will come back to this point in the second example.

26.5.1   Meta-Analysis for Example 1 Using R Package Meta

As already mentioned above, R function metabin can be used to conduct a meta-analysis of binary outcomes.

```
m.ex1 <- metabin(event.e, n.e, event.c, n.c, data = Fleiss93,
            studlab = paste(study, year), sm = "OR")
```

The arrow "<-" is used to generate an R object m.ex1 containing the results of the meta-analysis. The first four arguments of metabin (number of events and observations in the two treatment groups) are mandatory. Other arguments can be used to define the dataset (arguments data and subset) or specify the analysis method (e.g. argument sm to define the summary measure and method to define the meta-analysis method). Here, we explicitly use the odds ratio as summary measure (**sm** = **"OR"**), because the risk ratio is used by default. Furthermore, argument studlab is used to define informative study labels (here a combination of study name and year of publication). By default, the Mantel–Haenszel method is used to combine the results (argument method = "MH") and therefore is not provided in the metabin command.

Again, the str function can be used to print the structure of meta-analysis object m.ex1.

```
str(m.ex1)
List of 123
 $ event.e      : num [1:7] 49 44 102 32 85 246 1570
 ...
 $ TE.fixed     : num -0.109
 $ seTE.fixed   : num 0.0331
 ...
```

We see that R object m.ex1 is a list with 123 elements of varying length. A list is an R object that can contain several other R objects as components, e.g. single values, vectors, matrices, or data frames, and is thus roughly comparable to a storage room hosting boxes of different sizes. In principle, list components – like boxes in a storage room – do not have to be related. However, components in our list m.ex1 share the property that they contain information on meta-analysis results. Here we show information on three elements from this list: the number of events in the aspirin group (variable event.e) and the logarithm of the Mantel–Haenszel odds ratio (TE.fixed, i.e. treatment estimate in fixed-effect model), with corresponding standard error (seTE.fixed). The meaning of all 123 list elements is described on the help page of metabin.

As before, typing the name of an R object will print it.

```
m.ex1
                 OR           95%-CI   %W(fixed)   %W(random)
MRC-1 1974   0.7197 [0.4890; 1.0593]        3.2          8.2
CDP 1976     0.6808 [0.4574; 1.0132]        3.1          7.8
MRC-2 1979   0.8029 [0.6065; 1.0629]        5.7         13.2
GASP 1979    0.8007 [0.4863; 1.3186]        1.8          5.4
PARIS 1980   0.7981 [0.5526; 1.1529]        3.2          8.9
AMIS 1980    1.1327 [0.9347; 1.3728]       10.2         20.7
ISIS-2 1988  0.8950 [0.8294; 0.9657]       72.9         35.8

Number of studies combined: k = 7

                        OR          95%-CI        z p-value
Fixed effect model    0.8969 [0.8405; 0.9570]  -3.29  0.0010
Random effects model  0.8763 [0.7743; 0.9917]  -2.09  0.0365

Quantifying heterogeneity:
 tau^2 = 0.0096; tau = 0.0982; I^2 = 39.7% [0.0%; 74.6%]; H = 1.29 [1.00; 1.99]

Test of heterogeneity:
    Q d.f. p-value
 9.95     6  0.1269

Details on meta-analytical method:
- Mantel-Haenszel method
- DerSimonian-Laird estimator for tau^2
- Mantel-Haenszel estimator used in calculation of Q and tau^2
  (like RevMan 5)
```

As we see, the list with 123 elements is not fully printed, but a user-friendly print layout is generated instead. First, results for the seven studies are printed, i.e. odds ratios with 95% confidence intervals and percentage weights from fixed-effect and random-effects models. Next, results of both fixed-effect and random-effects meta-analyses are followed by information on between-study heterogeneity. Details at the end specify that the analysis used the Mantel–Haenszel method in the fixed-effect model and the DerSimonian–Laird estimator of the between-study variance in the random-effects model.

A forest plot can be produced using the forest.meta function, which is called using the following command:

```
forest(m.ex1, comb.random = FALSE,
       lab.e ="Aspirin", lab.c = "Placebo",
       label.left = "Favors Aspirin",
       label.right = "Favors Placebo")
```

Only the first argument – a meta-analysis object generated with **meta** – is mandatory to produce a forest plot. The other arguments are used to show only results for the fixed-effect model (comb.random = FALSE) and to enhance the forest plot, which is shown in Figure 26.2.

The Peto method is also available in R function metabin using argument method = "Peto". Instead of a new metabin call, a more concise way is to use the update.meta function.

```
update(m.ex1, method = "Peto")
. . .
```

	OR	95%–CI	z	p-value
Fixed effect model	0.8968	[0.8405; 0.9570]	–3.29	0.0010...

A meta-analysis based on the inverse-variance method can be conducted in the following way:

```
update(m.ex1, method = "Inverse")
. . .
```

	OR	95%–CI	z	p-value
Fixed effect model	0.8969	[0.8405; 0.9571]	–3.28	0.0010...

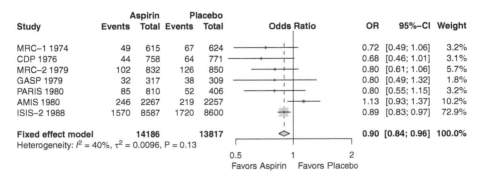

FIGURE 26.2   Forest plot for aspirin meta-analysis [5] using the forest.meta function from R package **meta**.

Results of the three methods are identical to the third decimal place in this meta-analysis due to the large sample sizes and number of events.

26.5.2   Meta-Analysis for Example 1 Using R Package Metafor

The Mantel–Haenszel method is also available in **metafor** in R function rma.mh. The command **args(rma.mh)** gives a listing of all function arguments and shows that the first four arguments of rma.mh are the four cell frequencies, i.e. number of events and nonevents in the two treatment groups. Accordingly, we can use the following command to conduct the meta-analysis:

```
m4.ex1 <- rma.mh(event.e, n.e - event.e,
                 event.c, n.c - event.c,
                 data = Fleiss93, slab = paste(study, year))
```

Argument slab defines study labels in this function. By default, the odds ratio is used as summary measure (argument measure).

The printout for a Mantel–Haenszel meta-analysis is different between **meta** and **metafor**. However, exactly the same results are calculated in both packages.

```
m4.ex1
Fixed-Effects Model (k = 7)

I^2 (total heterogeneity / total variability):  39.67%
H^2 (total variability / sampling variability): 1.66

Test for Heterogeneity:
Q(df = 6) = 9.9461, p-val = 0.1269

Model Results (log scale):

estimate      se     zval      pval     ci.lb     ci.ub
 -0.1088  0.0331  -3.2876   0.0010   -0.1737   -0.0440

Model Results (OR scale):

estimate   ci.lb    ci.ub
  0.8969  0.8405   0.9570
Cochran-Mantel-Haenszel Test:  CMH=10.7107, df=1, p-val=0.0011
Tarone's Test for Heterogen.:  X^2= 9.9788, df=6, p-val=0.1255
```

Here, results are printed both as log odds ratio and odds ratio, with "ci.lb" and "ci. ub" denoting the lower and upper limit of the 95% confidence interval. In addition, results for the Cochran–Mantel–Haenszel and Tarone's test are given. On the other hand, results for individual studies are not reported.

A forest plot can be produced using the forest.rma function, which is called using the following command:

```
forest(m4.ex1, transf = exp, showweights = TRUE)
```

The resulting forest plot is shown in Figure 26.3. Again, only the first argument – a meta-analysis object created with **metafor** – is mandatory. Results would be printed as log odds ratios without argument transf and argument showweights is used to

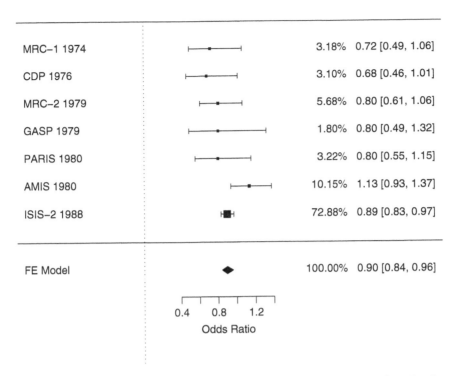

FIGURE 26.3   Forest plot for aspirin meta-analysis [5] using the forest.rma function from R package **metafor**.

print percentage weights for individual studies. In comparison to Figure 26.2, number of events and participants as well as heterogeneity information are not printed; however, several arguments are available to modify both forest plots – see the help pages of R functions forest.meta and forest.rma for more information.

The Peto method is implemented in **metafor** in a separate function called rma.peto. Accordingly, this function has to be used instead of the update function.

```
rma.peto(event.e, n.e - event.e, event.c, n.c - event.c,
        data = Fleiss93, slab = paste(study, year))
...
Model Results (OR scale):

estimate     ci.lb       ci.ub
0.8968       0.8405      0.9570
```

The inverse-variance method is implemented in another R function called rma.uni (or rma), which is a generic function for meta-analysis based on the inverse-variance method. This function can also be used for meta-regression. Using the command args(rma.uni) we see the long list of arguments. In the following command we provide the number of events and participants as input to the rma.uni function and use argument method = "FE" to calculate a fixed-effect meta-analysis:

```
m4.ex1.iv <-
  rma.uni(ai = event.e, n1i = n.e, ci = event.c, n2i = n.c,
```

```
          data = Fleiss93, slab = paste(study, year),
          method = "FE", measure = "OR")
m4.ex1.iv
...
estimate      se     zval    pval    ci.lb    ci.ub
 -0.1088  0.0331  -3.2828  0.0010  -0.1737  -0.0438...
```

We see that results are only reported on the log scale. In order to print the odds ratio, we can use the predict function:

```
predict(m4.ex1.iv, transf = exp)
   pred    ci.lb    ci.ub
 0.8969   0.8405   0.9571
```

Here, "pred" corresponds to the odds ratio in a meta-analysis using the inverse--variance method and "ci.lb" and "ci.ub" to the corresponding lower and upper limits of the 95% confidence interval.

In summary, R packages **meta** and **metafor** provide exactly the same meta-analysis results, but they are printed using different layouts.

26.6 BETA-BLOCKER IN PREVENTING SHORT-TERM MORTALITY AFTER MYOCARDIAL INFARCTION (EXAMPLE 2)

Our second example is the classic meta-analysis of trials of oral beta-blockers to prevent short-term mortality after myocardial infarction. The data are from Table 6 in Yusuf et al. [6] and are included in dataset dat.yusuf1985 of R package **metafor**.

We use the get and subset functions to extract data from the meta-analysis of short-term mortality.

```
yusuf85 <- get(data(dat.yusuf1985))
tab6 <- subset(yusuf85, table == "6")
str(tab6)
'data.frame':  22 obs. of  7 variables:
 $ table: chr   "6" "6" "6" "6" ...
 $ id   : chr   "1.1" "1.2" "1.3" "1.4" ...
 $ trial: chr   "Balcon" "Clausen" "Multicentre" "Barber" ...
 $ ai   : int   14 18 15 10 21 3 2 NA 19 15 ...
 $ n1i  : int   56 66 100 52 226 38 20 NA 76 106 ...
 $ ci   : int   15 19 12 12 24 6 3 NA 15 9 ...
 $ n2i  : int   58 64 95 47 228 31 20 NA 67 114 ...
```

This dataset consists of 22 studies and provides information on the number of deaths in beta-blocker and control group (variables a_i and c_i) and the number of patients per group ($n1_i$, $n2_i$). We see a value of NA (not available) for each of these numbers, which means that information is missing.

26.6.1 Meta-Analysis for Example 2 Using R Package Meta

We use the Peto method to analyze these data in the same way as in the original publication. Therefore, we suppress the printout of results for the random-effects model
(argument comb.random = FALSE). Note that by using the Peto method (method =
"Peto" in metabin) the odds ratio is used as summary measure. We use the summary
function to suppress the printout of individual study results.

```
m.ex2 <- metabin(ai, n1i, ci, n2i, data = tab6,
                 studlab = trial,
                 method = "Peto", comb.random = FALSE)
summary(m.ex2)
Number of studies combined: k = 18

                           OR         95%-CI       z p-value
Fixed effect model 0.9332 [0.7385; 1.1792] -0.58  0.5623

Quantifying heterogeneity:
 tau^2 = 0 [0.0000; 0.2029]; tau = 0 [0.0000; 0.4504]
 I^2 = 0.0% [0.0%; 21.4%]; H = 1.00 [1.00; 1.13]

Test of heterogeneity:
     Q d.f. p-value
 10.83  17  0.8654

Details on meta-analytical method:
- Peto method
- DerSimonian-Laird estimator for tau^2
- Jackson method for confidence interval of tau^2 and tau
```

Although the dataset consists of 22 studies, only 18 studies are combined in the meta-
analysis. Information on studies that are not included in the meta-analysis, i.e. studies
providing a weight of 0%, can be extracted using the following command:

```
subset(as.data.frame(m.ex2), w.fixed == 0) [, 1:9]
```

	event.e	n.e	event.c	n.c	incr.e	incr.c	studlab	TE	seTE
8	NA	NA	NA	NA	0	0	Snow 1	NA	NA
12	0	9	0	8	0	0	Pitt	NA	NA
15	0	16	0	13	0	0	Hutton	NA	NA
19	0	11	0	11	0	0	Yusuf	NA	NA

First, the as.data.frame function generates a dataset from the meta-analysis object
m.ex2. Afterwards, the subset of observations with 0% weight (w.fixed==0) is
extracted and only the first nine variables are printed ([, 1:9]) in order to show
only the essential information. We see that the study Snow 1 does not provide any
information on short-term mortality, as both number of deaths (event.e, event.c)
and patients (n.e, n.c) are missing. The other three studies provide information on

short-term mortality; however, the number of events is zero in both treatment groups, yielding an inestimable treatment effect (TE), i.e. log odds ratio and corresponding standard error (seTE).

The same information about zero events and missing data could also be derived from the forest plot shown in Figure 26.4. The four studies with 0% weight are printed at the bottom of this plot, which is sorted by decreasing weight in the fixed-effect model; missing values are printed as ".". The forest plot in the layout of Review Manager 5 was generated using the following R command:

```
forest(m.ex2, layout = "RevMan5", sortvar = -w.fixed)
```

26.6.2   Meta-Analysis for Example 2 Using R Package Metafor

Analyzing the short-term mortality data is also straightforward using R package **metafor**.

```
m4.ex2 <- rma.peto(ai = ai, n1i = n1i, ci = ci, n2i = n2i,
                   data = tab6, slab = trial)
Warning messages:
1: In rma.peto(ai=ai, n1i=n1i, ci=ci, n2i=n2i, data=tab6,  :
   Tables with NAs omitted from model fitting.
2: In rma.peto(ai=ai, n1i=n1i, ci=ci, n2i=n2i, data=tab6,  :
   Some yi/vi values are NA.
```

Study	Experimental Events	Total	Control Events	Total	Weight	Odds Ratio Peto, Fixed, 95% CI
Norris	21	226	24	228	14.5%	0.87 [0.47; 1.61]
Barber	14	221	15	228	9.7%	0.96 [0.45; 2.04]
Clausen	18	66	19	64	9.5%	0.89 [0.42; 1.90]
Snow 2	19	76	15	67	9.3%	1.15 [0.53; 2.49]
Multicentre	15	100	12	95	8.3%	1.22 [0.54; 2.74]
Balcon	14	56	15	58	7.8%	0.96 [0.41; 2.21]
Fuccella	15	106	9	114	7.6%	1.90 [0.81; 4.42]
Lombardo	8	133	11	127	6.3%	0.68 [0.27; 1.72]
Barber	10	52	12	47	6.1%	0.70 [0.27; 1.79]
Wilcox 1	8	259	7	129	4.6%	0.53 [0.18; 1.59]
Wilcox 2	6	157	4	158	3.5%	1.52 [0.43; 5.34]
Briant	5	62	4	57	3.0%	1.16 [0.30; 4.50]
Kahler	3	38	6	31	2.8%	0.37 [0.09; 1.50]
Thompson	3	48	3	49	2.0%	1.02 [0.20; 5.29]
CPRG	3	177	2	136	1.7%	1.15 [0.19; 6.83]
Ledwich	2	20	3	20	1.6%	0.64 [0.10; 4.07]
Gupta	0	25	3	25	1.0%	0.12 [0.01; 1.25]
Tonkin	1	42	1	46	0.7%	1.10 [0.07; 17.87]
Snow 1	.	.	.	.	0.0%	
Pitt	0	9	0	8	0.0%	
Hutton	0	16	0	13	0.0%	
Yusuf	0	11	0	11	0.0%	
Total (95% CI)		**1900**		**1711**	**100.0%**	**0.93 [0.74; 1.18]**

Heterogeneity: Tau^2 = 0; Chi^2 = 10.83, df = 17 (P = 0.87); I^2 = 0%

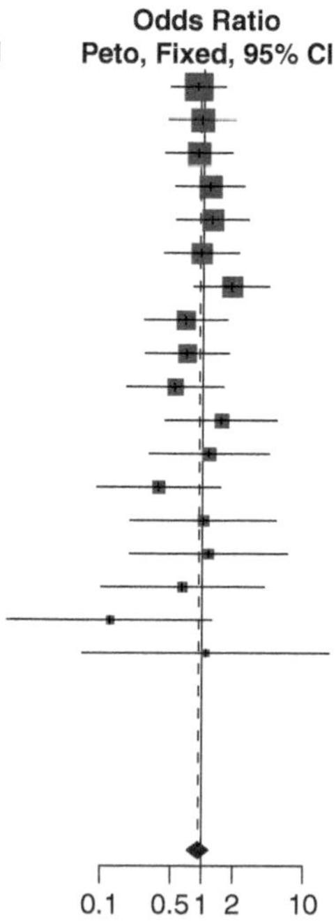

FIGURE 26.4   Forest plot for beta-blocker meta-analysis [6] in Review Manager 5 layout using the forest.meta function from R package **meta**.

Execution of this command results in two warnings. The first warning states that studies with missing values in the corresponding two-by-two table are omitted from the meta-analysis. The second warning states that some estimated treatment effects (yi), i.e. log odds ratios, and corresponding variances (vi) are missing.

The printout of m4.ex2 reports that 21 of 22 studies in the dataset have been included in the meta-analysis. However, the heterogeneity test with 17 degrees of freedom (df) reflects that only 18 of these 21 studies contributed to the meta-analysis.

```
m4.ex2
Fixed-Effects Model (k = 21)

I^2 (total heterogeneity / total variability):  0.00%
H^2 (total variability / sampling variability): 0.64

Test for Heterogeneity:
Q(df = 17) = 10.8275, p-val = 0.8654

Model Results (log scale):

estimate       se      zval      pval     ci.lb    ci.ub
 -0.0692   0.1194   -0.5794    0.5623   -0.3031   0.1648

Model Results (OR scale):

estimate    ci.lb    ci.ub
  0.9332   0.7385   1.1792
```

A function as.data.frame is not available in R package **metafor**. Accordingly, we construct our own dataset using with and data.frame to print information on studies that do not contribute to the meta-analysis (i.e. with missing variance vi.f identified using the is.na function).

```
with(m4.ex2,
      data.frame(event.e = ai.f, n.e = ai.f + bi.f,
                 event.c = ci.f, n.c = ci.f + di.f,
                 slab, TE = yi.f,
                 seTE = sqrt(vi.f))[is.na(vi.f), ])
```

	event.e	n.e	event.c	n.c	slab	TE	seTE
8	0	NA	NA	NA	Snow 1	NA	NA
12	0	9	0	8	Pitt	NA	NA
15	0	16	0	13	Hutton	NA	NA
17	0	11	0	11	Yusuf	NA	NA

This command results in a very similar output as given above for R package **meta** and identifies the same four studies that do not contribute to the meta-analysis. Based on this printout, we see that **metafor** reports the number of studies with non-missing data (including studies with double zeros, even though giving them 0% weight in the meta-analysis), whereas **meta** reports the number of studies contributing to the meta--analysis (excluding studies with double zeros). Regardless, both R packages provide the exact same results for this meta-analysis using the Peto method.

26.7   META-REGRESSION – INFLUENCE OF DISTANCE FROM THE EQUATOR ON TUBERCULOSIS VACCINE EFFECTIVENESS

Subgroup analysis and meta-regression can be conducted with **meta** and **metafor**. As subgroup analysis can be seen as a special case of meta-regression with a categorical covariate, we only have a closer look at meta-regression. Subgroup analysis and meta-regression with **meta** and **metafor** are described in more detail in [1, 4] and in Chapter 10 of this book.

Colditz et al. [7] evaluated the overall effectiveness of the Bacillus Calmette-Guerin (BCG) vaccine against tuberculosis. This is a classic example for meta-regression [8], with distance from the equator as an effect modifying factor. The BCG data with 13 studies is part of the **metafor** package.

```
bcg <- get(data(dat.colditz1994, package = "metafor"))
bcg$ablat
[1] 44 55 42 52 13 44 19 13 27 42 18 33 33
bcg$year
 [1] 1948 1949 1960 1977 1973 1953 1973 1980 1968
[10] 1961 1974 1969 1976
```

Primary interest lies in the variable ablat, which contains information on the absolute geographic latitude, i.e. absolute distance from the equator. In a second meta-regression, we will also consider the publication year. In order to get a more sensible interpretation of the intercept in the second meta-regression, we center variable year around its mean value.

```
bcg$year.c <- bcg$year - mean(bcg$year)
```

Meta-regression can be conducted with the metareg function in the **meta** package and the rma.uni function in **metafor**. Actually, metareg is a wrapper function that calls the rma.uni function internally to do the calculations.

The metareg function expects a meta-analysis object as the first argument and covariate(s) used in the meta-regression as the second argument. Therefore, we have to start by conducting a meta-analysis in the usual way without any covariates.

```
m.ex3 <- metabin(tpos, tpos + tneg, cpos, cpos + cneg,
                 data = bcg, sm = "OR")
```

This meta-analysis object can be used as input to the metareg function.

```
m.ex3.mr <- metareg(m.ex3, ablat)
m.ex3.mr
Mixed-Effects Model (k = 13; tau^2 estimator: DL)

tau^2 (estimated residual heterogeneity): 0.0480 (SE = 0.0451)
...


Test for Residual Heterogeneity:
QE(df = 11) = 25.0954, p-val = 0.0088

Test of Moderators (coefficient(s) 2):
QM(df = 1) = 26.1628, p-val < .0001
```

```
Model Results:
          estimate      se     zval     pval    ci.lb     ci.ub
intrcpt     0.3030   0.2109   1.4370   0.1507  -0.1103    0.7163
ablat      -0.0316   0.0062  -5.1150   <.0001  -0.0437   -0.0195...
```

This printout is generated by the print.rma.uni function from **metafor**. The first line reports that the DerSimonian–Laird method (DL) was used to estimate the between-study variance (argument method in rma.uni command). The "Test of Moderators" shows that absolute geographic latitude is a strong modifier of the effectiveness of the BCG vaccine. The intercept corresponds to the log odds ratio for the effectiveness of the BCG vaccine at the equator. The influence of a one-degree change in absolute geographic latitude is given in the line starting with ablat. The negative value −0.0316 translates into a stronger reduction of positive tuberculosis cases with increasing distance from the equator.

The "Test for Residual Heterogeneity" clearly shows that the absolute geographic latitude does not explain all heterogeneity between study results. This can also be seen in the bubble plot shown in Figure 26.5, which was generated using the command bubble(m.ex3.mr). Despite the remaining heterogeneity, a clear tendency of a stronger effect of the BCG vaccine with increasing distance from the equator is visible in this figure.

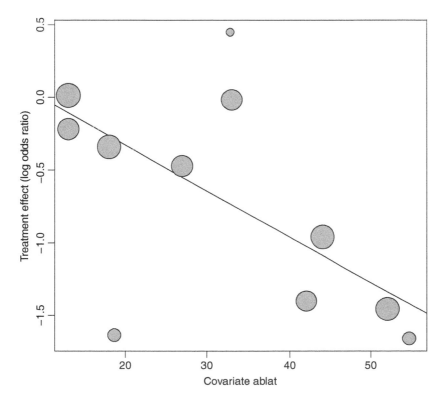

FIGURE 26.5 Bubble plot for meta-regression of BCG vaccine dataset [7] using the bubble. metareg function from R package **meta.**

We get exactly the same meta-regression results using the following command based on rma.uni from **metafor** with argument mods to define covariate(s), i.e. moderator variable(s).

```
rma.uni(ai = tpos, n1i = tpos + tneg,
        ci = cpos, n2i = cpos + cneg,
        data = bcg, measure = "OR",
        method = "DL", mods = ablat)
```

Due to the remaining heterogeneity, a next analysis step could be to consider a second covariate in the meta-regression. In the BCG dataset, publication year is a natural candidate to evaluate whether the effectiveness of the BCG vaccine changed over time.

```
metareg(m.ex3, ablat + year.c)
Mixed-Effects Model (k = 13; tau^2 estimator: DL)

tau^2 (estimated residual heterogeneity): 0.0667 (SE = 0.0652)
...
Test for Residual Heterogeneity:
QE(df = 10) = 25.0121, p-val = 0.0053


Test of Moderators (coefficient(s) 2,3):
QM(df = 2) = 20.6855, p-val < .0001
```

Model Results:

	estimate	se	zval	pval	ci.lb	ci.ub
intrcpt	0.2210	0.3010	0.7342	0.4628	-0.3689	0.8108
ablat	-0.0295	0.0085	-3.4906	0.0005	-0.0461	-0.0129
year.c	0.0046	0.0124	0.3694	0.7118	-0.0197	0.0288...

As we use the covariate year.c instead of year, the intercept corresponds to the effect of the BCG vaccine in a study conducted at the equator in 1966 (the average value of year), which seems more sensible than a study conducted in the year 0 BC. We see that the effect of absolute geographic latitude does not change very much and that publication year does not seem to be an independent prognostic factor. Worryingly, the residual between-study heterogeneity in this analysis is even larger than in the meta-regression only considering absolute geographic latitude. This should serve as a warning not to over-fit and over-interpret the available data [8]. Based on a general rule of thumb, one needs 10–20 observations (studies) for each covariate in a (meta-)regression. Accordingly, the inclusion of a second covariate in the meta-regression in the BCG dataset with 14 studies might seem adventurous, like entering uncharted territory. To assist the user in such an endeavor, R package **metafor** provides R functions with regression diagnostics [4] in order to sail around the most dangerous reefs.

26.8   EVALUATION OF BIAS IN META-ANALYSIS – TESTS FOR SMALL-STUDY EFFECTS AND TRIM-AND-FILL METHOD

Various sources of bias can threaten the validity of meta-analyses. This topic is discussed in detail in Chapters 4 and 5. Here, we show how to produce a funnel plot using R and how to conduct statistical tests for funnel plot asymmetry (otherwise known as small-study effects). In addition, the trim-and-fill method [9] to adjust for small-study effects is applied, which, although a simple and ad hoc method, has gained popularity over the last two decades. We briefly comment on more advanced (and typically more appropriate) statistical methods to adjust for small-study effects in an overview of other R packages for meta-analysis later in the chapter.

Funnel plots can be created with the `funnel.meta` function in R package **meta** and `funnel.rma` in **metafor**. Statistical tests for small-study effects are available in the `metabias` function in **meta** and the `regtest` and `ranktest` functions in **metafor**. The trim-and-fill method is implemented in R functions `trimfill.meta` and `trimfill.rma.uni`. Here, we will only describe R functions in **meta** for the sake of brevity.

Typically, the first step to evaluate bias in meta-analysis is to generate a funnel plot. A funnel plot for the first example of trials of aspirin after myocardial infarction can be created with the `funnel.meta` function. The first argument of this function is a meta-analysis object. Other important arguments of this function are `yaxis` to change the y-axis in the funnel plot and `contour.levels` to produce contour-enhanced funnel plots [10]. The command **funnel(m.ex1)** creates the funnel plot shown in Figure 26.6. Despite being based on only seven studies, this plot shows some indication of funnel plot asymmetry, as the two largest studies are closest to the null effect, i.e. an odds ratio of 1.

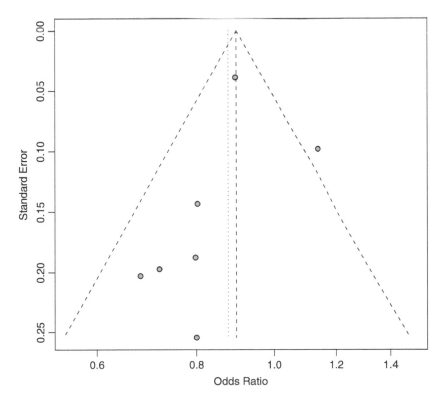

FIGURE 26.6 Funnel plot for aspirin meta-analysis [5] using the `funnel.meta` function from R package **meta**.

The metabias.meta function can be used to test formally for funnel plot asymmetry, and provides several linear regression and rank correlation tests for funnel plot asymmetry (argument method). This function considers recommendations for examining and interpreting funnel plot asymmetry in meta-analyses [11]. Regression tests are preferred over rank correlation tests due to their larger power. The classic Egger regression test [12] is used for all but binary outcomes. In this case, the Harbord test [13] is used, which is a modified regression test based on the efficient score, also called score function, and its variance. By default, a test is only conducted if the number of studies is at least ten, a widely recommended minimum number of studies [11].

The command **metabias(m.ex1)** produces an informative warning that the number of studies is smaller than recommended to conduct a test for funnel plot asymmetry. We can conduct this test using argument k.min, as mentioned in the warning message.

```
metabias(m.ex1, k.min = 5)
Linear regression test of funnel plot asymmetry

Test result: t = -0.92, df = 5, p-value = 0.3991

Sample estimates:
    bias se.bias intercept se.intercept
 -0.7259  0.7878   -0.0593       0.0690

Details:
- multiplicative residual heterogeneity variance (tau^2 = 1.7042)
- predictor: standard error of score
- weight:    inverse variance of score
- reference: Harbord etal. (2006), Stat Med
```

The P value shows that no clear indication of funnel plot asymmetry (small-study effects) exists in this meta-analysis. However, this conclusion is based on a rather small number of studies. Therefore, in a sensitivity analysis, we apply the trim-and-fill method to the aspirin meta-analysis despite a nonsignificant test for funnel plot asymmetry.

```
print(trimfill(m.ex1), digits = 2)
                      OR         95%-CI %W(random)
MRC-1 1974          0.72 [0.49; 1.06]        6.7
CDP 1976            0.68 [0.46; 1.01]        6.4
MRC-2 1979          0.80 [0.61; 1.06]       10.7
GASP 1979           0.80 [0.49; 1.32]        4.4
PARIS 1980          0.80 [0.55; 1.15]        7.2
AMIS 1980           1.13 [0.93; 1.37]       16.5
ISIS-2 1988         0.89 [0.83; 0.97]       27.9
Filled: PARIS 1980  1.05 [0.72; 1.51]        7.2
Filled: MRC-1 1974  1.16 [0.79; 1.71]        6.7
Filled: CDP 1976    1.23 [0.82; 1.83]        6.4

Number of studies combined: k = 10 (with 3 added studies)

                      OR         95%-CI      z p-value
Random effects model 0.92 [0.83; 1.03] -1.40  0.1622
```

```
Quantifying heterogeneity:
 tau^2 = 0.0102; tau = 0.1011; I^2 = 37.4% [0.0%; 70.1%]; H = 1.26 [1.00; 1.83]
Test of heterogeneity:
     Q d.f. p-value
 14.37    9  0.1099

Details on meta-analytical method:
- Inverse variance method
- DerSimonian-Laird estimator for tau^2
- Trim-and-fill method to adjust for funnel plot asymmetry
```

Three studies were added to the aspirin meta-analysis (see lines starting with "Filled:"). As the trim-and-fill method adds studies to the meta-analysis, the use of a fixed-effect model – which by construction has a smaller confidence interval by adding studies – is not a sensible choice. Accordingly, the `trimfill.meta` function only reports results for the random-effects model. This sensitivity analysis indicates that the evidence for a benefit of aspirin from the seven trials may be less robust than the main analysis indicates: the effect is smaller and no longer statistically significant.

26.9   OTHER STATISTICAL METHODS FOR META-ANALYSIS IN R PACKAGES META AND METAFOR

We now give a brief overview of some additional statistical methods available in **meta** and **metafor**; see also the next section for further statistical methods implemented in **metafor**.

26.9.1   Handling of Zero Events in Meta-Analysis of Binary Outcomes

We have seen in Example 2 that studies with zero events in both groups do not contribute to a meta-analysis using the Peto method, i.e. `metabin` in **meta** and `rma.peto` in **metafor**. This is the general meta-analysis approach for the odds ratio and risk ratio, which are not defined for zero events in both groups. Likewise, in **meta** and **metafor**, studies with zero events in both groups get 0% weight in a meta-analysis using the Mantel–Haenszel method. For the inverse-variance method, `metabin` also by default excludes studies with double zeros (see argument `allstudies`), whereas `rma.uni` includes studies with double zeros in the meta-analysis (argument `drop00`). Accordingly, this default of `rma.uni` should be changed in meta-analyses with double zero studies!

An increment of 0.5 is typically added to cells in studies with a zero in one group – also called a *continuity correction* – in order to include these studies in a meta--analysis with the odds ratio or risk ratio as summary measure. This increment can be changed using argument `incr` in R function `metabin` and argument `add` in the `rma` functions. Furthermore, the user can decide whether to add the increment only to studies with a zero in one group (default) or to all studies – either in general, or only if at least one study has a zero in one group; see arguments `allincr` and `addincr` in `metabin` and `to` in the `rma` functions.

There are subtle differences between **meta** and **metafor** in the handling of studies with a zero in one group in the calculation of meta-analysis estimates. For the Mantel–Haenszel method, by default `metabin` – like Review Manager 5 – applies a continuity correction (see argument `MH.exact`), whereas `rma.mh` uses the exact Mantel–Haenszel method (argument `drop00`). For the Peto method, a continuity correction is not necessary in studies with a zero in one group. Accordingly, R functions in **meta** and **metafor** do not apply a continuity correction in this situation. While this behavior can be changed in **metafor**, all arguments concerning the continuity correction are ignored in **meta**, which provides the unmodified Peto method only.

26.9.2   Advanced Methods for Meta-Analysis of Binary Outcomes

A distinctive and frequently overlooked advantage of binary endpoints is that individual participant data (IPD) can be extracted from a two-by-two table. Accordingly, statistical methods for IPD, i.e. logistic regression and GLMM, can be used in a meta-analysis of binary outcomes [14, 15]. These methods are implemented in the `rma.glmm` function in **metafor**. Again, these methods are also available in the `metabin` function of **meta** (argument `method = "GLMM"` and argument `model.glmm`) by calling the `rma.glmm` function internally.

26.9.3   Meta-Analysis for Outcomes Other than Binary Outcomes

In this chapter we have focused on the meta-analysis of binary outcomes. This can be conducted with a single function in **meta** and four functions in **metafor**. Thus, the **meta** package follows the first part of the Three Musketeers' motto "one for all" in this setting, whereas the metafor package follows the second part "all for one," as the various meta-analysis methods for binary outcomes (Mantel–Haenszel, Peto, inverse variance, GLMM) are implemented in dedicated R functions.

The Three Musketeers' motto is reversed in **meta** and **metafor** for meta-analyses of other outcomes. The **metafor** package provides a single function for other outcomes; see the help page of `rma.uni` function. On the other hand, several meta--analysis functions exist in **meta** for specific outcome types:

- `metabin` – meta-analysis of binary outcomes.
- `metacont` – meta-analysis of continuous outcomes.
- `metacor` – meta-analysis of correlations.
- `metacr` – meta-analysis for outcomes from a Cochrane review.
             (internally calls `metabin`, `metacont`, and `metagen` functions).
- `metagen` – generic inverse-variance meta-analysis.
- `metainc` – meta-analysis of incidence rates.
- `metamean` – meta-analysis of single means.
- `metaprop` – meta-analysis of single proportions.
- `metarate` – meta-analysis of single incidence rates.

26.9.4   Estimation of the Between-Study Variance

The DerSimonian–Laird method is the most commonly used estimator for the between-study variance. However, a large number of alternative estimators have been proposed over the last decades [16]. These are implemented in meta-analysis functions in **meta** by the argument method.tau and in the **metafor** package by argument method (see the help pages of metagen and rma.uni).

26.9.5   Hartung–Knapp Method – Alternative Method for Meta-Analysis

Hartung and Knapp developed an alternative method for meta-analysis [17, 18], which was extended to meta-regression by Knapp and Hartung [19]. This method is referred to as the Hartung–Knapp method in R package **meta** (argument hakn in meta-analysis functions) and Knapp–Hartung method in the **metafor** package implementing this method in the rma.uni function for meta-analysis and meta-regression (argument test = "knha").

26.9.6   Prediction Interval

A prediction interval [20] can be calculated in meta-analysis functions of the **meta** package using argument prediction. These intervals are implemented in **metafor** in R function predict.rma. Forest plots with a prediction interval can be generated using argument prediction in forest.meta and addcred in forest.rma (see the help pages for examples).

26.10   OVERVIEW OF OTHER R PACKAGES FOR META-ANALYSIS

An up-to-date summary of R packages for meta-analysis is available online for CRAN packages (https://cloud.r-project.org/web/views/MetaAnalysis.html). Here, we briefly describe a selection of R packages for more advanced meta-analysis methods.

26.10.1   Bias in Meta-Analysis

Tests for funnel plot asymmetry (small-study effects) and the trim-and-fill method have been described in this chapter. More advanced methods to evaluate bias in meta--analysis are available, with **metasens** [21] providing the Copas selection model and the limit meta-analysis and **selectMeta** [22] providing various selection models, e.g. the parametric model by Iyengar and Greenhouse. Rosenthal's fail-safe N method is also available in R (**metafor, MAc** [23], **MAd** [24]), although its use is not generally recommended.

26.10.2   Network Meta-Analysis

Many network meta-analysis methods are based on a Bayesian approach using the Markov Chain Monte Carlo (MCMC) method [25]. Typically, these Bayesian analyses are conducted in WinBUGS, OpenBUGS, or JAGS. A number of interfaces from R to WinBUGS and similar MCMC software exist, such as the **R2WinBUGS** package [26]. Van Valkenhoef et al. have published the **gemtc** package [27] using BUGS or JAGS that conducts network meta-analyses based on a Bayesian hierarchical model. Another Bayesian approach is implemented in the **pcnetmeta** package [28] using JAGS.

Over the last couple of years, R packages for meta-analysis using frequentist methods have been published. The **netmeta** package [29] is a user-friendly implementation of the methods by Rücker [30] and Krahn et al. [31]. Distinctive features of **netmeta** are a function to produce a net-heat plot [31] and a function for ranking of treatments in a network meta-analysis [32]. The **netmeta** package and its application are described in the Use-R! book on meta-analysis with R [1]. Methods for network meta-analysis are also available in the rma.mv function of **metafor**.

26.10.3   Multivariate and Diagnostic Test Accuracy Meta-Analysis

Methods for multivariate meta-analysis are provided by several R packages. For example, **metafor** with the rma.mv function and **mvmeta** [33] provide fixed-effect and random-effects models with various methods to estimate the between-study covariance matrix. Both packages also provide functions for multivariate meta-regression. The **xmeta** package [34] makes available multivariate meta-analysis methods and tests and adjustment methods for bias in multivariate meta-analysis.

Diagnostic test accuracy (DTA) meta-analysis modeling sensitivities and specificities is a special bivariate case of multivariate meta-analysis. Accordingly, R packages for multivariate meta-analysis can be used in principle for basic analyses. However, it is more convenient to use R packages specifically developed for DTA meta-analysis, which also provide common plots like received operating characteristic (ROC) or summary ROC curves. The **mada** package [35] provides both univariate methods and the bivariate meta-analysis model by Reitsma [36]. The **meta4diag** [37] package implements Bayesian methods for DTA meta-analysis.

R packages **mvmeta** and **mada** are described in the Use-R! book on meta-analysis with R [1].

REFERENCES

1. Schwarzer, G., Carpenter, J.R., and Rücker, G. (2015). *Meta-analysis with R*. Cham: Springer.
2. R Foundation for Statistical Computing. (2017). *R: A Language and Environment for Statistical Computing*. www.r-project.org.
3. Balduzzi, S., Rücker, G., and Schwarzer, G. (2019). How to perform a meta-analysis with R: a practical tutorial. *Evid. Based Ment. Health* **22**: 153–160.
4. Viechtbauer, W. (2010). Conducting meta-analyses in R with the metafor package. *J. Stat. Softw.* **36**: 1–48.

5. Fleiss, J. (1993). Review papers: the statistical basis of meta-analysis. *Stat. Methods Med. Res.* **2** (2): 121–145.

6. Yusuf, S., Peto, R., Lewis, J. et al. (1985). Beta blockade during and after myocardial infarction: an overview of the randomized trials. *Prog. Cardiovasc. Dis.* **27**: 335–371.

7. Colditz, G.A., Brewer, T.F., Berkey, C.S. et al. (1994). Efficacy of BCG vaccine in the prevention of tuberculosis: meta-analysis of the published literature. *JAMA* **271**: 698–702.

8. Thompson, S. and Higgins, J.P.T. (2002). How should meta-regression analyses be undertaken and interpreted? *Stat. Med.* **21**: 1559–1573.

9. Duval, S. and Tweedie, R. (2000). Trim and fill: a simple funnel-plot-based method of testing and adjusting for publication bias in meta-analysis. *Biometrics* **56**: 455–463.

10. Peters, J.L., Sutton, A.J., Jones, D.R. et al. (2008). Contour-enhanced meta-analysis funnel plots help distinguish publication bias from other causes of asymmetry. *J. Clin. Epidemiol.* **61**: 991–996.

11. Sterne, J.A.C., Sutton, A.J., Ioannidis, J.P.A. et al. (2011). Recommendations for examining and interpreting funnel plot asymmetry in meta-analyses of randomised controlled trials. *BMJ.* **343**: d4002.

12. Egger, M., Davey Smith, G., Schneider, M. et al. (1997). Bias in meta-analysis detected by a simple, graphical test. *BMJ.* **315**: 629–634.

13. Harbord, R.M., Egger, M., and Sterne, J.A.C. (2006). A modified test for small-study effects in meta-analyses of controlled trials with binary endpoints. *Stat. Med.* **25**: 3443–3457.

14. Stijnen, T., Hamza, T.H., and Ozdemir, P. (2010). Random effects meta-analysis of event outcome in the framework of the generalized linear mixed model with applications in sparse data. *Stat. Med.* **29**: 3046–3067.

15. Simmonds, M.C. and Higgins, J.P.T. (2016). A general framework for the use of logistic regression models in meta-analysis. *Stat. Methods Med. Res.* **25**: 2858–2877.

16. Veroniki, A.A., Jackson, D., Viechtbauer, W. et al. (2016). Methods to estimate the between-study variance and its uncertainty in meta-analysis. *Res. Synth. Methods* **7**: 55–79.

17. Hartung, J. and Knapp, G. (2001). On tests of the overall treatment effect in meta-analysis with normally distributed responses. *Stat. Med.* **20**: 1771–1782.

18. Hartung, J. and Knapp, G. (2001). A refined method for the meta-analysis of controlled clinical trials with binary outcome. *Stat. Med.* **20**: 3875–3889.

19. Knapp, G. and Hartung, J. (2003). Improved tests for a random effects meta-regression with a single covariate. *Stat. Med.* **22**: 2693–2710.

20. Higgins, J.P.T., Thompson, S.G., and Spiegelhalter, D.J. (2009). A re-evaluation of random-effects meta-analysis. *J. R. Stat. Soc. Ser. A* **172**: 137–159.

21. Schwarzer, G., Carpenter, J.R., and Rücker, G. (2021). *metasens: Statistical Methods for Sensitivity Analysis in Meta-Analysis.* R package version 0.6-0. https://CRAN.R-project.org/package=metasens (accessed 21 February 2022).

22. Rufibach, K. (2015). *selectMeta: Estimation of Weight Functions in Meta Analysis.* R package version 1.0.8. https://CRAN.R-project.org/package=selectMeta (accessed 21 February 2022).

23. Del Re, A.C., and Hoyt, W.T. (2018). *MAc: Meta-Analysis with Correlations.* R package version 1.1.1. https://CRAN.R-project.org/package=MAc (accessed 21 February 2022).

24. Del Re, A.C., and Hoyt, W.T. (2018). *MAd: Meta-Analysis with Mean Differences.* R package version 0.8-2.1. https://CRAN.R-project.org/package=MAd (accessed 21 February 2022).

25. Salanti, G., Higgins, J.P.T., Ades, A.E. et al. (2008). Evaluation of networks of randomized trials. *Stat. Methods Med. Res.* **17**: 279–301.

26. Sturtz, S., Ligges, U., and Gelman, A.E. (2005). R2WinBUGS: a package for running WinBUGS from R. *J. Stat. Softw.* **12**: 1–16.

27. van Valkenhoef, G. and Kuiper, J. (2020). *gemtc: Network Meta-Analysis Using Bayesian Methods.* R package version 0.8.8. https://CRAN.R-project.org/package=gemtc (accessed 21 February 2022).

28. Lin, L., Zhang, J., and Chu, H. (2020). *pcnetmeta: Patient-Centered Network Meta-Analysis.* R package version 2.7. https://CRAN.R-project.org/package=pcnetmeta (accessed 21 February 2022).

29. Rücker, G., Krahn, U., König, J., Efthimiou, O., and Schwarzer, G. (2021). *netmeta: Network Meta-Analysis using Frequentist Methods.* R package version 1.3-0. https://CRAN.R-project.org/package=netmeta (accessed 21 February 2022).

30. Rücker, G. (2012). Network meta-analysis, electrical networks and graph theory. *Res. Synth. Methods* **3**: 312–324.

31. Krahn, U., Binder, H., and König, J. (2013). A graphical tool for locating inconsistency in network meta-analyses. *BMC Med. Res. Methodol.* **13**: 35.

32. Rücker, G. and Schwarzer, G. (2015). Ranking treatments in frequentist network meta-analysis works without resampling methods. *BMC Med. Res. Methodol.* **15**: 58.

33. Gasparrini, A., Armstrong, B., and Kenward, M.G. (2012). Multivariate meta-analysis for non-linear and other multi-parameter associations. *Stat. Med.* **31**: 3821–3839.

34. Chen, Y., Hong, C., and Chu, H. (2021). *xmeta: A Toolbox for Multivariate Meta-Analysis.* R package version 1.3-0. https://CRAN.R-project.org/package=xmeta (accessed 21 February 2022).

35. Doebler, P. (2020). *mada: Meta-Analysis of Diagnostic Accuracy.* R package version 0.5.1. https://CRAN.R-project.org/package=mada (accessed 21 February 2022).

36. Reitsma, J.B., Glas, A.S., Rutjes, A.W.S. et al. (2005). Bivariate analysis of sensitivity and specificity produces informative summary measures in diagnostic reviews. *J. Clin. Epidemiol.* **58**: 982–990.

37. Guo, J., and Riebler, A. (2018). *meta4diag: Meta-Analysis for Diagnostic Test Studies.* R package version 2.0.8. https://CRAN.R-project.org/package=meta4diag (accessed 21 February 2022).

CHAPTER 27

Comprehensive Meta-Analysis Software

Michael Borenstein

Comprehensive Meta-Analysis (*CMA*) is a computer program for meta-analysis that was developed with funding from the National Institutes of Health in the United States. The program was initially released in 2000 and has been updated on a regular basis since then. As of this writing, the most recent major update was in 2021, and new releases are scheduled for the next few years.

CMA features a spreadsheet view and a menu-driven interface. As such, it allows a researcher to enter data and perform a simple analysis in a matter of minutes. At the same time, it offers a wide array of advanced features, including the ability to plot the distribution of true effects, to compare the effect size in subgroups of studies, to run meta-regression, to estimate the potential impact of publication bias, and to produce high-resolution plots. The program is designed to work with studies that compare an outcome in two groups, or that estimate an outcome in one group. It is not intended for network meta-analyses nor for meta-analyses of diagnostic test accuracy.

27.1 MOTIVATING EXAMPLE

To illustrate the program, we will use a meta-analysis of 17 studies that assessed the utility of St. John's wort (*Hypericum perforatum*) for treating depression. In each study, patients who suffered from depression were randomly assigned to either *Hypericum* or placebo, and researchers recorded the number of patients that responded in each group, based on improvements in the Hamilton Rating Scale for Depression (HRSD). An odds ratio greater than 1.0 indicates that St. John's wort was helpful. An odds ratio of 2.0, for example, would indicate that treatment doubled the odds that a patient

Systematic Reviews in Health Research: Meta-Analysis in Context, Third Edition. Edited by Matthias Egger, Julian P.T. Higgins, and George Davey Smith.
© 2022 John Wiley & Sons Ltd. Published 2022 by John Wiley & Sons Ltd.
Companion website: www.systematic-reviews3.org

would improve. The original analysis was performed by Linde et al. [1, 2]. Here, we use the subset of 17 placebo-controlled trials that provided data for all moderators, as discussed by Viechtbauer [3]. Our goal in this chapter is to provide a sense of the look and feel of the program. For the reader who would like to carry out the analyses, a video of this analysis and a PDF with step-by-step instructions are available at http://www.Meta-Analysis.com. This chapter is not intended to provide any medical advice. For that, one should consult the original papers.

27.2 DATA ENTRY

Figure 27.1 shows the data-entry screen. For each study, we enter the study name into column A and the summary data into the columns labeled B. The program computes the odds ratio, log odds ratio, standard error, and variance for each study, and displays these in the columns labeled C. We have also entered data for a series of moderator variables in the columns labeled D, including the type of depression diagnosed (Dx), the baseline HRSD scores (Baseline), and the dose of the *Hypericum* extract (Dose). Dose is computed as daily dose (in mg) times study duration.

In this example, the user has elected to enter the events and sample size for each group and has chosen to display the odds ratio. However, the user may elect to enter data in more than 100 formats and to display any number of effect-size indices. The data may be entered directly into CMA or copied from another program such as Excel™.

To run the analysis, we click Run Analyses on the toolbar.

27.3 BASIC ANALYSIS

Figure 27.2 shows the basic analysis screen. A tab at the bottom (E) may be used to switch between fixed-effect and random-effects meta-analyses. The fixed-effect model is appropriate when all studies come from the same population and are identical in all

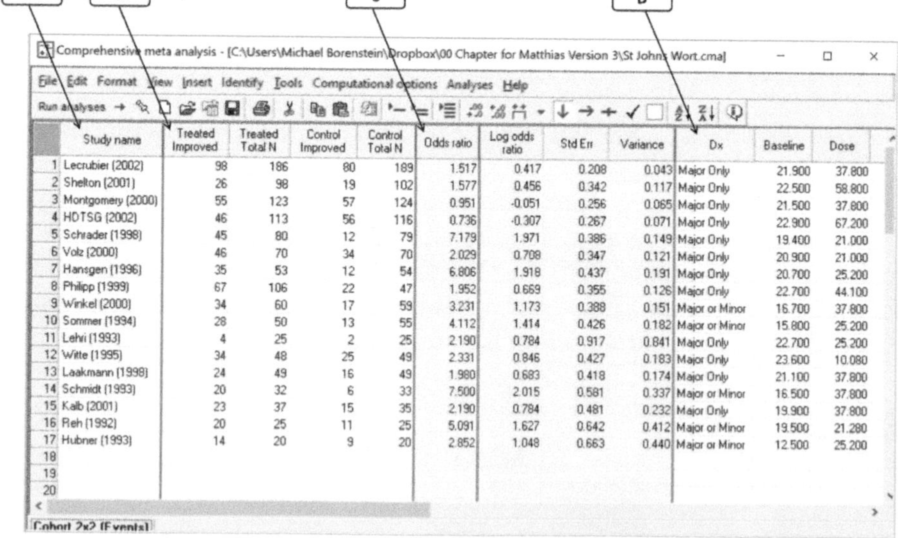

	Study name	Treated Improved	Treated Total N	Control Improved	Control Total N	Odds ratio	Log odds ratio	Std Err	Variance	Dx	Baseline	Dose
1	Lecrubier (2002)	98	186	80	189	1.517	0.417	0.208	0.043	Major Only	21.900	37.800
2	Shelton (2001)	26	98	19	102	1.577	0.456	0.342	0.117	Major Only	22.500	58.800
3	Montgomery (2000)	55	123	57	124	0.951	-0.051	0.256	0.065	Major Only	21.500	37.800
4	HDTSG (2002)	46	113	56	116	0.736	-0.307	0.267	0.071	Major Only	22.900	67.200
5	Schrader (1998)	45	80	12	79	7.179	1.971	0.386	0.149	Major Only	19.400	21.000
6	Volz (2000)	46	70	34	70	2.029	0.708	0.347	0.121	Major Only	20.900	21.000
7	Hansgen (1996)	35	53	12	54	6.806	1.918	0.437	0.191	Major Only	20.700	25.200
8	Philipp (1999)	67	106	22	47	1.952	0.669	0.355	0.126	Major Only	22.700	44.100
9	Winkel (2000)	34	60	17	59	3.231	1.173	0.388	0.151	Major or Minor	16.700	37.800
10	Sommer (1994)	28	50	13	55	4.112	1.414	0.426	0.182	Major or Minor	15.800	25.200
11	Lehri (1993)	4	25	2	25	2.190	0.784	0.917	0.841	Major Only	22.700	25.200
12	Witte (1995)	34	48	25	49	2.331	0.846	0.427	0.183	Major Only	23.600	10.080
13	Laakmann (1998)	24	49	16	49	1.980	0.683	0.418	0.174	Major Only	21.100	37.800
14	Schmidt (1993)	20	32	6	33	7.500	2.015	0.581	0.337	Major or Minor	16.500	37.800
15	Kalb (2001)	23	37	15	35	2.190	0.784	0.481	0.232	Major Only	19.900	37.800
16	Reh (1992)	20	25	11	25	5.091	1.627	0.642	0.412	Major or Minor	19.500	21.280
17	Hubner (1993)	14	20	9	20	2.852	1.048	0.663	0.440	Major or Minor	12.500	25.200
18												
19												
20												

FIGURE 27.1 Data-entry screen. *Source*: Biostat, Inc.

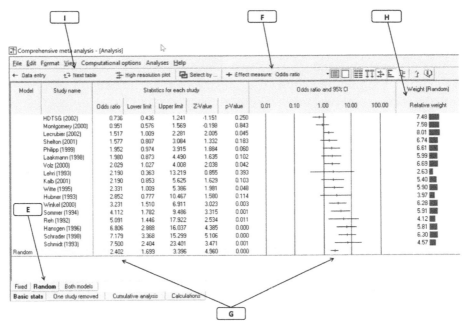

FIGURE 27.2   Basic analysis screen. *Source*: Biostat, Inc.

material respects. The random-effects model is appropriate when these conditions are not met [4] (Chapter 9). In this example, where studies were performed in different populations, we have selected the random-effects model.

In the toolbar (F) we have selected "Odds ratio" as the effect-size index. Using this toolbar, we could switch to the risk ratio, the risk difference, the standardized mean difference, and an array of other effect-size indices.

27.3.1   What is the average effect size?

The program (G) displays the combined effect size as 2.402 and the confidence interval as 1.699–3.396. Since this is a random-effects meta-analysis, this tells us that the average odds ratio in the universe of comparable studies is estimated as 2.402, and probably falls in the range of 1.699 to 3.396. The Z value of 4.960 and the corresponding P value of <0.001 test the null hypothesis that the average odds ratio in the universe of studies is precisely 1.0. We can reject the null, and conclude that the true average odds ratio is greater than 1.0 – that the treatment is helpful. At the right (H) the program displays the relative weight assigned to each study when computing the combined effect size.

27.3.2   How much does the effect size vary?

The *average* effect size represents a substantial clinical improvement. But to understand the potential utility of this intervention, we need also to know how much the effect size varies across populations. Is the intervention consistently effective, or is the impact trivial in some populations and exceptional in others? Is the intervention always beneficial, or is it sometimes harmful?

To address these questions, we can click a tool on the menu bar (I) in Figure 27.2 and display the tables shown in Figure 27.3. The statistics at the left of Figure 27.3 (J) are the same as those in Figure 27.2 and address the *average* effect size. The statistics at the right of Figure 27.3 (K) address the *variation* in effect size across studies, as follows.

We can test the null hypothesis that all studies share a common effect size, and that the variance in observed effects is due entirely to sampling error (see Chapter 9). The test statistic Q is 55.6116 with 16 degrees of freedom and a corresponding P value of <0.001. We conclude that the herbal remedy's effect is stronger in some populations than in others. However, the important question is not whether the effect size varies *at all*, but rather *how much* it varies [5, 6]. We turn to that now.

To get a general sense of the dispersion we can start with the forest plot (right of center in Figure 27.2), where the observed odds ratios vary from roughly 0.75 to 7.50. However, only some of this dispersion reflects variation in true effects (the variation that we care about), while the rest reflects variance due to sampling error. The I^2 statistic is the ratio of V_{TRUE} to $V_{OBSERVED}$, and as such it provides some context for understanding the forest plot. When I^2 is low, the variance in the forest plot is mostly due to sampling error. When I^2 is high, the variance in the forest plot provides a reasonable estimate for the variance of true effects. Here, I^2 is around 75%, so the forest plot provides a reasonable estimate of how the true effect size varies across populations. (There is a common belief that I^2 tells us how much the effect size varies, but this belief is incorrect. As above, I^2 is a proportion, not an absolute value. The correct interpretation is the one presented in Chapter 9 and in [6, 7].)

The program displays T^2, the variance of true effects (0.3462), and T, the standard deviation of true effects (0.5884). When the effect size is a ratio (as it is here) these statistics will always be displayed in log units (this is true for all programs).

While most reports of meta-analyses tend to highlight the statistics outlined above, none of these statistics directly addresses the question "What is the expected range of true effects for populations similar to those in the analysis?" To address this question, the program (at the bottom of Figure 27.4) reports: "The true effect size in 95% of all comparable populations falls in the interval 0.65 to 8.90." This is called the 95% prediction interval. If we were asked to *predict* the true effect size for any one population (selected at random from all populations comparable to those in the analysis), we would *predict* that the odds ratio for that population would fall in the interval 0.65–8.90. And

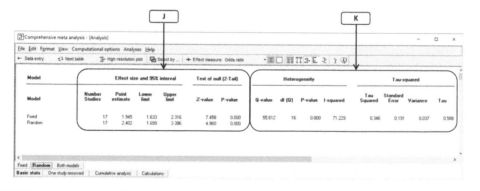

FIGURE 27.3   Average effect size (left), variation in effect size (right). *Source*: Biostat, Inc.

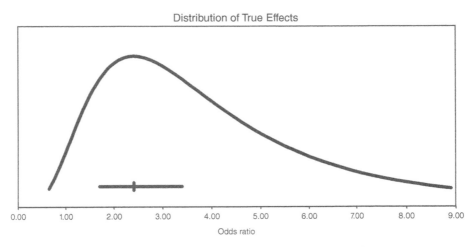

The mean effect size is 2.40 with a 95% confidence interval of 1.70 to 3.40
The true effect size in 95% of all comparable populations falls in the interval 0.65 to 8.90

FIGURE 27.4   Plot of true effects and prediction interval.

if our assumptions are correct (including the assumption that the effects are normally distributed in log units), our prediction would be correct 95% of the time.

The program also plots the distribution of true effects as shown in Figure 27.4. The endpoints of this plot (0.65 and 8.90) correspond to the prediction interval, but the plot itself yields additional information about the distribution. It shows that the treatment will be harmful in only a small minority of cases. Additionally, while the treatment will be helpful in the vast majority of cases, the extent of this impact varies widely. In most cases the odds ratio falls in the range of 1.0–5.0, but there are some cases where the treatment increases the odds of improvement more than eightfold. As mentioned, the distribution is assumed to be symmetric in log units. It appears to be skewed because the plot uses the odds ratio rather than the log odds ratio on the x-axis.

27.4   HIGH-RESOLUTION PLOT

We can click the menu button labeled "Hi-resolution plot" to create the plot displayed in Figure 27.5. Menus allow the user to extensively customize the plot and then export a copy directly to Microsoft Word™ or PowerPoint™.

27.5   SUBGROUP ANALYSIS

At this point we have established that St. John's wort is more effective in some populations than in others, and we might want to identify factors associated with the magnitude of the effect. One possible factor is the nature of the population. Specifically, some studies enrolled patients with major depression only, while others enrolled patients with major or minor depression. We want to compute the odds ratio separately for each subgroup of studies, and then to compare the two values.

St. John's Wort for Depression

Study name	Statistics for each study					Odds ratio and 95% CI
	Odds ratio	Lower limit	Upper limit	Z-Value	p-Value	
HDTSG (2002)	0.736	0.436	1.241	−1.151	0.250	
Montgomery (2000)	0.951	0.576	1.569	−0.198	0.843	
Lecrubier (2002)	1.517	1.009	2.281	2.005	0.045	
Shelton (2001)	1.577	0.807	3.084	1.332	0.183	
Philipp (1999)	1.952	0.974	3.915	1.884	0.060	
Laakmann (1998)	1.980	0.873	4.490	1.635	0.102	
Volz (2000)	2.029	1.027	4.008	2.038	0.042	
Lehri (1993)	2.190	0.363	13.219	0.855	0.393	
Kalb (2001)	2.190	0.853	5.625	1.629	0.103	
Witte (1995)	2.331	1.009	5.386	1.981	0.048	
Hubner (1993)	2.852	0.777	10.467	1.580	0.114	
Winkel (2000)	3.231	1.510	6.911	3.023	0.003	
Sommer (1994)	4.112	1.782	9.486	3.315	0.001	
Reh (1992)	5.091	1.446	17.922	2.534	0.011	
Hansgen (1996)	6.806	2.888	16.037	4.385	0.000	
Schrader (1998)	7.179	3.368	15.299	5.106	0.000	
Schmidt (1993)	7.500	2.404	23.401	3.471	0.001	
	2.402	1.699	3.396	4.960	0.000	

0.01   0.1   1   10   100

Favours Pbo   Favours Tx

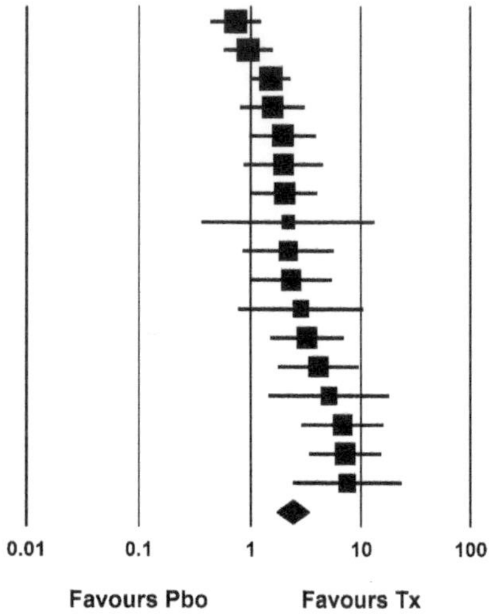

FIGURE 27.5   High-resolution forest plot.

We return to the analysis screen and use the "Computational options" menu to "Group by > Dx." The result is displayed in Figure 27.6.

First, we assess the mean effect of treatment for each subgroup of studies. For studies that enrolled patients with major depression only (L), the combined odds ratio is 1.969 with a 95% confidence interval of 1.375–2.819, a Z value of 3.697, and a P value of <0.001. For studies that enrolled patients with major or minor depression (M), the combined odds ratio is 4.207 with a 95% confidence interval of 2.218–7.978, a Z value of 4.400, and a P value of <0.001. Thus, we can conclude that *Hypericum* is more effective than placebo in each subgroup.

Next, we want to compare the effect size in the two subgroups. That is, we want to ask if the treatment is more effective in studies that include patients with major or minor depression than in studies that include patients with major depression only. Again, a button on the menu bar (N) allows us to switch between the plot in Figure 27.6 and the details in Figure 27.7.

The screen in Figure 27.7 shows two sets of analyses. The section at the top is labeled "Fixed-effect analysis." We would use this section if all studies within a subgroup shared a common true effect size. The section at the bottom is labeled "Mixed-effects analysis," which allows that the true effect size may vary across studies within subgroups. In our example, the studies within each subgroup are sampled from different populations of patients, and so we will be using the latter section.

The combined odds ratio for the Major Only subgroup is 1.969 with a 95% confidence interval of 1.375–2.819, while the combined odds ratio for the Major or Minor subgroup is 4.207 with a 95% confidence interval of 2.218–7.978 (O). To test the difference between the two effect sizes we may use a Q test. The Q value for this difference is 4.113 with 1 degree of freedom and a P value of 0.043 (P). We conclude that the treatment is more effective in the subgroup of populations we have called "Major or Minor" as compared with those we have called "Major Only."

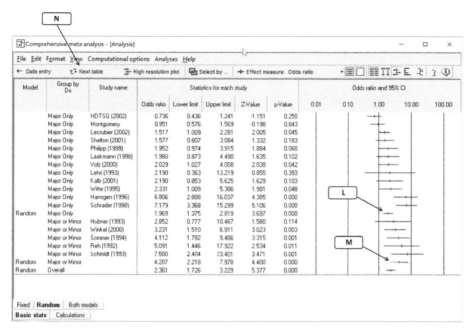

FIGURE 27.6   Impact of treatment as a function of subgroup (Major Only vs. Major or Minor).
Source: Biostat, Inc.

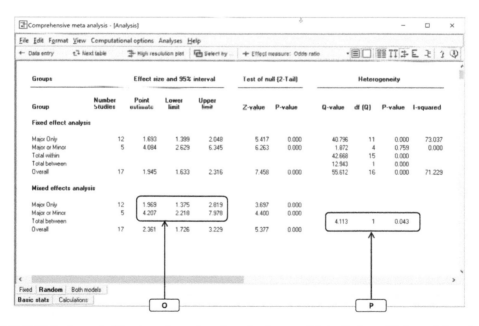

FIGURE 27.7   Impact of treatment as a function of subgroup (Major Only vs. Major or Minor).
Source: Biostat, Inc.

It is important to recognize that (with rare exceptions) subgroup comparisons in a meta-analysis are observational by nature and cannot prove a causal relationship. In this example, it is *possible* that *Hypericum* is more effective in the "Major or Minor" studies because the extract is more effective with these kinds of patients, which *would be* a causal relationship. But it is also possible that *Hypericum* was more effective in the "Major or Minor" studies for other reasons. For example, it is possible that the

"Major or Minor" studies employed a different dosing schedule than the "Major Only" studies, and it is the dosing schedule (rather than the diagnosis) that was responsible for the larger effect in these studies.

27.6   META-REGRESSION

In a primary study, we may use regression analysis to study the relationship between covariates and outcome. Similarly, in a meta-analysis we may use regression to study the relationship between covariates and effect size. In this case, the procedure is commonly called meta-regression (see Chapter 10). In a primary study the unit of analysis is the *individual*, with covariates and outcome measured for each *individual*. In a meta-analysis, the unit of analysis is the *study*, with covariates and outcome measured for each *study*. However, with some modifications, the full arsenal of procedures that fall under the heading of "regression" in primary studies is also available in meta-analysis.

In the current example, we want to see if *Hypericum*'s effect is related to the level of depression at study entry (Baseline) and/or the mean dose employed in the study (Dose). On the main analysis screen (Figure 27.6) we select "Meta-regression 2" on the "Analyses" menu. We define a regression with these two covariates, and the program displays the results in Figure 27.8. The results based on the random-effects model are shown

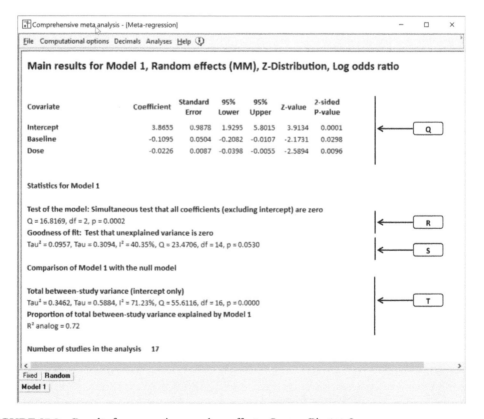

FIGURE 27.8   Results for regression, random effects. *Source*: Biostat, Inc.

here. The user may also choose to use a fixed-effect model, though this is generally not recommended (see Chapter 9).

The table at the top (Q) displays the relationship between each covariate and effect size when all other covariates are held constant. For example, the coefficient for baseline score is displayed as −0.1095. This is plotted in Figure 27.9, where we see that the treatment is more effective when baseline depression is moderate and less effective when baseline depression is more severe. Concretely, as the baseline depression score increases from 13 to 23 (points U–V on the regression line), the impact of treatment drops from 1.68 to 0.59 in log units. These values are computed using the Eq. Y = 3.8655−0.1095 (Baseline) − 0.0226 (Dose), which is displayed on the plot. The regression line is drawn using the simple mean for Dose, which is 33.59 mg. As noted, the plot is scaled in log units. The odds ratios corresponding to points U and V are 5.38 and 1.80, respectively.

The table (Q) provides additional details for the relationship between baseline score and effect size, with Dose held constant. As noted, the coefficient for Baseline is −0.1095. The confidence interval for the coefficient is −0.2082 to −0.0107. A test of the null hypothesis that baseline score is not related to effect size yields a Z value of −2.1731, and a corresponding P value of 0.0298.

As noted, in Figure 27.8 the table at the top (Q) displays statistics for the *unique* impact of *each* covariate. By contrast, the other sections displays statistics for the *joint* impact of *all* covariates.

In the section labeled "Test of Model" (R), we test the null hypothesis that *none* of the covariates explains any variation in effect size. The Q value for this test is 16.8169 with 2 degrees of freedom and a corresponding P value of 0.0002. We reject the null hypothesis, and conclude that at least one of the covariates is related to effect size.

The section labeled "Goodness of fit" (S) addresses the residual variance. The variance of true effects about the regression line (T^2) is 0.0957, and the standard deviation

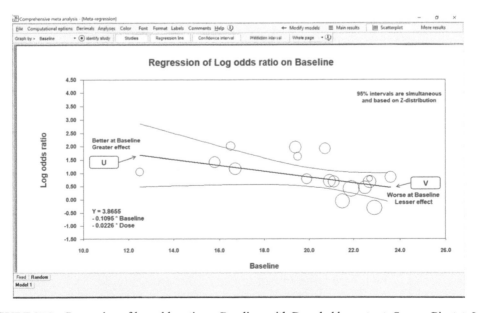

FIGURE 27.9 Regression of log odds ratio on Baseline, with Dose held constant. *Source*: Biostat, Inc.

of true effects about the regression line (T) is 0.3094. The I^2 statistic is 40.35%, which tells us that some 40% of the observed variance about the regression line reflects variation in true effects rather than sampling error. The test for heterogeneity yields a Q value of 23.4706 with 14 degrees of freedom and a corresponding P value of 0.0530. We conclude that the model does not fully explain the variation in effects. Finally, the program displays R^2 as 0.72, which tells us that the covariates are able to explain some 72% of the initial variance in true effects.

The program offers a number of options for regression. It allows the user to include categorical covariates in the model. In this case, the program will automatically create a set of dummy variables to represent the covariate. It allows the user to select either the Z-distribution or the Knapp–Hartung adjustment [8] for computing confidence intervals and P values (see Chapter 9). It allows the user to estimate T^2 using either the method of moments [9, 10], maximum likelihood, or restricted maximum likelihood. It allows the user to define sets of covariates (for example the linear and curvilinear impact of dose) and to assess the impact of the full set with other covariates held constant. It allows the user to define multiple prediction models and then compare them with each other.

As was true for analyses that compared subgroups, the relationships explored in meta-regression (with rare exceptions) are observational rather than causal. In this example we attempted to identify the relationship between baseline score and effect size while controlling for dose, but there may be other confounding variables that we have not considered [11].

27.7   PUBLICATION BIAS

To address the potential impact of publication bias, we can select "Analyses > Publication bias" on the main analysis screen, to display Figure 27.10. The two plots in this figure show the effect size (on the x-axis) by the standard error (on the y-axis). The large studies appear at the top and the smaller studies appear toward the bottom.

The upper plot shows the studies that are actually included in the analysis. A vertical line denotes the average effect size (W). If the effects are normally distributed, we would expect half the studies to fall on either side of the line. However, as we move toward the smaller studies, we see a cluster of studies toward the right (X) and no corresponding studies at the left (Y). One possible reason for the asymmetrical funnel plot is that the studies toward the left were not statistically significant, and therefore were not published and did not find their way into the analysis. In that case, the combined odds ratio is based on a biased subset of all actual studies and overestimates the true average effect size. (Under this model we expect less bias in the larger studies, since these will be statistically significant even with smaller effects.)

In some cases, the trim-and-fill method [12] may be used to remove this bias. The method employs an iterative procedure to identify the studies that may be missing. It then "creates" these studies and inserts them into the analysis. These are displayed here as filled circles (Z) which are the mirror image of the actual studies (AA). We can use all the studies (actual and imputed) to compute an adjusted estimate of the mean effect size. The initial estimate of the combined odds ratio (in log units) was 0.87 (AB), but the

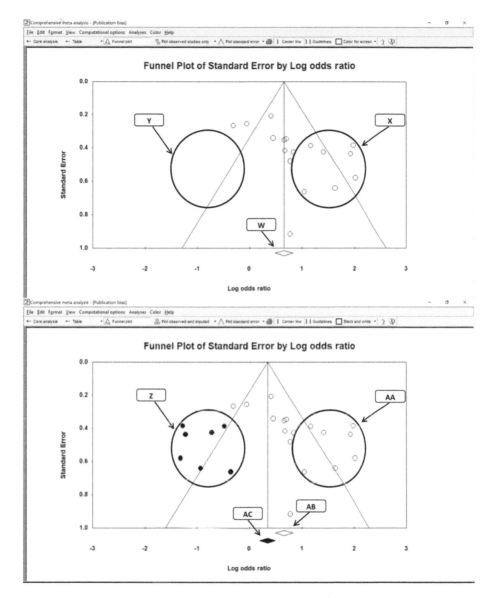

FIGURE 27.10   Funnel plot and adjustment based on trim and fill. *Source*: Biostat, Inc.

adjusted value (included the imputed studies) is 0.40 (AC). In odds ratio units, the initial estimate was 2.40 and the adjusted estimate is 1.49 (displayed by the program on another screen). If the asymmetry was due to publication bias, then this adjustment yields an estimate of the unbiased effect size. Note that there are reasons other than publication bias that may explain or contribute to asymmetry in funnel plots (see Chapter 5).

CMA also features other methods that are typically used to test and/or adjust for publication bias. These include the Egger test of the intercept, the Begg and Mazumdar rank correlation test, and Rosenthal's Fail-safe N [13, 14]. The program can also generate a text report that explains how to interpret the results for each of the publication bias procedures.

27.8   ADDITIONAL FEATURES IN COMPREHENSIVE META-ANALYSIS

The first step in conducting a meta-analysis is to compute an effect size and variance for each study. Many programs will perform this computation automatically when the data are in the form of 2×2 tables, or in the form of means and standard deviations for each group, but not for more complex data formats. By contrast, CMA will allow the user to enter data in more than 100 formats. For example, the user can enter data as events and N in each group; or as an odds ratio and its confidence interval; or as a log risk ratio and its standard error. Or, the user can enter means and standard deviations for two independent groups; or the pre and post scores for a pre/post study; or the P value from a *t*-test for two independent groups; and so on. Critically, the user may use a different format for each study. Thus, if one study reports means and standard deviations for two independent groups, a second reports a P value based on two independent groups, and a third reports pre and post scores for a pre/post study, the user may enter data for each study in its own format. The program will apply the appropriate formula for each format to compute the effect size and its variance, and then include all the effects in the analysis. The program allows the user to select from an array of effect-size indices, including the odds ratio, risk ratio, risk difference, mean difference, standardized mean difference, correlation, hazard ratio, and prevalence, among others.

In the motivating example, each study provides one row of data. CMA also allows for the possibility that some (or all) studies will provide more than one row of data. There is an option for studies to report data for two or more outcomes, based on the same subjects. In the analysis, we could elect to look at either outcome alone. Or, we could tell the program to create a synthetic outcome that incorporates both measures, taking into account the fact that the two outcomes are not independent of each other.

Similarly, we can enter data for an outcome recorded at two or more timepoints, which allows us to assess the impact at each timepoint and to see if the effect size changes over time. We can enter data for two or more independent subgroups within studies, and then run the analysis using either subgroup or study as the unit of analysis. Finally, we can enter data for studies that employed one control group and multiple treatment groups.

27.9   TEACHING ELEMENTS

The program incorporates a number of features intended to make the computations as transparent as possible. On the data-entry screen, the user enters summary data and the program displays the effect size and its variance. Double-click on the computed values and the program will show how those values were computed. On the analysis screen there is also a tab labeled "Calculations," which opens a window onto the calculations.

The program is also able to generate a report that explains the meaning of the various statistics. For example, the section on heterogeneity reads as follows:

> *The* Q *statistic provides a test of the null hypothesis that all studies in the analysis share a common effect size. If all studies shared the same true effect size, the expected value of* Q *would be equal to the degrees of freedom (the number of*

studies minus 1). The Q-value is 55.612 with 16 degrees of freedom and P < 0.001. Using a criterion alpha of 0.10, we can reject the null hypothesis that the true effect size is the same in all these studies. The I^2 statistic is 71%, which tells us that some 71% of the variance in observed effects reflects variance in true effects rather than sampling error. τ^2, the variance of true effect sizes, is 0.346 in log units. T, the standard deviation of true effect sizes, is 0.588 in log units. If we assume that the true effects are normally distributed (in log units), we can estimate that the prediction interval is 0.648 to 8.897. The true effect size in 95% of all comparable populations falls in this interval.

27.10   DOCUMENTATION

A manual is installed with the program. Each module in the program features an interactive guide that will walk the user through that module. Additionally, the website offers an array of PDFs and videos that show how to enter data, run the analysis, and then interpret the output. In each case we also discuss how to report the data. The program's algorithms are discussed in the text *Introduction to Meta-Analysis, Second Edition* [15]. Key chapters from this text may be downloaded free on the website. A manual for meta-regression is also available for download.

27.11   AVAILABILITY

The program's website is http://www.Meta-Analysis.com. The program may be downloaded and run for free as a trial. The website lists rates for licenses. There are discounts available for nonprofit institutions and for students. The program is free for short-term workshops in meta-analysis, and is available at a discount for semester-length classes in meta-analysis.

All materials relevant to this chapter can be accessed at http://www.Meta-Analysis.com or at www.systematic-reviews3.org. This includes a PDF with step-by-step instructions for performing the analyses in this chapter, and the data file. Questions should be sent to Info@Meta-Analysis.com.

Another program on the website is CMA Prediction Intervals. Researchers who are using Revman, Stata, R, or other software for their meta-analysis can use this software to plot the prediction intervals and distribution of true effects, as shown in Figure 27.4.

ACKNOWLEDGMENTS

Development of the program was funded by the National Institutes of Health in the United States under the following grants: MH052969 (Computer program for meta-analysis in mental health), AG021360 (Combining data types in meta-analysis), AG020052 (Publication bias in meta-analysis for mental health), AG024771 (Software for meta-regression), DA019280 (Forest plots for meta-analysis), AG029029 (Software for meta-analysis of diagnostic tests), and DA029351 (Software for meta-analysis with correlated outcomes). As a matter of policy, NIH does not endorse any product or software.

The program was developed by Michael Borenstein, Larry Hedges, Julian Higgins, and Hannah Rothstein. We gratefully acknowledge the contributions of Doug Altman, Betsy Becker, Jesse Berlin, Michael Brannick, Harris Cooper, Kay Dickersin, Sue Duval, Roger Harbord, John Ioannidis, Jeff Valentine, Spyros Konstantopoulos, Mark Lipsey, Mike McDaniel, Fred Oswald, Terri Pigott, David Rindskopf, Stephen Senn, Will Shadish, Jonathan Sterne, Alex Sutton, Steven Tarlow, Thomas Trikalinos, Jack Vevea, Vish Viswesvaran, and David Wilson.

REFERENCES

1. Linde, K., Mulrow, C.D., Berner, M., and Egger, M. (2005). St John's wort for depression. *Cochrane Database Syst. Rev.* **2**: CD000448. https://doi.org/10.1002/14651858. CD000448.pub2.

2. Linde, K., Berner, M., Egger, M., and Mulrow, C. (2005). St John's wort for depression: meta-analysis of randomised controlled trials. *Br. J. Psychiatry* 186: 99–107.

3. Viechtbauer, W. (2007). Accounting for heterogeneity via random-effects models and moderator analyses in meta-analysis. *J. Psychol.* 215: 104–121.

4. Borenstein, M., Hedges, L.V., Higgins, J.P.T., and Rothstein, H.R. (2010). A basic introduction to fixed-effect and random-effects models for meta-analysis. *Res. Synth. Methods* 1 (2): 97–111.

5. Higgins, J.P.T., Thompson, S.G., and Spiegelhalter, D.J. (2009). A re-evaluation of random-effects meta-analysis. *J. R. Stat. Soc. Ser. A Stat. Soc.* 172 (1): 137–159.

6. Borenstein, M. (2019). *Common Mistakes in Meta-Analysis and how to Avoid Them*. Englewood, NJ: Biostat.

7. Borenstein, M., Higgins, J.P.T., Hedges, L.V., and Rothstein, H.R. (2017). Basics of meta-analysis: $I2$ is not an absolute measure of heterogeneity. *Res. Synth. Methods* 8 (1): 5–18.

8. Knapp, G. and Hartung, J. (2003). Improved tests for a random effects meta-regression with a single covariate. *Stat. Med.* 22 (17): 2693–2710.

9. DerSimonian, R. and Laird, N. (1986). Meta-analysis in clinical trials. *Control. Clin. Trials* 7 (3): 177–188.

10. DerSimonian, R. and Laird, N. (2015). Meta-analysis in clinical trials revisited. *Contemp. Clin. Trials* 45 (Pt A): 139–145.

11. Borenstein, M., Hedges, L.V., Higgins, J.P.T. and Rothstein, H.R. *Meta-Regression - Multiple Regression in Meta-Analysis*. Englewood, NJ: Biostat (in press).

12. Duval, S. and Tweedie, R.L. (2000). Trim and fill: a simple funnel-plot-based method of testing and adjusting for publication bias in meta-analysis. *Biometrics* 56: 455–463.

13. Rothstein, H., Sutton, A.J., and Borenstein, M. (2005). *Publication Bias in Meta-Analysis: Prevention, Assessment and Adjustments*. Chichester: Wiley.

14. Sterne, J.A.C., Sutton, A.J., Ioannidis, J.P.A. et al. (2011). Recommendations for examining and interpreting funnel plot asymmetry in meta-analyses of randomised controlled trials. *Br. Med. J.* 343: d4002.

15. Borenstein, M., Hedges, L.V., Higgins, J.P.T., and Rothstein, H.R. (2021). *Introduction to Meta-Analysis*, 2e. Chichester: Wiley.

Index

N.B. – Images on separate pages are displayed in **bold**, entries in of text set in boxes and tables are shown in *italics*.

Systematic Reviews in Health Research: Meta-Analysis in Context, Third Edition. Edited by Matthias Egger, Julian P.T. Higgins, and George Davey Smith.
© 2022 John Wiley & Sons Ltd. Published 2022 by John Wiley & Sons Ltd.
Companion website: www.systematic-reviews3.org